Ancient Cure

DECEPTIVE GLOBAL PHARMACEUTICAL ESPIONAGE

John F. Derr, RPh, FASCP

Ancient Cure:
Deceptive Global Pharmaceutical Espionage
Copyright © 2024 by John F. Derr, RPh, FASCP

ISBN: 978-1962497817(sc)
ISBN: 978-1962497824(e)

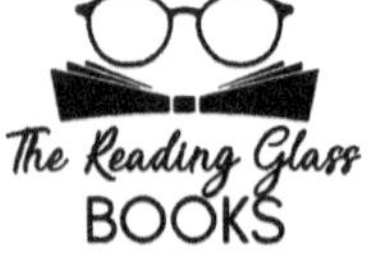

The Reading Glass Books
1-888-420-3050
www.readingglassbooks.com
fulfillment@readingglassbooks.com

Table of Contents

STOVER PARK, PENNSYLVANIA

Jean Paul Koenig, Ph.D. pulled around the circle drive and headed back down the driveway to Stover Park Road. At the end of the driveway J.P. turned left. He was increasing speed on the blacktop when the lights of a car immediately behind him suddenly came on, surprising J.P. They were halogen lights and they blinded him for a few seconds. The other car was so close to his car that he was sure the driver was intending to ram his vehicle from the rear. J.P. stayed with the speed limit of 35 mph. The road curved right and then became a straight shot to Tomickon Hill Road, which would take him to the small town of Point Pleasant and Pennsylvania Route 32 where he would turn south to New Hope.

J.P. and his tail made their way towards Point Pleasant. He was sure the car was the Lexus that had followed him to Doylestown. J.P. decided to change his original route back at Point Pleasant. He knew there was another road through the park. He made a quick decision to turn left instead of the normal traffic flow to the right. He hoped that he could lose the tail in the tight turns of the Point Pleasant and driving north instead of the expected southern direction to the highway back to New York City.

The car was right behind him as he slightly increased his speed. J.P. crossed the bridge over a creek and hit the brakes swinging the wheel into a sharp left-hand turn. His rental car fishtailed and he turned the wheel to the right to counter the cars spin. The car straightened and J.P. accelerated north on Cafferty Road with the park canyon on his left.

The pursuer had anticipated that J.P. would make a right turn on to route 32 and was taken by surprise by J.P.s sudden left turn. He quickly tried to change to a right hand turn almost crashing into the street light at the intersection.

J.P. looked in the rearview mirror and saw the lights of the other car swing in an arc and then disappear. The driver had taken a 360. This was J.P.'s opportunity to get as far ahead of his chaser as possible. He floored the gas pedal.

As J.P. neared the next turn, he took his foot off the gas pedal. The car did not slow down. The car acted like it was on cruise control. He checked the cruise control switch and found that it was off. He hit the brake pedal but the car only slowed a little. It seemed as if his foot was on the gas pedal and brake pedal at the same time. He used both feet on the brake pedal and pressed down with all of his leg strength. The car started into a skid. He checked the skid rotation by turning the wheel the opposite direction as he had done when he made the quick left turn in Point Pleasant. He glanced first at the speedometer, 70 mph and then in the rearview mirror, two bright headlights.

He suddenly came to the realization that something was wrong with the gas pedal. It was stuck in the accelerated position and the car was increasing speed. J.P. knew that he wouldn't be able to safely negotiate the expected upcoming tight turns in the park road at more than 40 mph. He had to get out of the car before the car launched into space and dove to the canyon floor.

It was twilight and he could barely see a tight curve ahead. J.P. decided to try and slow the car down by glancing off the sides of the highway guardrails and then try to make the curve. His thoughts turned to a plan of making the first curve using the guardrail and then jumping out of the car as it glanced off the trees growing along the road before it would probably go airborne into the canyon. He glanced down at the speedometer. The numbers only went to 85 mph and the car was pegged at the 85 mph position. He reached down and unfastened his seatbelt.

He made the first curve just like a pinball making its upper curve before hitting the bumpers. The car left the highway. He opened the driver's door just before he hit the trees. The first tree tore the door from the car giving him freedom to jump as the car glanced off enough trees to slow it down in order for him to make the jump. He was headed west and the fading sun illuminated a fairly clear trail through the trees to the canyon's edge. The now destroyed rental car continued to carom off the trees with glancing blows as it made its way to the edge. The car was going slower, but not slow enough. He hit the brakes hard and tried to keep the car in a straight line and out of a skid on the wet forest undergrowth. J.P. pulled on the emergency brake. He felt the brakes lock and smelled the burning emergency brake as it grabbed hold. He knew he must exit the car, but when.

He saw the canyon edge ahead and suddenly, too late, he saw a large dead tree three quarters buried in the soil lying across the cars path.

The car hit the submerged tree and became airborne. The impact of the vehicle hitting the tree threw J.P. violently out of the vehicle. The car was about ten feet off the ground when J.P. took his leave of the car. He hit the ground hard on his left shoulder and knee. He bounced, rolled, and stopped suddenly braced against a rock, hitting both his head and rib cage on the rock. He could not catch his breath and his head was spinning, but he was still conscious.

He could hear his car hitting trees that were growing out of the walls of the canyon as the car continued towards bottom of the canyon. Then, there was deadly silence. A second later there was a tremendous explosion as the car hit the creek bed. J.P.'s hazy night vision turned red as the sky was lit with a gasoline fireball. His head began a swimming, dizzy sensation. His last thoughts before becoming unconscious was, how in the hell did he, a skier from Mammoth Lakes, California, get wedged against a rock in a small county park outside Doylestown, Pennsylvania?

2:00 A.M., MONDAY, JANUARY 16

MAMMOTH LAKES, CALIFORNIA

Three months earlier in the calm and peaceful village of Mammoth Lakes, California on the eastern slopes of the Sierra Nevada Mountains, J.P was in the twilight zone between deep sleep and waking.

It was the strangest thing he had ever felt. His phone was ringing yet every time he reached for the handset it moved just a bit further away. At first he felt himself becoming angry and then increasingly helpless as he tried in vain to answer the moving telephone. He knew that if he could just somehow pick up the handset and stop the incessant ringing his sense of helplessness would soon pass.

"Oh," he muttered to himself as his eyes snapped open and he realized that he had been in a deep sleep and the phone was actually ringing.

"Open connection" he spoke activating the self-connecting software. "Huh," he grunted.

"J.P.? Jean Paul is that you? Hello? I'm trying to reach Jean Paul Koenig. This is Dr. Phillip T. Bradsmith calling."

"Huh, what? Phillip? What the fuck are you doing calling me? Do you have any idea what frigging time it is?" J.P. growled as he sat up.

"Ah, yes, I must have reached my dear old friend, J.P. No one else I know in the civilized western world would dare speak with such vulgarity to someone that they have scarcely seen or talked to in five years."

J.P. was silent. He was still thinking about the dream he had been having when the ringing woke him. He had found the dream disconcerting, but he forced himself to refocus on the present.

"Phillip, it's always such a pleasure to hear from you...how is that? Does that better suit your sensitive self?" he remarked in a slightly sarcastic tone.

"Well, it is a start, I suppose." Phillip paused. "J.P., I need your help and please don't ask me to explain. I need you to come to New York City on the earliest possible flight."

J.P. lay there trying to comprehend just what it was that Phillip wanted from him. In the thirty-one years that he had known Phillip, he had never known him to reach out for help. They had first met when both joined James Pharmaceutical Company as sales representatives in Southern California. J.P., following a five-year stint of active military service as an officer in the Navy and Phillip just after college. Although they began working at James Pharmaceutical the same year, Phillip was five years younger than J.P.

After two years in field sales, J.P. was selected for a position in the New York City home office. He was promoted on a fast track and after three years became vice president of the James' marketing division.

The same year that J.P. became a vice president, Phillip was promoted to regional director of sales for Southern California. A few years later, J.P. asked Phillip to join him in the home office. Phillip had jumped at the opportunity. They worked closely together for five years before J.P. decided to move off on his own. Phillip had stayed at James working his way up the corporate ladder. Just a few years ago, he finally landed the position of CEO and president, following the death of the company's founder, Gunther F. "Doc" James.

During those years, J.P. was active in the Selective Naval Reserve serving as commanding officer of numerous naval units until he was promoted to the rank of Captain a year a head of his class. In the twilight of his Naval career he was appointed Code 03, Strategic Planning for the Naval Readiness Command for the southwest USA located in San Diego. As Code 03 J.P. helped to form a think tank made up of Senior Naval Officers called the Command Management Action Group (CMAG). CMAG was an elite group of Reserve Officers which studied specific issues assigned by the Readiness Commander. The assignments varied in scope and lead to many interesting adventures. When Captain Koenig moved from the Selective Reserve to Stand-by Reserve status, he and the other officers of CMAG remained associates and secretly worked on projects for corporations.

J.P. knew that if Phillip was to the point of practically begging him to come to New York, he must be in dire need. He knew full well that he would make the trip to New York City, but not before he made Phillip squirm just a little bit.

"You know, Phillip, I'm a busy guy. I have a publisher breathing down my neck because I've already missed my deadline to get the next section of my manuscript to him and, oh by the way, the snow skiing here is the best it has been in years. Besides all of that, it's pretty nervy after five years of no contact to call a guy in the middle of the night and ask him to fly 3,000 miles with virtually no explanation as to what it is that you want from me."

"J.P., the world, as we know, abounds in business books. I feel confident in my belief that the delay of publication of your latest book is not likely to tip Wall Street onto its collective ear. As for my depriving you of whatever pseudo-sexual pleasure you derive from launching yourself down the face of a mountain at frightening speeds—I would ask you to consider growing up."

Phillip's voice lowered slightly as he said, "And finally, regarding my request for you to fly here with no explanation, I can only tell you that I really prefer not to give the reason over the phone. Please say you'll come."

"Yep. Okay. With any luck at all I should arrive by early evening. Do you want me to meet you at The Spectrum of Medicine?"

"Yes, of course. Thank you, J.P."

"Yeah, yeah. Okay, I'm on my way," J.P. gave the disconnect command.

J.P. lay there for another few minutes making one of his mental lists of everything he needed to do before leaving on a trip.

"Open connection to Mountain Aviation Services." After nearly twenty rings the overnight attendant finally answered.

"Mountain Aviation, this is Paul," the voice on the other end said rather curtly.

"Paul, it's J.P. Listen, buddy, sorry for the short notice, but I've got an emergency here. I need you to gas the Lear and get it ready. I'm leaving for LAX in about an hour."

"Uh, sure, J.P. You want me to file for you?"

"Yeah, thanks, that'll help a lot. See you soon," he again gave the disconnect command.

He swung his legs over the side of the bed and leaned forward so that his elbows rested on his knees. He was tired, but he felt certain that he would be able to make the trip to Los Angeles to catch a flight to New York City. He thought back to his last contact with Phillip.

It was just after Phillip had been promoted to CEO and president. He had called him to congratulate him on his promotion to the top position that he had aspired for so many years. Phillip T. Bradsmith, Ph.D., only J.P. knew that the "T" stood for Thaddeus. Phillip refused to answer the question when anyone asked about his middle name. In fact, he was so sensitive about the name, Thaddeus, that he marked the middle name square on his employment application form that his middle name was an initial.

Phillip was an instant pharmaceutical CEO success. Executive search firms were always dangling "opportunities" in front of him to lure him away from James. He would usually investigate the new opportunity and sometimes he even interviewed for the position. But in the end, Phillip always felt that James Pharmaceutical was the best place for him. Over the years, Doc James had always taken care of him and he felt a compelling sense of loyalty to his mentor.

J.P. reminded himself that he had better get moving and thought about calling his longtime friend and infrequent lover, Annie, to tell her that he was leaving town and ask her to keep an eye on the house, but then he thought better of it. He knew Annie would not be amused if he called her at 2:00 a.m., particularly since she had probably just gotten to bed after closing her bar and grill. Whenever J.P. traveled, Annie would collect his mail, make sure the heat was still working, and forward any seemingly important local messages. He decided he would call her when he arrived in New York.

He raised his 6'1" muscular frame to a standing position and began packing for the trip. Mid-way through the packing, he ran a hand through his coarse beard and decided he would shave it off. He didn't know what Phillip had in mind for him, but he felt he should probably make himself look a little more "business professional" as they say at Harvard Business School.

J.P. was no stranger to business. While working at James Pharmaceutical, he had managed to find the time to complete an MBA. After his departure from James he had spent the next twenty years establishing three start-up healthcare companies, written dozens of business books, consulted for a number of corporations on strategic planning, and provided the leadership for CMAG. Through it all he still managed to complete the requirements for a Ph.D. in business administration. Over the years, while amassing a personal fortune, he had developed a reputation as a futurist, a strategist, and a successful entrepreneur.

Since retiring to Mammoth Lakes two years earlier, he divided his days between his writing, consulting, CMAG and the pursuit of his passion for snow skiing. He loved the snow, the mountains, the tall lodgepole pines, and everything else that made up Mammoth Mountain and the town of Mammoth Lakes.

He felt that Mammoth Lakes provided him with the right mixture of youthful hope and mature experience. The area was peaceful and quiet except on the weekends when the LA crowds increased the village's population from 4,000 to nearly 57,000 and during an earthquake.

After he packed his bag, he walked through his house quickly making sure that everything was as it should be if he was going to be out of town. It occurred to him then that he didn't really know just how long he would be gone. He told himself again that he had to be sure that he called Annie when he got to New York City. He went into his study and opened a drawer that was set into the lower half of the floor to ceiling bookshelves. He removed a small gift-wrapped box and returned to the kitchen. He kept a number of small gifts wrapped and ready-to-go for hostess gifts, forgotten birthdays, or whatever impromptu emergency might arise. He scrawled out a note on a piece of paper:

"Annie—Sorry for the short notice. Back soon. Help yourself to the hot tub. Thanks, J.P."

He hesitated for a second, wondering if he should have signed it, "Love, J.P." and then thought better of it. He left the box with the note sitting on his kitchen counter. He picked up his bag and headed for the garage.

JAL FLIGHT #330 FROM TOKYO TO LOS ANGELES

The gentleman in sitting in 3B had done his best to stay awake for the trip to Los Angeles. Sometimes, on other trips, he had succeeded in making it all the way without falling into a deep sleep and experiencing his recurring nightmare. On this flight, he had tried to remain awake to avoid the dream, but he had fallen asleep during the movie. The nightmare always began whenever he flew. First came the dream, a recurring movie of a life event that he had played out many times before, both in dreams and in reality. The dream always turned nightmarish and then the outward physical effects would consume him. He would begin to experience difficulty in breathing, certain that his seatbelt was slowing tightening and cutting off his supply of air. At the point of hyperventilation, the muscles of his abdomen would begin to spasm. He always managed to force himself awake long enough for the next sequence to start. His vision would blur and color red and then he would move to a semi-coma state.

On this flight, consciousness returned when the air pressure in the first class cabin changed and the pilot announced the flight was committed to final approach and would land in Los Angeles in twenty minutes.

The same recurring dream had haunted him for twenty years. It happened almost every time he fell asleep on a long flight. To anyone sitting next to or near him, he looked as though he were in a sound sleep with deep breathing. For him, it was a terrifying experience. Over the years he had spoken with medical specialists about the problem, but there never seemed to be an easy explanation, much less an answer for his condition. They always recommended a battery of tests to determine the origin, but he never agreed to any testing.

He felt that he had, thus far, lived with the strange phenomenon and he could live with it in the future.

He pushed the flight attendant call button on the armrest. He was pleased to see that it was the same flight attendant that had been on many of his trans-pacific flights during the past year. He thought he had seen her in the galley when he boarded, but a different flight attendant had served him throughout the flight.

She handed him a hot towel and spoke softly in Japanese, "How do you feel, sir? Your sleep seemed troubled. I considered waking you, but I felt I would be intruding." She took the towel from him after he had refreshed himself and handed him a glass of water.

He noted her name on her uniform. "Thank you, Reiko. Please speak English, I want to get back into the habit of speaking English as soon as possible."

She had noted his name from the passenger manifest. *"Hai,* I mean, yes, Nacheda-san. I understand," she replied with a smile. "I am surprised to see you again so soon. Are you still commuting once a month from Japan to the United States? If so, it seems to me that you're a week early."

"Yes, it is an unexpected trip, but nothing too important. I'm just earning more JAL frequent flier miles which, for some reason, I never seem to have time to use," Nacheda responded in a low voice.

Nacheda thought to himself that he should learn to be a bit more discreet. It would not pay for someone in his position to leave such an easy trail for others to follow.

Nacheda recalled the events of the previous day when he had been called into Dr. Nakasone's office. Dr. Nakasone had sternly reminded him of the reason why Bandai Pharmaceutical Company had employed Nacheda in the first place. Namely, to identify a pharmaceutical company in the United States that had a compatible research program.

Twenty years ago, the Japanese Pharmaceutical Association (JPA) had set a 10-year industrial goal. The goal was to establish Japan as a major player in the U.S. pharmaceutical marketplace. The twenty years had quickly pasted and Japanese companies were still only minor players.

Just last week, the President of the JPA had announced to the members of the association and news media that, "As of today, with our advanced technology and ideal work ethic, Japan should have earned at least a twenty percent share of the U.S. market, not three percent."

In their meeting Nakasone had reproached Nacheda, "You don't even have a beginning, Mr. Nacheda. The Europeans have succeeded in establishing themselves in the U.S. and we have failed. You have had a year in which to succeed in finding a US company for Bandai Pharmaceutical and you have failed. You said you were experienced and that you could do what no other person has done and you have failed. The JPA sits on its philosophical behind even as the American pharmaceutical companies negotiate them to death. Japanese pharmaceutical researchers die old men researching their outdated chemicals or herbals as the Americans continue to make billions of yen selling our people their pharmaceuticals. We have failed to defend our market and we have failed to penetrate the U.S. market where so many other Japanese industries have been successful. You have failed Bandai Pharmaceutical, Nacheda-san. You have failed us all."

The plane's cabin pressure increased as the plane descended towards its landing in Los Angeles. Nacheda pinched his nose shut with his fingers and blew to clear his ears...in doing so also blew out the memory of Nakasone's voice.

Reiko sat a glass of water down on the armrest of his seat. "Five minutes until we land."

Nacheda focused on his agenda for this trip. He would meet with his U.S. team the next morning at the Westwood Village condo. He hoped, with all his heart, that they would have good news for him, but he harbored doubts.

"Is it possible that I will fail to complete my project this time?" Nacheda asked himself. "No, I cannot fail." He had never allowed anyone to call him a failure. No one. Dr. Nakasone will be proven wrong. He thought of his native Japanese culture and smiled. His reaction was exactly the reaction Dr. Nakasone would expect from him after his Monday morning scolding.

Bandai Pharmaceutical Company was founded in 1960, just when Japan was realizing that it had to join the world trade market and break out of the bounds of U.S. post-WWII occupation. The U.S. had encouraged Japan to rebuild and General MacArthur had laid the groundwork. By 1960, it was up to the Japanese industrialists to take control. Dr. Nakasone had been the director of cancer research for Dai Nippon Pharmaceutical Company located in Osaka. After years of struggling in a small research section of a giant Japanese corporation where he received little to no recognition, Nakasone had decided to take the unusual, ambitious path and break with tradition and start his own company. Nacheda felt pride when he thought of what Dr. Nakasone had accomplished on his own.

Nakasone had worked with the Tokyo banks and received the funds to purchase a small, failing chemical company located in Bandai in the Fukushima Prefecture in upper Honshu. Bandai was a quiet village known mostly for its snow skiing on the 1819-meter Bandai Mountain. Nakasone had formed a research team and, since 1960, had consistently pursued cancer research at a time when other pharmaceutical companies worldwide had stopped research and moved to the more lucrative product classes of antibiotics and hypertensives.

At that time, even in the U.S., basic cancer research had essentially been given to the American Cancer Society, the National Institutes of Health, and universities. There wasn't enough profit in pharmaceutical products earmarked for treating the elusive disease of cancer. This wasn't a purely financial decision. Researchers really didn't know very much about what caused cancer. Cancer came in many forms and the treatment of the disease was extremely complex. To date, the best a researcher could expect from a new cancer chemical entity was arresting the spread of the disease.

In 1960, Dr. Nakasone re-named the failing chemical company Bandai Pharmaceutical Company. Dr. Nakasone retained the small core of people who had tried desperately to make a success of Bandai Chemical.

Dr. Nakasone knew that he would have a unique organization and that the organization had to be able to survive for many years of research in order to develop a new class of cancer pharmaceuticals. From the beginning, Nakasone's biggest challenge wasn't only to attract the best pharmaceutical research minds from Tokyo, Osaka, and Kyoto, but he had to keep the researchers happy after relocating a long distance from the mainstream of Japanese pharmaceutical power. He knew that when researchers chose to join Bandai it was a career limiting decision and that the other pharmaceutical companies would ostracize them.

Nakasone's business philosophy wasn't all that different from other Japanese industrial executives and leaders. He believed in the team concept, but he also had a deeper belief in the respect that one human should provide another. Respect didn't have to be earned in Nakasone's world. It was given from the first moment of employment.

The Bandai area had been the perfect place for Dr. Nakasone to implement his management philosophy. The village of Bandai was a short four-hour train ride from Tokyo. In Japanese distances, Bandai was close to the metropolitan area of Japan, but not so close that the sprawling Tokyo dragon would swallow up the picturesque village and choke it with its congestion, smog, political corruption, and expensive lifestyle. Dr. Nakasone routinely referred to the Tokyo dragon as the neutron bomb of the 21st Century. Nothing is destroyed, but all dies.

Bandai was still a quiet village and had much of the charm of old Japan. Nacheda loved Bandai, as did the majority of the researchers and workers that he had hired.

Bandai Pharmaceutical Company was successful in Dr. Nakasone's mind. But Tokyo bankers always wanted more return on their investment. They were not totally unhappy with the performance of the company, but they were far from satisfied. As a result, Dr. Nakasone had to take a great deal of personal grief from his pharmaceutical peers. First, he had broken the Dai Nippon loyalty code by leaving the company; second, he had become a viable competitor in several target market segments; and third, he had achieved success in the village of Bandai, not Osaka, Tokyo, Kyoto, or Yokohama.

Dr. Nakasone wanted to expand his company's success and reach for the sky. He wanted success to show the other pharmaceutical companies that, compared to their strong-arm management methods, other philosophies could nurture success.

He had hired Nacheda a little more than one year ago. Nacheda was to provide Bandai Pharmaceutical Company with the strengths that would enable them to deal with the Americans. The strengths that Nakasone lacked because he had chose to locate in Bandai and out of the mainstream of power and business intelligence. There were always good and bad results to every decision. Over the years, Bandai Pharmaceutical had developed into a company with one of the top bioengineering research programs in the world. They had made great strides in their research, but product and revenue successes had been mediocre. Product success had to be earned in the marketplace and assistance had to be purchased from the outside. Thus, into Bandai Pharmaceutical and Nakasone's life entered Nacheda. His only purpose was to find an American pharmaceutical company to target.

When Dr. Nakasone met Nacheda he had immediately taken a liking to him. Nacheda was young by comparison, mature, and confident, but most importantly to Nakasone, he was also humble. He was aggressive, but cautious. Factors which Nakasone admired. Nacheda knew Americans, but not in a way most Japanese knew Americans. He knew Americans in a way that Nacheda would not openly speak about.

Nakasone also knew more about Nacheda than he would ever let on. A friend had given Nacheda's name to Nakasone. A man much respected and who had access to Nacheda's military personnel records and to his post war rehabilitation records.

Nacheda had served with the American forces in Vietnam and Cambodia. He was one of only twenty young Japanese men who had been specially trained by the Japanese government as a secret unit positioned to watch the Southeast Asia War centered in North and South Vietnam. Nacheda, as well as the other nineteen men, were required to report back to the Japanese government what they judged to be present and future threats to Japan. Since participation in warfare was illegal in Japan, Nacheda and his group existed under a secret agreement between the Japanese government and the U.S. Departments of State and Defense. The Central Intelligence Agency had been their sponsor, ensuring that they were adequately trained, equipped, and supplied for whatever they might encounter Southeast Asia.

In plain everyday terms he had been a spy for Japan. His mission was to assist in ensuring that Japan was isolated from becoming involved in the war. Yet, if necessary, Japan would be prepared to be involved. Nacheda hadn't known who the other nineteen spies were, nor did he care to know. He just knew that they were also somewhere in Southeast Asia.

In 1971, Nacheda was captured by the Vietcong and had spent the next two years in the POW camp that American prisoners called the Hanoi Hilton. The Hanoi Hilton was the old prison named Hoa Lo, which translated means place for cooking fires. The prison was constructed with thick walls to withstand the cannon balls of Chinese guns during the past Vietnamese wars with China. Prisoners tried but did not usually succeed in escaping from the Hanoi Hilton.

There were a number of buildings in the prison complex. Some were three stories high. They were connected by walkways. Open areas surrounded the buildings. The small six-by-nine foot cells had cracked and disintegrating cement walls. They were bare except for carved names of inmates of different cultures and the dates that they had existed. The doors were made of heavy wood with two large metal hinges on the passageway side. There was a wooden bar in the middle that assured the door could not be opened unless the guard removed the bar. Food was shoved under the door in a porcelain pan.

In the cell there was a wooden bed with a thin, bare mattress. A light blanket was used for warmth. There was a chipped porcelain pot where he could relieve himself which, at certain times when the food caused him to have dysentery, could be quite often. There was a specific time when the pans were emptied. The prisoners tried to time their visits to the pot as close to the time of pickup as possible. His uniform was a cotton sweat suit that was changed weekly. Cleaning of the sweat suit, if cleaned at all, was with a course soap that caused itching and rash.

In the time before his capture and while he stayed at the Hanoi Hilton, Nacheda grew to know Americans and to respect them for what they represented. He knew Americans continued to fight even though they did not understand or respect the fact that Congress nor the U.S. citizen had neither declared nor approved this war. Nacheda learned to speak and think as an American. He had learned that, in both the jungle and prison, he had to acclimate himself to the environment if he were to survive.

In prison, Nacheda's Japanese culture helped him cope with the solitude, but it wasn't enough to carry him through the ordeals of hardship and isolation. He couldn't tolerate being in complete solitude while being surrounded by American prisoners who managed to communicate with each other about their personal thoughts and lives. It took a year, but he was gradually Americanized. Looking back on the experience, he didn't remember the exact day of his conversion because it happened very slowly. He had begun to secretly communicate with the other prisoners and over time they had accepted him. When he had returned to civilization and his war wounds had healed, Nacheda became a man of two countries. In Japan he was Japanese and when he was in the United States he was an American. Most Japanese didn't understand this split loyalty, but it was understood by Dr. Nakasone.

JAL flight 330 touched down at LAX and started its long taxi to Bradley International Terminal. The large plane docked and the pilot hit the switch that sounded the pong in the cabin. Nacheda unbuckled, stood up, retrieved his briefcase from the overhead compartment, and began to leave the aircraft. At the door he thanked Reiko and left the plane.

Reiko watched Nacheda's lanky body walk down the exit ramp. He was tall for Japanese. Although he always wore loose-fitting clothing, it was not hard to tell that he was physically fit and muscular. His face was very handsome, with cheek bones set unusually high and eyes not as narrow as most Japanese men. Reiko had been very observant of Nacheda during their infrequent in-flight conversations. She thought that Nacheda was a man that she would like to know better, but even in today's world, she felt that Japanese culture made it difficult for a woman to make the first move in a relationship. The man had to do the asking and Nacheda didn't seem to be interested in Reiko.

She turned away from watching Nacheda and went back to the task of saying good-bye to the other passengers. She rationalized her disappointment by thinking that he was just too busy and preoccupied with his work to notice her. Besides, she could not spend anymore time thinking about something that wasn't to be. Her American friends had asked her to a party in Venice Beach later in the evening. She had a 48-hour layover and intended to have fun and not pine over a Japanese businessman passenger.

Nacheda proceeded through the international terminal and on to U.S. customs. He had nothing to declare, but it still took two hours. After clearing customs, he proceeded to the car rental area. Most Japanese businessmen relied on being picked up by associates, but Nacheda wanted to maintain a low profile and he wanted his freedom. He caught the shuttle to the off-site location where he would pick up his car.

Nacheda didn't notice the Asian man standing outside the baggage claim exit. The man closely watched every movement Nacheda had made since leaving customs. When Nacheda got on the shuttle, the man spoke into a handheld scrambler phone. After acknowledging his associate's message with the handset, a second man, who was sitting in a nondescript white Honda, started his car, and drove to the off-site lot where he parked on the street and waited to pick up the surveillance of Nacheda.

After picking up his car, Nacheda drove straight to his condo in Westwood Village. He loved the atmosphere of UCLA and Westwood Village and was pleased that he had chosen it as the center for his operations.

When Nacheda opened the door to his condo in Westwood Village he was met by his team leader, retired Marine Corps Colonel

Skip Howard. Skip had served in Vietnam from 1966 to 1973 as a Marine intelligence officer. He was a highly decorated combat veteran and had worked together with Nacheda in the jungle. Skip lost track of Nacheda in 1972 and tried in vain to locate him for several months. He had finally given up and decided that Nacheda was MIA. It had been impossible for Skip to even think of the possibility that Nacheda might be dead.

In 1973, Skip was wounded in one of the final skirmishes of the war. He ended up at the Naval Hospital in Saigon. Following his release from the Hanoi prison, Nacheda was sent to the same hospital. Their reunion took place in the hospital cafeteria. It was a happy albeit subdued occasion and they made every effort never to lose track of one another again.

When Nacheda received the Bandai mission from Dr. Nakasone, Nacheda contacted Skip immediately. Skip was working in The Pentagon as an executive assistant to an Assistant Secretary of Defense. After Nacheda explained the Bandai project and pleaded with him to join as his head of intelligence for the project, Skip jumped at the opportunity. Skip had already set a date for his retirement from the Marine Corps, so he was able to join Nacheda and begin forming the project team. Together they chose the nondescript condo in Westwood Village.

To kick off the project, the previous February, Skip and Nacheda had met with their assembled project team near the Dallas-Fort Worth Airport for a weekend of briefings. Nacheda told them about Bandai Pharmaceutical Company. He explained that his mission was to find an American pharmaceutical company that marketed products in a market segment that was compatible with Bandai Pharmaceutical research efforts. The team would be rewarded as a team if they were successful. Following the Dallas meeting, they all agreed to participate on a part-time basis. All five would continue to work in their present positions, which added another layer to the cloak of secrecy that Nacheda desired for the team.

The team that Nacheda and Skip had formed went back many years to shared military experiences in Vietnam and afterwards.

Their professional credentials included the head of nursing of Baylor University Hospital in Houston; a lawyer who specialized in healthcare law; a retired neurosurgeon; the editor of the *New England Journal of Medicine*; and a bio-geneticist. Nacheda had agonized for some time over whether he shouldn't just hire people with intelligence gathering backgrounds, but finally opted for a wide variety of professionals with medical and healthcare backgrounds. He felt that he and Skip knew enough about being spies to steer any cloak and dagger issues that might arise.

Skip and Nacheda began to discuss the activities since the last meeting of the team and to plot out the next day's work. Nacheda told Skip about his early Monday morning meeting with Nakasone. Skip was sympathetic, but knew as well as Nacheda that Nakasone had good reason to be angry. They had spent more than 45,000,000 yen of Bandai Pharmaceutical money over the last eleven months. If they failed, it was almost inevitable that, in the long-term, Bandai Pharmaceutical Company would also fail. Bandai would have to sell out to one of the large Japanese pharmaceutical companies. The sale would be set up by one of the Tokyo banks without Dr. Nakasone's approval. If this happened, it would be a sad day, indeed, for Dr. Nakasone, Bandai Pharmaceutical, and the city of Bandai. Nacheda and Skip both knew that Dr. Nakasone would in turn make it a sad day for Nacheda as well. Nakasone was a very poor loser. Their discussions revolved around ways to turn up the urgency levels of the group and whether Skip could forecast any new breakthroughs.

"Well, there has been a ton of data moving to the consoles over the last couple of weeks," Skip said. "It seems that our team has turned up the intensity on their own or there has been a lot of activity in the marketplace since the holidays. AIMS has been grinding away, continually working on the newly transmitted data. Who knows what AIMS will come up with after massaging all the new data." Skip laughed, "Hell, with eleven months of information, the AIMS will either find us an answer or burn itself out trying. Now, let's cut for some dinner. I have more work to do this evening before midnight when team member 8 is planning to perform tune-up routines on AIMS."

Number 8 was the silent member of the team. Only Skip and Nacheda knew the identity of team member 8. Skip was the only person who had actually met member 8. AIMS stood for Artificial Intelligence Management System and was a very sophisticated computer application that sifted through hundreds of online databases analyzing information using algorithms developed by the team. Dr. Nakasone had left nothing to chance in investing Yen to obtain what he wanted. At some point in the analytical process AIMS would present conclusions. To date, there had been no conclusions.

4:30 P.M., MONDAY, JANUARY 16

SPECTRUM OF MEDICINE BUILDING, NYC

The security guard looked down his list of James approved visitors. He then asked for J.P.'s driver's license. The guard was heavy set and outfitted in a light blue colored police-like uniform. His hat was set slightly back and seemed a bit small for his head. He looked to be in his fifties. A slight band of moisture rested on his upper lip from the exertion of carrying his girth. The lobby temperature was comfortable, certainly not hot enough for perspiration. The plastic nametag on his shirt told J.P. that the guard's name was Robert King. The guard took J.P.'s license and examined it very carefully. He looked from the license to J.P.'s face and back to the license again. Then he held up the license at an arm's length in front of J.P. and stared at both the picture and J.P. at the same time.

Apparently satisfied, the guard returned J.P.'s license and said, "Dr. Koenig, welcome to James Pharmaceutical Company and the Spectrum of Medicine. Please use the executive elevator to your left. Dr. Bradsmith said that you are to go directly to his office on the fiftieth floor."

J.P. turned and began walking towards the elevator. The guard moved from behind the security station and began to walk along with J.P. The guard asked, "Dr. Koenig, is this your first trip to the Spectrum of Medicine?"

J.P. continued walking and replied, "Yes, Mr. King, it is." He continued, "Do you have a fear of elevators?"

"No," J.P. answered confidently. "Sir, are you afraid of heights?"

J.P. stepped into the elevator. He was beginning to lose his patience over what seemed to him was quickly becoming an interrogation. "All right, Mr. King, what is this? Why am I being interrogated? I have passed your inspection and I'm an approved guest." J.P. tried to be polite, "I believe I had better be getting up to Dr. Bradsmith's office. He is expecting me. So if you will please excuse me "

The doors began to close. The guard tried to keep the door from closing by waving his chubby hand between the doors. The door continued closing while he urgently said, "But, but, Dr. Koenig.. " The elevator doors closed on his words.

J.P. pushed the button for the thirth floor and turned his back to the doors. He caught a quick glimpse out the heavy glass back of the elevator of the New Jersey Palisades as the elevator began its rapid ascent. J.P. had a sense of rapid acceleration although time seemed to be moving very slowly. The closest analogy he could make was the feeling of going over the top of the tallest roller coaster. He viewed the rapidly receding ground from the glassed wall section of the elevator. He actually began to feel that his legs would buckle. He felt certain that he was experiencing a g-force of two. He realized then that the guard had been trying to warn him about the executive elevator. Even before the elevator arrived at the thirth floor, he began to wonder if there was an alternate means for getting back down to the lobby.

Finally he heard the familiar ding as he arrived at his destination. J.P. stumbled from the elevator, somewhat disoriented and off-balance. He started to fall to the floor of what appeared to be an office lobby, he put his hand out to the wall to steady himself.

Once he felt steadier, he brushed off the dark double-breasted suit that he had put on several hours before in Mammoth. He always believed in playing the role in which he was cast. Phillip expected to see the clean shaven executive J.P. in a business suit, not the bearded Mammoth writer, teacher, and consultant dressed in West Coast business casual. He walked towards a door at the far end of the lobby with a gold plate plaque engraved with "Dr. Phillip T. Bradsmith."

As he walked, he glanced around the lobby. He felt his confidence coming back since the lobby was empty and it didn't appear that there had been any witnesses to his acrobatics. He noted the photographs and murals that were hanging on the walls. He concluded that the room contained the history of James Pharmaceutical Company. It was a historical museum in modern décor. Light in the room was supplied by recessed lighting that duplicated the glow emitted from the afternoon sun streaming through the windows. J.P. figured that there must be a sensor that balanced the lighting between the outside and inside according to the time of day and amount of actual sunlight. The effect was warm and calming. It was in direct contrast to the personal stress of the elevator ride. But, J.P. remembered old Doc. James had a weird since of humor and player of practical jokes.

The walls were filled with memorabilia of ninety-nine years of James history. The history was dominated by three major portraits. The largest was a painting of the founder, Dr. Gunther F. James. Under his portrait there was a gold plated plaque, which read:

Dr. Gunther Frederick James Founder of James Pharmaceutical Company Born 1879, Stuttgart, Germany Died 1949, Sheepshead Bay, Long Island, New York President and Chairman, 1906-1949

On either side of the founder were two additional paintings. One was of the Doc James that J.P. had known and the other was of Phillip. He looked at these slightly smaller paintings and read their plaques.

Gunther Frederick James, Jr., Honorary Doctor of Philosophy Born 1924, Sheepshead Bay, Long Island, New York Died 1996, Sheepshead Bay, Long Island, New York President and Chairman, 1949-1996 You could easily see that Doc James was the son of the founder. Their sharp facial features were the same. The founder had a large beard and the son a full moustache. They shared the same faraway look in their eyes. The eyes portrayed the vision they had for James Pharmaceutical. Both men had been tall for their eras. Doc James was six feet tall, but he always gave the illusion of being well over six feet. Both men had square, but not large shoulders. Their hair was dark and eyes were pale blue. The faraway look didn't hide the kindness that showed in their faces.

The founder looked like he was in his eighties when his portrait was painted, but young Doc James looked like he was in his early sixties. He had always looked younger than his age. He had been married four times.

J.P. looked to the founder's left and saw the portrait of his friend.

Phillip T. Bradsmith, MBA, Doctor of Philosophy Born 1948, Ojai, California President and Chief Executive Officer, 1996—

Phillip looked as J.P. had last seen him before he took over the presidency. He was robust. His 6'4 stature showed the physical conditioning of the man who had played rugby well into his thirties. He had the tan of a Californian, blond hair, and brown eyes. His jaw was square and determined. His eyes showed the understanding of a teacher. Phillip looked liked a corporate president. The other two men resembled grandfathers.

There was one more portrait that was hanging all by itself on the wall panel to the right. It was slightly larger than Phillip's portrait and was of a woman. The plaque read:

Mrs. Evelyn Preston-James Born 1957, Scarsdale, New York Chairperson of the Board, 1996—

J.P. had never met the fourth and last Mrs. Doc James. The last time he had seen Doc James was in the old James offices on First Avenue. He vaguely remembered the wedding picture sitting on Doc's desk. In the picture the former Miss Evelyn Preston of Scarsdale, New York and Wellesley University was standing next to Doc James. They had been married in 1985. She was thirty-three and he was a young sixty-one when they married. J.P. had been invited to the wedding, but at the time he was starting a new company on the West Coast and could not get away. The employees of James thought it was great that Doc was marrying a young, intelligent woman to be with him in the remainder of his years.

J.P. studied her portrait. He thought Mrs. James was a handsome looking woman. Mrs. Evelyn Preston-James, as she insisted on being called, had class. J.P. could tell that from the expression on her face. He supposed that any woman born in Scarsdale and educated at Wellesley would be expected to have class. Other than that, he could deduce no other insights from the portrait.

Mrs. Evelyn Preston-James had made it to the top. Chairperson of the James Pharmaceutical Company Board of Directors. He looked back and forth at the two portraits and wondered how Phillip and she were getting along.

As he continued through the lobby, J.P. noticed the various plaques of patents hanging on the wall. He had seen the plaques in the old First Avenue offices. They illustrated the 25 patents that James had been granted for work in herbal pharmaceutical compounds. Herbal pharmaceuticals were the past strength of James and also the hope for its future. This strategic strength was in contrast to the current trend of pharmaceutical development. Herbs were not thought of as the future and had, for the most part, been replaced by synthetic pharmaceuticals in the 60's and 70's. In the 80's and 90's all progressive, successful drug companies strove to develop their products from the bio-genetic engineering class of pharmaceuticals. Doc James was attempting to make the transition from herbs to bio-genetic engineering when he died. In the recent pharmaceutical industry periodicals there had been numerous articles describing Phillip's continuing attempts to pull James into the 21st century.

Phillip did not want to give up the past herbal heritage, but he had to show the financial community and physicians that James, Inc., was a company to be reckoned with well into the 21st century. J.P. again wondered if Mrs. Preston-James was helping or hindering Phillip in his challenge to change the company.

He reached Phillip's door and turned the handle to open it. Just inside the door was a second lobby. This room was dominated by a large mahogany reception desk. Janet Williams sat behind the desk. Janet had been Phillip's secretary and now executive assistant since he had become president. Now in her late thirties and a mother of two children in high school, J.P. thought that she still looked great. Her long black hair framed her face. She hated short hair and always kept hers as long as possible even when styles were short. Her figure wasn't thin or heavy. J.P. guessed that she was the same weight as when he last saw her.

Janet made a quick glance from her desk at J.P. "Hello.. .may I help you?"

"Janet, you look as great as ever," J.P. said as he crossed the room towards her desk. "How is the family?"

Suddenly, with recognition, Janet's face lit up. She pushed her chair back and jumped up from her desk. She ran around the side of the desk and threw her arms around J.P.'s neck, kissing him on the mouth.

"My God, J.P., is it really you? You look wonderful. Why didn't you tell us you were visiting, I'd have sent a limo. How are you?" She kissed him again.

"Whoa, Janet, hold on. It's great to see you too, but this is more of a welcome than I bargained for," J.P. said laughing.

Janet smiled and said, "It is such a wonderful surprise to see you again,

J.P. I couldn't help myself." She paused, "And by the way, how come you don't write or call?" Her smile widened.

"Well, for a guy who has retired twice in the last ten years, I manage to stay busy." He noted that Phillip must not have told her about the phone call or the trip to New York. That seemed a little strange to J.P. Generally, Phillip told her everything, or at least he had done so in the past.

J.P. asked her, "How is Bill, Sr., and the rest of the family?"

"Everyone is fine. The twins, Linda and Bill, Jr., are seniors in high school and preparing for college. Both are very bright and want to stay close to home. They've been accepted to Princeton. It's expensive, about $100,000 per year for the two of them, but we'll get through it. I just hope they are able to find some way to tear themselves away from their anticipated social activities to study and finish in four years. The expenses are going to be particularly tough with Bill's new job."

Janet noted the look of shock on J.P.'s face and answered his question before he had time to ask. "I'm sorry, you didn't know that Bill left James, did you?"

"No, I didn't. What happened?"

"Bill left James a little over a year ago. We knew that with Phillip as president, it would be very difficult for Bill to rise any higher than executive vice president of business development. Phillip's strategy isn't to acquire or license new products. The strategy is to develop all products internally. So Bill became discouraged and when an opportunity presented itself a year ago, he left James and took a position as president of a high tech start-up company.

"Phillip tried to get him to stay, but Bill felt it would be better to solve a potential depressing situation by taking a new opportunity. The company is developing exciting new technology in clinical testing instrumentation. Bill had to take a cut in pay, but he received stock options for a 10% share of the company. The company, Clintec, is funded by venture capital."

"And how are things going after a year?" J.P. asked.

"It's been rough. The company isn't profitable and they have cash flow problems, but everyone has high hopes," she replied. "But what about you? What brings you to Doc James' Spectrum of Medicine?"

J.P. was desperately trying to think of something to tell her, when the door to Phillip's office flew open. Phillip took a step towards J.P. and Janet and then stopped with a startled look on his face. In the next instant he realized that it was, in fact, J.P. and he smiled and continued forward taking J.P.'s hand in his and then hugging him.

"By God, Janet, why didn't you tell me that Jean Paul was here? What brings you to this cold, miserable climate? Is it too warm for you in California?"

"I had just asked him that same question. Just before you busted in on our private conversation, Dr. Bradsmith," Janet said with more than a little bit of reproach in her voice.

"Yes, well, I do apologize, Mrs. Williams. I will try harder in the future to contain my enthusiasm when I see an old friend whom I haven't seen for some time. Please do continue your *private conversation* while I visit one of my staff. I should return in ten minutes. Will that be sufficient?" Without waiting for a response he turned and walked out towards the elevators.

"I see there's not much that has changed around here," J.P. said with a smile after Phillip disappeared into the outer lobby.

"No, I learned a long time ago how to handle him. If I'm meek, he'll run all over me. If I beat him to the punch, he usually backs down," she said proudly.

J.P. and Janet continued their conversation for a few more minutes before he excused himself to wait in Phillip's office. J.P. hoped that Phillip hadn't noticed the surprised look on his face when he saw him. Phillip wasn't the same man that J.P. remembered from a few years previous, nor was he the man in the portrait in that outer lobby. Phillip had aged dramatically. His blond hair was receding and there were gray streaks in the hair at his temples. In J.P.'s estimation he looked to be nearly 20 pounds heavier than when he had last seen him. It occurred to J.P. that all in all he still looked the part of a dignified executive and most people who saw him every day would not have noticed the changes. J.P. wondered if the change in his physical appearance had anything to do with whatever had prompted Phillip to call him to New York.

J.P. looked around the office. It was an executive office, not the office of the president of a large pharmaceutical company. It was large, but not too large and more functional than auspicious. Phillip's offices were never for show, but rather designed for work. The décor was modern metal with wood furnishings. This seemed to blend nicely with the steel and smoked glass of the building. Windows were on two sides of the corner room and bookshelves on the third. In front of the bookshelves was a full-length couch. His desk was in the center facing the door with the windows at his back. In front of one of the windows and behind the desk was a credenza. There were two doors on the side from which he had entered. The windows were ceiling to floor. They had the same hue that he had seen in the outer office and lower lobby. Again he felt warm and welcome.

He walked to the second door. It was unusual looking. There was a window built into the door that allowed you to see into the next room. Judging by its tint, J.P. guessed that this was a one-way mirror. J.P. looked through this window and saw that it was a conference room, which probably doubled as a boardroom.

The room was large by most standards. Two large pictures hung on one wall. One was a picture of the old James headquarters and the other of the Spectrum of Medicine. There was a door along the wall with the pictures that J.P. assumed was the entry from Janet's office for visitors. J.P. entered the conference room and looked at the wall that separated the room from Phillip's office. On one side of the door hung pictures depicting Phillip's career with James as well as his honors and degrees. On the other side was a ceiling to floor bookshelf. The books on the shelves were old Physician Desk References and old pharmaceutical books.

J.P. smiled when he realized that this was more than the James conference boardroom. It was also Phillip's ego room. J.P. imagined that when Phillip had visitors who didn't know him, he would probably leave them in the conference room for a few minutes. He probably watched them through the one-way mirror in the door. If the visitor examined the pictures and the books they would know a little about Dr. Phillip T. Bradsmith, Ph.D., the man that they were about to meet. If the visitor just stared out the window, Phillip probably assumed they didn't care to know about the man with whom they were dealing. This afforded Phillip the opportunity to take advantage of the situation by knowing a little more about his visitor if he needed a negotiating edge.

J.P. returned to Phillip's office. He noted the computer on the mahogany desk and remembered how he had dragged Phillip into the world of personal computers. Stacks of papers were on the credenza in what seemed to be disarray, but he knew that this was Phillip's way of working. Phillip always knew what every piece of paper contained and where it was located in the stacks. Along another wall was a large video screen. Just in front of that was a small conference table. This was definitely Phillip's office, not the office of Doc James. Doc James' office would have had an antique décor.

It was curious. Doc James had been a visionary, made frequent decision changes, and preferred old style surroundings. Phillip was a decision-maker, confident in his implementation of other peoples' visions, and preferred modern, simple, functional surroundings. The differences in business styles and talents were why James was finally on its way up in the pharmaceutical marketplace. In truth, a little slowly, but a slow upward trend was preferable to a flat or downward trend.

A few days before, Jack Husted mentioned in his *Wall Street Journal* column that, "Dr. Phillip T. Bradsmith was fulfilling the vision that the James boys had always had for their company. Maybe one day soon, we will finally know what Dr. Bradsmith was talking about when he used the words, a "Magnitude of Change" at the opening of the James Spectrum of Medicine building." On that day, the stock went up \$5 per share for about twenty-four hours and then came back down to \$60 where it had been bouncing around for two years.

J.P. walked over to one of the windows and stared west in the direction of the New Jersey side of the Hudson River. In the distance, late afternoon clouds shrouded the Watchung Mountains. The sun had set behind the mountains and the clouds were a light shade of pink from the last rays of sunlight. He looked at his watch and saw that it was just past 5:00. The New York City commuters' working day was coming to a close.

"And I'm just getting started," he said quietly to himself.

J.P. saw the office door open in the window reflection. He slowly turned around from the window and beheld the face of a worried man.

Phillip motioned him to sit down at the small conference table. J.P. moved from the window and sat down at the table. Phillip walked over and took a seat on the opposite side. He was staring off in the direction of the window, saying nothing.

J.P. finally took the initiative, "OK, Phillip, why the call?"

Phillip turned his head and looked straight into J.P.'s eyes. The vigor and confidence that J.P. had known in his friend's stare was replaced now with a look of dark dread.

"Jean Paul, I need your help." He continued before J.P. could say anything, "No, don't say anything J.P. Not yet. Not until I finish my story. You will probably say that I am crazy or that Old Doc James' ghost has been walking the corridors of this building. So please, hear me out and then you can make your decision as to my mental state. After your diagnosis, Dr. Koenig, you can decide whether you can, or even want to help me." A slight grin appeared at one corner of his mouth and then quickly disappeared.

"As you know," he leaned back in his chair slightly and again turned his head to stare out the window. "James' released the drug Lifeal for antiarrhythmia use four years ago. We positioned the product as a preventive or prophylaxis to ventricular fibrillation. This disease is estimated to kill more than 1,000,000 last year. If we use a low death rate of 6%, the number of people walking around with cardiac arrhythmia is almost thirteen million…thirteen million. These patients have to take a pharmaceutical one or more times per day. This is a huge market.

The pharmaceuticals used in the treatment of cardiac arrhythmia are simply that, a treatment, they don't cure the disease. Patients are not generally diagnosed with cardiac arrhythmia until they have experienced an occurrence of sudden disruption in their heart's rhythm. Once diagnosed, the patient is placed on a course of an anti-arrhythmia pharmaceutical.

"There are a number of different ways to prevent the reoccurrence of cardiac arrhythmia, but nothing currently available on the market can prevent the initial onset." Phillip moved his chair closer to his desk and stared intensely into J.P.'s eyes. "We believed that Lifeal had the necessary properties to prevent the first occurrence of fibrillation. You see Lifeal works on the heart's atrioventricular or AV mode by modulating its activity.

"Based on our clinical studies we profiled a patient who would likely be the most susceptible to a cardiac arrhythmia. We then promoted Lifeal as the best course for this type of patient. We couldn't say that Lifeal was a preventative of cardiac arrhythmia because we didn't yet have FDA clearance for the prophylactic indication. We hoped... .we believed that physicians would find out the unique properties of Lifeal for themselves, but our strategy hasn't worked. Lifeal's primary ingredient is derived from an alkaloid of the Indonesian Alstonia Spectabilis tree, more commonly known as the Devil Tree. We have a patent on the compound. At any rate, as I've said, our prophylactic strategy hasn't worked. Physicians refuse to prescribe on a projected occurrence of a disease based solely upon a documented patient profile provided to them by a manufacturer." Phillip smiled slightly for the first time since they had set down, "Physicians can be so uncooperative that way. And, by the way, the FDA still has not given us clearance.

"Thus, Lifeal is classified in the group of cardiac arrhythmia compounds as just another treatment. The large pharmaceutical companies who make the leading treatment products have the marketing strength to keep James from earning a reasonable market share. Lifeal grows, but slower than what we have forecasted or what we require for working capital to support our research programs.

"Truthfully Jean Paul, Lifeal is a good product, not great perhaps, but certainly better than its market performance. I'm sure time will prove me right on this.of that I have little doubt." He paused. "Have you heard of Husted, of the Wall Street Journal? Have you read any of his reports of James?"

J.P. nodded. He was puzzled that Phillip didn't seem to remember that Jack, Phillip, and he had all been friends years before. He had known Jack Husted since he first arrived in New York City to work in the James corporate headquarters. J.P. started to say something, but then decided to let Phillip continue.

"Well, Husted can go to hell with that conservative, narrow-minded view that he expresses in his column. Lifeal will prove itself in the marketplace, given time. Given the time.that I suppose is the hook, J.P. I don't know how much time we have before things really run afoul."

J.P. finally spoke, "What do you mean, Phillip? Not enough time before what?"

"The James board has been on my tail for the past year. They want a better performance from the James stock. The current stock price languishing at $60 is not their idea of success. Particularly when their stock options are at

$50." His face took on an angry expression. "Damn this board's nonoperating attitude. If I listened to those parasites on the board about how to run James, we would be mired down in problems of our own creation rather than those created by our competition. If you haven't yet heard or figured it out, the board sides nearly unanimously with Mrs. Evelyn Preston-James. I am in a constant battle to get anything, in terms of business, past the board. I'm certain that she will attempt to make a bold move at this year's annual meeting in May. Jean Paul, if she continues with outdated and selfish strategies for James it will almost certainly destroy the company. I believe she will do almost anything to get control of the company away from me and then implement a litany of short-range plans that will increase share prices, but not the value of this company. Along with her overall attempts to manipulate the stock, she continues to increase the dividends for her own benefit. I certainly don't have to tell you that increasing dividends cuts into the working capital for research.

"Jean Paul, Lifeal isn't all we have going for James. In the course of our research and work with the various derivatives of Alstonia Spectabilis tree bark, we have made a remarkable discovery in terms of herbology. Don't laugh, I know, some research analyst in the investment community would say that we have been holding on to our traditional herbal research strength too long. Well, believe it or not, we have made a breakthrough. I don't have time to go through the specifics now, but if you decide to help me, you will learn more about our new Alzheimer's compound called JPC138.

"As you may imagine, if we have a genuine breakthrough in a cure for Alzheimer's, James will be one of the hottest pharmaceutical companies with both the investment community and the medical marketplace. We will finally bring in a winner and achieve that elusive 'magnitude of difference' I so flippantly spoke about years ago that no one will ever let me forget. The James Board knows we have a new compound and that it has potential to become the greatest boon to mankind since penicillin, but they don't understand the clinical or financial possibilities. I have purposely withheld some pieces of the entire picture for fear that they might try to take advantage of the situation by hyping the stock. I am convinced that this would ultimately prove a disaster for JPC138 before we can properly prepare the public for disclosure of our discovery. I've taken great pains to ensure that everyone that is or has been associated with the discovery of JPC138 has been sworn to secrecy. Which reminds me."

Phillip got up from his seat and walked back over to his desk to retrieve a piece of paper. J.P. noted with some concern that Phillip never straightened upright as he walked from the conference table to his desk. He walked back to the conference table and laid the paper on the table, pushing it towards J.P.

"As a precaution, Jean Paul, I would like for you to sign this confidentiality agreement. I have every confidence that I can trust you, but I had better do this just to keep a paper trail, as they say."

J.P. signed the document without reading it. He had signed hundreds of confidentiality agreements over the years and knew they all said the same thing and rarely held up in court. He pushed the document back over towards Phillip.

Phillip spoke, "I am sorry that it is taking me so long to finally get to the point. I wanted you to have the background that I've just given you in order for you to fully understand the ramifications of what I am now going to tell you." He paused for a long moment. "Jean Paul, someone is stealing James' secrets. I don't know how, why, or even what, but I do know someone, or perhaps it is more than one person, is stealing from us."

J.P. had begun to grow impatient with the meandering fashion with which Phillip was finally getting to the point of his summons.

That combined with the fatigue from his long day of travel caused him to respond to Phillip with an edge in his voice.

"Oh come on, Phillip! Just spit it out, what are you really saying? Is someone stealing product and reselling it to pharmacies? If that's it, what the hell do you need me for? You could solve this by hiring better security at the plant."

Phillip answered calmly, "Please, Jean Paul, just listen. It isn't that simple and I don't know whether I can even correctly explain all of my fears." He leaned forward with his elbows on the conference table and his chin resting in the cradle of his two thumbs. He rubbed his temples with his forefingers as he put his thoughts together.

J.P. studied Phillip's posture and realized that his old friend, a consummate business leader, was obviously in the throes of something much deeper than common thievery. J.P.'s voice took on a quiet and concerned tone.

"Okay Phillip, what the hell is going on here?"

Phillip lifted his head and looked directly at J.P. "I called you because you are the only person I feel that I can truly trust and aid me in a situation that could easily be a harbinger of death for this company." He paused and a slight smile came to him. "I know I am sometimes overly dramatic, so I will leave it you to come to your own conclusions about the situation.

"Last fall we rewrote our strategic business plan. We being, myself and my staff. We felt that since Lifeal had not lived up to its potential after four years on the market, we should take some time to make an out-of-the-box study of our entire operation. The strategic planning process was one of the best in which I had ever been involved. It was good planning, nothing was sacred and everything was on the table. We took input from all over the company. My personal staff worked overtime flushing out new ideas. It was an exciting process as we all were working on the same agenda, to make James a better company. The board, quite naturally, wasn't very excited because I did not fully involve them and they were more than a bit peeved at my long-term efforts when they think I should be focused on the short-term. Nevertheless, we worked the real issues and came up with what I felt were excellent strategies and tactics to turn problems into opportunities. To use an old favorite phrase of yours, we were planning to pro-act against threats, both internal and external.

"When the 21ˢᵗ Century Plan, as I preferred to call it, was completed last November, I made six copies. The original was placed in my safe along with one computer disk containing the entire plan. I distributed the six copies to my COO, Joe Marshall; Brian Smith, CFO; Dr. Helmut Wahlters, senior vice president of research; and Amanda Hays, whom you will meet soon. She's the vice president of marketing. A copy also went to Henry Sanberg, vice president of professional relations, and the final copy I retained to use as a working paper.

"Six copies, Jean Paul. After the plan was completed I saw to it personally that it was purged from all electronic media, save for the one CD. Mind you, I'm not paranoid. I just wanted to make absolutely sure that I had control of the plan. Each of the five staff members with copies of the plan had their own focused departmental plan backing up the 21ˢᵗ Century Plan. The 21ˢᵗ Century Plan was considered company secret."

J.P. shifted slightly in his seat, trying to fathom exactly where was the problem.

"As I mentioned," Phillip continued, "the 21ˢᵗ Century Plan contained our long-term strategy. What I failed to mention was that it also contained a comprehensive explanation of the areas where we currently have major corporate problems. Details of potential situations with regulatory, research, toxicology, and marketing. All issues that turned up during our study...veritable snakes in the proverbial woodpile you might say. The plan also contained a very detailed overview of how we arrived at our breakthrough with JPC138 and what we are planning to do to exploit the technology. When I made the determination to make hard copies of this comprehensive plan, I did so hesitantly, but release it I did to five trusted corporate officers."

"Damn, Phillip, what the hell were you thinking? Were you planning to publish it as a manifesto in the New York Times? Okay, that aside...what's the real problem? Phillip continued without acknowledging J.P.'s sarcasm, "In last Friday's mail I received an envelope postmarked from Doylestown, Pennsylvania. Inside the envelope were a letter and a copy of a page from James' 21st Century Plan. The letter was from a pharmacist named G. Kuhn."

Phillip picked up a piece of paper that had lying on the table next to him and handed it to J.P.

KUHN APOTHECARY 44 East Court Street Doylestown, PA 18901 January 10th

Phillip T. Bradsmith, Ph.D. President

James Pharmaceutical Company Spectrum of Medicine Building Upper Westside Commercial Center New York, NY 09010

Dear Dr. Bradsmith,

A belated Happy New Year. I hope you have a very successful year. You do not know me, but I am a strong supporter of James Pharmaceutical Company. I own a small apothecary in Doylestown. It is not large, but I compete well against the large chains that are located in the shopping malls. I am writing to you because of the attachment to this letter.

Last Thanksgiving, while I was cleaning my coin operated copy machine I found the attached page marked "secret". I guessed it might be a page from a James business plan. I wasn't entirely sure because the words didn't make any sense. I recognized the name, James Pharmaceutical, of course and since it was marked "secret" I thought you would want it returned.

Whoever made the copy had apparently not noticed that two copies had been made. It's an old copy machine and sometimes it hiccups and makes two copies of a page. This has never bothered me too much since it never registers on the counter so my customers are never charged for the extra copy. If they get an extra copy for free, they're happy which in turn makes me happy.

The page was jammed inside the machine. It must have been the last page of whatever it was that the person was copying. I make that assumption ofcourse on the fact that if it were any other page the customer would have noticed the jam and brought it to my attention. I have to get that machine fixed some day.

I apologize for the lateness in sending this back to you. I found the page around noon when I was closing up to go home for Thanksgiving dinner with my family. I was in a rush to get home and threw the page on the pile of paperwork that seems to grow exponentially on my desk.

I realize I am rambling. It's one of my weaknesses. Anyway, the page was forgotten and misplaced until yesterday when I began to close my books for yearend.

Good luck to you and your new product, Lifeal. I know the prescriptions aren't as high as you would like them to be, but give the product time and don't give up on the prophylactic concept. It is good to see James coming through with new products again. We pharmacists are all with you and hope that James can survive the invasion from Japanese companies. Tokyo is a long distance to call for drug interaction assistance!

Again, have a happy and prosperous New Year. If you ever visit Doylestown, please stop by and say hello. You are always welcome.

Sincerely,

G. Kuhn, Pharm. D.

J.P. handed the letter back across the table to Phillip. "Phillip, what are you so excited about?" he asked. "So one of your trusted five wanted a spare copy or became careless and left the plan lying around for someone else to borrow and make a copy. We both know that strategic plans don't do anyone else any good. If your competitors did get hold of the plan they would likely figure it was planted misinformation. If someone tried to sell it to any other

U.S. company, the competitor would blackball that person and give you a phone call. You know as well as I do that strategic plans can change."

As J.P. continued to talk and rationalize the situation, he became less certain of his confidence in his assessment that nothing bad would come of the duplicated plan. It dawned on him suddenly what the long build-up to his reason for being there was about. J.P. was about to say something when Phillip slammed his fist on the table.

"Goddamnit, Jean Paul, don't you get it? There is a section in that plan that contains a detailed analysis of Lifeal and JPC138. Some person or persons has access to the family jewels and I cannot sit here and honestly say whether it's friend or foe. It has been two months since the plan was copied. I certainly haven't noticed any unusual activity among my executive staff. Do the thieves have anything in progress? What will they do with the information? Just think of the damage that this information could do if it fell into the hands of someone like Jack Husted. What do you think the FDA would do if they had a copy of all of our problems?

"Jean Paul, I need your help! This is driving me crazy. I spent the entire weekend thinking of the worst scenarios possible. I don't even recall any of the discussion from this morning's executive staff meeting. I was too busy looking at each of my staff attempting to ascertain who among them might be plotting against me or this company."

J.P. leaned forward slightly in his seat. "Phillip, I have to be honest with you. I think you may be tilting at windmills here, but I can't give you an honest opinion until I see what was in the 21st Century Plan. Maybe, as an uninvolved third party, I can determine whether the information would be valuable to a competitor and therefore damaging to James."

Phillip got up and walked across the room to his personal safe. While it wasn't hidden, it was recessed into the wall. He pressed his palm against the reader unit and waited until one of the two red lights above the safe turned to green signifying that the unit had made a positive recognition. He then placed his right index finger into a hole located in the center of the security lock and tapped out a numeric code on a cipher pad. The safe opened with a soft hiss as the pressure changed in the safe.

"Jesus, Phillip what do you keep in there...launch protocols for a ballistic missile strike?"

"Well, one can't be too careful nowadays, can one?"

J.P. noted that the irony of what Phillip had just said seemed lost on him as he reached into the safe and brought out a one-inch binder. He walked back across the room and handed the binder to J.P.

"Please sit here and read the plan. I will do some work at my desk," Phillip said as he walked back around to his desk and began working at the computer.

J.P. looked over the document. It was glued with a slight break in the soft cover about "from the edge. Buried in the glue were five recessed screws. J.P. could see the screw heads on both sides of the binder. Interestingly there were no grooves on the heads to facilitate a screwdriver or anything else. J.P. opened the publication and wondered how anyone could make a copy without completely destroying the book. Although, he reflected, today's handheld scanners could scan in the document.

J.P. read and studied the plan for nearly two hours. He first skimmed the plan to get the macro view and then read it more slowly to analyze the microelements. He had written down a list of additional material he would need from Phillip to continue his study.

J.P. closed the plan and looked up. Phillip was still working at his computer, probably answering e-mail. If there was one thing that J.P. did not miss in the corporate environment was dealing with daily landslide of electronic messages. J.P. glanced at his watch, which read 8:00 p.m. At that moment Phillip looked up from what he was doing.

"So, old friend...how is it going? Find anything interesting?"

"First, Phillip, I have to compliment you. You have come a long way in the time since we last worked together in terms of writing strategic plans. This is very well written and more importantly it is clear enough that it can be understood by anyone and implemented. I dare say that if you were killed on the road tonight whoever followed you would be able to carry on nicely. Of course, the flip side of that is you've written such a great plan that any competitor with a copy has a blueprint for success in this business and possible insights into destroying James Pharmaceutical."

Phillip's face took on the dark expression he'd shown earlier. "Yes, I know. Hopefully now you can better understand my concerns regarding this errant page that turned up in Doylestown. My greatest fear is that someone close to me, a member of my immediate staff, is the culprit."

J.P. rubbed his eyes as his lack of sleep began to take its toll, "I know it looks bad, Phillip, but let's wait a bit to see if we can figure out who and why before we start jumping to conclusions. Now then, there are a few more materials that I'll need to see before I can come to any real conclusions and tomorrow morning is fine. Do you think it would be possible to put the documents on this list onto a portable hard drive that I can take back to Mammoth for a few days of careful study?" J.P. walked across the room and handed Phillip the list.

Phillip took the list from him and looked it over. "I don't see why not, if I can't trust you, I am in serious trouble. Let's see here, a copy of the employee confidentiality agreement, a copy of the company standards and policies, departmental versions of the 21st Century Plan for marketing, production, and research, a copy of our FDA filing for Lifeal.research and clinical results for Lifeal. and the research plan for JPC138. Well, there's nothing here that should present a problem in obtaining. I'll have this for you first thing tomorrow morning."

J.P smiled, he could see Phillip's mood lifting again, "For the rest of this evening, I'd like access to your personnel department files. May I use your computer to access those records?"

Phillip turned back to his computer and typed in a few access codes, "There, it's all set for you. Do you have a plan of attack, Jean Paul?"

"A plan is forming, but give me until tomorrow morning to put a proposal together."

"Very well. Do you have a place to stay tonight?"

J.P. looked around him, "If you don't mind, your couch looks very comfortable. Knowing your work ethic I'm certain you've spent a few nights sleeping in your office."

"Indeed I have and, yes, it is very comfortable. There is a full bath with shower over there." Phillip pointed across the room to the wall with the bookshelves. He reached under his desk and pushed a button. A section of the bookshelves swung outward, revealing a bathroom.

"All the things you'll need are in the bathroom including a clean set of sheets and a blanket. There's also a small refrigerator in there with soft drinks and a couple of those frozen pasta dinners. The microwave is on top of the fridge. Now, unless you require me for anything more, I believe I'll depart for the evening."

"Give Sandi a hug for me. See you tomorrow morning."

"I will. Thanks again, J.P.," Phillip said as he picked up his brief case and left the office.

J.P. sat down at Phillip's desk and stared at the computer screen. He smiled to himself as he realized he had almost spoken a command for the computer to respond before he remembered that it wasn't his custom MAC at home. His home MAC was a new prototype he got from a fellow he knew at Apple. I was complete with built in complete voice recognition. J.P. would have to input his requests to Phillip's computer the old fashioned method, manually. J.P. touched the mouse and the screen suddenly displayed the entire James organizational chart. He clicked on one of the organizational boxes and a sub-organization dropped onto the screen complete with names. He clicked the top organizational box and Phillip's personnel record filled the screen. He continued reading through five levels of employees, taking a few notes, but mostly mentally noting interesting facts that stood out about people. He was looking for historical connections or possible connections between members of different departments or management levels.

Around, 11:00 p.m. fatigue finally caught up with him and he prepared himself and the sofa bed for a night's rest.

SPECTRUM OF MEDICINE BUILDING
NEW YORK CITY

J.P.'s internal alarm clock woke him at 5:00 a.m. He lay still for a few minutes gathering his thoughts and trying to remember where he was. Finally, he swung his legs over the side of Phillip's converted couch, walked to the desk and located the hidden switch that opened the bathroom door. The bathroom light spilled out into the office giving the furniture a surreal appearance in the otherwise dark room. J.P. turned on a desk lamp and by its light finally located a light switch for the room on a wall near the door to the outer office. He converted the bed back into a sofa and headed towards the bathroom to prepare for his day.

After shaving and showering, J.P. dressed and began hunting around for a coffee maker. He found it near Janet's desk in the outer office. He filled the coffeepot with water from the cooler, poured the water into the coffee maker, added fresh grounds, and turned the machine on. He stood staring at the coffee maker until its cycle finished and poured him a cup of coffee. Now he was ready to get started.

He walked back into Phillip's office and sat down in front of Phillip's computer. J.P. typed out a point paper that covered Phillip's concerns:

Jean Paul Koenig, Ph.D.

13 Snow Run Drive Mammoth Lakes, CA 93546

PERSONAL AND SECRET

FOR DR. PHILLIP T. BRADSMITH'S EYES ONLY

To: Phillip T. Bradsmith, Ph.D.

From: Jean Paul Koenig, Ph.D.

Subject: 21st Century Plan Point Paper

Reference (a) 21st Century Plan

Enclosure (1) Contract

OBJECTIVE

The objective of the project you have asked me to evaluate is to determine who is stealing or attempting to steal James Pharmaceutical Company, Inc. (JPC) technology and for what purpose.

CONTRACT

Enclosure (1) is a contract between Jean Paul Koenig, Ph.D., (Koenig) and JPC.

INITIAL FINDINGS

After an initial review of the JPC 21st Century Plan, it is evident that there is a strong possibility that some of James' current products (Lifeal), products in research, and long-term strategies have been compromised and are targets for corporate espionage by an unknown party or parties. This preliminary conclusion is based on the following findings and assumptions:

- *A page from one of six copies of the secret JPC 21s Century Plan was found in a Doylestown pharmacy copy machine.*

- *The new James compound labeled JPC138 is a revolutionary pharmaceutical research concept and is therefore, an excellent candidate for pharmaceutical espionage.*

- The 21st Century Plan was comprehensive in all respects, especially in the description of current and future potential problems. Should this information fall into the hands of certain competitors or others wishing to do JPC harm, it could adversely affect JPC and, in some cases, could provide certain competitors, in the global pharmaceutical marketplace, unfair advantages. There is the remote possibility that some of the information pertaining to regulatory issues could be taken out of context and used to blackmail James.

PLAN OF ACTION AND MILESTONES WEEK OF JANUARY 16

- Contract: Koenig and JPC sign the attached contract.

- Information: Information requested January 16 to be provided to Koenig in electronic format no later than January 17.

- Assistant: Identify a qualified assistant for Koenig on January 17.

- Review of Data: All data will be reviewed and analyzed from 18 to 22 January. The findings will be analyzed by Koenig and presented to Dr. Bradsmith on Monday, 23 January at 7a.m. in his office.

QUESTIONS/MATERIAL

I would like the following questions answered:

- Has the Board approved the 21st Century Plan and signified who opposed and who favored the plan?

- Gross margins on Lifeal have declined since product release. Why?

- What are the marketing reasons for Lifeal's weak penetration of the anti-arrhythmia marketplace?

- Who is on the JPC138 research team?

- Cash reserves are low. How is JPC going to acquire enough working capital to complete and launch JPC138?

J.P. finished typing his point paper and drained his fourth cup of coffee. He saved the report to the hard drive and then printed a copy. He gathered his things up from Phillip's desk and returned to the bathroom to finish dressing. As he was adjusting his tie, he thought he heard movement in the office. Deciding that it must be Phillip he walked into the office and saw Janet standing behind Phillip's desk studying his papers. Janet jumped when she saw J.P. and he detected what he interpreted to be a guilty look on her face.

"Good morning, Janet."

"J.P., you startled me. Did you have a good rest?" She continued without waiting for his answer, "I was just straightening up Phillip's desk to see if what he might have left for me to do today. Is there anything I can do for you today?"

"Thanks very much for asking. I really don't know what I may need. I need to talk with Phillip first. Just so you know, I'm planning to leave around noon."

As he spoke, J.P. watched Janet's body language. He wasn't sure whether she had seen the secret report or whether it mattered even if she did. She seemed nervous and was standing behind the desk with her hands folded in front of her.

J.P. smiled at her and said, "We didn't finish our talk yesterday. How are things going?"

Janet returned the smile, "Things are going okay, all things considered." "I don't mean to pry Janet, but what do you mean by all things considered?"

"Well, how about if I get myself a cup of coffee and we can sit and talk for a few minutes."

"Great. I have until Phillip arrives. Be warned though, that coffee is a bit on the potent side."

Janet seemed to relax a bit, "I remember full well your coffee, J.P. and I will give my cup a heavy shot of cream. Do you want a refill?" "Please," J.P. said as he handed her his cup.

She walked around the desk and out of the office. J.P. turned to look out the window. The morning sun was lighting the eastern sky. He sat down on the couch and waited for Janet, who returned with a mug of coffee in each hand and a small dish with a Danish resting atop each mug.

"I bought these on my way to work this morning. As I recall you're rather partial to a Danish in the morning."

J.P. smiled at her, "Thanks, Janet."

Janet sat down at the opposite end of the couch, turned slightly to face him, and crossed her legs. J.P. waited for her to open the conversation, but she couldn't seem to find the words. Finally, she spoke.

"Well, J.P., I'm afraid my problem is very complicated and because of the interactions between people I love and care for, I've no one to talk to about my situation. It's a combination of problems starting with Bill's startup company, our two teenage kids that are about to go off to college, Bill and Phillip being at odds with each other, and of course Phillip's fight with the James' Board of Directors. I feel as though I'm being pulled in many different directions and everyone is depending upon me to provide them strength. The things that used to make me happy, my job, Bill's enthusiasm about his work, my family, and Phillip's vision for James are now making me unhappy."

J.P. wanted to pursue what she was saying to see if he could be of help, but this wasn't the best moment to do so. He most of all wanted to pursue her statement about Bill and Phillip being at odds. As far as J.P. knew they had always been the best of friends. He didn't feel this potential conflict had anything to do with the copied plan, but he had to explore every possibility. He decided to assure Janet that he wanted to help, but not right then.

"Janet, I'm sure whatever the adversities of the situation are, you'll work them out in the long run. Look at what you and Bill have been able to accomplish in your lives. You both should be very proud." The expression on Janet's face told him that he wasn't doing a good job of postponing his assistance. "Janet, I know what you have to say is real and I hope I can help you, if that only means listening, but I'm sure you can see that I don't have time today to give you the focus you deserve. Please don't think I don't care, because I do. I'll tell you what, when I come back, you and I will have a long lunch together. You can tell me what Bill is up to then."

"Sure, I'm sorry I didn't mean to turn this into a counseling session. I'd love to have lunch with you. So, you are coming back?"

J.P. raised his gaze from his Danish and looked Janet in the eye. The fact that she had asked him that meant she hadn't read his point paper to Phillip.

J.P. began to relax a bit and told her, "I'm certain Phillip will provide you with the answers to all of your questions. It's nothing spooky, I just think he should explain since I'm a James outsider."

"First of all, you could never be considered a James outsider, at least as long as you still have friends here," she said laughing.

Just then Phillip burst through the door, "Good morning, friends. Another great James day in Gotham City." J.P. was surprised at how happy he seemed. It was quite a contrast to the dark mood he had exhibited yesterday. "I really don't know how I can be so cheerful in the morning after riding up on the damn express elevator. Doc James must have been mad when he contracted for a launch platform cleverly disguised as an elevator."

"Phillip, why the hell don't you slow that elevator down? Can't they put a speed governor or something on it? I'm just happy you didn't see me fall out of it when it hit the fiftieth floor yesterday."

Phillip and Janet both laughed. "Oh, don't be so sure, Jean Paul," Janet said pointing to a video screen built into Phillip's desk, "Look over there. I have one at my desk too. We see everyone come out of that elevator. In fact, Phillip has devised a six point scoring system based on the person's acrobatics. Yesterday, even though I didn't recognize you, I watched you leave the elevator. You scored a very respectable 5.5."

Phillip said, "I think Doc James had the elevator installed so he could throw his visitors off guard. You know, make the person ill at ease and on defense during the meeting. You must remember, he prided himself on never making anyone wait to see him. He also set up booby traps for each new visitor. Do you remember when he used to rig the door handle of his office so that it would not work properly? It was a handle like you would see on a pair of French doors. If you didn't push down on the handle with just the right pressure you could stand there rattling the door for minutes before he would let you in."

Janet spoke up, "I remember a trick he used to place vendors on the defensive. He would put a heavy chair just inside his office door. When the vendor finally opened the door, he or she would run straight into the chair. The surprise and impact sometimes literally took their breath away."

They all had a good laugh reminiscing about Doc James and his tricks.

J.P. thought it was good to see Janet and Phillip having a good time, particularly during what seemed to be a stressful period for both.

Janet was the first to become serious. "Well, I'd better get to work so J.P. can catch his early plane. See you gentlemen later," she said as left the office, closing the door behind her.

"What did she mean, early plane? Why the hurry? My God, am I in so much trouble that I can't possibly be helped?"

"Whoa, slow down, Phillip. It's all in my report. To tell you the truth, I don't know whether you're really in trouble or not. I've a great deal more homework to do before I can be certain of anything. My gut tells me that there is something going on here at James. What that is, I cannot possibly tell you right now. We'll figure this thing out."

Phillip's mood became dark and very serious again. "As I mentioned yesterday, I don't know how much time I have to figure this thing out. Mrs. Preston-James is trying to push me out. I'm certain of her intentions. She wants to run James Pharmaceutical Company her way and she knows that as long as I'm president and CEO that will never happen. She has certainly stacked the Board of Directors against me and by doing so has jeopardized the future of James. I can't figure out if this is a personal vendetta against me or if she is simply power hungry. Whatever her reasons, I believe the missing copy of the 21st Century Plan is part of her overall scheme to discredit me and eventually gain complete control over this company. You know what's funny about all of this? I'm convinced she believes she deserves complete control and that her management style, whatever form that might take, would be better for this company in the long run."

"Phillip, what the hell does she want from James?"

"Ah, yes, I've thought that through several times, trying to second guess her motives and gain insight as to her strategy she since made her first move a few years ago by replacing two of Doc's oldest friends on the board, Franklin and

Morgan. That was my first indication that her maneuvering to take control of the board might be part of a much bigger scheme. I've come to the conclusion that, in the short term, she wants to drive the stock price up to obtain a higher multiple of earnings per share. I don't know whether her primary reason is to sell some of her 10% share of James, merge, or sell James outright. She certainly doesn't need the money. There are 50 million shares outstanding. That places her holdings at five million shares. At today's price she's worth $85 million. We pay $1.15 a year in dividends so her annual income from dividends is $5,750,000. I guess my biggest fear of her motives lie in the fact that she doesn't exhibit, outwardly at least, the slightest bit of loyalty or obligation to James or James' customers.

"She's never talked to me about what she wants to do with James, if anything. In fact, she doesn't talk to me at all except to tell me that I am going too slow with the research and introduction of JPC138 and that I've failed with Lifeal."

"How much time do you have," J.P. asked?

"I really believe she will make her move to replace me at the April board meeting. She'll then make her major move to control James at the annual shareholders meeting in May. The proxy statements will be mailed after the board meeting the third week in April. If I am correct, we have three months to figure out her plan and to implement our own plan to counteract her actions and save James. That is, with your help of course."

J.P. paused before answering. He didn't want to give Phillip any false hopes about what he might actually be able to accomplish.

"Phillip, before I can give you a definitive answer, I really need more time to digest the 21st Century Plan and the other material I've asked for in my point paper. I will say this much. If you do have a problem, I will help you to resolve the issue or issues leading to the solution. As far as why I want to catch an early flight today, I would rather do my initial homework at home in Mammoth. I didn't bring anything with me on this trip. My body has not had time to figure out what time zone I'm standing in so if I can catch the noon flight back to LA, my body won't know that I ever left California.

"I've written a point paper on the situation as I know it today. I've also attached a suggested contract between James and myself. Why don't you read this document and then we'll discuss our situation and what we should do next."

Phillip picked up the report from where it was lying on the conference table and walked back over to his desk to begin reading. J.P. moved over to the window to witness the beautiful morning coming to life. He looked across the Hudson River and watched as sun bathed the New Jersey Palisades in its brilliant light.

"I can find no problem with any parts of the report, Jean Paul. As usual, you are very thorough and honest, which of course is why I wanted your help on this. And I'm especially appreciative of the fact that you did not jump to any premature conclusions. This morning I'll draft answers to all but one of your questions. As for the question on marketing, you will have to ask your assistant.

"I'm planning to assign Amanda Hayes, my vice president for marketing, as your assistant. Amanda is a widow, which I'm certain is of little consequence either way to you, but I can assure you that she is completely trustworthy. Despite the fact that she is one of my youngest executive staff members, I would, without hesitation, entrust her with my professional life. She knows nothing of this current problem. I will ask her to come to my office this morning and give her a brief rundown about you and the reason you're here. I'll leave it entirely up to you to fully brief her on the situation. It is my plan to continue normal operations of James Pharmaceutical just as we were doing before I received the letter from Doylestown last Friday. Amanda will continue her function as VP of marketing. If there is anything you require that should be handled through me, just ask. I will tell Janet as much as I feel she needs to know. You will, as you have already done, provide only me with a copy of your reports. Are these conditions acceptable?"

"Yes," J.P. replied, "except Ms. Hayes. What if we don't hit it off? Do I have a choice in the matter of choosing my assistant? I don't wish to challenge your judgment, Phillip, or maybe I do, but how wise is it to have one of the suspects working with me on this?"

Phillip smiled, "As I've told you, I trust her completely. I'm positive she isn't the person who made the copy. I'm sure that she'll be completely acceptable to you. She is without a doubt one of the most intelligent and perceptive staff members that I have here.. .a real find you might say.

"I'll tell you what, sit down at my desk and read through the files I've brought up on my screen. It's Amanda's entire personnel record including her resume. I will ask her to come to the conference room on the other side of my office. I'll inform her that you will be helping me with a special project. After a short time I'll call you into the conference room and you can discuss marketing with her. After your discussion, you can give me your decision as to whether she can fill the position of your assistant, though I seriously doubt there will be any hesitation on your part. As for whether she will even want to be your assistant, I'll let her decide about you on her own. Now then, I would suggest a role or cover story to use while you are working on this project. Any thoughts on that?"

"Yes, let's use my knowledge of James and business strategies to work on the market positioning of Lifeal and JPC138. My credentials will hold up under the closest scrutiny. I'll be the president's assistant working with Ms. Hayes. The only question I have is whether Ms. Hayes will take the cover as an insult to her marketing abilities."

"Perfect," Phillip exclaimed! "Although I can't speak for Amanda, I think she'll be okay with the set up. She knows of your reputation and I'm certain she'll be very excited about the opportunity to work with the infamous, or is it notorious, Jean Paul Koenig. Now then, peruse her record and I'll call her up to the conference room." As an afterthought he added, "Shall I have Janet make your plane reservations

"Yes, please, the noon flight from JFK. Also, would it be possible to arrange a helo ride from here so I can stay longer? This would save me a long cab ride along the GCP."

"Yes, of course, consider it done. Although I know the real reason for wanting a helo isn't the cab ride. You're just scared to ride that elevator back down to the lobby. Afraid your testicles will disappear back into your body cavity?" Phillip laughed with a loud guffaw and without waiting for an answer, walked out of the office.

J.P. sat reading Amanda Hayes personnel records as he had actually done the night before when he was reviewing the records of the entire executive staff. He was no less impressed with her credentials the second time through. Her work and education history read like a how-to manual for succeeding in business: Undergraduate degree in business from UCLA; MBA from Universtiry of Southern California less than two years later; steady upward job performance as sales manager, district sales manager, product manager, product director, director of market planning, and her current position, vice president of marketing...all over a period of ten years.

He closed the record on the screen and walked over to the conference room door. He looked at his watch. 9:00 a.m. He had to be out of there in an hour or so if he was going to catch the noon flight to LA. He wanted to be in LA early enough to file his flight plan to Mammoth Lakes and make the twohour flight in daylight. He didn't like landing at the Mammoth Airport at night as it was dicey at best.

He peered through the small one-way peephole in the door and saw Phillip and Amanda sitting at the conference table. Phillip was facing the door with Amanda facing away. He reached for the doorknob and twisting it, burst into the conference room. Phillip was quick to recover.

"J.P.," he said as he stood up, "we were just talking about you. How good of you to join us.

Amanda Hayes had jumped up from her seat but remained facing away from J.P. and stood rigidly, almost at attention.

"I'm sorry if I startled you. Phillip, I've finished reading the materials you provided to me." J.P. started towards the two, "Hello, you must be Amanda Hayes."

As he said this, she turned around and faced him. She extended her hand to shake and J.P. caught his breath. She was certainly beautiful. Green eyes and red hair set against flawless pale skin. "Steady boy," he thought to himself as he took her hand.

"Dr. Koenig, this is a real pleasure for me to meet you. I've heard so much about you. Your reputation precedes you whether you like it or not.

You're something of a marketing legend. The MBA program at USC uses several of your books as reference material."

Phillip broke in, "Well, Mandi, I would tell you about his other activities in the recent past, but then he'd likely have to kill both of us." She gave Phillip a quick look, not comprehending what he meant.

"Ms. Hayes, please excuse Phillip. He somehow finds the fact that I've been doing consulting work amusing. But, thank you for your kind comments about my books, it's good to know someone is reading that dribble. Phillip speaks very highly of you and has told me you're doing a great job in marketing products for James."

J.P. quickly deferred the personal compliments and began his interview. Phillip had said that she had done a great job, but that wasn't entirely true when it came to Lifeal. He wondered if she would comment on the point that he had made about her successes in marketing.

Her face became serious and she immediately answered, "I appreciate your compliment, Dr. Koenig, but I'm afraid the jury is still out on the success of Lifeal. I've not done very well with Lifeal because the sales have never reached the potential this product deserves in the clinical marketplace. I take the blame because I'm responsible. We are presently developing a new Lifeal strategy and I certainly welcome any help you can provide."

J.P. looked behind her at Phillip who was grinning. "I'm sure we will have a chance to discuss Lifeal. What about JPC138? Have you developed a marketing program for the new product?"

She turned to look at Phillip, who gave her a slight nod of his head. J.P. liked that. JPC138 was a secret product, and she had look to Phillip for guidance in answering his question proving that she only provided information when it was necessary and to people that had a need to know.

J.P. began to feel that Phillip had indeed made the right choice.

She turned back towards J.P., "We, that is marketing, have been directing the development of this product from its inception. Prior to the discovery of JPC138 we had identified a number of clinical disease entities for which we wanted R&D to develop new products. JPC138 is the first product from our strategic R&D plan and has great promise in a number of the identified clinical areas. At this point, we have identified Alzheimer's disease as the primary market segment. At this point in the product's development, we aren't entirely sure in which Alzheimer's target market segment to position the product. We're remaining flexible since that particular TMS is so broad. And, of course, R&D doesn't seem to be moving as fast as marketing wants it to move." She stopped and then stated matter of factly, "We will wait to do more market positioning of this research compound until it enters stage three clinicals."

As far as J.P. was concerned, the interview was over and he had his assistant, "Please call me J.P."

"Fine, J.P., please call me Mandi."

Phillip began explaining to Mandi the circumstances of J.P.'s visit and what he was trying to accomplish. She sat quietly and listened. When Phillip finished, he asked if she had any questions.

She paused and then in a very serious tone said, "Since you've asked me, I'm not quite clear on what problem we may have here at James. My own instinct tells me that there is an undercurrent dissatisfaction in the way things are going with the events surrounding both Lifeal and JPC138." Mandi turned to look directly at Phillip and made a minor apology, "These events, or happenings, aren't really serious problems, Phillip. I can't even be more specific, so I concluded they didn't warrant your immediate attention. I was going to look into them myself, but, now that J.P. is on the team, I welcome his help. I'm sure you both know more about what's happening than you are telling me and that's okay. I understand the need for secrecy. I do look forward to working with you, J.P. I understand, from Phillip, that you have a question you would like answered today. I'll get on it right away. I'm also led to believe that you are headed back to California today, but will return to New York next Monday. Is that correct?"

"Yes,"

"Will you gentlemen please excuse me? I must get back to work. I'll see you at the staff meeting today Phillip. And you, J.P., next Monday. California, eh? Must be nice. I'll fax the answer to your question to your home tonight. Bye." With that she turned and walked out of the room.

"Well," Phillip broke the silence, "what did I tell you?"

J.P. didn't answer. He just stared at the door through which she had departed.

At exactly 11 a.m., with a rush of cold wind and the unmistakable sound of helicopter blades thrashing the winter air, the JFK shuttle landed atop the Spectrum of Medicine Building. The co-pilot jumped down from his seat and opened the rear starboard door for J.P. As J.P. climbed into his seat, the copilot handed him a headset that helped block out the noise and would be used to communicate once they were in the air. The ground attendant slid the door closed and prepared to launch the helicopter.

The headset crackled as the co-pilot spoke to J.P. "Good morning Dr. Koenig. All set for take off?"

"As ready as I'll ever be in one of these things," J.P. responded weakly.

With that the pilot communicated with the attendant, gave him a thumbs-up, and lifted off the building making a 90-degree turn to head south along the Hudson.

"Dr. Koenig, hi, I'm Mike Jensen, your pilot. Did I detect a bit of apprehension on your part?"

J.P. chuckled slightly, "Morning, Mike, not with flying, I'm a pilot myself. I just don't like helicopters. Figure that if God had intended for helos to fly he'd given them wings."

The pilot turned his head slightly to look at J.P. and smile, "I see a fixed wing jet jockey eh!, well, we'll make this as painless for you as possible. Our ETA to JFK is about 15 minutes, there will be a car to meet us and run you over to the passenger terminal."

"Great. Thanks."

As they flew, J.P. looked out at the crystal clear sky hung over the city.

He looked back to the left as the Manhattan skyline diminished.

As they set down on the tarmac at JFK, J.P spoke into the mic, "Okay, thanks guys. Always happy when I'm able to cheat death."

The two pilots turned in their seats and gave him a quick wave goodbye.

WESTWOOD VILLAGE, CALIFORNIA

Nacheda looked around at Skip's constructed room where the task force members were now seated. The room inside the condominium was set up to resemble a Pentagon war room. Nakasone had given Nacheda a free hand with expenses and Nacheda, in turn, had given Skip a free hand in developing the computer intelligence system. Because of Dr. Nakasone's financial investment in the project, Nacheda didn't really blame him for his impatience or for scolding him the day before.

Westwood Village seemed like the ideal location for the war room. Skip had paid "scouts" to survey the area and its activities and to their surprise discovered that there was other corporate intelligence activities taking place there. Westwood offered anonymity. No one in the complex seemed to even notice Nacheda's once a month task force meeting where participants were sometimes sequestered for two or more days.

Skip picked up the remote hand control unit for the Artificial Intelligence Management System, or AIMS, and touched the upper right button. All six of the computer consoles came to life. Members of the task force sat behind their own computer console. Each console was programmed specifically to the assignment of the individual. Although each of the consoles had its own monitor, the screen of the active console was fed to a 3 foot square flat screen mounted on the wall for the entire group to see. Skip's console fed to a 5 foot square wall screen and was known as the decision console, or as he referred to it, the DC. All of the other computers were networked to the DC and to a satellite via an extremely complex data scrambler that Skip himself had designed. This enabled the task force members to access the information stored in the main computer when they were at home by means of a black box and a specially encrypted key to turn the box on.

It occurred to Skip that he was probably being too cautious, but the technology was available, so why not use it? Skip was the AIMS coordinator and sat between consoles #3 and #4 where he could retrieve any information he desired from the other six consoles, generate new information, and come to conclusions. Incoming information was always analyzed against the information that was already stored in the data warehouse. Another feature of AIMS was SAM. SAM stood for strategic analysis manager and was a computer-generated persona who presented summary information and conclusions to the group based on hard data. The team had not seen much of SAM because to this point, there had been no need to come to any conclusions.

The war room was 30 feet long and 10 feet wide. Skip had taken care to ensure that the walls were specially coated to prevent electronic eavesdropping and the windows were treated with a film that virtually repelled any visual or electronic means of spying.

Nacheda recalled Skip commenting during the war room design phase, "You know we redesigned the National Command Center in here, and, as far as I know we don't even have a crisis. All we'll be doing is analyzing data and then turning it into conclusive information and business intelligence. We're working with pharmaceuticals, not plotting World War III."

Nacheda explained to his friend that the world of corporate knowledge, intelligence, and strategies was, in fact, World War III. Most corporations were actively involved in market warfare and, without the means of acquiring business intelligence, a company would not able to compete. Nacheda smiled and informed Skip that he had spent too much time sitting behind a desk in the Pentagon and that he had much to learn about how the real world worked.

Nacheda admired military intelligence officers because they were very important to a satisfactory solution to a situation, although they often had little, in the way of information to work with or enough time to properly find the information they needed. Yet they were always expected to make the correct recommendation.

Following the team's December meeting, Skip had remarked to Nacheda, "Would you please tell me what the hell you've gotten us into? We have access to more data and information than I've ever seen in my life, but where's the substance? Where's the solution? We keep a room of very intelligent people locked up in here with what I'm certain is the most sophisticated computer network in the world and for what? We've been at this now for ten months and there's nothing we can really call a solution."

Nacheda sensed Skip's growing frustration, "Patience, Colonel. The answer is in the information, but it is not yet in sight. Perhaps the January meeting will provide us with a New Year's gift. When it is time, the answer we seek shall reveal itself."

Following that December meeting, Nacheda had left Westwood Village to return to Bandai. Skip had remained at the condo to massage the information and coordinate incoming data from team members. Although they never spoke of the possibility of failure, both knew that Nacheda's optimistic feeling was becoming weaker with each passing month.

Now the team was meeting for the eleventh time. It was January and they had only one more month to accomplish their mission. Everyone was comfortably seated behind his or her console. Skip pressed another button on the AIMS hand control, which brought down the room lights. The radiant light from the computer monitors produced an eerie glow in the room.

Skip announced, "Okay, gang, we've been at this for eleven months now, and we have yet to arrive at a solution or develop a new strategy. Our current strategy has not been effective. Today, I don't want a long summary, but let's each give a brief update on our current status. Five minutes each. Okay, down the line. Console One, Terri."

Everyone looked up on the wall at the three foot square screen which read:

CONSOLE #1, UNIVERSITY STAGE ONE CLINICAL STUDIES, TERRI CRUTHERS.

Terri began her summary, "In the past eleven months, we've analyzed 536 new pharmaceuticals currently in stage-one clinical studies. 413 have been classified as inappropriate for us because they don't offer any advantages over other products within the same pharmaceutical product class. Seventy-one of the remaining 123 products are classified as too early to determine the clinical value, but, so far none of these look very exciting. The remaining 52 products look promising. I tell you all, I'm not trained as a futurist, and the titration of these 52 products was not an easy task. I have however chosen five products to evaluate and each meets the criteria which you now see on the screen." Terri hit a few keys and the criteria appeared on the screen:

- Clinical indication that can provide patients with a better quality of life.

- New chemical compound.

- Patent rights undefined so there is an excellent chance for a patent on the compound or one of its derivatives.

- A product with mysterious and/or unexpected clinical results.

- Excellent chance that the compound has additional undetermined indications that could open up new clinical markets.

- Clinical trials that are being initiated or sponsored by a small-tomedium sized company.

- Clinical trials which seem to be under-financed.

- A better than average chance that the product and/or company could be acquired.

- A possibility of a new class of pharmaceuticals.

Terri paused, giving the team a chance to read and absorb the criteria, and then continued, "The following are the five products I've identified as possible candidates for the Bandai project."

Terri typed in a command and five pharmaceutical compounds were shown on the screen:

1. DY321
2. JPC138
3. PH631
4. BQ519
5. SK3H4

Skip hit a command key on his AIMS handset and the data from Terri's computer was transferred to the data warehouse server. Skip looked over at Console Two and said, "John." The monitor quickly changed and showed John King's responsibilities: CONSOLE #2, PATIENT SEARCH, NIH GRANTS, AND ASSOCIATION GRANTS, JOHN KING.

John King was, by nature, a quiet person. As a rescue helicopter pilot in Vietnam, he never said much. He had always lived by the philosophy that his actions spoke louder than his words. He had a reputation as one of the Navy's finest rescue pilots, who doggedly pursued every avenue to complete his mission, often under intense fire. All pilots who flew missions over Southeast Asia respected him. During the war, if a fighter pilot went down over land or water, the first prayer that came to his lips was, "Please Lord, send the King."

Following his service, John chose law as his new career. Upon graduation from Indiana University, he chose healthcare law as his specialty, mostly because he thought he might be able to make an impact. Over the years, he waged a silent but relentless battle to keep a fair balance between physician talent, the patients' access to quality healthcare, government regulations, and the insurance third-party pay industry.

John had not written his report for the task force nor had he downloaded the information from his home computer. He was accustomed to dictating letters and chose to dictate his report using the audio transcriber capability of AIMS.

"In the past year, over 1,100 patents on pharmaceutical products and their derivatives have been filed with the U.S. patent office. I'm sorry to report that, based on our task force criteria, none of these products show any promise as a candidate for the Bandai project. The NIH had their budget cut and very few new research grants have been issued over the last few years. With the FDA approval criteria, it takes longer to prove pharmaceutical efficacy and therefore, research projects take up to 100% longer. This means each research project requires more funding than what had been budgeted.

"I've evaluated the medical area focused on health oriented associations and research funds and where they have been investing their money. To this point, I have not come up with anything that we would consider unusual. Thank you."

Skip hit the handset key and John's digitized short report was added to the DC computer.

Skip nodded to Cap at Console Three and the screen displayed: CONSOLE #3, CLINICAL REQUIREMENTS AND SIDE EFFECT ANALYSIS, DR. JEREMY MCKENNSEY.

"Well y'all, the first thing I want to state is this, I sure wish we would get a break," he said in his unmistakably Georgia drawl. "Nothin' has changed in my camp, I haven't anything to break this log jam."

He pressed his computer's command key and the five diseases the team had chosen to study were listed on the video screen:

1. AIDS
2. Hypertension
3. Breast Cancer
4. Prostate Cancer
5. Alzheimer's

The five had been chosen based on a rating system that took into account a number of variables including:

- Health rating
- Unique side effect of pharmaceutical

- Quality of life to the patient

- Projected number of patients with the disease in the year 2020

- Number of products currently on the market in the clinical category

- Number of research compounds presently being studies within the category

During the first meetings the team had come up with this unique rating system. This was an advantage of the six-computer system. All of the data from the six computers was analyzed and then converted to information. The information was then sent to the decision computer where artificial intelligence took over. The responsible individual had developed each of the six subject computer scripts. Then six computer artificial intelligence consultant programmers were contracted to take the task members script and convert it to computerized information. Team member #8 then programmed AIMS that took the intelligence information from the six individual programs and programmed it for the DC in such a manner that the DC could come to conclusions.

The team now focused on Cap's rating table. The health rating indicated the importance of the disease in the present and future health of humanity. Each of the ratings used over 100 comprehensive data points plus the artificial intelligence capability of the DC.

"Now then, as for what we'll call the unique side effect category," Cap said, "the answer has always been a tough one for this ol' boy. There are, in my estimation and I assume in your own estimation, five side effects that can be considered detrimental to a product's indications. That is, indications that are currently being used or tested for in the laboratory or clinic. What could be an advantage for one indication could be a disadvantage for a yet undetermined indication. Four side effects are repeated from previous meetings. The fifth is new." The five side effects came up on the screen:

1. ACCELERATED HAIR GROWTH

2. DORMANT SPERM PHENOMENON

3. BONE GROWTH STIMULATION

4. LIBIDO ENHANCEMENT

5. EXCESSIVE MENTAL ALERTNESS

Cap continued, "We have discussed the first four. The number five side effect is intriguing. Excessive mental alertness." He paused for effect. "Now, this is something that I know we need more of in many parts of the south, but as far as

I know this has never popped up in any of the other data we've looked at over the past year. We've seen hyperactivity, but never excessive mental alertness. Skip, I have to be real honest with you here, I don't know what this means to our goal of a rapid solution. It could be a breakthrough or just a diversion. I studied the matter, but could not come up with a recommendation. I know we have discussed the other side effects at previous meetings. How about some help? Do any members of this astute team have any pertinent knowledge of excessive mental alertness?"

Skip affected Cap's drawl and replied, "Cap, just you wait one minute here while I get this here DC to do what it was designed to do."

Skip entered a combination of keys on his handset and waited for DC to shift the keyboard control. He became very intense as he worked the keyboard, moving information and intelligence from computer to computer, most of the moves from memory. Abruptly he stopped and the team waited a full 10 seconds before anything happened. Suddenly, the DC wall monitor did an instant refresh and started a sequence of words rolling across the screen.

SEARCH TOPIC: EXCESSIVE MENTAL ALERTNESS METHODOLOGY:

All global medical dictionaries were searched as well as the medical literature for the last twenty-five years. No reference to the combination of the words forming the term "excessive mental alertness" was found in the search. Finding no such reference in the 25-year history, a search backward in time was made from prior literature. The first medical reference to the term was found in the October 15, 1898, *Singapore Times*. A wealthy British subject, on a hunting trip to Indonesia, became seriously ill. The man was taken to an Indonesian native batak house. It was reported that for three days, a tribal shaman gave the subject an indigenous drug. After returning to Singapore, the man developed a high fever, a dark yellow rash, and severe hallucinations. At the urging of friends, he checked himself into Queen's Hospital.

The video screen refreshed itself and new text appeared:

NEW MEDIA SEARCH: Singapore British Crown Colony start date October 1, 1898. Keywords: British subject, hunting trip, and Indonesia. Located: *Singapore Times,* October 6, 1898, p3, c2, Sir Darwin Thomas Gains.

Upon returning from a two-week hunting trip to Indonesia, British subject Sir Darwin Thomas Gains demonstrated an intellectual power that he, heretofore, had not shown. "To say the least," a friend commented, "good old Dars had turned into a genius overnight. He ran about quoting the likes of Plato and Aristotle. By God, we thought he was going to think himself to death. He would jump up from his chair and begin quoting, then run to another chair, sit down, and start a brilliant new sequence all over again. It would have been humorous except for the dreadful look on his face. We finally convinced him to visit Queens Hospital." At press time Sir Darwin remains in hospital.

CONTINUING SEARCH: *Singapore Times,* October 15, 1898, Obituaries Sir Darwin Thomas Gains, Esq., of 33 South Banister Rd., Upper Sussex, England, died at Queen's Hospital at 3:00 a.m., this morning from dehydration caused by what his physician termed excessive mental alertness. He was 48 years old. His wife, Melissa, and five children in Upper Sussex, England, survive. CONTINUING SEARCH: *Singapore Times,* October 15, 1898, p6, c4 How Sir Darwin Thomas Gains Spent His Days Before Hospital Friends who had been on Sir Darwin's hunting trip to Indonesia tell the story about how he suddenly took seriously ill from a mysterious source. The medical knowledge of the hunting party was quickly exhausted and they were preparing to carry Sir Darwin back to civilization when one of the hunting party baggage bearers volunteered to go for help. Without instructions from the group he disappeared into the jungle. When he returned a short time later he convinced the members of the hunting party to transport Sir Darwin to a tribal shaman located at a native long house not far from their camp. Sir Darwin was treated by a medicine man of an unknown tribe. The hunting party spent three days camped near the house located in the interior of Indonesia. After one day at the house the members of Sir Darwin's party had resolved themselves to his eventual death from mysterious illness. On the third day, Sir Darwin awoke and was hungry. Either the shaman's drugs had begun to show dramatic results or the disease had run its course. Sir Darwin regained his full capabilities the same day and the entire party walked out of the jungle and returned to Singapore.

Skip hit a button on his handset and the DC monitor went blank. "So, Cap, there's your answer…your one answer. There appear to be no additional references to excessive mental alertness. So, do we have anything, or not?"

Nacheda at Console Six rose from his seat and walked over to Cap. "Well, Cap, what do you think? Do we have something?" Nacheda's voice betrayed his eagerness for a breakthrough.

Cap sat quietly for a moment. He knew everyone was looking for an answer and if he weren't careful they would deduce an answer from any seemly relevant information. He knew one thing was for sure, he didn't have any answers, only more questions.

"Y'all know me about as well as I know myself and you know that I do not, will not, jump to quick conclusions. All we have here are questions." He paused and leaned back in his chair. "What we have here is one reference in a century-old newspaper clipping of events surrounding a mysterious death, and the use of three words, 'excessive mental alertness'. The same three words have shown up in my recent research. Does this mean anything? As far as I can tell here, my friends, what we have is an unusual nothing. Now then, I suggest we all go out and get some food before I slip into insulin shock from a lack of nourishment."

There was a pause in the war room. Everyone was looking for an answer and it certainly wasn't lunch. Nacheda turned and walked back to his own chair where he sat slumped down so far that his shoulders were nearly even with the arm rests. After a few seconds, the members of the team set their computers to stand-by, rose from their seats, and walked towards the door.

"Good move, Cap," Joe said quietly.

Cap moved towards the door. His face showing deep thought. For nearly a year he had been feeding Console Three information on side effects and nothing had come of his actions. Now, finally, there was something. Yes, it was a little unusual, but at least it was something to think about. It could also have been a fluke and he needed time to think through this new development. Was it a side effect that only shows up once every hundred years? A century side effect, he wondered? Terri came up beside and hooked her arm through his.

"What are you so deep in thought about, old man?" she whispered.

Cap looked into her lovely face at those brilliant green eyes he had known for so many years. When they had worked together in the operating room, he had so loved to look into those green eyes as they peered at him over the top of her surgical mask.

Cap leaned closer and whispered in her ear, "Wouldn't you like to know! I just might be thinking of one of those wild nights we had a couple of decades ago."

Terri's face took on a slight flush. She squeezed his arm and they led the team out of the condo for lunch in Westwood Village. As the team walked across the commons towards Alice's Restaurant, they didn't notice the man in the dark suit who followed them at some distance. He gave no outward appearance of having any active interest in the group. As the group clustered around the entrance to the restaurant, the man stopped and bent down near a brick planter to tie his shoe.

After they were seated inside at a large round table in Alice's, Nacheda leaned over towards Joe Berger to his right and said, "How are you doing, Doctor?"

"Hey, old buddy, just great," he responded in what Nacheda referred to as Joe's GI voice. "Just great. Really looking forward to a breakthrough on this project. Guess I'm getting a little restless for results. So how are you holding up, Nacheda-san?"

Nacheda always enjoyed Joe's manner of speech. Joe, following his release as a POW, had become what could only be termed a professional student. He was now a Ph.D. and a world-renowned expert in the field biogenetic engineering. Somehow that didn't fit with the voice and it always made Nacheda smile.

"I am holding up well, Joe, but I agree, we need results," Nacheda answered. "On the bright side, I have a funny feeling we're close to something."

"Nacheda-san, what are you going to do when we do have something?" Joe asked seriously.

"My objective will be to accomplish the leg work to follow-up on our leads until we uncover a specific company that will make the best target. Once we know that, I'll take direction from Dr. Nakasone. I have to give him a thorough report before next Monday. I will then take his direction, that is, assuming he still wants me on the project. Like you, Joe, he is very restless about the lack of any real progress. And, what will you do when this project is over?"

"Well, life in the San Juan Islands is never bad. I have a couple of real interesting NIH research grants coming up for review. John was right. There are not many grants out there, but I've managed to be the lead investigator on two bioengineering cancer grants. If we don't hit a homer at this meeting, I might have to ask you to release me as a free agent. I know that puts you in a bad position and believe me I don't want to let you down, but I've got to get on with my life. These NIH projects are too exciting to pass up. If I don't take one of them, they'll go to someone else and I'll be out in the cold. The University of Washington lives on these grants and they don't take kindly to one of their Ph.D.'s letting them slip through their fingers."

Joe's words hit Nacheda hard. He often wondered when the team would begin fragmenting. A year was too long. It occurred to him that perhaps the criteria were too restrictive. Nacheda decided that if the team didn't come up with something substantive, he would make a decision based on the data currently available to identify a company.

"I understand, Joe. Let's keep our hope up for today. If nothing comes up today, let's talk before you go back to Anacortes."

"I'm sure we'll score, Nacheda-san," Joe responded cheerily.

The man who had followed the group across the commons had entered the restaurant and taken a seat at the bar. His back was to the group, but his eyes watched the group closely in the mirror behind the bar. He caught the attention of one of the task force members. Their eyes, in silent recognition, stayed locked for a few seconds. He spun around on his barstool to face the group. As he did the task force member with whom he made eye contact asked the waiter for more ice water. The man turned back towards the bar and looked down into his drink. The signal that would have told him that the group had reached a "significant conclusion" had not been passed.

Nacheda turned to his left and asked Mary Christian how she was doing in her professional life.

"I'm doing fine, thank you," she responded. "Being editor of a prestigious publication like the New England Journal of Medicine is just what I've always wanted. Healthcare is so dynamic." She paused briefly and then said, "You know, Nacheda-san, it's looking like we may be heading towards a resolution of some sort to our task here and there's something I've always wanted you to know. Before you were captured in Vietnam, you probably lived in fear, not knowing when you might get shot. When I arrived as a correspondent for the Christian Science Monitor the war had wound down. It was a safe war for me. As far as the media correspondents were concerned they had won our Vietnam War. We felt we had fairly represented the conscience of the American people and had finally convinced politicians to quit the war. So we had won the war. We didn't think about how those of you who were fighting the war felt about what we were doing or about the dead and captured. All that was important was the fact that we had caused the war to come to an end.

"I was wrapping things up for the Monitor and looking for a final human interest story when I met you guys at the naval hospital. I lived the real war vicariously by listening to all of your stories. But I never felt the war and the mixed internal feelings of your terror." She paused again. "I did not fight the real war, yet I had selfishly felt that I had won. In retrospect, I guess I feel a little ashamed of my behavior and selfish feelings."

Nacheda with a caring tone, said, "Ah, but Mary, you did nothing to be ashamed of, you and your colleagues simply presented what you saw there. And who knows, the media may have saved thousands of other lives on all sides by bringing to light the horrors and seemingly aimless direction of that mess. And, of course, you won a Pulitzer Prize for your story about us. In fact it was your piece that gave me the idea of forming our present team." He thought back to the article in which she concluded that different perspectives, personalities, and backgrounds had a strong and positive effect on a team. She had used the team she got to know at the hospital, but she felt it would equally have applied to a field squad of soldiers or Marines that fight as a group. Almost a year ago, Nacheda had recalled Mary's "Mixed Bag of Warriors" article and that had given him the idea to bring as much of the group together as possible to work on the Bandai project.

Mary's article also pointed out that a group required a strong leader to achieve this unique group effect. Skip was that strong leader.

Nacheda continued, "Mary, you're an excellent journalist, therein lies your reward, don't you think?"

"Yes, I know, I just felt that I had missed something in Vietnam in how I presented the situation with the Monitor articles." She smiled and lowered her voice, "You know, even though I might complain, I love being an editor now. Knowing what is happening in the world of medicine and knowing that I've an influence on medical care and the publishing of clinical results is really rewarding. Plus, my monthly meeting with your…our mixed bag team provides me with the real thrill of exploring the cutting edge of a few developments in healthcare. I am sorry for the long answer to your question. I am doing fine in my professional life and thank you, Nacheda-san, for including me in your team."

"My pleasure, Mary. Your perspective is invaluable and your support material plays a very important role in forming the ultimate picture of the product or products we will target."

When they had finished their lunch, the group returned to the condo and took their respective seats. Skip turned to Console Four, "Well, Mary, we have a few mysteries going for us today. Do you have anything to link up any of this?"

The monitor on the wall displayed:

CONSOLE #4, LITERATURE SEARCH, TOXICOLOGY AND PATHOLOGY.

Mary's responsibility was to initiate and complete literature searches to determine whether any article tied in to the findings of the three team members that presented before her. One of the reasons she was at Console Four was to give her time to search all the healthcare journals for the product group that was being discussed. While the others were making their presentations, Mary was listening and typing key words into her console. Through satellite links, Mary had access to every major medical and pharmaceutical library in the world.

Mary began her presentation, "Although I usually prefer to type my own material, Skip, I would like to input the system through the audio transcriber."

"Very well," Skip replied.

"Thank you. I've analyzed the five unique side effects Cap mentioned this morning. There was some interesting literature activity on the side effects of dormant sperm phenomenon and bone growth stimulation, which I'll go through in a minute.

"There were the usual reprints on stimulation of hair growth but they were on every part of the human body except the male scalp. One paper from Europe mentioned a menopause product that seems to accelerate the growth of hair under the arms and on the legs. Depilatory companies in the US would love to place a little of that product into the female diet to stimulate their sales." Mary paused for laughter that didn't come. "Guess my joke wasn't very funny."

"Well, Mary, as you know we have a pact never to laugh at your jokes," Skip said. It was true. Mary tried very hard to be funny and quite often she was very funny, but the group had a silent code to never laugh at her jokes.

Mary continued, "Libido enhancement still seems to be associated with emotional issues and are not necessarily physiological, which would require a pharmaceutical product. Of course Viagra™ is an exception to the pharmaceutical statement. You all know it is not a libido effect but a product that increases blood flow. It seems when a person experiences increased libido he or she is usually too sick to exercise or enjoy the result.

"The side effect of excessive mental alertness is a new one. I didn't have a chance to search beyond what was done by Skip this morning. If the team agrees to go ahead with exploring this new side effect, I'll do more homework when I return to my office.

"Now as for the background on the dormant sperm phenomenon. This side effect was noted in two clinical papers. One was in the Journal of Obstetrics and Gynecology and the other in France's LaFemme Media. The OB-GYN article documented a side effect associated with a product called Diet-Level. The clinician found a sub-group of 25 couples who had been taking Diet-Level as an appetite suppressor and, at the same time, they were also trying to become pregnant.

"The couples had tried most of the accepted fertility techniques and had stopped because of the lack of satisfactory results. They did continue to take Diet-Level. In every case, one menstrual cycle after each of these 25 couples stopped using Diet-Level they became pregnant. All twenty-five. An amazing correlation." As Mary spoke, the screen continuously provided formula and other technical information on Diet-Level. The information stopped on an abstract of a clinical paper on Diet-Level. Mary continued, "The director of public relations of Pharmatec, Inc., the manufacturer of Diet-Level, stated in a press release just this month that their research department was looking into the reported so-called dormant sperm phenomenon. The press release concluded by stating that Diet-Level is a unique low-dose diet control product that works gradually to suppress the appetite.

"The company claims Diet-Level adjusts the individual's food craving to a nutritional level that sustains their individual physical activity regimen." Mary paused for effect and then quipped, "Which, by the way, I think is BS. Pharmatec reports that Diet-Level has had extensive toxicity and pathology studies on any possibility of an adverse effect on pregnant women. It was found to be very safe and therefore it wasn't required by the FDA to carry a restriction for women in their fertile years.

"Diet-Level has been very successful because women don't have large weight gain and loss swings. The weight loss is gradual and the weight loss remains as long as the woman takes a maintenance does of Diet-Level. One interesting side note is that the product apparently does not work as well for men trying to lose weight. I suppose that would explain why LaFemme Media picked up on the phenomenon. What we might have here is a contraceptive side effect on an over the counter diet product. That combination is a marketers dream when you consider that this is also a product that requires a maintenance dose that obviously has some effect on the reproductive system."

Mary went on to discuss the last unique side effect. "As you know, all internally ingested bone growth stimulation products have had a systemic effect. This systemic effect causes growth stimulation in all skeletal bones not just the specific bone that is being targeted by the surgeon. The surgeon wants to stimulate growth of a specific broken bone so it will heal faster with a reduced traumatic effect on a patient's life habits. Currently, specific bone growth stimulation requires an invasive technique of surgery or an injection of a pharmaceutical directly into the targeted bone.

"The article reporting the side effect of bone growth stimulation is from Sweden. The article is about an ointment, which is currently being applied topically on the epidermal layer before a plaster cast is constructed around a broken limb. Its approved indication is to prevent fungal growth under the plaster cast. The article concluded that one of the side effects was a stimulation of bone growth causing the healing to be quicker than when the ointment wasn't used. In a double blind study, the healing process of the broken bone was much faster when the ointment was used than when the ointment was not used. This can be visually demonstrated by showing a sequence of x-rays taken from the reported study."

The monitor refreshed and showed a sequence of a number of x-rays showing side-by-side broken femurs healing on a split screen. Each femur xray had a clock so the viewer could see the healing time. One side of the screen showed a femur of a patient that had used the ointment and the other a patient's femur that had not used the ointment. The limited data sample obtained from this one study clearly illustrates that there was a faster healing of the bone when the ointment was present.

"The ointment is a combination of an anti-inflammatory, anti-fungal, antipyretic, and antibiotic. The ingredients are commonly used except for the anti-fungal, which is a derivative of Fungizone. The paper doesn't go further except to state that the authors don't know if the side effect was caused by the combination of the ingredients or one of the ingredients having a different than anticipated pharmacological effect in the therapeutic environment caused by the cast material, the ointment, and the patient's body chemistry. The somewhat closed environment with body heat could very well change the properties of the ointment. I'll try to find out more about this situation."

Mary concluded, "Not the greatest report, Skip, but there are some interesting points. I'm sorry, but I don't see any clear or definitive links between my work and the work of the others on the team."

"No need to apologize, Mary," Skip said. He pushed the button sequence that converted her verbal report to digital. Her presentation and the digitized video were transferred to the DC.

"Dr. Joe, you're up. Anything on your end?"

"Thanks, Skip," Joe answered. Joe cleared his deep, resonant voice. The wall monitor displayed:

CONSOLE #5, FUTURE PHARMACEUTICALS.

He typed in several commands and the words on the monitor were replaced with the subject BIOGENETIC ENGINEERING. "I want to brief you on two classes of pharmaceuticals. The first is in the category of biogenetic engineering. As you know, this is my main suit. I'll do my best not to put you to sleep.

"What I would like to ask the team to look for is any situations where a DNA chain is being changed. We...that is, the University of Washington... have been investigating products that are candidates for DNA alterations for the last five to ten years. In the industrial sector, Genentec and Amgen have continued to lead the way to commercial bio-genetically engineered products, but at great research expense and time. The agricultural sector is working with changing the DNA of food products to increase per year per acre crop yields.

"With the information I've been feeding our computer and with the DC combining information from the other consoles in conjunction with artificial intelligence, we have been able to arrive at some preliminary conclusions. I believe, and luckily the computer agrees, that we should be looking into more crossover between agriculture and pharmaceuticals. As you will see by the following video demonstration, changing the DNA of an ordinary corn seed can make a dramatic change in the mature plant and the plant's subsequent seeds." The monitor showed the DNA structure of corn. In a subsequent of change of the DNA, one of the chains was deleted and replaced by a different chain with a subtle difference in its structure. The screen was cleared and replaced by two kernels of corn. The kernel on the left looked the size, texture, and shape of a normal kernel of corn. The kernel on the right was about twice the size, more round, and pitted.

"As you can see, there is a dramatic difference between the two kernels. Not only in the size which is about twice that of the original kernel, but the nutritional food value of genetically altered corn on the right is more than two times that on the left. A true synergistic effect, but as in most cases of genetic engineering there are other changes." The monitor screen changed and showed two ears of corn.

One was normal and the other was almost a perfect sphere. The image on the screen caused the team to begin laughing. The new corncob resembled a yellow unpopped popcorn ball.

"By God, it's a nature-manufactured popcorn ball," Cap guffawed.

Joe quickly spoke up to quell the laughing. "Yeah, okay, it is pretty funny, but please consider the expense required to harvest such a physically different product. Even though the crops of the new cornball increased crop yields, the expense of re-tooling to harvest the new shape outweighed any beneficial gains. The point here is that altering DNA is extremely difficult and expensive and in most cases, the new product is unpredictable to the researcher. The new product has to be completely evaluated, from its chemical composition to the costs of the technological transfer from R&D to the consumer.

"Still, when success comes, and in a very few cases, success does come, the product is extremely valuable to mankind and can be very profitable for commercial concerns involved.

"I believe there is a new line of bio-genetically engineered pharmaceuticals on the horizon and more will be possible when plants are bio-genetically changed by DNA bombardment. These new products could be used as pharmaceuticals and not as food substances." The monitor cleared and he continued.

"The second class of pharmaceuticals I want to discuss is a long-range product and is highly controversial." The monitor displayed the words, PRENATAL CHROMOSOME. Joe continued, "This class of pharmaceuticals changes fetal chromosomes to prevent certain diseases from occurring in a child's future. In the past, fetal treatment has been done through intravenous injection of systematic chemical pharmaceuticals or by surgery. An historical example of systemic treatment is the use of a drug in the early '70's on pregnant women who tested for an Rh-negative blood type. Women with the Rh-negative factor have had a history of giving birth to what was then called a blue baby or Mongoloid. Intervention with this drug greatly reduced the odds of the woman giving birth to a Mongoloid baby.

"In the '80's, surgery on the fetus was conducted to correct some organ complications such as heart deformities even before the fetus heart was fully developed. Today, the class of pharmaceuticals I'm talking about gives us the ability to prevent any number of problems simply by giving the fetus an injection in its early stages of development. The fetus will be tested for chromosome deficiencies by taking a blood sample. This is a common procedure now for other reasons and has no adverse side effect to the mother or fetus. The fetus blood is run through a battery of tests. Those tests along with three generations of parental history will be compared with known value ranges using a sophisticated software program that has been developed. As an example, this class of pharmaceuticals could prevent such diseases as AIDS from being passed from mother to fetus and could put an end to multiple sclerosis, which is hereditary.

"Now then, this treatment is controversial because the next question you will undoubtedly ask is whether this theory can be carried to the next stage. Could we change the child's sex or make the child more beautiful?" Joe stopped and thought for a second, "The answer is a definite, yes. That is why this class of pharmaceuticals is controversial and is being developed, shall we say, somewhat covertly.

"There are some terrible diseases plaguing civilization, and who can predict the future? In the future, these diseases must be cured before the baby is born. As an example, my sister who has MS would not be living a costly painful life, with little to no quality, if there were a way to have prevented MS before it developed. Why shouldn't we use the knowledge and technology that we have to ensure that every child has best opportunity to live a full and productive life?"

The room fell quiet. Joe had never demonstrated this level of passion. Skip asked quietly, "Joe? Hey, buddy, you okay?"

Joe looked down at the floor and then said, "Yeah. I'm fine, thanks. As I said, this class of pharmaceuticals is going to be controversial, but I believe these products will offer the possibility of successfully eradicating diseases like AIDS. Because of their promise for society, I believe over time that these drugs will become more acceptable. I don't have a timeframe for any new products. I've brought up the subject of Prenatal Chromosomes because there are products currently on the market with fetus side effects. Some of these products could be developed into specific Prenatal Chromosome products. We may be closer than we realize. Look at Thalidomide. It went back into clinical trials several years ago and has been found to be very beneficial in the care of non-pregnant AIDS patients." Joe turned to the group and smiled. "Anyway, Skip, I thought you should enter this information into the computer.

"Again as a reminder, since it is in the press daily, I have considered stem cell research, but have concluded the politics around this research limits products for at least 10 years."

Skip began pressing buttons on the handset to download Joe's information into the DC. "Well now, it's time for our benefactor and his report. Nacheda-san, please enlighten us on Bandai technology."

Nacheda hit a few keys on his keyboard and the monitor screen read: CONSOLE #6, BANDAI INTERFACE.

Nacheda began speaking in his grammatically perfect American English with only the slightest trace of a Japanese accent. "As you know, my role in this astute group is to inform you on the research activities of Bandai Pharmaceutical Company and to input the computer with this information. In the past months, I haven't been able to add much to our process, but today I have important information from Bandai. As you know, Dr. Nakasone doesn't trust the satellite transmissions, no matter how many security loops we have in place. I have therefore brought my report with me on specially encoded CD." He inserted the CD into the drive of his console. The access light blinked and the wall screen refreshed itself. The familiar Bandai logo appeared and Nacheda began his presentation.

"Skip, I would also prefer to use the audio transcriber for my presentation."

"Fine," Skip said as he initialized the transcriber program.

Nacheda continued, "As we have discussed many times, Bandai has spent a great deal of money in biological research. The major emphasis of this research has been on developing a method of isolating and extracting pure active ingredients from sources found in nature. Experiments have been done on both animals and plant material. In the 1980's there was a high level of interest in the possibilities of developing pharmaceuticals from ocean life. Although this research is ongoing and great strides have been made, you don't hear much about this research in popular media. This is likely due to the fact that most of these programs are long-term and the media is only interested in what it can find, report, and resolve in the short-term.

"Bandai is one of the companies that continues to work on the ocean life programs while still exploring other sources of herbals on land. In the past month, Bandai has made a remarkable breakthrough in isolating natural ingredients from plant life. As I'm certain most of you know, when an active ingredient is removed from the host source it is almost always altered in some way or another or, even worse, it contains contaminants. A pharmacologist can be as careful as possible using all of today's technology, but isolating a pure ingredient is almost impossible. This lack of pure ingredients in the pharmaceutical contributes to the incidence of unwanted patient side effects.

"Through a complex method of magnetic resonance extraction, Bandai has been able to extract pure ingredients with virtually no alteration in their biological structures. Bandai has filed notice of this exclusive process through the proper international channels.a patent if you will. Basically, the process changes the desired active ingredient's polarity from the host product's polarity. The result is that the active ingredient springs free of its host. Once the desired active ingredient isolated from the host, its polarity is switched back to normal and is available in its pure state.

"As you might expect, when used in the manufacture of a pharmaceutical, the pure active ingredient doesn't present the side effects that the same active ingredient had when isolated using more traditional methods. We don't have the process completed for commercial production, but Bandai believes there will not be any problems in scaling up the process, to isolate kilogram quantities within a reasonable amount of time. So what we have here is, as you Americans say, a whole new ballgame."

Nacheda paused and then said, "This concludes my report for today."

Skip punched a few buttons on his handset and Nacheda's oral presentation and the information from the CD was added to the DC.

Skip pushed his chair back from the console and rose to address the group. "Okay people, as you know it will take at least an hour for the AIMS program to convert the data and information into intelligence and then use artificial intelligence to come up with any summaries, correlations, and or conclusions. I therefore recommend that we adjourn to the living room for cocktails and some really great microwave snackies that I recently came across in the store. You can thank me later." The team stood up and moved as a group into the living room. Skip stayed behind and keyed in some commands to the DC before leaving.

Nacheda lagged behind the rest, "What do you think, Skip?"

"I really don't know and I'm hesitant to get too excited, but I do feel good about today's session. We've had some interesting stuff in here today. I'm starting to believe we may actually be on to something. We've been looking for a paradigm shift and we may actually have one when we analyze today's presentation as a whole. What do you think, friend?"

Nacheda looked at Skip and said, "I must say that I do not like your choice of the phrase paradigm shift. I'm not looking for an entirely new direction or model. I'm looking for an ending. Still, I do have a good feeling about this session."

The two men left the war room and walked to the living room to join the other team members. After one hour exactly, the green light over the door to the war room went on. This signaled that the DC and AIMS had finished their job of analyzing the data and information.

Skip's voice broke in over the din of conversation in the room. "Okay.

Looks like the computer has come up with something. Please finish your drinks and let's reassemble in the war room in five minutes."

After the team had returned to the war room and taken their respective seats, Skip asked, "Is everyone set? Let's wrap this up as quickly as possible. You all know what happens next. We'll hear the computer's summary and then hand out assignments for the February meeting. Let's pray we come up with something substantive this evening.

The lights in the room automatically dimmed for the summary session.

From somewhere in the darkness came a faint, "Amen."

Skip picked up his handset and keyed in a sequence of commands. The large wall-mounted monitor brightened and a computer-generated image appeared. The image of a masculine head to just below the shoulders was named SAM for Strategic Analysis Manager. SAM's appearance was a surprise and there were a number of gasps from members of the group. Usually, the summary session was just text and numbers. SAM had appeared only twice before when he had concluded that they were not doing a very good job.

"I'm sure you all remember SAM. SAM, say hello to the team," Skip commanded.

SAM began to speak, "Good evening to the team." SAM had been programmed with a voice that sounded very much like that of Basil Rathbone. SAM's voice and appearance were so realistic that the team members had to think twice not to respond, "Good evening" back to him. SAM's image reflected a look of wisdom. The face had very high cheekbones and reddish-blond hair combed straight back. He looked to be a very handsome man in his forties. There were crows feet around the corners of his eyes and fine wrinkles across the forehead. His programmer was the unseen team member #8.

SAM continued, "You have certainly provided me with a great deal of new and valuable information today. Thank you." His eyes shifted slightly and took in everyone in the room. "I worked on your input for sixty-one minutes and thirty-three point four seconds. I apologize that I've not had the opportunity to talk to you for a while, but I've not had very much information to analyze until today.

Well, I'm certain you all want to get home so let's get on with the conclusion."

The wall monitor went dark for a second and then lit up again with a line chart that graphically mapped the artificial intelligence computing times for each of the previous eleven meetings. The time has gone from less than one minute in the first month to 46 minutes in September. It then dropped to between 14 and 33 minutes over the last three months and illustrated the team's failure to generate new data and information. There was a nice upward line showing computing time for the current meeting.

SAM continued, "Your information has allowed me to come to a macro conclusion. From this macro will come some very important actions which will require completion prior to the February meeting. In short, I have concluded that today's summary is a significant event." There was a quick gasp from one of the team members. "Due to the fact that the information I have heretofore been given wasn't substantive, I have not had the opportunity to make any conclusions before tonight.

"After I receive the information I will be requesting from you today I will analyze the situation. By the February meeting, I project a better than 90% chance that I will have at least one correlation lock-on. There is a 67.3% chance that I will have two correlation locks." SAM paused.

"On the monitor you will see in turn the summary of each of your presentations. Terri you have identified five compounds."

The wall screen changed to show the five compounds that Terri had identified earlier:

1. DY321
2. JPC138
3. PH631
4. BQ519
5. SK3H4

"John, you had no up-to-date data. This is understandable since we have, up until now, not identified a specific target product. John, you will have to wait while others are working.

The wall screen changed to show:

PATENT AND GRANTS—NONE IDENTIFIED

SAM continued, "Cap, you identified five side effects which you felt were significant."

The wall monitor showed:

ACCELERATED HAIR GROWTH DOMANT SPERM PHENOMENON BONE GROWTH STIMULATION LIBIDO ENHANCEMENT EXCESSIVE MENTAL ALTERNESS

"Mary, you cam up with two areas in your medical literature search."

LITERATURE SEARCH

DORMANT SPERM PHENOMENON

JOURNAL OB/GYN PAPER

FRENCH <u>LAFEMME MEDIA</u>

BONE GROWTH STIMULANT OINTMENT

"Joe, you also had two areas of future pharmaceuticals."

FUTURE PHARMACEUTICALS

PLANT DNA

PRENATAL CHROMOSOME TREATMENT

"And, finally, Nacheda, you had one area to report."

EXTRACTION OF THE PURE ACTIVE INGREDIENT OF A PRODUCT OF NATURE

"While you were away from the room for sixty-one minutes and thirtythree point four seconds, I analyzed the data and information you supplied me today. I have reached the following macro conclusions that will require additional work in order for me to come to a micro conclusion and identify the best product and company for Bandai.

"From Terri's report we find compounds DY321 and BQ519 are biogenetic and have no correlation. PH631 is herbal and ties in with the ointment in Mary's literature search and Cap's side effect of bone growth stimulation.

This is a three-way correlation. Good! SK3H4 is an herbal and ties in with Cap's dormant sperm phenomenon and Mary's articles on Diet-Level. Again, a three-way correlation. Good! Plant DNA ties in with herbs JPC138, PH631, and SK3H4 because herbs are plants. The plant DNA also ties in with Cap's excessive mental alertness because the product from Indonesia that caused the excessive mental alertness was an herb.

"This is a nine-way correlation. Excellent! Nacheda's pure active ingredient extraction is also plant and herbal related. This makes it a ten-way correlation. Outstanding!" SAM's face again filled the wall monitor. His skin appeared to dark brown although the race of the image was otherwise indistinguishable. Although his face, particularly up close, was definitely masculine, #8 had programmed him with many feminine gestures and expressions that made him a very unique individual.

SAM, in a very low voice, said to the group, "As I stated earlier, we have something but we require more information. Let me summarize my macro conclusion." The screen darkened momentarily and then brightened with:

MACRO CONCLUSION INVESTIGATE HERBS, PH631, JPC138, AND SK3H4 DO A COMPREHENSIVE MEDICAL INVESTIGATION INTO: DORMANT SPERM PHENOMENON BONE GROWTH STIMULATION EXCESSIVE MENTAL ALERTNESS RESEARCH PLANT DNA BOMBARDMENT SAM concluded his summary of the situation, "What you have hit upon is the field of herbal pharmaceuticals and what DNA bombardment might do to the pharmacological properties of the herb. At Bandai, they have found a way to isolate the pure active ingredient once the DNA of the herb has been altered.

"You are closer than you have ever been to finalizing your mission. Before we meet in February, I want you to provide me with additional information to analyze. At the February meeting there is a better than 90% probability that we will have a lock on and a possible conclusion to your project. My plan is to provide you the identification of a product and company. Good luck with your acquisition of the additional information."

The wall monitor went blank and the room became silent, except for the noise of the laser printer as it printed one copy of SAM's report for Nacheda. The silence only lasted for a few seconds, then the tension broke, and the team began giving one another high fives and laughing.

Nacheda was the first to get everyone's attention, "Thank you all very much. You've all saved my bacon." Everyone laughed. Nacheda thought to himself that perhaps now Nakasone would be happy, though he knew in his heart that Dr. Nakasone could never be happy. He added quietly, "At least temporarily."

Skip was the only member of the team who wasn't celebrating. When Joe said, "Let's go back over to the bar and have a drink to celebrate," Skip jumped in.

"Everybody hold it just one minute, we are not finished. I know we have made one giant step forward but the game isn't over and SAM, or maybe I should say Simon as in the children's game, could order us to take two steps backward if we don't do our homework between now and the February meeting." The room was again quiet.

Joe muttered, "Leave it to Skip to pull us back to reality."

Skip smiled, "Not that I'm not happy but, let's itemize what we have to do before February and maybe we can wrap up this mission within the one year time span that was given to Nacheda-san." Everyone sat back down at their console. They knew Skip was right.

Skip gave out the assignments. First, he warned them not to discuss anything from today's meeting with anyone. In their future investigation and information gathering they were not to arouse any attention to the task force or the target product compounds. They were to operate alone and concentrate on the areas SAM had mentioned in his macro conclusion. They were instructed to down link their information to AIMS as it was obtained.

Skip concluded, "Again, you are not to draw attention to any aspect of our project. The project now has a top-secret classification. Only Dr. Nakasone is to be briefed on the macro conclusion. Any questions?" Skip looked over the group. "Nacheda-san, do you have anything you want to say?"

"No, Skip. You said it all. I want to thank all of you for the work you have already done and for the work ahead of us. Dr. Nakasone will be very pleased with our results. I look forward to our February meeting. If you have any problems or questions please call Skip. In most cases, he can help you with the issue or he will always know how to reach me. I'll see you in four weeks."

The team began leaving the condo. Some hung around for a little while and talked. Within thirty minutes they had all left except for Skip and Nacheda.

As the team left the condo, the man who had sat at the restaurant bar watched from the street corner for his contact. Once his contact emerged from the condo he followed at a short distance until both walked into the main section of the UCLA/Westwood complex. The contact walked clockwise around the center block. The man walked around the block in the opposite direction. When they met each other on the far side of the block, the contact spoke three words, "Outstanding. Close. February." And they both continued their walks. The man returned to the street corner across from the condo. A new person had picked up surveillance of the condo when the first man had moved off behind his contact. The surveillance team didn't want to lose sight of Nacheda while they were making contact. The man who had followed the contact passed the three words to his partner who moved off to make a phone call.

Since the time in Japan was 2:00 p.m., Wednesday afternoon, Nacheda phoned Dr. Nakasone and told him he would have good news upon his return. The project wasn't over, but large gains had been made and the February meeting looked good for a conclusion. He asked permission to meet with Nakasone early Friday morning in his office. Nakasone agreed, thanked him for the good news, and hung up.

Nacheda and Skip had a few drinks and then went out for dinner. They went to bed early. Skip in the master bedroom and Nacheda on the sleeper sofa.

The surveillance of the condo and Nacheda continued throughout the night.

SPECTRUM OF MEDICINE BUILDING NEW YORK CITY

Peggy McCleary, Ph.D, Director Lifeal Research was a 35 year old beautiful single woman with Pharmacy Doctorate from Rochester School of Pharmacy and a Doctorate in Herbal Sciences from Columbia University thanks to the James educational program for bright researchers. She had grown up in Lake Placid, New York where her father was the owner of McCleary Apothecary and her mom ran a nursery, Through her dad she gained an appreciation of the roll of pharmacy in healthcare and through her mom gained a love of plants and herbs.

While Peggy was in her final year, almost 10 years ago, her pharmacology professor invited an outside speaker to lecture for three days on herbal plants and their potential pharmacological properties. Allen Stevenson Strong was a Ph.D. from James Pharmaceutical Company in New York City where he was the director of genetic herbal sciences. Dr. Strong's curriculum vitae read like a roadmap for anyone aspiring to a successful career in the pharmaceuticals industry. Peggy had never heard of a herbal profession in the pharmaceutical industry. Dr. Strong's lecture caused an awakening in Peggy. A marriage between her two professional loves, pharmacy and botany.

At the end of the lecture, Dr. Strong gave a short sales pitch for James.

He explained some of the work that was being done at James.

"Old Doc James," he had said, "has been, is, and always will be a fanatic of plants and herbs and their impact on medicine. While the rest of the pharmaceutical industry has embraced genetic engineering and other chemical synthetic products, Doc James has continued to conduct research programs in herbal pharmaceuticals. The other companies dropped their herbal programs after it seemed that every possible medicinal plant and herb had been ground up, tabulated, and/or emulsified to discover whether it would be the next wonder drug.

"Better pharmaceutical possibilities came along and away went the research money the other companies had allocated to herbal research. But, Doc James wouldn't give up on plants and herbs. He had a strong personal theory that advances in genetic engineering would eventually bring both the sciences of genetics and herbal alkaloids into a new class of pharmaceuticals. He felt that genetic engineering could alter the plants' or herbs' DNA structures and create totally new families of pharmacologically active products that would gain the classification of 'wonder drug'.

"Despite shifts in conventional wisdom and the attention Wall Street has lauded on what it perceives as the now and forever more industry leaders, Doc James refused to let go of his idea of a merging between the two sciences.

After graduating, Peggy contacted Dr. Strong about a position at James.

Dr. Strong had explained, "we're working on a new class of pharmaceuticals that is so secret I don't have full access to the total project. At times I feel like I'm on the Manhattan Project, although ours would be called the Sheepshead Bay Project, I suppose."

Peggy, said, "Huh? Why Sheepshead Bay?"

He smiled, "I'm sorry, let me explain further. Sheepshead Bay is an inlet off the Atlantic Ocean in Long Island Sound. Doc James grew up there. His father founded the original company there in 1896. After moving the majority of the company to New York City, he retained all of his favorite and secret research projects in the remote Sheepshead Bay laboratories."

After four years as a researcher for James Pharmaceutical, Dr. Strong suggested to Peggy that she take a sabbatical and get her masters and Ph.D. in herbal sciences at Columbia University. Her pharmacy doctorate wasn't based in a masters program in research, so she had to earn the masters before she could earn her Ph.D.

Now, over ten years after she had joined James, Peggy was a major researcher and in charge of the Lifeal program.

Peggy looked at her watch as she stepped into the employee elevator to ride to the research offices on the 40th floor 8:30 AM. She inserted her plastic card into the security slot to access floors 40-49 that housed the James' Research Laboratories.

James did not conduct potentially harmful or explosive research at the Spectrum of Medicine building. Any experiments or research that could be potentially hazardous were done at the Sheepshead Bay Laboratories. Most of the research staff and clean programs had been moved to the Spectrum of Medicine Building when it opened. The long-term herbology programs and animal studies were still done at Sheepshead Bay where it was easier to take care of the animals. Peggy had worked in Sheepshead Bay when she first joined James as Dr. Allen Strong's assistant. After earning her Ph.D. she moved her major research to the Spectrum of Medicine labs where they had the most modern analytical research instruments in the world. Helmut Wahlters, SVP of Research had made sure the best equipment had been purchased before Doc James died and the decision was left to another CEO, whom, he was certain, would be less informed about these matters.

The elevator doors opened to the research reception desk. "Good morning, Dr. McCleary," said the receptionist. "You already have three new phone messages that I've forwarded to your e-mail. Dr. Wahlters would like to see you at four regarding the Lifeal project. The meeting reminder is on your computer meeting schedule."

"Thank you, Kathy," Peggy answered as she walked towards her corner office. She was in the quarter of the research floor aptly called the Lifeal wing. She hung her heavy winter coat in the closet, sat down at her desk, and switched on her computer. She saw the three phone messages that Kathy had mentioned, noting that all three were low priority. She donned a lab coat and walked down the hallway to obtain a status report on the Lifeal studies in preparation for her meeting with Wahlters at 4:00.

After meeting with her group to get the latest rundown on Lifeal, Peggy worked on her projects until a few minutes before her meeting. She arrived in Wahlters' office at exactly four o'clock, but as usual, Helmut wasn't there. Peggy smirked as she looked around his office. He was never on time. It was his reputation.

In truth, Helmut Wahlters wanted to be late and make people wait for him. He enjoyed making his visitors wait. He felt that his position as director of research was a critical one that demanded respect and that respect was properly shown by waiting for his entrance. When asked why he was always late to meetings, he would always answer, "I don't attend meetings at the stated time because everyone else is always late and that is disrespectful. I get nervous when people don't show respect and make me wait to start a meeting. Therefore, I ensure everyone is in attendance, then I make my appearance."

Peggy was always on time for meetings. Helmut knew this and still he would make her wait for at least five minutes. She looked around his office.

The walls and shelves were covered with the usual mementos that one finds in corporate executive offices. In fact, everything that she could see was James Pharmaceutical related with the exception of his university degrees.

Helmut Wahlters had attended Heidelberg University in Germany for his undergraduate and post-graduate studies, as well as his doctoral program. After earning his Ph.D. in pharmacology, he had worked at the Heidelberg University-associated Heidelberg Cancer Institute as a research scientist until 1970. Doc James lured him away from academia research that same year.

Peggy had been in Wahlters' private office both in the Spectrum of Medicine and in the old offices in Sheepshead Bay. Helmut always maintained a nice, efficient workspace, but it always seemed to be devoid of warmth. He was taciturn, which many in the company interpreted as uncaring coldness. Peggy had always thought of him as a good boss, teacher, and researcher. She was proud to be at James and to work with him. She looked at her watch and saw that it was 4:15. When she looked back up, Helmut was standing in the doorway.

"Sorry I'm late, Peggy, please forgive me." he asked. He had a firm voice, but spoke very softly. He often told friends and associates that he expected people to listen to him, not hear him.

Wahlters smiled and gestured for Peggy to sit. He moved around behind his desk and sat down. He placed his folded hands on the desk. His eyes were focused on the hands. "Peggy," he said, still looking down at the desk, "I'm very concerned about some of the side effects we're seeing with Lifeal. I want for you to expand your toxicology and pathology research into the areas where these new side effects are possibly manifested. Please provide me with a research protocol on this subject early next Monday morning. I wish to present it at Dr. Bradsmith's eleven o'clock executive staff meeting that morning. Do you have any questions?"

Peggy knew that with his question asking if she had any questions meant the meeting was over. She rose from her seat, saying, "No, Helmut. I agree completely with your assessment of the situation. I'll have the protocol completed on Friday for you to study over the weekend. If you have any questions, you can always call me at home. That will allow us enough time to make any changes prior to Monday's meeting."

"Thank you. That's an excellent idea. Friday afternoon it is." Helmut stood up and formally shook Peggy's hand.

Wahlters watched her leave his office. He liked it that she worked hard and always made time to ensure the job was done correctly. She was a good researcher and, as far as he could tell, a good person.

He looked down at his desk. Things were not going well for him. Everything seemed to take longer than he thought it should. Research was moving at a much slower pace than when Doc James had been in charge. Phillip was too much of a businessman in Helmut's opinion. Phillip's heart was for James, but he just wasn't doing it correctly. Phillip, only the month before, in a desperate effort to shore up Lifeal had ordered several research projects into a temporary inactive status. Phillip emphasized to Wahlters that it was only a temporary measure, but to Helmut it might as well have been permanent. He would be seventy years old in two years and he wanted to finish some of those important projects.

Suddenly, to emphasize the point to himself, he slammed his large fist down on his desk making a loud bang. Everyone just outside his office looked up with surprise.

Back at her desk, Peggy leaned back and thought back at the abupt end of the meeting. I have been working directly for him for years and he still shakes my hand. Wow, she thought and now back to work. She brought up the Lifeal side effects file on her computer. The file was split into three subfiles titled, Package Insert, Not Relevant, and New.

The side effects listed in the Package Insert sub-file were not really the problem. They had all been detected during the original clinical studies. All had been completely investigated and were included in the filing that had been approved by the FDA. Included in the files "Not Relevant" category were those side effects that were judged as not being caused by Lifeal. As an example, there was a skin rash reported by one of the clinical patients. It was determined that this was neurodermatitis. It turned out that the patient had been very scared about taking a new pharmaceutical and a rash had broken out.

Although Lifeal had not directly caused the neurodermatitis rash, it had been a factor that had to be reported. This category had to be watched because it was possible that a seemingly irrelevant side effect could become relevant over time. This change in classification could happen if the side effect occurred more than once and was found to be directly caused by Lifeal.

The third category, "New", was the most important category following FDA approval. Side effects directly related to Lifeal that occurred after the official clinicals had been completed were essentially classified as "surprises." In pharmaceutical products, when it takes up to fifteen years to obtain FDA approval, there aren't supposed to be any surprises. Surprises cause products to be recalled by the

FDA or, at minimum cause a corporate letter to be written to all physicians explaining the new side effect. Advertisements placed in medical journals had to explain the new side effect, and sometimes the FDA required that the new side effect be outlined by a black box. Recalls could signal the end of a product's success or the beginning of a product's failure. Recalls not only stopped product sales, but the marketing costs of producing new literature and destroying the obsolete promotional materials was in the millions. Whatever the penalty, a recall was the kiss of death for a pharmaceutical product. The regulatory rules were not wrong. It was the way the FDA and the pharmaceutical industry worked together. Companies worked very hard to prevent recalls by investigating every unusual side effect. The companies wanted to know everything about their products not only to protect themselves, but also to protect the patient using their products.

One of Peggy's responsibilities was to watch over the reported side effects. She was presently investigating two that could be classified as either 'not relevant' or 'new'. The ultimate classification was dependent upon the outcome of Peggy's investigations. That was why she had wanted to get back to the lab. Blurred vision and tingling in the fingers were the two new side effects.

She also was monitoring one of the minor side effects, hyperactivity, which had actually been listed in the package insert.

As the number of prescriptions increased for Lifeal, the number of side effects increased as well. The specific number was important, but a more important number was the percentage of patients reporting each specific side effect in relation to the number of patients taking Lifeal. The rate for the two new side effects had increased slightly over the last two months.

When a new patient was placed on a pharmaceutical his dosage had to be titrated and then adjusted to determine the correct pharmacological dose for his body chemistry. Sometimes this titrating process temporarily resulted in an increase in certain side effects due to a slight overdose as the long-term dosage regimens were determined.

Unusual side effects had to be reported to the FDA and the manufacturing company by the patient, the pharmacist, the physician, or all three. The word "unusual" was subjective. Many side effects were not reported because they were not "unusual." Peggy had to ensure that all "unusual" side effects were reported and investigated. The FDA did not have the staff to police all of the companies and their products. They relied on researchers like Peggy and presidents like Phillip to do their own policing.

She looked at her watch and saw that it was 5:15. She decided to leave for the day. Tomorrow she would draft a report on these side effects and also start working on the side effect protocol for Helmut.

2:45 P.M., TUESDAY, JANUARY 17

LOS ANGELES INTERNATIONAL AIRPORT

J.P.'s plane touched down softly at LAX and taxied to the assigned terminal gate. He gathered his things and made his way to the ground transportation lanes near the baggage claim area. He had made a call to the private aviation service at the airport using the Airphone on the plane. He gave the service his flight number so that someone would meet him to drive him around to the commercial side of the airport. He also asked that they file a flight plan for him on his return to Mammoth Lakes.

After performing his pre-flight checks, he checked in with air traffic control and began to taxi to his assigned runway. As he waited in the queue for his turn to take-off, he glanced at his watch and saw that it was 3:30. J.P. smiled, it was his favorite time of the day to fly. Finally, his turn came and he ran the engines of the Lear to full throttle and began rolling down the runway.

After being airborne for a few minutes, his headset came alive. The air controller vectored him to a heading of 080 degrees at 10,000 feet. J.P. banked slowly to the right and headed over the mountains of Los Padres National Forrest to the Antelope Valley. His flight plan took him along a course that followed the Los Angeles Aqueduct to China Lake, and then north up the throat of the Owens Valley.

The flight up the Owens Valley was always one of his favorites. He often used route 395 as his navigational guide as it led him to Mammoth Lakes Airport. He often tried to visualize the track bed from the old Carson and Colorado Narrow Gauge Railroad that was an outgrowth of the Virginia and Truckee. Time and the desert winds were gradually washing away what the Owens Valley residents used to call their slim rails through the sand. The long defunct line had run from

Keeler, California to Carson City, Nevada. The name Colorado had come from optimistic intentions of running the line all the way to the Colorado River that made up the Arizona and California state line. Eventually, the gold ran out and the Southern Pacific Railroad bought the line only to later tear it out.

To his right was the Bristol Cone pine forest, where a person could find the oldest living things on earth. Some of the trees were thousands of years old and still growing. The combination of altitude and climate enabled the trees to grow at an extremely slow rate. Some of the trees were more than 5,000 years old.

"Bishop tower, this is Lear 13 checking in. Course is zero, zero, zero at angels ten, over."

"Lear 13, Bishop, is that you, J.P.? Over," was the reply from the Bishop air controller.

"Bishop, Lear 13, you pegged it. Hiya Pete. Clearance to Mammoth, over."

"Roger Lear 13, permission granted, over"

"Bishop, Lear 13, roger permission granted. Thanks. Out."

J.P. banked left and continued along route 395 the remaining 40 miles to Mammoth Lakes Airport. The winter sun was off to the left. In the winter, this leg of the flight from Los Angeles wasn't too bad because the sun was in the southwest. In the summer, it was dangerous with the sun more in the pilot's eyes. Landing at Mammoth Airport was tricky enough without adding the pressure of being temporarily blinded by the sun.

The landing strip at Mammoth is lined up north to south with a 15 knot right-to-left crosswind the norm. For a pilot, the runway was just beyond a rocky hill. The plane had to clear the hill and then set down almost immediately onto the runway. With the constant crosswind and other potential environmental conditions, flying in and out of Mammoth was always exciting for J.P.

He began to set himself up for landing. To his left was Mammoth Mountain, an extinct volcano and some of the best skiing in North America. It last erupted hundreds of years ago when it blew off the northeast half of the cone. In the dusk, he could see the last skiers coming down off the cornice. The setting sun formed a halo around the summit. The shadow of the mountain was creeping down the slopes. Its path was blocking the warm sun and would slowly turn the top of the packed snow to crusty ice. The lifts had stopped around 4:30 and he could make out skiers moving down the face in a line. Probably the ski patrol making their final sweep of the day to ensure there were no skiers left on the mountain.

After taking in the view of his adopted home, he wondered why he was contemplating a new consulting project. Phillip, Mandi, and James Pharmaceutical Company seemed to be in a totally different world. It wasn't that he disliked the business world of New York or Los Angeles, he just preferred Mammoth. He muttered to himself, "I should be on the ground making my last run of the day instead of up here swaying in cross winds and trying to figure out who stole a goddamned strategic business plan."

"Lear one-three, Mammoth approach, say again, over." The controller's voice echoed in J.P.'s headset and snapped him back to the present. He had forgotten that he had switched his radio to hot microphone. It was a trick he had learned after making a number of landings at Mammoth. The landing frequently required both hands, so after clearing Bishop, he would switch to hot mic just in case he needed assistance in the course of his final approach.

"Mammoth, Lear 13, sorry there Jake, it's J.P. and I guess I was thinking out loud. Request permission to land. What are the crosswinds, over?"

"Crosswind is 5 knots moving right to left on your approach. Please be aware that those winds are shifting frequently to a head wind and gusting to 30 knots. Permission granted, over."

"Roger, on short final."

He made a quick check of his altimeter to make certain that it was set for the airport altitude of 6,500 feet. He made a soft landing on the snow-cleared runway and taxied to his hangar at the northeast corner of the airport. He secured the plane inside the hangar and checked-in with the air operations building. After passing instructions for maintenance on the jet to the mechanic on duty, he left the building and started for home.

Snow was piled on either side of the roadway to six or seven feet. This winter, Mammoth Lakes has experienced an early and nearly continuous snowfall. Although the snowfall of the previous few winters had not been the best for skiing, this year was looking much better for skiers.

He loved the snow, the mountains, the tall lodgepole pines, the sun, Mammoth Mountain, and the town of Mammoth Lakes. All of these provided him with just the right amount of fuel for what he termed his outer and inner selves. Mammoth Lakes residents had just the right mixture of youthful hopefulness and mature experience that J.P. liked.

As J.P. drove along his thoughts turned back to his present business with James Pharmaceutical Company. He quickly chased them from his mind, deciding that there was plenty of time to think about work. He turned off the main road and headed up Mountain View Road before turning into his driveway. He pushed the button to open the door of his underground garage and drove into the garage. He noted that in the 38 hours that he had been away there had been no new snowfall. The drive was still clear of snow.

J.P. had lived in Mammoth for seven years, ever since he left the presidency of his own start-up company. The variety of challenges that had excited him before then had become repetitive. Whenever he got the urge to rush headlong back into the fray of the daily business world, he simply looked out his window at the face of the mountain and then patted himself on the back for having the great fortune and good sense to move to Mammoth Lakes and live in the shadow of Mammoth Mountain. He constantly reminded himself that there was no other place on Earth that he would rather live.

His house was on a wooded corner of a residential area of single family homes. He was only two blocks from the ski lifts. He had three bedrooms downstairs and a large great room upstairs on the second floor to maximize the impact of the view. The large second floor room had glass walls and redwood decks on three sides. The house had been situated so as to make maximum benefit of the sun.

Once J.P. was in his house, he moved quickly to his bedroom and changed out of the flight suit he had put on in Los Angeles. He pulled on a pair of jeans, boots, a loose flannel shirt, and a wool sweater.

After changing his clothes, he climbed the stairs to the upper floor two at a time and emerged into the great room. The large room was sparsely furnished with only a sofa, an overstuffed chair, a home theater system, a stereo system, and a floor to ceiling bookcase. Among the books in the case was his collection of Great Western Books, which he never seemed to find time to read until he moved to Mammoth Lakes. He had even founded the Mammoth Great Western Books discussion group.

Although the idea of a Great Western Books discussion group wasn't particularly original, it was new to the Mammoth area. Once word began to spread about the group, He found there was more interest than he had thought possible. The group often met at his house whenever he was in town.

J.P. retrieved a cocktail glass from the dishwasher and opened the freezer door to retrieve his bottle of Stolichnaya vodka and a tray of ice cubes. He then sat down on the deep leather couch and used his handset to select a classical CD to play.

The music swept over him and filled the room. He stared into his glass of vodka, rolled his wrist and swirled the ice cubes in the viscous frozen Stoli. The silver liquid seemed to adhere to each cube and then slowly flow back to the bottom of the glass. The music that was playing was Prokofiev's *Romeo and Juliet.* All thoughts seemed to leave his mind except for the strains of music. He began to feel himself drift away.

Suddenly, he felt a strong jolt as the house shook and the Stoli sloshed over the rim of the glass onto his right hand. His mind snapped back to the present. He looked at his watch and noted the time. He decided it must have been about three-point-four. Living life on the Richter Scale was just how it was when you chose Mammoth Lakes as your home. J.P. had, over the years, grown adept at estimating the strength of quakes to within two or three tenths. He realized that he must have dozed for a short time. Prokofiev's music still filled the room. He reached for the remote and turned the CD off.

It was 10 PM, he figured he had just enough time to head over to Annie's Bar and Grill for a late supper and conversation. He went down to the garage to get back into his four wheel drive, when he suddenly felt a pang of guilt about the project he had been working on before he had received Phillip's phone call. He went back upstairs to his office where he opened the door, turned on the room lights, and then just stared at his desk. His custom computer sat on the desk staring back at him. His desk was covered with books, reprints, and business magazines. He thought it would probably be a while before he got back to writing on his latest business book, "The Strategic Continuum." He decided the James project took precedence and would only last a few months at any rate. Then he could get back to the book. He dreaded telling his publisher about his decision since he was already behind in delivering the book to the editors. He told himself that spring was the best time to write business books and he would be able to complete the book then he figured he would wait until morning to clean off the desk and begin the James project.

J.P. closed the office door and walked back down to the garage where he started his vehicle, backed out, and proceeded down the mountain to Annie's. He made a right turn at the Whiskey Creek Restaurant and drove the remaining two blocks to Annie's Bar and Grill.

Annie Wilson owned, managed, and was the bartender of the place since her father had died fifteen years before. Her father had named the bar after his only daughter when Annie was born. Sam Wilson had told the *Mammoth News Reporter* that after Annie was born he just didn't feel that the name Sam's Bar and Grill was appropriate. Annie's mom, Shirley, had left Sam, her daughter Annie, and Mammoth Lakes when Annie was seven years old. Shirley never seemed to fit in with Mammoth, Annie's Bar and Grill, or with any of Sam's friends. She had come to Mammoth in the nineteen sixties from Orange County to be a ski bum. Sam had lived in Mammoth all of his life— one of the true natives of Mammoth. Sam and Shirley met on the backside of chair #3, fell in love, and married. Annie came along and shortly thereafter the relationship began to sour. After Shirley left her family and Mammoth behind, no one ever heard from her again.

Annie was J.P.'s best friend. There were times when they were both friends and lovers, but mostly they were just very close friends. Annie had an uncanny way of keeping J.P. grounded. She would sit and listen to him talk himself out of most any situation from business opportunities to relationships. At the right time she would interject a few extremely well chosen pearls of wisdom that shed new light and most often led to a solution.

He parked in the snow plowed parking lot. There were only a few other cars in the lot. It was mid-week and that meant that Mammoth was relatively dead compared to the weekends. To the LA crowd that emigrated on the weekends, Annie's was known as a local's bar. That made it almost taboo to be seen there if you were from LA. To the Mammoth locals, Annie's was the best place for food, booze, and good conversation.

J.P. entered Annie's through the old, thick redwood door on the front and was nearly knocked over by the warm air that came from inside. There was only one large room. The bar stretched the entire length of the left side of the room. The right side contained the original solid wood tables for four. There was a small dance floor in a corner near the front.

The floor was solid oak. It was buckled in places with age and use and gave a comforting squeak as you walked across it. The walls were California redwood. At the far end of the room was a large walk-in fireplace. In the fireplace there burned what could only be called an inferno.

Annie had one of the few wood-fueled fire permits in the Mammoth Lakes area. Several years before wood burning fires had been banned. The smoke and soot had gotten so bad that something had to be done to prevent the possibility of a near-continuous state of smog alert. The volcano heated homes and businesses in the village. Heat from geothermal wells was pumped up from the Earth's depths to the geothermal plants located in the valley below Mammoth. There the steam was converted to dry heat, forced up to the village by large turbines driven by the geothermal pressure from the wells. Once the village converted to geothermal heat, the Mammoth Lakes air became clear again. The local government allowed a few places to keep their open fireplaces burning, one of which was Annie's.

J.P. walked up to the end of the bar closest to the door. Since he tended to prefer colder rooms, the end of the bar closest to the door was about as close as he wanted to get to the roaring fire. Annie spotted him as soon as he came through the door and ran around the end of the bar to give him a kiss. "How are you, J.P.?" she asked as she looked deep into his eyes.

When J.P. first met Annie her deep searching looks annoyed him. As he grew to know and love her, he found out that this was the way Annie could tell whether you were telling the truth. She had a sixth sense about people lying. It seemed to him that her beautiful gray eyes could look straight into his soul.

Annie had auburn hair and a deep facial tan that never seemed to fade. Her eyes had a natural squint that came from living her life under the mountain sun. Her complexion was smooth, which one might not expect from a person who was used to living out of doors in the harsh mountain climate. Annie took care of herself; of this there was little doubt.

"I'm doing very well, thank you, my dear," J.P. replied looking straight back into Annie's eyes. They hugged and then broke apart. Annie moved back behind the bar and reached down for the freezer door. In a flash she came up with his Stoli. J.P. smiled when he saw the bottle. He stood at the bar since there were no barstools in Annie's. If you drank at the bar, you stood. When you sat at Annie's tables you ate, drank, played chess or backgammon, or talked skiing or town gossip.

"So, where the hell did you go in such a hurry Monday morning, J.P., to LA?" Annie asked. Annie and J.P had an agreement that she never asked too many questions about where he was or what he was doing. That came from his working with the Navy CMAG. If he could tell her, he would. If he couldn't, she didn't press. She would look after his place in his absence and wait for him to return.

"LA and then to New York City," he replied. He noticed that she was overly polishing a glass beer mug, which betrayed her nervousness over his sudden departure and return.

Annie had never liked J.P. working for Navy as the CO of CMAG and constantly reminded him of that fact. She always told him that people that are secretive about their work live in a different world and that he didn't belong there. He always pointed out to her that they had an important job to do and they were pretty darned good at doing it. Once, after CMAG had completed a covert project, the deputy director of the CIA had approached J.P. about joining the agency to head their new economic intelligence branch. Doing so would have meant that J.P. would have had to relocate to Northern Virginia and endure the rigorous background investigations to gain CIA credentials.

J.P. had considered it for a short time and finally turned down the proposition. He enjoyed the on and off work of CMAG and the freedom to do other consulting work. He told Anne that there were other challenges in life. Annie approved of J.P.'s decision, but she still did not like it when CMAG was in charge of J.P.'s life.

"Well, I wasn't on a CMAG assignment, if that's what you're worried about. I got a call from an old friend of mine, Phillip

Bradsmith. He's the CEO of James Pharmaceutical Company... the one I used to work for a long time ago. Anyway, he called me at two in the morning and asked, nay, he instructed me to come to New York City to give him a hand with a little problem they may or may not have brewing."

"Well, that was the fastest damn trip to New York City I've ever seen, J.P. Out and back in what, a day and a half? So was it a false alarm or did the great J.P. solve all of the world's problems in matter of a few hours?"

He smiled and looked down at the bar, "Nope. Actually, I wasn't prepared physically to stay any longer. I had only packed one pair of underwear and a toothbrush. So I brought all the background and research back home with me to think about. You weren't worried about me, were you? Did you miss me, Sweetie?" J.P. asked, half laughing. Annie's face showed that she didn't appreciate his humor at her expense. Because they were both so close and lived alone, they always took the time to check up on one another. "I'm sorry, Annie. That wasn't fair. Am I forgiven for not letting you know about the trip?"

Annie answered with a quick, "Yes," and returned his smile before setting the highly polished mug down and moving to the other end of the bar to serve a customer.

When Annie returned to J.P., he was staring at the bar thinking about the James project. While he had given Phillip no reason to think that he would not take on the project, he could still turn it down. He had learned that he didn't have to take on everything that was asked of him. He was a free man, free of the corporate politics and could pick and choose what he wanted to do with his life.

Annie picked up another beer mug and began polishing it, though a bit more calmly than before. "Tell me about your trip and your new project."

J.P. without looking up from the bar, said, "Well, I don't know that it is my new project just yet. I'm not entirely sure that I want a new project at this stage." He explained the basic outline of what he was doing without too much detail. He had, after all, promised Phillip that he would keep the nature of the project a secret. He concluded his explanation by saying, "I've got some work to do over the next few days. I plan to go back to New York on Sunday and give Phillip my answer on Monday morning. By then, I should have a much better picture of the situation."

J.P. realized that he had been overly serious in the last few minutes of their conversation. He looked up from the bar, glanced around as if to see who might be listening, and beckoned Annie to come closer. When she did, he whispered in her ear, "How about fixing me a bowl of chili and mug of Old Mammoth Dry?"

She turned her head to whisper in his ear, "J.P., you bastard. You know I'll eventually get what you're doing out of you. Behave yourself and go sit at a table and I'll bring your chili."

The scent of her perfume raised his spirits somewhat. She blew a short breath into his ear, giddily touched her tongue to his ear lobe, and backed away from the bar. As he stood there at the bar relishing their intimacy, she drew a chilled mug of Old Mammoth Dry. She walked back over to where he stood and set the mug down in front of him with a loud bang. Nearly an inch of beer flew out of the mug and onto the bar. She smiled slightly and said, "Oops," before turning to wait on another customer.

J.P. picked up the mug and was about to take a swallow when a loud voice from the back of the bar said, "J.P., where the hell have you been? I nearly froze my balls off waiting for you for two days at Climax and you never showed up."

J.P. gave Annie a knowing wink, and began walking back to the group of men seated around a card table. "Hal, you old coot. You don't have a set of balls big enough to freeze much less stand at the top of Climax for more than 30 seconds." The group around the table broke out laughing. Climax was the toughest run off the crest of Mammoth Mountain. The run was nearly 1,000 feet straight down the face.

J.P. sat down at Hal's table. There were also three locals seated there, all of whom worked year round in Mammoth. They were all in their late thirties, tan, and very physically fit. They made their livings on the slopes. "Take a fifth player," he asked?

"After that derogatory remark about my manhood, J.P., I'm not too sure I want to play poker with you. What do you boys say?" Hal asked.

"Set your ass down, J.P. Your money is better than Hal's IOU's," remarked Mammoth's own Austrian ski instructor, Fritz Wagner.

J.P. looked over at Annie. She saw that he was settling in and gave him a quick wink.

"So there, Dr. Koenig, you never did answer my question, where the hell have you been?" Hal asked again.

J.P. did his best to fend off Hal's question without having to go through the long explanation again, "New York City to see a man about a horse. Any more questions? No? Good, deal the damn cards."

"Yeah, come on deal the cards, Hal. Um, J.P., what you want to go to see Big Apple for, eh?" Fritz asked. Fritz spoke perfect English when he so chose, but was careful to keep his Austrian accent for his students, particularly the female students. Not many in Mammoth knew of the intellectual side of Fritz, that he had a Masters from Oxford and a Ph.D. in Philosophy from University of Vienna.

Annie placed the bowl of chili off to the side of J.P.'s stack of poker chips. He thanked her and picked up the stack of crackers she had also left with the chili. He placed the entire stack of crackers in the palm of his left hand and smashed his right fist into the stack sending small crumbs all over the table. He then dumped the cracker crumbs into the chili and stirred the coagulated mess.

The other players, knowing of his habits with crackers had scooted their chairs back from the table in order to be free of flying cracker debris. No one said a word. All, at one time or another, had determined that there was no changing J.P.'s habits and had resigned themselves to live with it.

"I was visiting an old business friend that needs some help, Fritz. That's about all there is to it, at least for right now. If anything does come of the trip I'll let you know." He looked over at Fritz as he spoke he added for the benefit of the rest of the group, "The weather in New York was clear, crisp, and cold."

J.P. looked at his cards and quickly added, "I've got three queens, what do you bums have?" The entire group threw their cards at him as he raked in his winnings of ten dollars. This was fun poker, not cut throat.

5:45 A.M., WEDNESDAY, JANUARY 18
MAMMOTH LAKES, CALIFORNIA

J.P. woke slowly to the music playing on the radio from a station originating from Bishop. He reached over to the home environmental control unit that had been installed on the right side of the headboard of the bed and touched the A.M. button. This initiated the sequence of events that always started his day when he was at home. The bedroom windows, open slightly for air during the night, closed shut. The geothermal heating unit came on and began warming the house. The small coffeemaker on the dresser next to his bed began gurgling. In another fifteen minutes the radio would shut itself off and televisions in the bedroom and bathroom would come on set to a cable news channel.

He had programmed the fifteen minute delay to allow himself time to sit up in bed, drink his first cup of coffee, and plan his day. He decided that he would spend a good portion of the day in his office reading the materials he had brought back from New York. He reached over to the environmental control unit and touched the button marked office. This would prepare the office for him.

After determining the days work, he thought over what he had to do between then and next Monday when he would be back in New York. He made a mental note to email Janet about a place to stay while he was in the city. Since he was probably going to be there a while, he would ask her to look around for a nice short-term apartment rather than a hotel.

He continued to sit in the bed and sip his coffee. He reminded himself to give Annie plenty of notice about watching the house while he was back east. His house was set up to run itself from a computer program with redundant back-up systems in case of electronic or mechanical failure. Still it was the unknown of what a strong earthquake could do to the house that worried him the most. He always felt better knowing that Annie was keeping an eye on things.

Suddenly, the radio shut off and the television came on. Despite the fact that he lived in a remote mountainous area, J.P. did his best not to lose touch with the world. He had a digital satellite system installed to bring in news and entertainment from around the world.

He had his *Wall Street Journal* delivered to Annie's Bar and Grill. If he was out of town, she would read it and then leave it on the bar for her customers. If he was home, sooner or later during the day, he would make the trek down to the bar to read it and any other papers that he found laying about the Grill. He even had a deal with the local postmaster to deliver his mail to Annie's when he was out of town. She would go through the mail, throwing out the junk mail and forwarding the remainder to wherever he was at the time. It was a comfortable and convenient arrangement and the fact that she was such a close friend made it that much better. He was sometimes concerned about asking her to do so much for him when he was out of town, but she never seemed to mind.

After showering, he put on a pair of sweats and moved upstairs to the kitchen for another cup of coffee and a bowl of oatmeal. He sat eating and watching the sunrise through the large window at the end of the room.

Finally, he walked to the back of the house where his office was located. As he entered the room, he spoke out loud, "Computer on." The screen on the desk suddenly lit up. A computer-generated female voice said, "Good morning, J.P. How are you this morning? You have received one high priority email since I was last activated. It is from James Pharmaceutical Company. Shall I display the email for you?"

"Yes, display on screen." He then began dictating to the computer the day's schedule. "Input. To do list. Item. Dictate email to Janet at James regarding apartment search. Item. Notify Mountain Aviation about Sunday departure and routine maintenance check on the Lear. Item. Reserve hangar space at LAX.

Item. Find a gift for Annie." J.P. paused and smiled, "Item. Ski my life away. Item. End the day consuming mass quantities of a distilled beverage made from potatoes and garnished with a middle eastern fruit. End list. Did you get that?" "Yes, J.P., a copy is printing now."

He smiled again. His computer was a next generation business computer with a voice activated artificial intelligence platform (VAAIP) that Apple built for him. This model, code named Mammoth MAC after the mountain, was a prototype that Apple had built and given to J.P. for a test drive. He appreciated the name recognition for Mammoth but the computer was anything but mammoth. It was basically a mouse incorporated keyboard and a screen. He thought VAAIP MAC pronounced "vap mac" would have been a better brand name but the CEO said the name when pronounced was too cute.

The CEO of Apple and J.P. had become friends after CMAG had solved a corporate espionage situation where a competitor was stealing Apple's leading edge technology in order to prevent Apple from gaining more market share. Thus far, he had no complaints and made monthly status reports to the CEO on the computer's operations and reliability. After his last report, the CEO had called him to thank him for his help in the trial. Apple would market the Mammoth into a closed market, selling only to the intelligence community. The CEO told J.P. that once the computer was in production he would switch out J.P.s prototype

There were times when J.P. felt a little silly talking to a computer, but it was somehow comforting having the voice respond to whatever request he made of it. He turned his attention to the email that had opened on the screen:

DATE: January 17

TO   Dr. Jean Paul Koenig

FROM: Amanda Hayes

SUBJ   Marketing Reasons for Lifeal's Poor Penetration of the Anti-Arrhythmia Market ENCL: Point Paper

1. I hope you had a safe trip home. I'm envious. I love California. I don't have many chances to visit as often as I would like.my trips are usually very short. I fly into LA for meetings and fly back the next day. When I do stay, I have to make compulsory rounds of visiting my parents and relatives.

Although I love them all dearly, it's not exactly what I would call a California holiday.

I have attached a point paper on the marketing question you had asked in your memo to Phillip. If you have any questions, please don't hesitate to call or email. I look forward to working with you on this project. If I can do anything for you, please let me know.

Sincerely,

Mandi

"Computer. Create new file folder entitled James on the hard drive and transfer the point paper attached to this email to that folder."

"Yes, J.P...it is done."

"Computer. Dictation. Email to Ms. Janet Williams, James Pharmaceutical Company, New York. Begin body. Janet, I plan to make my way back to New York on Sunday. Would appreciate your making flight reservations for me from LAX on Sunday morning, sometime between 8:30 and 10:00 and I guess it should be an open return. Prefer first class, aisle seat. Will likely need a hotel room for at least one night. For the longer term, would appreciate anything you can do to find me a suitable month to month lease on a small apartment located not too far from the Spectrum of Medicine Building. It doesn't have to be anything too fancy and furnished for a bachelor.. .that is to say, functional for working in the evenings and simple cooking. Will need a computer. It doesn't have to be too fancy, but it has to be a high end MAC and a removable hard drive. Also I need an independent dedicated digital line for working on-line. I don't want anything that is already in place. This should be a new install with the line registered to a different phone exchange if it's ISDN. Thanks, Janet, look forward to seeing you next week and having lunch together. Warmest, J.P.

"Did you get all that?" J.P. asked.

"Yes, J.P. Shall I transmit the email now?"

"Yes, please do." He grimaced whenever he used the word please in connection with commands to the computer. He dictated three other emails, one to Amanda, or Mandi now, thanking her for her prompt response to his questions. He told her that he was very much looking forward to working with her. He smiled when he thought about her and said to himself, "Yep, I'm definitely looking forward to working with you." He also dictated emails to the commercial aviation services at Mammoth Lakes Airport and LAX.

When he had finished with most of his administrative duties for the day, he settled down to learning all he could about Lifeal and James. He took out the CD that Phillip had given him and transferred the information from the CD to the newly created James file on his hard drive and then broke the CD into multiple fragments in the CD shredder.

"Computer. Open the James file. And inform me of the time of day on a half-hourly basis."

"Yes, J.P." Within seconds the screen displayed a list of files: James Confidential Agreement James Code of Conduct Compartmentalized 21st Century Plans Marketing Research Report on Lifeal 21st Century Plan FDA Filing for Lifeal Clinical Results for Lifeal James Personnel Files Lifeal Point Paper

J.P. realized he would miss the utility of his Mammoth MAC computer when he was away in New York. It had provided such good service to him over the last couple of years that he had been using it. The computer knew his voice and only his voice. If someone else tried to turn the computer on, it would not comply. If it was on and another voice gave it a command, the computer would shut down and immediately sever its connection to whatever server it was connected to at the time. Annie had a small metal box located in her Mammoth Lakes Bank safety deposit box. Inside the box was an adapter that she could plug into one of the ports on the front of the computer which allowed her to issue a sequence of keyboard commands that would provide her with limited access to certain files.

He had taken this precaution in the event something happened to him. If he didn't check in with the computer at pre-determined intervals, the Mammoth MAC would call Annie at home and give her instructions. It would then become slaved to Annie's voice pattern after she provided answers to specific questions that the computer would ask.

Annie thought the entire scheme was madness when J.P. first talked with her about it. Regrettably, she didn't realize the sensitivity of much of the information that he was protecting. As further security for his corporate clients, he had established a second satellite link to another server storage system that scrambled data into a nearly impossible to read jumble only unscrambling it when he downloaded it into his Mammoth MAC. He was never so nai've as to think that all of his precautions were failsafe, but he was doing the best could protect his clients' information.

He looked at the James file list and decided that he would read and study the 21st Century Plan and compartmentalized backups. Thursday and Friday, he would study Lifeal. Saturday, he would draft a status report for the Monday meeting with Phillip.

He intended to spend the first few weeks in New York interviewing the key managers in the research, operations, and marketing departments. After reading the compartmentalized backup plans, he prepared discussion questions. He decided that he would email Mandi the questions for dissemination to the respective managers. This would provide them with the time to work on the answers. He wasn't interested in having the managers write their answers. He wanted to give them plenty of time to think about and study their answers. Mostly, he wanted to personally observe them as they presented the information. Experience had taught him that when discussing sensitive issues, an individual presentation provided better insights into what the person was actually thinking.

He decided to begin with Phillip's answers to the five questions he had posed to him:

"Question 1. Board Approval of the 21st Century Plan: Yes, the Board had reluctantly approved the 21st Century Plan. I say reluctantly because the vote was close. Evelyn and five of her six board cronies said nay. The seventh said yea. That gave the yeas a vote of seven to six. You should have seen the look on her face when one of her handpicked board members switched to my side. Her Board majority still has the power to stall the implementation of the plan. This will become clear when you read my answer to question 5.

Question 2: Gross Margin Decline. Why?: J.P., I have been studying this issue for a year but, admittedly not as intently as required. It was very astute of you to see the subtle decline in gross margin from 78% to 76%. Two points on a gross margin of 78% doesn't seem like very much but it equates into a large quantity of margin dollars. The answer to the question lies in the cost of the bulk raw plant material. I am sure you will get a better handle on this situation when you question the Operations Division. You will find an unsatisfactory answer to the higher material costs in the compartmentalized plan for the Operations Division. The Operations Division does not seem to be overly concerned with slight dilution in margin. This, of course, is unsatisfactory.

As an aside, I have run a number of "what if" studies using our computers here at James. The answer was very clear. With Lifeal's lower than planned sales rate combined with the noted higher cost of goods, the sales will not produce enough working capital to allow us to implement the necessary research plan to bring JPC138 to market in a timely manner. I refer to you my answer to Question 5. I hope you can help me get a better grasp of this issue.

Question 3: Lifeal Status: Amanda will supply the answer.

Question 4: Key Research Reports on JPC138: The project leader is the senior vice president of research, Dr. Helmut Wahlters. Under him is Dr. Allen Strong, who runs the JPC138 day to day research program. Under Allen there are a number of bright pharmaceutical researchers. Helmut is a bit stuffy, very bright, and an experienced researcher, and very familiar with herbology. He is getting close to retirement and I think he is not very agreeable with some of my plans for the future of James. He is slightly out of date with the real world of biotech pharmaceuticals, but in the case of JPC138 this is somewhat to our advantage. He has a wealth of experience with herbal technology which some consider being passe. His knowledge, when combined with biogenetic engineering, provides James with a unique capability.

Allen Strong is an excellent pharmaceutical scientist. He is the bridge between the old established herbology and new genetic engineering. Both researchers and their teams are very capable of completing the work on JPC138 given the time and resources. Again, I refer you to the answer to Question 5.

Question 5: Cash Reserves: Working Capital Report. J.P., you have hit on one of the tender spots in our plans for a successful James future. When we released Lifeal, James had to have a financial product winner. The company had spent millions on Lifeal research as well as other derivative compounds which, for one reason or another, were dropped from research as they made their way through the James step by step screening process. I repeat, James had to have a winner. We thought we had the winner in Lifeal with a follow on big winner in JPC138.

We launched Lifeal with our most comprehensive and expensive marketing campaign in the history of James. In retrospect, even though this was a large launch budget using James standards, it was minuscule compared to the promotional monies spent by bigger companies when they launched their cardiac products. We deluded ourselves into thinking that since we had spent so much money on the launch, we would have quick success. In fact, we depended on the Panglossian financial success and the resulting increase in working capital. Of course, to use Voltaire's words from *Candide,* "the best of all possible worlds" was not to happen. The Panglossian financial model didn't happen and, even though the JPC138 toxicology and pathology expenses were on schedule and on budget, the total research project was behind schedule.

James is in extremis for working capital, we are in fairly good shape today, but later this year, if Lifeal and other products don't come through with above projection performances, we will have to drastically cut all expenses. This will have the result of postponing Lifeal's growth and JPC138's clinical release. James has the capability of raising additional working capital, but at a cost to the current business and control of the company.

The working capital required to increase the marketing programs of Lifeal and to continue the research on JPC138 could come from a number of sources:

Co-marketing of Lifeal with a pharmaceutical company who has a surplus of cash. This would lower our Lifeal marketing expenses, but a large percentage of our direct sales would be reduced to royalties. This would have the end result of lower Lifeal margin dollars and loss of full participation in the big "Lifeal win." The up side win is a higher market penetration of the arrhythmia market with a prevention or prophylactic indication.

Sell equity in James. A new James preferred or common stock offering would raise equity capital, but the legal and brokerage fees are expensive (you should know, you have taken enough companies public) and our stock is not a glamour stock with the boys on Wall Street. In fact, one "mental giant" investment research analyst recommended that James should think seriously about initiating a reverse stock split to increase per share value.

Acquisition of a company with cash reserves and new products to add to the James aging product line. If you know of any company with compatible product line, with too much cash, and wants to be acquired by James, please let me know.

Merge with another pharmaceutical company. It seems like merging is still in style, but this is the opposite of #3. Someone is looking to merge to supplement their own product line. To date, we haven't received any offers.

Be acquired by a US or foreign chemical company. Similar to #4. No offers to date.

At this point you might ask, why isn't James more active in the financial market trying to obtain answers about the availability of a working capital situation?

The answer lies with the board. Mrs. James will not even hear of acquiring working capital assistance from any source. I'm sure it's part of her plan to force me out of James. So the direct answer to your question #5 is: No, as things stand at this point, we don't have enough cash reserves to fully implement the 21st Century Plan. I'm presently holding departmental meetings to cut expenditures, freeze head count, and cancel or postpone future programs. My strategy is to do everything possible to protect the future of both Lifeal and JPC138.

I don't want to sound negative and lay a heavy psychological weight on your shoulders, but if Mrs. James has her way, or the project you're working on proves to be a disaster, it will be very hard on both James and me personally. The board will see to it that the fault is laid at my feet and request that I leave the company. As you know, I hate giving up on something I really believe in and I really believe in James and the 21st Century Plan.

J.P. leaned back in his chair. Off the top of his head he could see three major problems. Two of the problems he had already uncovered. First were the difficulties between the board and Phillip. Second was the lack of working capital. Finally, the third problem, Lifeal's cost of goods, was unexpected. He decided he would look more closely into this problem as he further analyzed Lifeal.

The Mammoth MAC announced, "Zero nine hundred." J.P. had set up his computer to work from military time.

"Computer, open the Research Department Plan. Prepare to take notes."

The only thing that J.P. saw in the plan that really caught his attention was an increase of several million dollars in projected costs associated with research into JPC138 derivatives. J.P. knew that this was Phillip betting on the yet-to-be-realized JPC138 success. The increase was offset by a reduction in funds for the development of potential new compounds from $37 million to $34 million which indicated to him that the up and coming compounds, presently in research, were not expected in the near term to produce any new dramatic commercial compounds. Further offsetting the decrease in the development budget was an increase in basic research. More basic research was planned for long-term growth and to feed the product development department with new compounds with a potentially brighter commercial value.

He noted that the total budget didn't reflect growth in the projected year and confirmed a shortfall in corporate working capital. Since the budget was reallocated rather than cut indicated a bold move with associated risk. If Lifeal continued to miss sales projections, there would not be enough margin dollars coming into James to cover the research program. If this happened, a specific program or perhaps marketing would take the hit. From what J.P. had seen thus far, Phillip had chosen not to reduce R&D programs any further and had left the overall R&D budget at its current level.

"Zero nine thirty."

"Computer, open the operations department plan."

He began reading the operations department portion of the plan. Most of the success of the 21st Century Plan was dependent upon two factors: the R&D schedule of product releases and the marketing unit forecast. Both of these areas brought into force the transfer of technology from R&D to the customer.

The James operations department had a sophisticated computer program that was used for value analysis. The program evaluated alternatives to lowering the cost of goods for products in the growth and mature stages of their product life cycles.

While the main corporate headquarters was located in the Spectrum of Medicine Building in Manhattan, the James production facility was still located in Brooklyn. After reading the operations department portion of the plan, it became apparent that if Lifeal was successful James would be stretched for production capacity to keep up with demand.

"If successful," he mused.

To provide more production capacity there had been scheduled a complete modernization of the Brooklyn manufacturing facility. Due to the slow growth of Lifeal sales and Phillip's decision not to spend the capital, the modernization had been postponed for another two years. The plan did contain Lifeal production improvements and JPC138 production start-up costs. These facility projects were budgeted over a number of years. If trends in sales of Lifeal improve, the success, if there was to be a success, would be very close to the same timing for the initial production quantities of JPC138, which could be a problem.

It seemed to him that there was a good possibility that the two products would require additional facilities and capacity during the same time period and not one project following the other project. The operations plan didn't reflect the possibility of simultaneous need and the associated capital requirement of conducting two major facility programs at the same time.

He didn't find any indication in the operations department plan that would indicate there was a problem with the Lifeal raw material supply.

"Ten thirty."

"Computer, open marketing backup plan."

He began read the marketing department's plan. The plan was not comprehensive and J.P. concluded that Mandi's objective had been only to summarize the product market plan in the overall 21st Century Plan. He wanted to read the actual product market plans rather than summaries, but decided that he would wait until he was in New York the following week.

"Eleven hundred."

J.P. felt somewhat frustrated. He had hoped he would see something in the plans that someone would want to steal. So far, he had seen nothing, except for a company that was beginning to show signs of trouble ahead.

"Computer, go to standby." The screen went dark. He stood up from his chair and moved towards the door. Before exiting the windowless office, he changed the environmental control to the maintenance mode, which shut down power to all outlets except of course the one that served the computer and reduced the temperature in the room to sixty-five degrees.

Back in the living area of the house, he sat back in a recliner and thought about what he had read that morning. It surprised him that he had not detected a valid reason for anyone to steal a copy of the 21st Century Plan. The board of directors was the only group that could be a viable threat to Phillip's projection of the James strategy and they already had access to the plan and didn't need to steal a copy. J.P. began to consider whether there might not be hidden issues that he had missed.

Lifeal seemed to be a product still in search of a market niche. Who would want information on Lifeal? So far the only thing Lifeal had going for it was surprisingly lagging sales. Knowing the product problems would give a competitor potential information to use against Lifeal, but the product still didn't appear to be a threat to the marketshare of any competitive product currently in the marketplace.

"Phillip doesn't need me to investigate possible corporate espionage, he needs to hire a goddamned marketing consultant for Lifeal," J.P. said angrily.

He thought about JPC138, but realized he didn't know enough about the compound to give too much thought to its potential or possible problems. His mind continued to search through everything he had read. The answer if there were to be an answer almost certainly lay in Lifeal and/or JPC138. There didn't seem to be anything else of interest to another company at the moment.

J.P. spent the afternoon doing what he loved to do the most, ski. He made four complete runs down Mammoth Mountain's 4,000 foot vertical drop stopping only when he began to tire. After returning home, he turned up the temperature of his spa that sat out on the deck. A one-way glass lined the side of the deck away from the house and assured the privacy of anyone using the spa. The glass wall also kept the cold mountain air off of the tub as a person sat neck deep in the swirling hot water. He moved through the house to the master bedroom where he removed his ski clothes and put on a robe. He returned back upstairs and poured himself a glass of Stolichnaya. He added two jalopeno-stuffed olives to the glass and then walked out onto the deck to the spa. J.P. removed his robe and quickly slipped into the hot, churning water. The warmth of the water soothed his tired body and the water jets kneaded his tired muscles.

He leaned back and took a sip of Stoli and began thinking of what or who could hurt or benefit James by stealing a copy of the 21st Century Plan. There was the James board. They might gain by discrediting Phillip, but not much more. But then again, they really didn't need to steal a copy. A competing company was certainly a possibility albeit remote, James was not, to the shareholders' regret, much of a competitive threat to anyone at present. Fuel for a potential takeover? That seemed to be a strong possibility in J.P.'s mind. He decided that he would make an effort to review the shareholders list to see if there was any unusual buying activity. He knew that review might also reveal a plan to discredit James and sell the stock short, which was also a possibility. A possible White Knight gamut? J.P. didn't consider this a viable possibility given the company's present situation.

He took another sip of Stoli, swishing the thick liquid around in his mouth. He rested his head back against the edge of the spa. The sun had set below the crest of the mountain and the sky was a magnificent reddish orange as the rays bounced off the cirus clouds. He closed his eyes and was just about to doze off when he felt a touch of cold on the top of his head. He quickly realized it was snow and opened his eyes to see Annie slipping out of a robe and sliding into the water next to him. The hot water and cold mountain air formed a swirling cloud across the surface of the water. J.P. watched as Annie slid the length of her tight, muscled nude body into the water. He knew that she worked hard to maintain herself in such great physical shape, sometimes rising at 5:30 a.m. to start her two-hour daily workout. He noted that despite the fact that it was January, her skin seemed to hold the tan that she developed every summer. He always wondered how she did that.

"J.P., you should be ashamed. Exposing yourself to the entire neighborhood…tsk, tsk, tsk," Annie said as she leaned over to kiss him on the cheek.

"Actually, it wasn't nearly so bad today. I only saw a pair of elderly sisters swoon when they spotted me," he responded, laughing. "You know something? You're goddamned beautiful. Have I mentioned that lately?"

Annie tilted her head back and laughed, "Yeah, yeah. I saw how you were ogling me as I innocently slipped into the water to warm my fair self." She batted her eyes at him. "You're such a lech.have I mentioned *that* lately? I am merely here as a friend anxious to hear about your trip to New York since we didn't get a chance to finish our conversation last night. Engaging conversation, that's all you're getting tonight, Buckoo!"

J.P. smiled and looked over at her. Annie raised herself in the tub just enough to expose her breasts on top of the water. He smiled and laid his head back on the side of the tub and closing his eyes, "Annie, Annie, Annie, you're such a tease! And I guess that's why I love you the way I do," he said as he opened his eyes to look back at her. "I'm really happy to see you. I'm glad you came over. I'm afraid I'm not in much of a talkative mood, but I do feel better having you here."

"Are you okay, J.P.?"

"Oh, I see…you're going to make me talk, aren't you? Yeah, I guess I'm okay. I'm just trying to sort through this James project. I don't want to let my friend, Phillip down, but so far, I figure that he doesn't really need me and I sure don't need multiple trips across the country to confirm that…especially when those trips are to New York City in freaking January. I would much rather be conducting cerebral masturbation on my Strategic Continuum book and sitting here in this spa with you."

He went on to tell Annie about the work he had done during the day and his sketchy conclusions. He spoke in generalities. He respected her opinions and her thought processes, but didn't see much point in giving her too many specifics. Phillip had, after all, stressed his desire for secrecy. J.P. concluded with, "That's about it, Annie, nothing too exciting. Any ideas?"

"No real ideas, J.P., just an observation. You don't have enough information. Give this a chance. It sounds to me as though you have a lot more research to do. Let it go for the moment and then come back to the alternatives. You're a clever lad. You'll figure it out. So, Big Boy, what's up with this Mandi chick? I saw that lecherous gleam in your eye."

J.P. smiled, took another sip of vodka, and leaned his head back, "Flattery will get you everywhere with me, Sweetie. I don't know, what's to tell? She's a very attractive and intelligent woman. We're going to be working very closely and it is the magical city of New York. However, there will not be much opportunity for romance. This looks to me to be a short project. Why? You jealous?"

Annie let out a loud, "Ha!"

J.P. continued, "You're right you know, I don't have enough information. Thanks for your observations." He started to stand up to leave the spa. "My Stoli is depleted. Have you had enough of soaking in chemically sanitized hot water? How about dinner, Annie? I have a couple of steaks and some salad. Not as good as your cooking, but definitely a distant second."

"Sounds too good to pass up."

After dinner they played three games of backgammon. Annie won two and J.P. won one, making their series even at 84 game each. Afterwards, they sat on the couch sipping wine and watching an old movie. They had not dressed and remained in their robes. Both kept drifting in and out of sleep.

Finally, Annie leaned over near his ear and said, "Do you have room for a friend tonight. I'm tired and I don't feel like dressing to go home."

"Shall I bring drinks?" J.P. responded.

"Nope, just warm bodies. Especially with the way you sleep with your windows wide open."

They moved downstairs to the master bedroom and crawled into the bed.

They were instantly sound asleep.

12:00 P.M., WEDNESDAY, JANUARY 18

LOS ANGELES INTERNATIONAL AIRPORT

Over breakfast that morning, Nacheda reminded Skip to follow up with the task force members to ensure that there were no delays in obtaining the intelligence material they would need for the February meeting and the beginning of the second phase of their project. He also suggested that Skip take a few days off before the project became very intensive and time consuming.

"Yeah, not a bad idea. I could use a break. In fact, I know just where I'll go," Skip had told him with a smile.

Later that day, Nacheda sat down in his first class window seat on board JAL 79 and thought about Skip's comment. He hadn't pursued the conversation with his friend, mostly because he was too involved in all that he had to do before leaving for the airport. Nacheda now wondered what Skip had in mind. Knowing him, Nacheda thought to himself, it'll involve work of some kind. He looked up to see Reiko walking towards him with a glass of orange juice.

"Good afternoon, Nacheda-san. How were your business meetings?" Reiko asked in Japanese.

"Fine, fine and how was your visit to Los Angeles? Enough parties and activities to keep you entertained?"

Reiko blushed slightly at the thought that he had assumed that she, being a flight attendant, was always partying on layovers. It surprised her that he would make that assumption.

"No, Nacheda-san, the layover was, as usual, uneventful. Most of my time was spent in my room at the Century City Plaza where all JAL crews stay in LA. I did a little shopping, but that's about it." Her voice took on a slight edge, "I'll talk with you later in the flight. I have to take care of the other passengers."

As soon as she moved away from him, she could feel the blush in her face fading. She was surprised at her reaction to his question. She felt she knew him well enough to know that there had been no hidden meaning in his words. Actually, she had always been very attracted to Nacheda. He was a nice looking and seemingly successful modern Japanese man. If only she could get him to pay more attention to her. She didn't want to be overt in her actions towards him as that would work against her if he harbored any traits of a traditional Japanese male.

She decided she would make every effort to get him to notice her on this flight. She thought she was already making a good start, she was certain she could feel his eyes on her back.

Nacheda watched Reiko's thin body walk up the aisle towards the passengers in the front row of the first class cabin. She wore her JAL uniform. Her long black silky hair fell almost to her waist. When she served the other passengers she would make a body movement that was more akin to a western curtsy than a traditional Japanese bow. That made him smile and he realized how much he enjoyed watching her.

He concluded that she was a beautiful Japanese woman and probably a very nice person to get to know personally. The only question was, how?

The plane's intercom system clicked on and one of the other flight attendants welcomed everyone on board JAL flight 79 en route Tokyo Narita Airport, followed by the usual airline safety precautions. Before long the 747 was airborne and Nacheda was on his way back to Japan.

Nacheda thought back over the task force's accomplishments of the past few days. For the first time in many months he was pleased with the results of the team. Over the last year he had come to doubt himself and his ability to accomplish Nakasone's mission. That self-doubt included not only himself, but also the abilities of his team. Now, in the course of twenty-four hours, everything had changed. Suddenly what seemed unattainable three days ago, the successful conclusion to Phase I, now appeared to be only a few weeks away.

Nacheda knew that Dr. Nakasone would push him even harder now. He would not recognize, share, nor encourage Nacheda's sense of accomplishment. Nakasone would push Nacheda for the quick completion of Phase I and then begin to push for the final resolution of Phase II. Nakasone was not necessarily an impatient man, but he felt that a person didn't work to their fullest potential without heavy-handed encouragement from a superior.

Phase II of the project would be more focused than the intelligence gathering of Phase I. In Phase II, the company identified would be thoroughly investigated and an insider identified who would become Bandai Pharmaceuticals' conduit. This would definitely be the most difficult portion of the project and Nacheda would not be allowed to fail. If he failed to find some in-road into the target company then the past eleven months of a perceived successful Phase I had actually been a failure.

His past experiences with American businesses had taught him to develop a contingency plan. He had to allow the possibility that he would not be able to find anyone in the targeted company to work with Bandai Pharmaceutical. He would be prepared with a secondary and even a tertiary target to pursue. Nacheda decided he should send an email to Skip and have him adjust the parameters of SAM in its search so that it would identify other targets.

Nacheda opened his laptop computer and began typing an email to Skip: TO: Skip FROM: Nacheda (somewhere over the Pacific) SUBJ: Phase II Contingency

SCRAMBLE CODE: MIKE NOVEMBER

Have been thinking back on last two days. Accomplishments excellent, but have determined that we require contingency plan in case we are unable to identify conduit into primary target. There is, of course, also the possibility that an old proverb applies to our euphoric sense of pending success, "what seems to be, is not what is."

Work with SAM to determine candidates that have a probability correlation of between 75%-90%. Believe we should have at least two other candidates.

Have SAM provide a detailed list of required information on new targets.

Disseminate the required information to the team members and explain to them the reasons for the request. Tell them this is a secondary priority to the tasks they were given at our meeting. If possible, they should provide you with information on contingency companies ASAP so you can feed SAM both the primary and secondary information before the next meeting.

Keep me informed of the results.

Don't cancel weekend plans to work on this contingency plan. Have fun....Nacheda

Nacheda re-read the electronic document. The plane was relatively empty so he didn't have to hide his screen from potentially dangerous competitive eyes. Nacheda entered a special command that scrambled the email in MIKE NOVEMBER code. The hard drive churned for a second. The scrambler changed the document shown on the screen from familiar letters and numbers to seemingly random symbols.

Nacheda pulled the plane's satellite telephone from its storage place in the armrest. He plugged in his phone line into the phone data port. The computer logged on with its specially built-in software ID. Within seconds the scrambled email was on its way to Skip.

Nacheda reached to ring the flight attendant button. Reiko saw the light go on for Nacheda's seat 3A. She informed the other flight attendant working in first class that she would take care of seat 3A's request. Because Nacheda's seat faced forward and the galley was behind him, he didn't see Reiko making her way up aisle to answer his call. Suddenly, there she was standing beside his seat. He felt at once pleased and somewhat embarrassed that she had answered his call. He was struck again by his attraction to her and didn't say anything at first, but sat there looking into her eyes.

"*Hai* dozo," Reiko said breaking the silence. She thought to herself that perhaps during this long flight she would be able to sit in the empty seat and talk with him during one of her long breaks. "How may I help you, Nachedasan?"

"I would like a glass of mineral water, please."

"Hai," Reiko replied. She turned and walked back to the galley.

Nacheda began planning Phase II in his head. It would most certainly be a difficult phase that would require Nacheda's special talents to see it to completion. There was much at stake here for both Nacheda personally and for Bandai Pharmaceutical.

When Reiko brought him a glass of mineral water their eyes met, but no words were spoken. He put thoughts of business and Reiko out of his mind and began thinking about dinner, an in-flight movie, and possibly sleep. He desperately hoped that the nightmares would not come again, but he knew that this was a shallow hope. The dreams were always there and at 36,000 feet he knew he would have to drink himself to sleep. He decided that three drinks and a typically boring movie would be all it would take to put him to sleep.

The meal was excellent and, much to his disappointment, so was the movie. The dinner wine and after dinner cognac warmed his insides. He enjoyed watching Reiko carry out her flight attendant duties. Their eyes met briefly every time she walked down the aisle. They would give each other a nervous smile and then look away.

Nacheda changed to the empty window seat next to him and drifted to sleep almost immediately after the movie ended. When Reiko walked past his seat and saw that he was asleep, she unfolded the blanket in the seat next to him and covered him with it. As she walked away she thought about how peaceful he looked and wondered if the nightmares that seemed to haunt him would return. She didn't know the subject of his dreams, but she had seen the manifestation of its terror on him. She had been frightened the first time that she had seen him go into what she could only describe as a terrorized, fitful sleep when he began thrashing about, muttering meaningless words, and perspiring profusely. She warned the other flight attendants not to be worried. It was a good thing that he always seemed to fly back and forth on days when the plane wasn't especially crowded so that no one sat next to him.

Although they were often on the same flight, she wondered who watched over him when she wasn't on board. "I'm sure he gets along perfectly well without me," she thought to herself. A twinge tugged at her heart. She actually enjoyed watching over him. It bothered her that there was the remotest possibility he could get along without her.

She smiled to herself, surprised at her feelings towards him. She would have to further explore this feeling that she felt for Nacheda. She most certainly felt an attraction for him, but was that all? She didn't feel love. Not love. She really didn't want to fall in love with this good looking pleasant man who didn't show any outward signs of knowing she was alive.

Reiko finished her duties and checked the passengers. The cabin was dark. The movie was over and all passengers were asleep, except for one woman who was reading. Reiko woke the other flight attendant working first class and informed her that it was time for her shift. She told Kumi that she was going to sit in 3B and sleep. Kumi looked at Reiko and smiled.

"Don't you smile, Kumi," Reiko said, "or read anything into my sleeping in 3B. You have chosen a few select seats next to handsome men yourself."

"Now, don't get angry, Reiko, I was only smiling. It's just that you have always gone out of your way not to sleep seated with a passenger. It's just a bit...ummm...out of the ordinary, that's all," Kumi said, still smiling.

Reiko looked at her friend whose face was bathed in the glow of the galley night-lights and decided there was no judgment in her remarks. She smiled back at Kumi, "You just mind the shop while I catch my deserved sleep."

"You go baby," Kumi replied in English.

Reiko made her way up the aisle to the third row and sat in the aisle seat next to Nacheda. She drew a blanket up around her neck to keep herself warm in the cool cabin and looked over at the man seated next to her. He appeared to be sleeping calmly with his head on the pillow against the window. Reiko raised her footrest and reclined her seat slightly. She tucked a pillow behind her head and closed her eyes. As she began to feel herself drifting off to sleep, she curled her legs so that her knees were close to his body. She found comfort in the warmth that radiated from him.

Nacheda had begun to dream and was entering the first stage of his strange affliction. It was the same dream every time. He was locked up in his cell at the Hanoi Hilton. The other prisoners were tapping their homemade shorthand code on the walls between the cells. Tap-tap.... taaap-tap-tap...tap taaap. The tapping never seemed to stop. Once, in his twilight sleep, he concentrated on trying to decode the tapping. He wanted to know if there was a message. His troubled sleep never allowed him to focus long enough to understand or decode the tapping sequences.

In his recurring dreams he was always walking back and forth across the square three-by-three meter cell. Every few seconds, he would hear screams from the distant interrogation wing.

It was a vivid recreation of his stay at the notorious POW prison. The Vietcong prison guards made sure all of the prisoners heard the screams of those being questioned. At first, he had fooled himself into believing that the screams were actually tape recordings used to scare the inmates. One day, however, he learned firsthand that the screams were not recorded when he received the first of many interrogations at the hands of his captors. He had tried to be brave and not scream, but found that screaming eased some of the pain. As hard as the Vietcong tried, they were never able to break Nacheda and make him tell why a Japanese army officer was in Vietnam on the side of the American war criminals. His captors were always careful to inflict their punishment on his body where injuries would not be easily detected. An electrode applied to the testicles was their favorite form of torture.

In his nightmares, it was always the same, back and forth....back and forth. He was an animal trapped in a tiny zoo cage. Why was he here? What had he done? This was not his war. It was not anyone's war save for the people whose land had absorbed and continued to absorb the blood of many nations.

Back and forth he paced inside of his cell in sandals that never completely dried from the constant oppressive humidity or when he stepped into a puddle. His sandals had been the perfect breeding ground for foot fungus.

The first six months of his imprisonment had been the worst. He had been unable to cope with the physical torture and the solitude. Sometime after six months though he began to change and accept his situation. Not that his life was any easier after the first six months, but he came to live each day, one day at a time.

Following his release, he tried to learn from the experience and to forget the torture, but the dreams never allowed him to forget. The dreams were always centered on the solitude and the mental and physical torture. Why the dreams continued after more than 20 years or why they only occurred when he was flying was something that neither he nor the military psychologists he had seen could determine.

Reiko felt Nacheda begin to shake. She knew the nightmare was returning. She took a chance and reached under his blanket and found his right arm and then his hand. His hand was cool and moist to her touch. The hand shook along with his entire body. She held his hand and squeezed it with a slight pressure.

Just as Nacheda began to feel himself slip into stage two, the most violent portion of the nightmare, he felt warmth moving from his arm to his hand. Although it was an alien feeling, it was not unpleasant and was in fact pleasurable.

He forced open his eyes and in his peripheral vision saw Reiko curled up in the seat next to him. He then realized that her hand was resting in his. It had been the warmth of Reiko's touch that had given him the strength to fight off the nightmare. She appeared to be fast asleep. He gently squeezed her hand and then fell into a calm sleep. The first calm sleep he had ever experienced while airborne.

Reiko had felt Nacheda's squeeze, but she was afraid to move. She felt him stop shaking and realized that she had succeeded in pulling him from the depths of his terror.

Later when Nacheda awoke and looked over at the seat next to him, it was empty. There was no evidence that anyone had been there. He felt rested. He knew the dream had come, but not the complete nightmare. He vaguely recalled holding Reiko's hand, but felt that he must have imagined her sitting next to him.

Nacheda rang the flight attendant call button. Reiko responded to his call looking refreshed and rested. Nacheda asked her for a cup of coffee. She returned with the coffee and a warm towel. He thanked her and took out his laptop to begin his report to Dr. Nakasone.

As the plane began its initial descent into the Tokyo, Reiko sat down next to Nacheda. "How was the flight," she asked in Japanese?

"Very restful. One of the best I have ever had." He paused. Nacheda didn't know how to ask the next question. His American cultural influences took over and he decided the answer was not to be direct. He asked in English, "Reiko, were you sitting in the seat next to me while I was sleeping?"

Reiko blushed and, this time, lowered her eyes and bowed her head. After a brief moment, she regained her confidence and raised her head to look at him. "I am sorry Nacheda-san. On many flights, I have seen your restless sleeps and I thought you might need a bit of comfort to help you sleep. I am very sorry that I have invaded your privacy. I promise I will never do this again."

Nacheda thought to himself, "Oh my, how truly Japanese." He decided he should explain.

"Reiko, can you remain for a few minutes?"

"*Hai,* Nacheda-san," she answered in a quivering whisper. "For no more than five minutes. I am so sorry."

"Reiko," he began in a very low and gentle voice. He felt a compelling urge to take her hand and return some of the strength she had given him during the night. He was concerned about jeopardizing her position with the airline though, for she would almost certainly be fired for showing such familiarity to a passenger. He would try to make his words substitute for his lack of physical action.

"Reiko, please. Both you and I have seen a great deal of this world and know that there are nearly as many cultures as there are stars in the sky. Each culture looks at a situation, or an emotion, from a different perspective according to custom. You and I know there is no real or absolute right to most philosophies. Right is what an individual feels within their own value system within the rules of society. Reiko, what you did as I slept last night might be considered by some outside of the bounds of the culture in which we were both raised, but, just possibly, this culture is outdated in today's world. At least outdated for the two of us."

Reiko raised her head and looked up at him. Nacheda went on noting that the sad look had left her face.

Nacheda continued, "You saw that I was troubled and you helped me through, what I can only call, one of my personal episodes. I appreciate what you did for me. I meant it when I said this was one of my best flights. I wish your cure was there to help me each time I have an episode." He smiled at her warmly.

Reiko wanted to ask him to explain about his episodes, but she knew that if he wanted her to know, he would tell her. She desperately wanted to know more about man, but she was afraid to ask. At any rate, the plane would be landing soon and she didn't know when their paths would cross again. In the past, his

Trans-Pacific flights had been very regular. This trip was a surprise and it was only by chance that they were on the same flight.

Reiko responded, "Thank you, Nacheda-san, for taking the time to explain your feelings. I feel privileged to have helped." She paused and decided to take what was for her a huge step in terms of culture, saying in a low voice, "Anytime you need my cure you are always welcome to ask." She began to rise from her seat.

Nacheda laid his hand on her forearm, "No, please don't get up just yet, one more minute, please." She sat back down and faced him. Nacheda continued, "I don't know your full name or where I can reach you. I would not like the person who has my cure to be anonymous. May I call you?"

Reiko's face brightened and her eyes had a moist look. She reached into her pocket and took out a piece of paper before rising out her seat. She pressed the piece of paper into Nacheda's right hand and said in a normal speaking voice, "Nacheda-san, it was good having one of our most important passengers on our flight today. I hope that we may be able to serve you again on your next flight to the United States or Tokyo. Please have a pleasant day."

With that, Reiko turned and walked back down the aisle to resume her duties. Nacheda turned his head and watched over the top of the seats as she retreated back towards the galley. He looked down at the piece of paper she had given him:

Nacheda, please call 3-533-0844 Reiko Watnabe

Nacheda felt himself flush. She wanted to see him again. He had been afraid to ask for fear of being turned down. Thus far, his life had been heavy mixtures of beauty, reward, intrigue, and violence. He was not very experienced in affairs of the heart. He sat for a time basking in the glow of Reiko's wish to see him again.

He was jolted out of his thoughts of Reiko by an air pocket as the plane changed altitude and began its final descent into Narita International Airport. First things first, I have to prepare for my meeting with Nakasone tomorrow. He slipped the paper with Reiko's telephone number into his wallet and prepared for the landing.

After retrieving his luggage and clearing customs, Nacheda caught the express train into Tokyo and then the early evening train to Bandai and home.

7:30 A.M., THURSDAY, JANUARY 19

WYCKOFF, NJ

Ralph Vandermere, senior partner in the twenty-year two-man criminal law firm of Vandermere and Patterson stared into the mirror on the wall above his bathroom sink. Ralph looked into the face that had peered back from mirrors for nearly sixty years. Ralph noticed things in the mirror today that he hadn't apparently paid much attention to before. The lines in his forehead seemed deeper than they did yesterday. He needed a haircut. His full head of gray hair covered most of his ears and was hanging slightly over the collar of his starched white shirt. He had an angular face with high cheekbones that caused his narrow chin to look even smaller.

He was dressed for court in a dark, double-breasted suit. He noticed for the first time that the tie he had chosen didn't blend very well with the dark material of the suit though he had worn that tie with that suit many times before and never given it a thought. He stared into his brown eyes and they seemed to look back at him. He looked through his eyes seeing into his own mind and it seemed he was able to visualize whatever he was thinking. Everything seemed so vivid. Much clearer than he ever remembered. It wasn't his imagination. Lately the phenomenon occurred each time he looked into a mirror.

What disturbed him most was that he couldn't attribute his newfound insight to anything in particular and he didn't like not knowing. He told himself that he shouldn't complain. His legal practice had been going extremely well since he had gained this mental clarity. The insight had not come on spontaneously, but seemed to emerge slowly and grow stronger over the past few weeks. It occurred to him that the initial onset of the insight seemed to coincide with his starting a new regimen of heart medication. His cardiologist and his pharmacist had told him to let them know if he had any reactions or side effects from the new drug.

"Is this a side effect?" he asked himself out loud.

The one thing that he did know for sure was that the tightness and fluttering in his chest had been greatly reduced. He felt much better now than he had in more than a year. His severe headaches had stopped for the most part. He really felt great except for the insight that seemed to grow daily and was beginning to worry him. That was the word he had assigned to what was happening to him, the insight. The insight had brought him amazing mental clarity and much improved memory. His legal cases were a snap. Suddenly his reputation as a superb criminal lawyer had grown and so had the rates that his firm was able to charge their clients.

His insights had started about eight months previously when Ralph had been diagnosed with severe cardiac arrhythmia. His cardiologist, Dr. Rosenberg, had tried a number of different pharmaceuticals to get Ralph's condition under control, with little success. Dr. Rosenberg had finally prescribed a new product that seemed to be working fine on the arrhythmia problem.

Ralph continued to look deep into his eyes. This insight had made him a better court lawyer. He was tireless. He felt that he could work non-stop for hours and still be sharp. He was constantly surprising judges, prosecutors, juries, and clients with his legal and practical knowledge. In fact, whenever required, he was able to recall any information that he had ever absorbed into his brain without the use of reference books or notes.

Ralph shook his head slightly to clear the vision of his eyes. He blinked twice and then turned to walk out of the bathroom and down the hall of his home to leave for work. He tried to be as quiet as possible so as not to wake his wife of thirty-five years. Once he was outside, he crossed the front of the house to the garage. Ralph pressed the button on the remote control and stepped back as the heavy wooden garage door swung upwards. After he started the engine of his BMW, he sat for a moment to allow the engine to warm and thought about his upcoming day in court.

Daniel Patterson, his partner, had accepted the current legal case because they both felt that once it reached court it would be over quickly. Their strategy was to obtain client cases that had projected long preparation periods as well as long trials. Staff could do the preparation while the partners' talents were used for court time. The more court time they could log at higher fees the higher the firm's profitability. Pretrial preparation for the current case had been done by pre-law college students from Rutgers. The pretrial depositions and background preparation had taken nearly a year.

It was pretty clear to both Ralph and Daniel that their client, Mr. Samuel Emmitt, had killed his accounting partner, Saul Bedlow, in self-defense. It seemed that in January of last year, Samuel and Saul decided to split their accounting partnership. Everything was going smoothly until one evening last February. Samuel and Saul had argued over how they would split their current customers. The row began after normal office hours and the office staff had made a hasty exit when the arguing started. The staff hoped that this would be the final chapter in the growing horror show that was the breakup of the partnership. Samuel and Saul had been talking about dissolving the partnership for years, but the percentage split and tax implications kept them from actually moving ahead with the dissolution. They had been partners for more than thirty years.

Each thought he deserved 70% of the practice.

They were in Samuel's office when the argument turned violent. They began throwing things at one another, mostly small accounting books that lined the shelves in Emmitt's office. Finally, Samuel picked up a large volume that contained statutes of the federal tax code. With both hands, Samuel threw the book and struck Saul directly in the face, knocking him backwards. As Saul fell his head struck the steam radiator used to heat the old brownstone where their office was located. Saul hit the radiator hard enough to leave three deep impressions in his skull. He died instantly.

The case would not have taken a year and Samuel might have gotten off with a suspended sentence for manslaughter had he not tried to cover up the accident. He explained to Ralph that he had simply panicked. He had pulled his partner away from the radiator, laid him in the coat closet, and then went home. Later that evening Bedlow's wife had called Samuel's home to ask if he had seen Saul. He told her no. He told her that when he had left the office, Saul had been at his desk completing spreadsheets. Samuel told her that he thought that Saul had mentioned that he was going into New York City in the morning to do some research on an account and might possibly have gone into the city that evening so that he could get an early start on his work. He then asked Mrs. Bedlow if Saul did in fact tell her he wouldn't be home that evening and perhaps she had simply forgotten. Samuel felt somewhat relieved when Saul's wife told him that now that she thought about it, she didn't really remember whether he had called tonight or last night. She thanked Samuel and told him she would call the hotel where Saul always stayed in the city to see if he was there.

After Samuel hung up the phone with her, he tried to push the evening's events from his mind. That night as he lay in bed his body began to shake uncontrollably as he realized the severity of what he had done. He didn't sleep at all that night. He returned to the office at around 4:00 a.m. to try to sort out the situation. He decided he would stick to his story that Saul Bedlow must have gone in New York. In order to substantiate his story, Samuel now had to make it look like Saul had been mugged and killed in the city. He devised a plan to drive Saul's body into Manhattan and dump him in a back alley somewhere north of the Wall Street district. It would look as though Saul had been mugged while walking. But first, of course, he had to get the body out of the closet and into the trunk of his car.

Samuel soon discovered his second mistake in how he had placed Saul's body in the coat closet. The evening before he had hastily laid Saul lengthwise across the closet opening. During the night, Saul's six-foot body had settled on the floor and with the initial onset of rigor mortis. His body was now tightly wedged into the bottom of the closet.

Samuel tried and tried for nearly an hour to get Saul out of the closet. He finally gave up resolving that he would have to break Saul's legs to free his body. Samuel began to panic again. He sat down at his desk and held his head in his hands. He considered running away and trying to disappear. He figured he could be long gone before any of the staff found Saul's body. After a few minutes he decided it was hopeless. He called his friend Daniel Patterson, the lawyer. After hearing Samuel's story, Daniel told him that he should turn himself in to the police and plead self-defense.

Once the case was in the open, the prosecutor's office wanted more than a self-defense verdict. They charged Samuel with murder in the first degree based on what they were going to prove was premeditated murder thinly disguised as self-defense.

The prosecutor claimed that Emmitt had premeditated the crime in order to get Saul out of the way. The prosecutors used the testimony of the staff who were witnesses to the many fights between the two partners. The partnership financial books were so convoluted that there was evidence of possible fraud and embezzlement. The business had become so entwined over the years that a reasonable split was impossible. Samuel's motive, said the prosecutors, was that he realized that they were never going to split the practice and he took things into his own hands. He killed Saul in order to obtain 100% of the practice. If Saul's murder wasn't premeditated, why had Samuel told Mrs. Bedlow that Saul had probably gone into the city?

Today, one year later, Ralph would begin the case for the defense. Ralph felt that he was more than ready for the upcoming legal presentation. Ralph slipped the car's transmission into reverse and backed out of his garage and down the driveway. He looked into the rear view mirror. He immediately took his foot off the gas pedal and stomped his right foot on the brake. He sat there staring into the reflection of his eyes in the rear view mirror. He was afraid to admit it, but things were getting worse. The insights took on a gorgonizing effect for him.

After a few minutes, Ralph shook his head again to force his mind back to reality. This was the first time a mere glance into a mirror had triggered the insight. Two weeks ago, in an effort to solve the problem, he had taken it upon himself to cut the dosage of the cardiac drug in half. He was now only taking a tablet every other day, rather than daily. He knew that he shouldn't have done this on his own, but he didn't have the time to see his physician or pharmacist. He was too busy preparing Samuel Emmitt's defense.

The, on the previous Friday, the headaches started to come back and last night he had trouble sleeping because his heart was fluttering. Before leaving for the courthouse that morning he had taken one tablet with his orange juice. He knew that he would take another the next day and put himself back on the prescribed regimen.

Ralph decided that a tablet every other day just wasn't doing the job. The insight had not gone away with the reduced dosage. Besides, to him, having the insight was better than the headaches, the heart fluttering, and a possible arrhythmia attack.

He turned onto Helena Street and proceeded downtown to his office.

8:00 A.M., THURSDAY, JANUARY 19
MAMMOTH LAKES, CALIFORNIA

J.P. made breakfast for Annie the next morning and then saw her out the door to her car. During the night a storm had come into the area from the northwest and there was an additional foot of snow on the ground. The gray sky was still depositing snow and the wind was very strong. HE helped her clear the snow from her car and then gave her a hug and a kiss.

He went back into the house and turned on the weather to get a forecast for the next few days. The forecast was for two stormy days and then clearing by Saturday.

"Yup, just in time for the LA crowds," he muttered.

He knew the storm would prevent him from skiing that afternoon. With the winds as strong as they were, most ski operations on the mountain were shut down for safety reasons. He thought to himself that he might be able to do some powder skiing on Friday, but today he would focus on James. He walked back through his house to his office to begin studying the toxicology and pathology sections of the Lifeal FDA filing.

"Computer, on. Report."

"Good morning, J.P. You have one email that was received at zero-sixhundred this morning from James Pharmaceutical Company."

"Open email."

The email was from Janet. She had made reservations for J.P. on an American Airlines flight from LAX to Newark Airport. She had also managed to locate an apartment for him and included the address. HE quickly glanced at the rest of the email before dictating an answer. He began his study of Lifeal. After reading for more than an hour, he came to the conclusion that the Lifeal toxicology and pathology studies were not relevant to the current low sales situation. There was nothing in the data to help the shortage of raw material problem or why Lifeal wasn't selling up to corporate or market expectations.

The toxicology study revealed no unusual problems at high, low, or normal doses. All three phases of the clinical trials for the drug had gone well enough except for one disappointing aspect. All clinicals were successful for treating arrhythmia, but no clinical connection could be made in preventing cardiac arrhythmia. The entire James clinical strategy had been to first prove the indication for the treatment of arrhythmia and second to establish Lifeal as a prophylactic against arrhythmia. More than $100 million had been spent on the effort towards approval of both indications.

In Lifeal's recommended dosage range the clinical studies didn't statistically prove any advantages over competitive products. This was verified when double blind clinical studies were conducted against the top three competitive products. There were no demonstrable advantages for Lifeal. James therefore could not justify competitive advantages of lower amounts of active ingredient per dose or less active ingredient per day or, even, fewer tablets per day. Put simply, James couldn't promote patient dosage conveniences or less patient cost.

Prescription prices were important to this class of pharmaceuticals. Usually, when a patient started to take a pharmaceutical to prevent cardiac arrhythmia, the patient would take the product for the rest of their life. The cost over the years mounts up. Lifeal's dose was one 100-milligram tablet per day.

The worst news that he came across in the reports was the conclusions on side effects. Lifeal had essentially the same side effects as all the products in this treatment category. If only it had fewer side effects than its nearest competitors, Lifeal would have had an important competitive edge.

He sat back in his chair and thought about what he had read. The findings must have been a difficult blow to James Pharmaceutical Company in general and to Phillip personally. The reports explained why it had been such an uphill struggle trying to convince physicians to prescribe Lifeal. There were no sustainable competitive advantages over the other products on the market. Every marketing person worth his salt wants a product with some competitive advantages. He concluded that, at this point in his study, there were no competitive advantages.

He told his computer to open the email that contained Mandi's point paper on Lifeal and a memo to J.P. He read the memo first.

Dear J.P.,

You don't know how hard it has been to write a point paper for a person who has a great respect for your reputation in strategic marketing. As I wrote the Lifeal point paper, I felt like I was writing a term paper for a grad school professor. I have to tell you, the feeling was strange, and it bothered me. If I'm to be your assistant on this project, I want to be an associate, not a student.

As you have probably already noticed, the attached point paper is only a couple of pages long. I am a firm believer that point papers should be as succinct as possible... hopefully, you agree. If you need more information, please ask. To give you a bit more information, I am also enclosing a comprehensive Lifeal Market Plan written by Frank Ascot, the Lifeal Product Manager.

It was a pleasure meeting you today and I look forward to us working together on this project.

See you Monday, Mandi

He said out loud, "Computer, open Lifeal point paper." He spent the next hour studying the paper and decided the summary and conclusion sections were the most important.

Summary:

The Lifeal Product was developed as both a prophylaxis against the onset of cardiac arrhythmia and maintenance against the reoccurrence of cardiac arrhythmia. The prevention indication was never approved. The main reason the FDA did not approve this indication was the inability of the cardiologist and pharmacologist to determine the patient profile of a candidate considered to be "susceptible to a cardiac arrhythmia event."

One of today's social objectives is to hold down patient pharmaceutical costs. Phase III clinical investigators determined that they couldn't develop a viable patient profile for susceptibility for cardiac arrhythmia. In the end, James' conclusion was that the FDA would in this case, judge the use of Lifeal as a prophylactic as "excessive medication". The FDA felt that physicians might prescribe Lifeal when there was no clear clinical justification. The lack of clinical justification by the clinical investigators for prevention of arrhythmia forced James to file with the FDA solely for the indication of long term maintenance from a reoccurrence of ventricular arrhythmia in a patient who already had an established history of the disorder/disease.

All of this, of course, placed Lifeal in direct competition with established products from companies with ten times the James marketing capabilities and budget.

Conclusion:

No competitive advantages.

Leaders of the market are entrenched and almost impossible to dislodge.

Majority of today's Lifeal business is from physicians approving refill prescriptions on patients to prevent a reoccurrence of cardiac arrhythmia.

Physicians approving refill prescriptions for patients already on an established maintenance product don't have a valid reason to change and move patients to Lifeal.

Lack of sufficient marketing budget prevents aggressive marketing campaigns to switch physicians from their present anti-arrhythmia products.

With the current Lifeal FDA approved indications, it will be difficult for James to capture more than an 11% market share of new prescriptions. The only refill prescriptions will be generated later from patients that were started on Lifeal. There will be minimal conversions to Lifeal from other pharmaceuticals unless the other product isn't having a positive clinical outcome or result.

Therefore, due to this situation, the Lifeal creative platform chosen by James is to focus on encouraging physicians to give Lifeal a try in patients that have had side-effect problems with their current prescribed maintenance pharmaceutical.

Suddenly, the computer generated voice announced, "Twelve o'clock, noon."

He had been so engrossed in reading that he had not heard the computer make any other half-hour announcements. He spoke out loud, "Computer, close the files and secure."

The computer responded, "Very well" and shut down.

Since he had decided not to ski, he still wanted to work out so he left his office and moved into the next room where his exercise equipment was located. While he was working on the Lifeal project he could hear the winds outside increasing in strength. He looked out the window of the workout room and saw that the snow was continuing to fall. He guessed that there had been another three feet of snow since yesterday.

He decided that he would run a half marathon today. He pulled his sweat pants off, revealing the running shorts that he had put on earlier that morning. He stepped onto the custom treadmill with its built-in satellite-ready television, CD changer, and computerized monitors that measured not only pace, distance, and heart rate, but also adjusted the room temperature after a few miles to keep the runner comfortable. The treadmill was produced locally and sold nationally by a company known as MARCI. J.P. was anxious for the next generation of treadmills to make it onto the market. He knew the designers at MARCI and they informed him that they had developed a prototype treadmill that used virtual reality combined with an artificial intelligence computer.

He pressed the play key of the CD changer that he had preloaded with three discs of Beethoven's piano music. He programmed the computer to run the half-marathon at a seven-minute mile pace. He pressed the start button and the surface beneath his feet began to move at a very leisurely pace, increasing steadily with each passing minute.

Annie thought it was crazy that J.P. ran on the treadmill during the winter. She was always quick to let him know just how boring she thought that was. HE explained to her that the running was as close as he got to spirituality these days and to leave him alone.

One and a half hours later, the treadmill began to slow for a cool down. As J.P.'s run became a walk he began to think about whether or not he really wanted to become involved in the James situation. He had done his best to hold off thinking about the Phillip's problem while he was running, but possible scenarios for what had happened kept entering his mind.

When the treadmill finally stopped he stepped off and took another drink of water. He looked over at the treadmill's computer screen. The screen showed the elapsed time of his run, his average speed, and a graphic comparison of past averages for this specific program. He noted that his average time was, as usual, nearly flat reflecting a steady performance.

He grabbed another bottle of water from the small refrigerator in the workout room and headed downstairs where he took a shower and then laid down for a short nap.

It was almost four-thirty when he went upstairs and began preparing an early dinner. He knew Annie wouldn't be stopping by that evening since it was ladies' night at Annie's Bar and Grill. Ladies' night was a fun night for local singles and couples who enjoyed dancing to country and western music.

After dinner, he poured himself a glass of Stoli and moved into the living room. He picked up a remote and pushed the button that lowered a five-foot entertainment screen down out of the ceiling. The screen served as both a high-definition television and a monitor for the computer he used for research. He switched the system to the computer mode. This was an older computer and didn't have the voice command capability of his MAC so he brought out a wireless keyboard from a cabinet along one of the walls. When the main menu appeared on the screen, he clicked on the research-shortcut button and typed pharmaceutical research in the box that appeared. Immediately, the computer's modem dialed up one of the nation's major pharmaceutical databases. Another box appeared on screen and J.P. typed the word herbal. Thousands of topics appeared on the screen.

"Well, looks like I'm going to be here a while," he murmured to himself.

For the next six hours he conducted his personal cram course on the history and use of herbs in medicine. Finally at 2:00 a.m., he decided to call it day and went to bed.

6:00 A.M., FRIDAY, JANUARY 20

BANDAI PHARMACEUTICALS COMPANY BANDAI, JAPAN

The sun was rising on a clear, crisp Friday morning in Bandai, Japan. Nacheda was already in his office looking through the presentation he would make to Dr. Nakasone in less than an hour.

At five minutes before 7:00, Nacheda walked towards Dr. Nakasone's office suite on the other side of the building. When he arrived outside Nakasone's office, Nacheda knocked.

"*Hai,* please come in, Nacheda-san," a voice said from inside.

Dr. Nakasone had an office in traditional Japanese style. His desk was low, perhaps one foot above the mat. He sat on the tatomi mat behind his desk instead of a chair. He had rice paper sliding doors on two sides of the office. One set of doors opened onto a beautifully manicured Japanese garden. Nacheda took off his shoes. As he entered, he had to bend low so that his head would not hit the upper frame of the door. He held his bowed position as he stepped up onto the tatomi mat and proceeded towards Dr. Nakasone's desk.

Still bowed, Nacheda addressed Dr. Nakasone, " *Ohayougozaimasu,* Dr. Nakasone-san." Dr. Nakasone stood and bowed, *"Ohayougozaimasu,* Nacheda-san."

Nacheda then stood up his full six-foot height. Nakasone motioned for him to sit at a small circular conference table surrounded by four sitting cushions. Nacheda waited for Dr. Nakasone to sit on his cushion before he sat.

After Nacheda had settled himself on the cushion, the door to the office opened and a female assistant entered carrying a tray. On the tray was a pot of green tea, two cups, and four breakfast cookies arranged on a plate. Nakasone thanked her and then said something else to her in a low voice that prevented Nacheda from hearing.

The woman replied, *"Hai douzo,"* and moved to slide back the doors that hid the sunlit garden from the room.

Nacheda felt that the gesture to open the room to the garden was a good sign. It was generally agreed among Bandai executives that Dr. Nakasone always wanted a pleasant atmosphere for fruitful meetings. Nacheda recalled the last meeting he had in this room, just one week ago when the garden doors had remained closed, the room somewhat darkened, and Dr. Nakasone issuing a stern reprimand to him for his lack of progress. Today things appeared much different, Nacheda began to relax slightly. As the assistant poured the tea, Nacheda looked outside at the garden. The garden was as beautiful in snow as it was when summer flowers gave the garden color. The snow contrasted nicely against the subtle color changes of grays and browns of earth, rock, and bamboo.

Nakasone spoke first, "The contrast of the snow against the rock is as striking as that between our last visit and today."

Nacheda replied, *"Hai,* Dr. Nakasone-san, what you say is very true." He picked up his cup and sipped some of the tea.

"How can circumstances so dark and dreary a mere six days ago brighten like the opening of the doors to my garden?"

Nacheda set his cup back onto the table. "The information from many sources, gathered over a long period of time have finally come together. This is much like the forming of your garden. The garden began as stone and earth. Time, patience, care, seeds from various sources, and the experience and knowledge of your gardeners made it into a painting. Our garden of information is near completion. The painting is clearly one of beautiful symmetries, yet one or two rocks are missing to complete our painting, but it is a small task to place those missing rocks. Today, I am here to assure you that we will have an answer after the February session."

Dr. Nakasone listened intently. When Nacheda had finished, he said, "You have done well Nacheda-san. Please provide me with the exact details of your meeting with the team."

Nacheda responded by handing him the report he had begun creating on the flight from Los Angeles. "Dr. Nakasone-san, this is the complete report of our meeting in Westwood Village. The report concludes that we have identified a number of new indications and pharmaceuticals that are herbal based and can be altered by plant DNA manipulation. The Bandai Pharmaceuticals active ingredient technologies will be very valuable to developing a new class of pharmaceuticals. There is some limited work being done in the United States on herbs and newer indications, but without substantive results. These efforts continue to be limited to the research laboratories. Large pharmaceutical companies require conclusive results in order to evaluate potential value. Without these conclusive results, they continue to concentrate on synthetic compounds and not herbs. Our technologies will provide the catalyst to make the DNA manipulation a success. The team is continuing to focus on the capability and products ofcompanies that will make the best targets for us. We are also looking for partners that would work well with us to bring the new class of pharmaceuticals to full clinical value."

As Dr. Nakasone listened, he tried to evaluate Nacheda's confidence level. He had been rough on Nacheda the week before and he wanted to make sure that Nacheda not only was reporting the good news, but that he genuinely believed what he was saying. "Nacheda-san, thank you. We will wait anxiously for the February meeting. Is there anything we can do help you ensure this project comes to swift and decisive conclusion?"

Nacheda was careful how he answered. He didn't want to have Nakasone become too involved in the actual running of the project. "I will be in contact with Colonel Howard every day. He will ensure that the other team members forward their new information as it becomes available."

Nacheda paused and then shifted back to the garden analogy. "We will require time to do the job correctly, Dr. Nakasone-san. We don't want to misplace one of the rocks in our garden. We are also being careful about how we gather the information so as not to alert competitors to our activities."

"I understand, Nacheda-san. What are your plans for the time between now and the meeting in February?"

"With your concurrence, Dr. Nakasone-san, I would like to learn more about Bandai Pharmaceuticals' isolation process technology. I will be better able to understand how this technology will play a role in acquiring our target. As of now, I only know the basics of this technology."

Nakasone smiled, "Ah, Nacheda-san, you have once again pleased me. I had already anticipated the need for you learn more of this technology. On Monday, I wish for you to begin working in research with Dr. Noguchi. We will now go to see him and explain your role."

Nakasone without another word rose from the floor. Nacheda, caught off-balance by this sudden turn of events quickly followed suit. They left Nakasone's office and put on their shoes before walking across the campus to the building that housed the research department.

Dr. Naksone introduced Nacheda to Dr. Noguchi. "Dr. Noguchi-san, this is Mr. Nacheda. He is on special assignment for us and will be working with you for two weeks beginning Monday. He is bright, but he is not a chemist. I want you to provide him with as much knowledge as he can assimilate about our herbal technologies. It is important for you to translate the information into words and actions that Nacheda-san can readily understand and ultimately translate into English. This project is vital to our future, Dr. Noguchi-san. Mr. Nacheda-san is playing a valuable role in Bandai Pharmaceuticals' future. Are there any questions?"

"No questions, Dr. Nakasone-san," replied Noguchi. "I am honored to play this important role in our future. I am sure that Mr. Nacheda-san will remind me to go slower or faster in my teachings according to his desires." Noguchi reached up to a bookshelf and removed two textbooks. "I would ask that Mr. Nacheda-san read these two books before Monday so that he could have a basic understanding of what we are doing here at Bandai Pharmaceuticals."

Nacheda took the books from Noguchi, looking into the man's kind face. He had heard stories about Dr. Matsuo Noguchi and his background. He was the grandson of the famous bacteriologist, Dr. Hideyo Noguchi, who did much of the early research on yellow fever. The grandfather eventually died of the disease he labored to eradicate while working in Africa.

Under the influences of his grandfather and father, who was also a doctor, Matsuo studied and became one of the most brilliant chemists in Japan. While he was attending Tokyo University, the Japanese Pharmaceutical Association (JPA) began to pay close attention to the progress of Matsuo. They had identified him as a valuable asset to their objective to become a force in the global pharmaceutical market. However, pharmaceutical companies were very disappointed when the dissertation for his Ph.D. was on the subject of active ingredient isolation. Isolation of active ingredients was never an issue in synthetic chemical pharmaceuticals. The JPA felt that he was reaching backwards to outdated technology and therefore, might not be the rising star they had hoped would propel Japan to the top of the global pharmaceutical industry.

After some consideration and debate, the JPA forgave Dr. Noguchi. They still felt he was a valuable future asset. All of the large companies in Tokyo still sought to hire him, but he chose Bandai Pharmaceuticals Company. This decision again angered the JPA and its members. The fact that he had joined Nakasone's breakaway company meant that his colleagues would forever ostracize him. He had been working for Bandai Pharmaceuticals for fifteen years now and had been invaluable to Dr. Nakasone and the growth of the company. He had written at least one scientific paper every year and held ten patents. The papers were all published in countries outside of Japan because in his own country, he wasn't recognized and was thought to be an embarrassment to his father and grandfather. To the people of Bandai and Bandai Pharmaceuticals, Dr. Matsuo Noguchi was admired as much as his father and grandfather.

"I would be honored to learn from you, Dr. Noguchi-san," Nacheda replied with some regret.

Despite the honor of working with Dr. Noguchi, he could not help thinking, "there goes my weekend." The three of them discussed the Bandai process for another thirty minutes and then left Dr. Noguchi's laboratory. Dr. Nakasone walked Nacheda back to the reception area where they said their good-byes. Dr. Nakasone advised Nacheda to get some rest and enjoy his weekend. He gave Nacheda a knowing wink, recognizing that he had been given homework to do over the weekend.

Nacheda left the Bandai Pharmaceuticals complex and walked to his car. As he drove back to his home, he took in the view of the surrounding mountains. He decided he was grateful to live there. It was so beautiful and offered so much in terms of outdoor recreation. Besides the extinct volcano, which offered great skiing, there were hundreds of small lakes and ponds as well as lush green forests.

There were only a few tourists in town. By tomorrow the city would be filled with thousands of people wanting to ski. Nacheda debated with himself as to whether he should call Reiko. He told himself that she was probably busy and at any rate he had two textbooks to read by Monday. Finally, he decided that he would call her and ask if she might be interested in coming up to Bandai to ski. After arriving home he opened his wallet to retrieve the slip of paper that Reiko had given him on the airplane. Her phone rang four times before he heard her voice on the other end.

"*Moshimoshi*," Reiko said.

Nacheda paused, he felt nervous. What if she turned him down? "*Moshimoshi*," he finally responded. "Reiko, this is Nacheda. I am calling from Bandai."

"Ah, Nacheda-san, what are you doing in Bandai?" Reiko answered. Her voice sounded so pleased to hear from him that some of Nacheda's apprehension began to wane.

"This is the location of my Japan office," he replied. "It is beautiful here. The sun is bright and the mountains are covered with snow. It is great skiing weather. Do you ski?"

"I love to ski, Nacheda-san," she replied with even more enthusiasm. "My first name is Masayuki, but many of my American friends call me

Mas. If you prefer you may call me Mas," he said in a soft voice. "Okay, Mas."

"Reiko, do you really enjoy skiing?"

"*Hai,* Mas. It is one of my favorite things to do, but the ski towns are always so crowded that it is difficult to find a place to stay."

He decided to go for it, "Have you ever skied Bandai?"

"No, but I have always wanted to ski the high mountains. Do you like to ski, Mas?"

"I try to ski as much as I can when I am working here," he paused.

"Did you want to ask me something, Mas?" she asked. She worked hard to stifle the giggle that was trying to come from her.

"I know it is somewhat presumptuous of me and also very late for me to be asking. But, would you like to come to Bandai this weekend and ski with me? I have two sleeping rooms and I would consider it an honor to have you as my houseguest."

Reiko answered immediately, further relieving Nacheda of any doubts he may have had about asking her to join him for the weekend.

"Mas, I would love to be your houseguest. It is not too late nor is it presumptuous of you to ask. I cannot think of anything that I would rather do this weekend. Um.how do I get to Bandai?"

Nacheda looked at his watch and saw that it was nearly noon. "There are three trains on Friday afternoon from Tokyo. They leave at three, five, and seven. It will take you four hours to get here if you take the three o'clock bullet train. The other two trains take two hours longer because of more stops. I will pick you up at the station. Will staying at my home be a problem?"

"No, of course not. I believe I can make the 3:00 train without any problem. It is only a 30-minute taxi ride from my home to the train station. I'll have to start digging out my skis and ski clothes. When would I return?"

"There is a noon train on Sunday. Do you think that will work for you? I have a great deal of reading to do this weekend in preparation for my Monday project. I will probably have to do some reading Saturday, but I just could not imagine not skiing this weekend and I did so want to see you again."

"The noon train on Sunday is fine. That will get me home in the evening, which is perfect. Will you call and make the reservations?"

"Yes, Reiko. I will call now and then call you back with the specifics." "Okay, great, I will start getting ready," she was so excited that she hung up the phone without saying good-bye.

Nacheda made the reservations and charged them to his credit card. He called Reiko back and gave her the information and told her he would meet her at the train station at 7:00. He filled the time between his last call to Reiko and the trip to the train station by shopping for food, drinks, and firewood and reading his textbooks.

The train was on time and when Reiko stepped off the train, Nacheda rushed to help her with her bags and skis. "Reiko, I am so glad you could come."

They stood looking at each other, afraid to touch. He had worn a dark clothing with a black turtleneck under a dark sweater. Reiko, on the other hand, had worn bright clothes. She wore tight jeans with a bright red sweater. Under her sweater she wore a bright yellow turtleneck pullover. She reminded him of a flower.

Reiko spoke, "Mas, thank you so much for asking me. I wanted to see you again and soon." She threw her arms around his neck and gave him a quick kiss on the cheek. Her sudden expression of familiarity, her kiss, perfume, and luggage almost toppled Nacheda over backwards. He was spellbound.

Reiko looked around the outdoor train platform at the landscape. The moon was bright so the outline of the mountains was visible even though it was dark.

"Mas, it is so beautiful. I can't wait until I see the mountains in the daylight. Let's go to your home. I am really hungry."

They drove in silence. Reiko was taking in all of the sights of the drive. Nacheda was wondering what the rest of the evening held in store. Reiko was certainly different from the other Japanese women he had dated. On the plane she was so Japanese, but here, now she seemed like a young American college girl. He had not thought about it before, but now he began to wonder. How old was Reiko? And what was their age difference. He guessed that she was in her early thirties. He realized for the first time that he was probably quite a bit older than her.

Dinner went well. After dinner they sat on the couch in front of the fire and talked about skiing. By midnight, both of them were yawning from the lateness of the hour, the wine, the food, and the leftover jet lag from the trip back from Los Angeles the previous day.

Nacheda rose from the couch, "Reiko, I have prepared my room for you and I will sleep in the guest room. If it is okay with you, I propose that we rise at 7:00 a.m. so that we can have breakfast and be skiing by 9:30."

"That is fine with me, but you didn't have to give up your room. I can sleep in the guestroom. You must be tired from your flight and I feel rested."

"No, I insist. You shall have my room. I will knock on your door at seven. If you will excuse me, I will use the bathroom first."

"That is fine, Mas. Please have a good sleep."

When Nacheda emerged from the bathroom five minutes later, Reiko was standing by the couch where he had left her. Reiko looked up at him and gave him a kiss on the lips. Nacheda put his arms around her and they kissed again. Her lips were full and moist. Their bodies pressed together. After a time, Reiko backed away.

"Thank you again for inviting me and for cooking such a wonderful meal. You are a gentle person and I really enjoy being with you." She turned and went into the bathroom, closing the door gently behind her.

7:00 A.M., FRIDAY, JANUARY 20
MAMMOTH LAKES, CALIFORNIA

J.P. slept in as long as he could and that was not very long. He had been an early-riser since his days in the Navy and he hated to think he was wasting part of a day by not being up with the sun. The early morning sun came through the curtains of his bedroom window and gave the room a warm feeling despite the fact that the open window had the room temperature at somewhere around freezing. The weather forecast on the news the evening before had predicted clear skies by morning. He smiled and thought to himself that they might actually be correct for once. He remembered the constant snowfall yesterday and thought about the fresh powder snow up on the mountain.

He reached up and hit the button that initiated the morning sequence to start his day and warm up the house. As the room began to warm, he finally came out from under his blankets and comforter. He was able to shower, dress, eat breakfast, and head out the door to the ski lifts in less than an hour. He had a deal with the ski patrol. They would let him go up on top of the mountain with them and not wait until the mountain was open to the public. All he had to do was show up at the lifts when they began their pre-opening checks on the equipment.

He put on his skies in the loading area of chair eight. As he bent down to fasten his boots he saw someone dressed in bright blue ski pants move behind him. Without looking up, he said, "Ah, Christie, good morning."

"J.P., how did you know it was me?"

"Who else would be up here so early in the morning and with such nice legs," he said as he stood up?

"You always say the nicest things, J.P."

Christie was warming up the motors for chair eight and had been shoveling away the snow from the chair-loading platform in front of the attendants' small warming hut. She typified what J.P. thought a young Southern California woman should be, 24 years old, long blonde hair, fine facial features, brilliant white teeth, and dark tanned skin. She lived in LA except for winters when she worked at Mammoth Mountain.

"How have you been, J.P.? I haven't seen much of you in the mornings this year."

"I'm fine, Christie. Is this thing ready to go?" "Yep. Get ready."

As the empty chair came around the flywheel, J.P. slid onto the lift chair. He yelled a thank you to Christie and started up the mountain.

He reached the top of chair eight and skied off the chair proceeding to the next chair and slope gradually making his way to runs around chair nine, his favorite part of the mountain. He paused at the top of the run. The upper lift safety operator, Mike, had already cleared the heavy snow from the top of the chair lift drop off. J.P. waved to him skied a short distance and stood poised at the top of the long stretch of whiteness that lay before him. Fine powder conditions were rare on Mammoth, but when was there, J.P. always made time to get out on the slopes.

He pushed off. The powder was deep. J.P. estimated that if the depth of new snow at his house was five feet, the new snow up on the mountain had to be at least eight to ten feet. Moving from side to side he flew as fast down the mountain as the snow would allow leaving behind a large snow rooster tail. He stopped halfway down the run and turned to look back up the slope. His ski marks were the only ones on that side of the mountain. He turned back around and finished the run to the bottom.

At the bottom, the lift operator met him and asked, "So, J.P., how was it?"

"Mammoth fine. We haven't had dry powder like this in years. This is going to be a great day."

He rode up chair nine, and then skied over to the mid-station where he caught the gondola to the cornice. The gondola ride to the top of the mountain gave him one of the best panoramic views of the Sierra Nevada Mountains to the northwest and the White Mountains to the east. Since he had already made a run down below, he would not be the first to go off the cornice, that distinction belonged to the ski patrol.

As the gondola continued to climb, he decided that he would ski all day. Tomorrow, LA skiers would invade the mountain. Like a lot of the other Mammoth Lakes residents, he did not ski on the weekends. He just couldn't stand the crowds.

He continued to ski throughout the entire day making countless runs down most of the black diamond runs of Mammoth. He finally decided to stop when he felt his well-conditioned legs began to weaken. He arrived back home at 5:30 and performed an hour of after-ski therapy in his outdoor spa. He was preparing dinner when the phone rang. It was Annie.

"J.P., hi. Do you think you can help me out tonight? The word must be spreading around LA that Mammoth has dry, fine powder. It seems that every skier in Los Angeles is headed up here now. I heard a report on the radio that the CHP is reporting that 395 is almost at gridlock at the Mojave turn. I'm afraid I'll need extra help tending bar. I know you have a great deal of work to do on your new project, but could you please help out?"

He didn't hesitate at all. Annie was always there for him when he required help. "When?" he replied with as much enthusiasm as he could muster.

"As soon as you can," Annie said with relief in her voice. "Okay, I'm on my way." J.P. knew that if the highway patrol said there was gridlock in Mojave, it was going to be a crowded weekend. He was glad that he would be able to help Annie. The James project could wait. He figured he would have all day Saturday to work.

He arrived at Annie's Bar and Grill in less than 30 minutes after her call. Even at the early evening hour of 7:15, Annie's was already half full of customers. As he looked around the room, J.P. realized he didn't, at first, recognize any of the customers. Finally, he noticed some regulars back in the corner having dinner.

He figured the LA ski reports on the radio with news of dry powder on the mountain must have encouraged people to leave work early and begin their trek to Mammoth. Usually, skiers from LA did not arrive at Mammoth until midnight or after on Friday night and then most went directly to bed. They were usually too tired to do much partying Friday night and they wanted to hit the slopes early on Saturday morning. Saturday night, on the other hand, was an entirely different story. The parties usually started early and lasted most of the night. Not much skiing was done before noon on Sunday and then around 2:00 p.m., the exodus back to LA began.

Annie saw him come in and she waved from behind the bar. Whenever

J.P. helped out, Annie always asked him to tend bar. He enjoyed the work until someone asked him for some exotic drink. It didn't happen very often, but when it did Annie took over.

"Hiya, handsome. Thanks for helping out. I owe you one," Annie yelled to him over the ever-increasing noise level of the crowd.

J.P. yelled back, "You owe me nothing, Annie. I owe a perpetual debt to you. I figure the debt I owe you will take a good twenty years before we're close to even."

J.P. wrapped a clean bartender's apron around his waist. He wrapped the long tie sash around himself twice and tied it in the front. He jumped immediately into action as more and more people came in. J.P. knew it would be a busy night, but he was having fun.

At around 11:00 p.m., he looked over at the man sitting at the far end of the bar nearest the roaring fireplace. At that end of the bar, the wall jutted out to form a cubbyhole. A person could stand at the bar and lean up against the wall. Since Annie didn't use bar stools, it was the only place to rest up against something unless it was another person.

By Annie's reckoning, a no bar stool policy had two benefits. It reduced the number of heavy drinkers who would take up bar space and slowly drink themselves into a stupor and it allowed more people to belly up to the bar to have a drink. When the bar area was packed, the customers were so tightly packed they would rest up against one another.

The man at the end of the bar was alone and had, to J.P.'s count, finished off three Japanese Asahi Dry beers. He had offered to switch him to a mug of Mammoth Dry, but he said that he was stuck on the rice beer. He told J.P. that for some reason Asahi never gave him a headache when he overindulged. He thought to mention that if you do not overindulge you probably will not get a headache from any beer, but thought better of starting a meaningless discourse that would distract him from the other more sober customers.

At this point the man hailed him for another beer. J.P. reached into the iced beer tub and brought out another Asahi Dry and walked it to the end of the bar.

"How are things going?" J.P. asked. The drink requests were starting to slow and he didn't feel as harried as he had before.

"Couldn't be better. You own this place?" the man asked.

"Call me, J.P. Nope, that lady over there in the blue denim dress, Annie, is the illustrious proprietress. You want any chow?"

"J.P., pleased to meet you. My name is Skip, Skip Howard," he said extending his hand to J.P. "Yeah, I think I will have some chow. What have you got on the menu?"

"Annie makes a great chili and also a great lean steak. The steak costs a bit more than usual, but it's low fat, low cholesterol, and great tasting. Comes from a special breeding farm near Sacramento. Annie orders it special. Kind of compares to Kobe beef, but nothing could be the same as Kobe."

"Okay, sounds great. I'll take a rare lean steak with fries."

J.P. turned to his left and yelled the order into the kitchen. He looked back to Skip. Skip was a big man and well built. He looked as though he regularly worked out, as his body appeared to be tightly muscle toned. He had cropped coarse, brown hair. He was wearing a suede leather jacket over a brown turtleneck pullover.

"You mentioned Kobe beef, J.P. You been to Japan?"

"Yeah, when I was an officer in the Navy and quite a few times since then on business. I remember the days when you could afford Kobe every night. Now, as I understand it, Kobe steaks are on the endangered list. How about you?"

"Not too much time in Japan. Most of my Far East experience was in 'Nam during the second non-approved war," Skip replied.

"I missed Vietnam, but I sincerely respect everyone who served there. Even after I left active duty and became a reservist, there was a few years that I couldn't wear a Navy uniform to and from my reserve ship because civilians would yell at us and tell us we should all be ashamed of ourselves. Some would even throw things at our cars. It was the uniform, it represented a colossal mistake in politics. People tend to forget that the military is merely an instrument of a politician's whim. Sorry, I know I'm probably preaching to the choir since you were there. So what do you do now and what brings you to Mammoth?"

Skip took a long drink from his bottle of Asahi. To J.P. it appeared that he was thinking about how he would answer the question.

"I'm working with a group of people investigating healthcare companies for... possible acquisition. Sort of a hush-hush project. I don't mean to make it sound so mysterious, there's really nothing special about any of it, but intellectually, it is very engaging. As for me being in Mammoth, I'm here to ski. I haven't skied in a good number of years and I heard the conditions up here are the best. The rumor around Westwood Village and UCLA was that everyone was going to Mammoth this weekend. The way things looked on the highway and in this bar, I'd say everyone did come up to Mammoth. Is it as good a mountain for skiing as they say, J.P.?"

"Great mountain. You'll enjoy yourself. There's a run for every ski level."

"Glad to hear it. Are you skiing tomorrow?"

"Nope. I don't ski when the LA crowd is on Mammoth Mountain. I don't mean to sound like a snob, but it just gets too crowded for my taste.

Also, I have work to do tomorrow. Come up some weekday, Skip, and I'll show you how to ski to exhaustion."

Skip asked, "Do you have a business card?" J.P. reached into his pocket and pulled one of his cards from his wallet. He handed Skip the card and Skip passed one of his. J.P. pushed Skip's card into his shirt pocket without looking at it.

The cook yelled through the pick-up window that Skip's steak was ready.

"Skip, you have to eat at a table. The bar is only for drinking. There's an empty table in the back to the right of the fireplace. On the table is a permanently mounted reserved sign. Someone may be sitting at the table even though they're not allowed. It's Annie's personal table so if someone is there you can tell them to leave. I'll bring your chow. Do you want another Asahi?"

"Thanks, I don't think there will be any problems clearing the table. Also, how about one of those Mammoth Dry's that you've been trying to push on me all night? Might as well get into the Mammoth mood," Skip said before turning away to make his way through the crowd.

J.P. pulled a Mammoth Dry from the ice tub and walked into the kitchen to get the steak and fries. He emerged from the serving door and looked towards Annie's table. Skip was seated at the table drinking down the last from his bottle of Asahi. There was a young man on the floor next to the table and a number of others gathered around the table staring at Skip.

"Trouble?" J.P. asked as he approached the table and set the food and beer down.

"Nah," Skip replied. "This young man's," he gestured at the man on the floor, "chair legs slipped out from under him and he fell down. You okay, buddy?" He looked down at the man on the floor.

J.P. could see that it was no small 20-something year old, the guy looked like a college athlete. He looked up at Skip and then at J.P. "Sure, mister. No problem. Chair slipped." He paused and then picked himself up off the floor. He brushed off his jeans and said sarcastically to Skip, "Thanks for breaking my fall," and then walked away to join his friends who had moved closer to the door.

Skip looked up at J.P. and smiled. "Some kids just can't sit straight. Sometimes they need a little help to sit up straight in their chair. Care to join me, J.P.?"

J.P. looked around the room and noticed that the bar crowd was beginning to thin. "I'll have to ask the boss. I'll be right back." He walked back through the kitchen. Behind the bar Annie was drawing a mug of draft.

"Business was good this evening, Annie," he remarked while placing his arm around her waist and giving her a gentle squeeze.

Annie smiled at him, "A very good night for both the bar and food business thanks in large part to your assistance. Who is the guy you've been talking to? Nice looking guy, by the way. Doesn't look like your typical LA executive wannabe."

"Watch out, Annie, your eyes are beginning to sparkle."

J.P. reached into his shirt pocket and gave Annie the card Skip had passed to him earlier. She read aloud from the card,

Skip C. Howard, Colonel, USMC Office of Naval Intelligence

The Pentagon, Rm 3E144 Washington, DC

Annie turned the card over and on the back was an address in Westwood Village, CA with a 310 area code telephone number.

"What did the Colonel have to say?" Annie asked.

"Colonel? Well how about that, he didn't mention anything about being a Colonel. When I asked him what he did for a living, he said he was working on a project of investigating healthcare companies for possible acquisition. Come to think of it, he did pause before answering my question about what he did. Seemed to think through his answer."

Annie laughed and said, "Well, J.P., we all have our dirty little secrets now don't we? He's a good looking man…is he married?"

"How the hell should I know? Go over and talk to him, Annie. He knows you're the owner. He didn't ask what I do for a living so I didn't volunteer the information. He probably thinks I'm a career bartender. Since he has some affiliation with healthcare, I didn't want him to ask me any questions about what I was doing."

"I see. By the way, if you want to go home, it's okay. My normal Friday night help and I can handle the remaining customers and clean up. I sure appreciated your help tonight. Any chance I can borrow you for a few hours tomorrow night, say from six to nine?"

"No problem," he replied.

Skip had been watching their conversation. J.P. gave him a wave and headed out the door.

7:00 A.M., SATURDAY, JANUARY 21

BANDAI, JAPAN

Nacheda awoke when his alarm went off at 7:00 a.m. Reiko and Nacheda ate a light breakfast, dressed for skiing, and walked with their skis to the shuttle bus that would take them to the ski tram. Not much was said between them, but they both felt something that they had not experienced with another person for a long time.

Bandai snow was excellent for skiing. They quickly discovered that they skied at the same experience level. They hardly qualified as experts, but both were experienced recreational skiers. They enjoyed one another's company, which was probably obvious to anyone who observed them.

When the skiing ended for the day, they stopped at the lodge for warm sake.

"Mas, what a wonderful day. I do not remember when I last had such a fun and exhilarating day. Thank you very much."

"You are welcome, but I must say that it was you who filled the day with light and happiness. And may I also say, you are a truly beautiful woman."

Reiko took Nacheda's compliment with grace, but didn't otherwise acknowledge it. "Mas, you have never told me what you do for a living and why you live in this heavenly place."

Nacheda looked down into his glass and told her, "I do not have an easy answer to your question, but I will try to give you as much information as I can."

Nacheda began telling her his story. The sun had not yet set when he began talking, but slowly set behind the mountains as he spoke. Finally, when he finished it was nearly dark outside the lodge. He had not told her the real purpose of his visits to Los Angeles, but he did tell her he was in healthcare acquisitions and was working on a special assignment for Bandai Pharmaceuticals Company. He told her that he had been in Vietnam, but not that he had been a prisoner of war.

Reiko sat patiently and listened intently as Nacheda told his story. He concluded by saying, "I apologize for talking for so long. My life is not very interesting, but I felt like talking. I hope you did not mind."

"Mas, you can't say that! Your life is very interesting. You have done so many things in such a short period of time. You did not say much about your two years in Vietnam. Frankly, I do not understand what a member of the Japanese Self-Defense Force was doing in Vietnam, but that is of little importance. If you do not wish to talk about it, I understand. I am interested though if you would like to discuss it."

He did not answer her right away and then replied, "I seldom speak to anyone about my experiences in Vietnam, let alone tell the full story. It was…it is…a very difficult subject for me. I do feel that I would like to tell you about my time there, but not at this moment. Perhaps later. It has been such an enjoyable day, I would hate to ruin it."

"Yes, of course," her voice betrayed disappointment.

Nacheda smiled at her and took her hand, "Reiko, you misunderstand. I want you to know of my time there, but later. First, let's go home and then I will take you to a fine Chinese restaurant." He laughed, "It has to be fine, it is the only Chinese restaurant in Bandai. Although Bandai is not Tokyo or Kyoto, we think we are just as good. Does this plan for our evening meet with your approval?"

Reiko loved his way of asking for her permission. He treated her as an equal, unlike many of the Japanese businessmen she had dated. She was beginning to enjoy this relationship very much. "Hai," she said, smiling at him.

Dinner conversation consisted of Reiko telling Nacheda about herself and her family. She was not from a samurai family, but her father had been very successful and was respected. He had been an electrical engineer for Mitsubishi. She had one brother who was also an electrical engineer. Her parents still lived in Tokyo. Reiko had gone to high school and college in Tokyo.

After dinner they walked home from the restaurant, holding hands. When they arrived home, Nacheda poured brandy and started a fire. They again sat on the couch in front of the fireplace, but tonight Nacheda had his arm around Reiko's shoulders and her head rested on his chest.

"Reiko, I want to try to explain my experience in Vietnam, but I will probably not be able to fully tell you how I felt or even how I feel today. It was a rough time in my life and sometimes when I think about those two years, I get upset. I do not want our evening to end unhappily. I have had such a wonderful day with you. But I feel very close to you right now and I want you to know everything about me. Although my time in Vietnam was very short, those two years have influenced and shaped my life for nearly thirty years. Do you still want to hear about this?"

Reiko raised her head and kissed him on the cheek. Nacheda reached around her waist with his right arm and pulled her close. They kissed softly and tenderly at first. Nacheda took her soft, delicate face in his hands, pulling her gently to him. He kissed along her jaw line, lingering for a second when he reached her ear. Reiko's hand moved up to his shoulder. She could feel the well-formed muscle beneath his shirt.

Nacheda kissed her full on the lips again, this time more passionately. The kiss lasted a long time. They did not want to break apart. After a while, their lips parted and Reiko whispered into his ear.

"I want to know all about you, Mas. I think I'm beginning to really fall for you. I knew when I first saw you on the plane that you were something special. Now I am certain that we are something special. If you don't want to talk, it doesn't matter."

Nacheda kissed her again and said, "No, it is very important that I tell you." Reiko nestled closer and placed her right hand on the inside of his left leg. Nacheda stirred, but disregarded his emotions and began his story.

"I cannot tell you everything. Some things that I was involved in are still classified and others are far too painful. I will try and give you a picture of my role in Vietnam and what that did to my life. First, I was with a special Japanese intelligence unit. Our objective was to observe the war and not become involved. As I'm certain you know, our constitution prohibits us from having a force capable of anything more than the defense of our borders. Still, our government felt that it was important to keep a watchful eye on what both the Americans and the communists were doing in the Pacific Rim. Of course, there was an economic side to this as well. We remembered only too well the amount of money that flowed through our nation during the Korean War and we did not want the war money for Vietnam to flow through Taiwan or the Philippines. Business from the American efforts in Korea, helped Japan to get back up on its economic feet. Business generated from America's involvement in Vietnam was seen by our government as a springboard to global industrial greatness. The government sought to ensure that it knew everything that was going on in Vietnam. So they sent me and four other intelligence officers into the country as observers.

"Before leaving, I had an eight-month training course in self-defense, intelligence gathering techniques, and Vietnamese and English language courses. I was a good student. I worked closely with the American intelligence services while I was there. I learned a lot from the Americans, particularly about their thoughts on freedom and life in general. We Japanese seem to feel that Americans do not have culture or any real philosophy of life. This is not true. Certainly they do not have the centuries of culture that Japan has enjoyed, but they do have a philosophy of individual freedom. Individual freedom of the mind, spirit, and the body. They feel very strongly about protecting that freedom.

"As the war moved along, it became a confusing morass of media hype, drug use, and the pet project of a confusing and contradictory American foreign policy. It was this lack of clear vision and the lack of support by the civilian population that cost America the war. They believed, or at least chanted it as a mantra, that they were fighting to defend the rice basket of the world and freedom for the people of South Vietnam. They believed they could do what the French had failed to do in nearly two decades.

The fire crackled from the gases stored up in the dry wood. Nacheda looked down at Reiko. The reflection of the flames gave her skin a warm glow.

He continued, "I spent fifty percent of my time in the jungle and fifty percent in Saigon. After I had been in country for about a year, I was given the opportunity to accompany an American Special Forces patrol conducting surveillance operations near a known Vietcong command center.

"I had been on many patrols and they were all dangerous, but somehow I always managed to fight my way out without getting hurt or being captured. When I was on a patrol, I was not supposed to actually fight. I was to be an observer. Whenever the patrol got into a firefight it was impossible to remain an observer. My life was as much in jeopardy as any other man there who was supposed to fight. The Vietcong certainly did not ask who was and was not an observer." Nacheda heard Reiko make a small giggle as she visualized the Vietcong asking who was and who was not an observer before conducting an ambush.

Nacheda paused for a second and then continued, "The enemy did not allow me to be an observer and, at any rate, in a firefight, I did not wish to remain an observer. Particularly when all around me men were being killed. On this particular patrol, I was captured. To this day I do not know how it all happened….everything went so fast. One minute we were fighting with the enemy in front of us and then before we knew it, we were completely surrounded. We were firing in every direction. We were caught in a clearing and the Vietcong kept drawing the circle tighter until we were forced to surrender.

"Once captured, the Vietcong did not know what to make of me.they hadn't expected to find a Japanese officer in that patrol. Our patrol had been reduced to ten men including myself. The rest of the patrol was Americans.

"They bound our hands and marched us into a rice patty. Without another word they summarily executed everyone in the patrol with a shot to the head except me." Nacheda's last sentence caught in his throat and tears welled up in his eyes. Reiko did not move. Nacheda took a couple of breaths in an attempt to regain his composure. He continued, "They bound my feet and hands with burlap and then pushed a pole between my bound limbs. I was carried out in that fashion, hanging from the pole like slaughtered pig.

They carried me to a processing station where I was put in chains and loaded onto a truck for transport to Hanoi and the prison that the Americans called the Hanoi Hilton.

"Reiko, I cannot go through the ten months I spent in the prison. Those memories are much too painful. It is also the source for the bad dreams you have seen when I fly. The dreams center on my capture and imprisonment."

When he paused again, Reiko looked up at him. Nacheda reached around and pulled her closer to him. They held one another very tightly for a long time. Finally, Reiko spoke, "What happened after prison?"

"At the end of the war there was an exchange of prisoners. I was transferred to an American Navy hospital in Saigon for three months. That is where I met some of the people I told you about earlier in the day.

"I came back to Japan after the war and decided to return to school for my advanced degree. I received my master's degree in political economics and business. I have been a consultant for many Japanese companies wanting to do business in the United States. My current work with Bandai Pharmaceuticals is the most rewarding that I have had because I am able to use my skills as a former intelligence officer in conjunction with my business experience to achieve an end and ultimately improve the quality of life for people everywhere."

Reiko looked into his eyes and smiled. Without a word she pulled him down to her.

5:45 P.M., SATURDAY, JANUARY 21
MAMMOTH LAKES, CALIFORNIA

J.P. had spent the day reviewing the history of herbal pharmaceuticals. He discovered that he had been incorrect in his belief that the era of plant medicine was past. Many products were still, to this day, herb-based and there were many new methods for isolating the medicinal active ingredient of plants. He also learned that while the research into herb-based medicines was still active and that the technologies for isolating active ingredients continued to grow, there were a number of other issues that sometimes got in the way.

He had read with much interest about the history of the Yew tree from which the bark was harvested to make a drug that could be used to shrink ovarian tumors by at least half. While the drug, Taxol, was not a cure there was evidence that it could extend life for months and maybe years. The company that developed the drug was required to work with various environmental groups that were working hard to protect the Yew tree from commercialization. They sought ways to extract the active ingredient in Taxol from the Yew needles rather than the bark. After a few years of some success with ovarian cancer patients, the drug was shown to be effective in the treatment of breast cancer and even with the AIDS-related cancer, Kaposi's sarcoma.

J.P. finally stopped reading when he remembered that he had promised Annie that he would help out that night at the bar and grill. When he arrived he was surprised to find that the place was packed. He put on his bartender apron and set to work handling the bar and filling drink orders from the tables. Saturday nights in Annie's Bar and Grill were always busy, but this night seemed particularly so. He thought that Annie's might actually break a one-night revenue record.

Annie always hired extra people for the ski weekends. Annie's objective was to handle as many customers as possible without sacrificing quality or the personal service for which Annie's was famous. Tonight Annie was scurrying around the tables talking to the customers, playing the role of owner and hostess.

At around 8:45, J.P. saw Skip come in the door. His face was a bright red. The weather on the mountain that day had been sunny and not too cold. There were a lot of skiers in the room who had gotten a little too much sun. Skip walked up to the bar where J.P. was standing.

"Hi, J.P. I see you have the watch again tonight."

"Well, good evening, Colonel. How was your day on the mountain?"

"A little crowded, but it was probably best that I had to wait between runs. I didn't realize how far out of shape that I've gotten since I left the Pentagon. I used run every day along the Potomac at lunchtime. Still, I gotta tell you that the ski runs were some of the best I've ever taken. I can sure understand why you live here. Have you eaten yet, J.P.?"

"Nope. And I'm hungry. Annie will cut me loose at 2100. Grab the reserved table and I'll join you in a while. Want a beer?"

"Sure. How about another Mammoth Dry."

J.P. passed him a mug of Mammoth Dry over the bar. Skip thanked him and then turned and disappeared into the crowd.

At 9:00 J.P. joined Skip at the reserved table. He brought two more mugs of Mammoth Dry.

"Skip, I'll let you in on another secret. Did you enjoy your steak last night?"

"I sure did. I could almost cut the meat with my fork. A Kobe steak could not have been any better. What did you have in mind for tonight?"

"Well," J.P. said as he took his first swallow of Mammoth Dry. "There is a little known secret about another steak that Annie serves. Do you trust me?"

"Trust a Navy officer? I don't know about that," he said laughing. "Yeah sure I trust you, order up."

"I took the liberty of anticipating your answer and ordered two steaks before I joined you." Annie walked up with a tray containing two plates with large steaks and a mound of sauteed vegetables.

"Here you are, two of my best steaks. Skip, I assumed that you like veggies, I know J.P. does." She put the plates down along with two more beers that she had brought along. J.P. noted that Skip was watching Annie closely.

Skip said, "Hmmmm, mystery meat. You gotta love that." He picked up his knife and fork, "Here goes."

They watched as Skip slowly chewed his first bite. He cut another piece. His face expressed deep thought as he finished chewing. He reached for the mug of beer and took a long drink. He looked over at Annie and J.P. who were waiting expectantly. Slowly a smile formed on Skip's face.

"Okay, what kind of steak is this? I have never had a steak that tasted quite like this. It's slightly sweet like it's been marinated. That's it, isn't it? Marinated beef?"

"Nope," Annie said. "Do you like it?"

"I'm not going to answer you until you tell me what kind of meat this is or at least what animal it came from," he paused and became serious. "Are you guys into exotic animal meats? If you are, this is not a joke. I don't go in for that kind of stuff." Skip started to push his plate away.

J.P. was about to say something when Annie spoke up, "No, honestly, Skip. This is not marinated beef and it is not what you would call an exotic animal. It was purchased here in California. How is the beer, Skip?"

"Don't change the subject, Annie," he replied a little humor coming back into his voice. "The beer was and is great. The combination of whatever this meat is and the beer was very pleasant to the palate."

"I see, just pleasant," Annie said feigning hurt. "Hear that, J.P.? Just pleasant, not great."

"Okay, yes it was great. Now what the hell is it," Skip's voice started to rise again.

J.P. started eating his steak. He decided that if Skip saw him eating then he would believe it was all right. After a couple of bites, he decided to at least give Skip a reason for the mystery, "Well, the identity of the steak is nothing very exciting, but Annie and I decided that we would have to clean our plates before she'll disclose the source of the steak." Skip started to argue. "Don't try and argue with Annie, Skip. I promised her I wouldn't tell and there is one thing I never do that is breaking a promise to Annie. So dig in and enjoy before the meat gets cold." J.P. continued eating and Skip reluctantly did the same. Annie smiled and went back to work behind the bar.

They watched her walk away. Annie knew that they were watching and she rolled her hips in a slightly exaggerated manner as she walked.

"Speaking of choice beef," Skip commented.

J.P. responded seriously to the words, "A fine woman I can handle, Skip. But referring to her as choice beef is out of bounds." Then he smiled, "She is a real friend and we protect and look out for one another."

"Are you and Annie a team?"

"If you mean lovers, no, we are just good friends."

"This is a nice little world you live in, J.P. The people are friendly and there are things happening that seem to show a bright future for the area. Is there any real hostility between the crowds that come up from LA and the locals?"

"Nah, not really. Most of the people that are referred to as locals originally came from LA. Annie is the exception. She was born and raised in Mammoth Lakes. The locals know that the folks from LA provide nearly 80% of their income. We have a few product industries here, but most people derive their incomes from the skiing, bicycling, and fishing. There's even an LA person on the city council."

"Sounds like a great place to retire," he paused. "Last night after you left for home, Annie and I had a chat. She said you are and I quote 'among other things' a business writer. Did you come here to retire or write?"

J.P. laughed, "Both really. Although I still have to travel quite a bit for research and consulting. Annie's reference to 'among other things' refers to consulting I do for business friends and the government. Still, it's always nice to be back home in Mammoth. Next time you're up, let me know and I'll have you over to the house."

"J.P., this is somewhat personal and I hope I'm not treading out onto a mine field here, but I.," he paused. "Hell, I feel like I'm back at the Naval Academy asking my roommate if I can ask his sister out on a date. Here goes, J.P., do you have any problem with my asking Annie out?"

J.P. was stunned for a second. He immediately regretted not answering Skip more quickly as his pause insinuated that there was more to his relationship with Annie than there actually was. Still, he couldn't help but feel a twinge of jealousy run through him.

"Hey, Skip, you don't have to ask my permission. Annie runs her own life. Like I said before, we're good friends and we support one another. It's up to

Annie as to whether or not she'll go out with you. I'm sorry if I gave you any other impression."

They sat in silence for a few minutes as they finished their beers. Annie, noting from her position behind the bar that they had finished eating, came over and joined them at their table. She brought two more beers.

Once Annie sat down, J.P. spoke, "Skip, we promised to tell you about our dinner, so I guess we should." J.P. leaned further over the table and took on a serious look. He took another drink of his beer. "There is an animal that is very prolific. The animal is so populous that it is hurting the agriculture of the country in which it is indigenous. It roams in the wild without fences. It doesn't eat a lot, but there are a lot of them. Their meat is very lean. In fact it is the best cardiac meat available, even better than the beef you had last night. There are two reasons that we did not tell you the name before dinner. Both reasons are emotional reasons, not chemical."

Skip looked from J.P. to Annie and back to J.P. again, "What do you mean emotional reasons?"

"The question is better answered by example. You ever notice on a restaurant menu how they never call dolphin meat what it is, rather they call it mahi mahi? Do you know why?

"Sure, because no one would eat it. Everyone would think they were eating Flipper. I suppose the same holds true with deer meat... nobody wants to eat Bambi." Skip stopped and then said, "Say, this wasn't some special Sierra deer, was it?"

"Nope, not even close."

"Okay, what is the second emotional reason?" J.P. noticed a slight edge in Skip's voice with his last question as though he was getting tired of playing guessing games.

"The second emotional reason is that the country whence this animal comes uses the meat for dog food."

Skip was growing increasingly impatient, "Okay, so what was it that I ate? Mule meat?"

"No, not mule, not deer, and not mule deer.it was kangaroo."

"Kangaroo," Skip shouted in amazement?

Annie spoke up, looking around the crowded room, "Skip, please keep your voice down."

"Kangaroo," Skip said in a whisper, "no shit, kangaroo?"

"There are over one million kangaroos in Australia and they have three babies going at the same time. Joey is in the pouch, another embryo is growing and will crawl out its way into the pouch as soon as Joey leaves. There is another fertilized egg ready in the fallopian tubes as soon as the embryo starts its trip to the pouch and so on. The gestation period is nine months, but it is almost continuous."

"Either the male or female kangaroo has got to be the horniest critter I have ever heard of, or they never heard of Planned Parenthood," Skip said, laughing.

J.P. continued the story, "Some enterprising Australians decided to start a kangaroo herd just southeast of Bishop, in the Owens Valley. You should see the size of the fences that are needed to keep in a kangaroo. The ranch is over 100,000 acres. The Aussies think they might have something and I agree. What do you think, Skip, would you have another kangaroo steak the next time you are up here in Mammoth?"

He didn't hesitate, "Yes, definitely. But next time you two want to introduce me to something new, let's dispense with the mystery game."

"Hey, if we had asked you to try a kangaroo steak, would you have said yes?"

"Probably, but with reservations.

J.P. chugged down the last of his beer and stood up from the table, "Well, kids, I'm sorry to break up the party, but I have to get home and get some sleep before tomorrow's trip to New York. I have to be up by 4:00 a.m. to fly to LA and catch the 8:30 flight to Newark."

Both Annie and Skip stood to say goodbye. J.P shook Skip's outstretched hand. "Skip, it was a pleasure meeting you. Hope to see you again, soon. And you.," J.P. said walking over to Annie, "I will, as usual, miss you. I'll call when I know my schedule."

He whispered in her ear, "See you, love, have fun."

Annie gave him a soft slug to the kidneys as he walked by on his way to the door.

6:00 P.M., SUNDAY, JANUARY 22

NEW YORK CITY

J.P.'s flight from Mammoth to LA had been routine, as was the airline flight from LA to Newark. In LA, he had parked his private jet at the commercial aviation terminal and left instructions for the mechanic to perform a routine maintenance service on the engines and then store it in the hangar.

Upon arrival at Newark Airport, he was very pleasantly surprised to find that Janet had thought to hire a limo to pick him up. After a full day of flying, the chauffeured limousine was a treat.

When he climbed into the back of the limo, he told his driver to head to midtown Manhattan. He realized he had barely looked at the email that Janet had sent to him in Mammoth and had no idea where the apartment was located. He began searching through his briefcase until he located a copy of Janet's email.

He leaned forward and said to the driver, "Driver, my destination is 348 Edgar Allan Poe Street....wherever the hell that is."

He sat back, bewildered by what he had just read. He had spent a number of years prowling around Manhattan, but had never come across a street named for Poe. He thought that there was some history behind naming the street and then reminded himself that he was in New York City and Edgar Allan Poe Street did not necessarily mean that it had any connection whatsoever to the famous poet author.

At any rate, he noticed that the driver seemed completely unfazed by the address. He simply turned his head slightly to the right and replied, "No problem, Dr. Koenig. I know where it is."

He sat back and watched out the window as the limo emerged from the Lincoln Tunnel and made its way to West End Avenue. The streets and sidewalks were surprisingly clear of snow and ice. He guessed that there had been a few days of warm sunshine since the last snowfall to dry up the pavement.

As the limo drove past the Spectrum of Medicine Building at 64th Street, he thought to himself that Edgar Allan Poe Street must be in the vicinity of the office. He began watching the street numbers climb. Finally, after passing 83rd Street, the limo turned left onto Edgar Allan Poe Street. The sign on the other side of West End Avenue read 84th Street. The driver drove to the end of the block, which was also the end of Edgar Allan Poe Street and stopped in front of an eight-story building. Since there were no other buildings between it and the Hudson River, he decided it must afford some spectacular views of Riverside Park, the river, and the escarpment of the New Jersey Palisades.

The building doorman opened his door. The cold, moist outside air filled the inside of the limousine as he stepped out onto the curb. He moved under the awning that extended from the front of the building where a space heater had been installed to warm the residents as they waited for a cab.

The doorman smiled as if he had known J.P. all of his life. "Good evening, Dr. Koenig. We were expecting you. My name is Charles and I have three messages for you. I'll bring your bags up for you." The doorman loaded the luggage onto a cart and led J.P. into the small lobby of the building.

The lobby was typical 19th Century New York City. A small counter, which resembled a hotel check-in desk, was off to the right side. Behind the desk, built into the wall, were pigeonholes for messages. On the left side was a floor to ceiling wall mirror probably placed there to give the illusion of a larger lobby. Everything else was wood except for the floor which was marble with an Oriental rug. Three artificial trees were strategically located to make things look bright and spring-like. The last two interior decorating items were straight-back chairs. They were probably used for those residents who required more warmth than the heaters under the awning outside provided. The single elevator was to the rear of the lobby between the desk and the mirrored wall.

Charles had gone behind the desk and brought out three envelopes from the pigeonhole for J.P.'s apartment. "Dr. Koenig, here are your three messages. The elevator is to the rear of the lobby. You are on the eighth floor. Up on the eighth floor there are two penthouse apartments. You will be staying in Penthouse South."

After Charles handed J.P. his messages, he pushed the cart loaded with luggage towards the elevator. The elevator was small and looked to be about 1920 vintage. The door was wrought iron design and had a large polished brass handle that Charles pushed down and with a flick of his wrist folded the door to one side. He then pushed back the chain door to the elevator and gestured for J.P. to enter.

"Please, Dr. Koenig. Please go on up to the eighth floor and I'll be up shortly with your luggage and key to your apartment."

As J.P. stepped into the elevator, he felt the small elevator box drop about three inches. He turned and gave Charles a startled look.

"Antique elevators, Dr. Koenig. The building's owner won't allow them to be changed. He says it adds charm to the building which, by the way, was built in 1907. Don't worry the elevator is in good condition. I make sure it is inspected monthly and it was completely rebuilt less than ten years ago." He reached around the elevator door and pushed the button marked, PH, for penthouse. "See you in a few minutes, sir."

The old elevator rose slowly making faint creaking sounds the entire way. At each floor there was a loud click and clank. He looked over at the elevator inspection certificate and discovered that it had been inspected within the past month.

He started thinking about the apartment above. Good apartments were always difficult to find in New York, particularly on short notice. He hoped that it would at least be habitable.

The elevator slowed noticeably as it passed the fifth floor. Finally, reaching the top floor, he pulled back the inner and outer doors.

As he stepped onto the firm floor, he began to wonder if he wasn't developing some sort of elevator phobia.

The thought of having to ride this elevator back down to the ground tomorrow morning and then fly to the top of the Spectrum of Medicine building to see Phillip was almost more than he could bear.

He closed the doors and the elevator began descending back to Charles. After a few minutes the doors opened and Charles stepped out wheeling the luggage cart behind him. He reached into the pocket of his coat, pulled out a key chain, and opened the door to Penthouse South with his master key.

J.P. walked into the apartment and was immediately pleased with his surroundings. Compared to his experiences in the lobby and elevator, he felt that had finally emerged through some sort of time warp into the lattertwentieth century. He was standing in a very large living room. The ten-foot ceilings consisted of molded plaster in symmetrical designs and cherry wood crown molding framed the designs perfectly.

The walls of the room were pained a pastel green. On the wall to his left was a home theater and stereo system. Whatever wall space was not taken up by the audiovisual equipment was floor to ceiling bookshelves. The opposite wall had a large fireplace. The room was sparsely furnished with a couch and coffee table in the center and a total of five speakers for the home theater system arranged around the room.

J.P. turned around to see Charles carrying the last of his suitcases in from the hall.

"Is there anything else I can do for you, Dr. Koenig?" Charles asked. "No, thanks. I appreciate all that you have done for me. I'm sure I can find my way around," he answered as he handed him a ten-dollar bill.

"Thank you, sir. If there is anything I can do for you please call me on the phone to the right of the door. It rings in the lobby and I respond right away, that is if I'm not doing something for another tenant at the time." Charles turned and walked out the door, shutting it behind him.

J.P. walked across the thick living room carpet to the three large windows. The view was southwest by his reckoning, down the Hudson River towards the James Spectrum of Medicine building. He noticed a bouquet of freshly cut flowers and a basket of fruit on the coffee table. He walked over and sat down on the plush couch. Attached to the outside of the basket of fruit was a note with his name on it. The envelope had a slight perfume scent. He tore it open and read the note inside.

> Dear J.P.,
>
> I hope you have found the apartment to your satisfaction. Janet mentioned to me that she had the task of finding you an apartment for the months you would be working at James. I have some dear friends who always go to Florida for the winter. On July 1st they return to the city for the summer and fall. I thought that you would like the way the apartment is designed, so I asked them if James could rent it for you. They agreed. I know this is not Mammoth, but it is as close as we can get for you in New York City. If you do not like the apartment, I am sure we can find you another place.
>
> When you get settled, if it is not too late, give me a call at (201) 5556793. Enjoy your new home.
>
> Sincerely, Mandi

J.P. set the note down on the coffee table and smiled. It occurred to him that if the rest of the apartment was anything like what he had already seen, she seemed to know him better than anyone else he had ever known. He surveyed the living room again as he stood up from the couch. There was a desk that he hadn't noticed before in a corner next to the door. On top was a computer that looked to be the same brand and model that Phillip had on his desk. He decided it was time to see the rest of the apartment.

There was a long hallway on the fireplace side of the room that led away into darkness. He turned on a light that illuminated the hallway and walked about five feet until on his left he came to a double door. When he opened the one side of the door he found a staircase. He closed the door and continued down the hall. The length of the hall was hung with beautiful oil-on-canvas replica paintings of Renoir and Monet. He knew the reproductions were likely the result of high-tech laser imaging and were virtually perfect reproductions of the originals that captured the vivid colors, surface texture, and even brushstrokes of the artists. After another ten feet there was another door. It opened into a nicely sized bedroom. He closed the door and continued down the hallway.

At the end, he found the kitchen. It was an elegant gourmet kitchen. Almost everything in sight was copper. He looked around for his favorite appliance, the microwave and located it on the counter in a corner.

On the other side of the kitchen was a swinging split three-quarter door. He went through the doors and entered one of the most elegant dining rooms he had ever seen. Two of the walls in the room were glass with a western view of the Hudson and the New Jersey Palisades. The southern view was the same as the view from the living room. There were stereo speakers in all four corners and the ceiling had a very large skylight. Drapes were bunched in the corners and he presumed that they could be pulled across the glass walls for privacy.

J.P. moved back down the hallway to the double doors and walked up the staircase. At the top he found himself standing in the master bedroom. It was magnificent. A huge room with a California king bed, which struck him as very unusual for New York. The headboard for the bed was against the north wall next to the staircase. One glass wall looked south. Along the west wall was a fireplace that tied into the flue for the fireplace in the room below. As he had found in nearly every other room in the place, there were four speakers in the corners. The master bath was done in a beautiful marble and contained every sort of bathroom fixture or convenience that one could imagine. There was a spa, a sauna, a shower, and a large Jacuzzi tub.

He walked back downstairs to the living room. He picked up a small bunch of white grapes lying in the basket of fruit and walked over to the desk. Next to the computer was a telephone and answering machine. The answering machine was blinking. He hesitated before pressing the playback key. He didn't know if someone from James had placed the answering machine there or if it actually belonged to the apartment's owners. Finally, he decided that since he was going to be living there for a while, he should see for whom the message was intended. He pressed play and heard Mandi's voice.

"Hi, J.P., how do you like the apartment? We were betting that you would love it. Janet and I had decided that this place would be perfect for you.

"The owners are a couple in their 40's and they love the outdoors and music, as you've probably already ascertained. The owner is a workaholic but he does like to work at home. He is an executive with a stock brokerage. They are a great couple and I hope that you will someday be able to meet them. Anyway, give me a ring once you 're settled. My number is on the card with the fruit. See you. Bye."

J.P. picked up the phone and dialed the number on the card.

"Mandi, hi, J.P. I wanted you to know that the apartment is perfect and miles beyond my expectations. I don't know how you read my mind, but it's perfect. Thanks very much."

"You're welcome, J.P. and since I know how great the place really is, I hope you will invite me over for dinner some evening when we do not have to work.

By the way, what are your plans for tomorrow? I've set aside all of next week to work with you."

"I will present a status report to Phillip tomorrow morning. Most of the next few weeks will be spent talking with the department heads. In my reading I came across a few items that require clarification. I still have no clue as to who made the copy of the 21st Century Plan or why. On the other hand, I really didn't think I would have an answer at this point, so I guess I can say I'm on track. I am up to speed on most of the macro issues. I have to dig into some more of the micro aspects, but there's still time to do that. Anything new happen at James since last Wednesday?"

"No, nothing, everything is calm. We are preparing for the January board meeting next Thursday. Rumor has it that Mrs. James is going to be really rough on Phillip. He requested that we prepare a comprehensive report on Lifeal. Although it was a great deal of work we pulled everything together. If we have time I would like for you to review it and perhaps share some of your creative ideas with me."

"No problem. I'd be happy to take a look at it. What time is Phillip's staff meeting tomorrow?" he asked.

"Ten o'clock."

"Great. I'll see Phillip at seven for an hour. How about meeting in your office at nine? We can go over the week's schedule."

"Good idea. I look forward to seeing you. Sleep well," Mandi said before hanging up.

J.P. hung up the phone and decided to work on his status report for Phillip. He was about to speak to the computer when he realized that this wasn't his computer and had no voice command system. He switched on the machine and began typing.

Date: January 24

To: Phillip T. Bradsmith, Ph.D. From: Jean PaulKoenig, Ph.D. Subj: Status Report

Recent Activities:

Reviewed the 21st Century Backup Plans and read history of pharmaceutical herbs.

Expected Activities of the Next Few Weeks:

With Ms. Hayes, interview the department heads on specific issues that I feel are important to the project.

Identified Issues:

Availability of Lifeal raw material Lifeal market plan

Conclusions:

None found at this point. Support Requirements:

No additional support required.

He read over what he had done. He knew that Phillip liked concise reports. He looked at his watch. It was only ten o'clock… seven California time. He watched a cable television movie and went to bed at midnight.

6:00 A.M., MONDAY, JANUARY 23

SPECTRUM OF MEDICINE BUILDING NEW YORK CITY

"Ah, good morning, J.P." Phillip asked as the executive elevator doors opened.

Phillip surprised J.P. by his personal welcome. He calmly stepped off the elevator and shook Phillip's hand. "And a very good morning to you, sir," he said with a smile.

The two men turned to walk back towards Phillip's office. "How were things in Mammoth?" Phillip asked.

"Things in Mammoth are pretty darn great. You know, Phillip, some time when your schedule permits you should join me in Mammoth for a few days of skiing. The snow and the slopes were perfect last week. I was able to get in several runs in-between my homework for James Pharmaceutical. The best surprise though was when I arrived back yesterday and saw the apartment that Janet and Mandi found for me on Edgar Allan Poe Street. The place belongs to friends of Mandi who spend their winters in Florida."

Phillip turned to look at J.P. as they entered his office. "I see. Two questions. Where in the hell is Edgar Allan Poe Street and second, when did you begin calling Mandi, Mandi? What happened to Ms. Hayes?" Phillip gestured for J.P. to sit down at the conference table. Phillip walked back to the outer office for coffee.

J.P. spoke up so that Phillip could hear him in the outer room, "Well, let's see, Edgar Allen Poe Street is really a one-block section of 84th Street between West End Avenue and Riverside. And second, it is still Ms. Hayes, I slipped." He smiled as Phillip returned with two mugs of coffee and sat down at the table with J.P. "Anything else you would like to know?"

"Yes, actually. I've been enormously curious about the consulting work you have done with the Navy. Anything you can tell me about that?"

J.P. looked down at his mug and then back up at Phillip. "Not really Phillip. The work of CMAG is, to put it bluntly, top secret. But there is some background information to your situation that I can give you because it is public information and therefore declassified. My Navy group became involved as it supported the CIA in a growing corporate espionage situation. We became involved as we were both civilian and military.

"In the early nineties the intelligence community with all of its various spy apparatus began to see a growing and determined increase in corporate espionage. It was particularly troublesome that most of the effort was coming from overseas companies.

"As vast as the intelligence community in the United States is, there was no one with the specific mission of tracking down or squashing foreign private efforts with the potential to destabilize the US and possibly the global economy. The first red flags went up when an aerospace contractor providing surveillance aircraft to the military inquired if it was possible for military intelligence to help them out with a problem they were having. Seems foreign aerospace companies bent on carting away little tidbits of information here and there were overrunning them. They had hired a private counterintelligence company to help, but the methods employed by the foreign companies and presumably their respective governments were so sophisticated that the private guys were soon in over their heads.

"As I'm certain you can well imagine, the military was absolutely the wrong entity to take on something like this, even though they probably had the greatest personal interest in getting this particular problem stopped. In the end, it wound up in the lap of CIA who immediately pushed it back to Justice and the FBI. The agency's thinking, and not incorrectly, is that because CIA has no law enforcement authority, there wouldn't be much that they could do. Another argument the agency put up was that the FBI had recently set up its own counter-terrorism division and since, in the agency's view, this was finally an issue of economic terrorism, the FBI should be handling it.

"The fee-bees, on the other hand, were quick to point out that they were up their necks in the counter-terrorism business and what they called real terrorism. The FBI has their hands full trying to track the movement of bomb or biological-carrying terrorists and thwart their entry into this or any other friendly country. They also dispatched an investigative team every time a friendly nation asks for help following a terrorist attack. So the last thing the FBI wanted was the additional mission of tracking down nefarious individuals stealing business secrets. They also felt that since the CIA already had the systems and field agents in place to combat this increasing threat, they were in the best position to keep their finger on the pulse of what foreign companies were up to here and abroad.

"Shortly after the squabble began, the media picked up on the story and began sowing seeds of panic among business groups. I'm sure you remember the entire hubbub."

Phillip nodded and said, "Yes, it increased my own paranoia by several degrees."

J.P. took a sip of coffee and said, "And with good reason. The pharmaceutical industry as a whole is the largest offender and conversely the most helpless victim. The issue finally made it to The White House where apparently the FBI and the CIA sat at opposite sides of the Oval Office pointing fingers and defending their respective rice bowls. In the end, the President forced them to agree to cooperate in the effort. The CIA uses its resources to keep tabs on what interest foreign companies may have in obtaining American business secrets. Once they identify a player, they turn that information over to the FBI, which then add their name to its growing list of terrorists to track.

"Because this was a fairly new mission for CIA, they enlisted CMAG to provide insights into what a company might have that a corporate terrorist would want." J.P. suddenly stopped not wanting to say anymore. "Well, anyway, that's it in a nutshell." J.P. pushed the short status report he had written across the table to Phillip.

"Well, it sounds as though I may have hired precisely the correct person for this job," Phillip said as he quickly read through the report. He looked up above the rims of his reading glasses and added, "But, then, I always knew that.

"J.P., I assume you received all of the information you requested from us when you were last here? Is there anything I can do for you this week?"

"Yes, to your first question and no, to your second question. Everything is on schedule." he made a point of changing the tone of his voice and said, "Phillip, I do feel there is something going on here at James. I know this statement contains both good news and bad news." He paused and Phillip looked back up at him. "I understand that you have a board meeting this week. Is there anything I can do to help you prepare for the meeting?"

"No, not at the moment. I feel confident that I can weather Thursday's storm. Under normal circumstances, I would ask you to join the meeting, but I think it will be better for us to keep you at a low profile until we know what is going on here at James. I would not want Mrs. James to think you and I were up to anything untoward."

"That's fine, Phillip. It's probably best to keep the element of surprise on our side so she doesn't have time to subvert our strategy. By the way, where is my office?"

"Ah, yes, there is an office on the same floor as Mandi's office. It is a corner office with a view of Central Park. I trust you won't spend your days counting clouds," he said with a smile. "There is already a nameplate on the door. Just turn left out of the elevator and follow the hallway around. The office is equipped with a networked computer. Should you require additional supplies, please let Janet know. I would like you to attend my Monday morning staff meetings. They start at 10:00."

J.P. rose from his seat. "Okay, I'll see you then."

He left Phillip's office and took the elevator down to the eighth floor to look for his office. He was pleased with what he found. The furniture was very modern looking. The top of the desk was semicircular in shape with no sharp corners. Behind the desk outside the windows that lined two walls of the office was a view of Central Park. He dropped his briefcase on the desk and hung his overcoat on the coat tree near the door, turned on the computer, noting that it was indeed a very adequate system equipped with the removable hard drive that he had requested.

After performing a cursory look through the computer's programs, he decided to look around the floor to familiarize himself with the layout. He found Mandi's office suite at the opposite corner of the floor. The outer office was empty so hne walked past the secretary's desk to the Mandi's office door. He knocked and heard her say, "Come in."

When J.P. first opened the door he didn't see anyone. He was looking at a view that swept down the Hudson to the Verrazano Narrows Bridge. He looked behind the door and saw Mandi's desk in the corner away from the windows. She had arranged her office to take advantage of the view.

Mandi smiled when she saw him and rose from her chair to greet him. "J.P., how good to see you again. How did you sleep in your new apartment?"

"It good to see you again too, Mandi." He paused. "May I call you Mandi?"

"Of course you may," she replied. He detected a slight blush spread across her face.

"Mandi, the apartment is outstanding. Thank you very much for making that happen."

"Well, I'm glad you like the place. I was a bit concerned that you wouldn't like the décor, I really don't know you that well. The Petersons, that's the name of the owners, are really great people. He is a successful investment banker in the high tech field. His name is Peter. I really don't know, what sort of a parent would name their son, Peter with a last name of Peterson? Lydia, his wife, is a successful entertainment attorney. They have a great time together wherever they go. Because Peter's field is a global market, they spend a great deal of time traveling overseas. They have a lot of fun and I am always just a little envious.

She walked over to the conference table near the window and invited him to sit down. Well, I think we should spend some time getting our project together.

Right. The information that both you and Phillip provided me was a good start. I have already seen Phillip this morning and given him my first weekly status report. he handed a copy of the report across the table. Here is a copy of the report. As you can see I'm still in the information gathering stage. I do feel there is something going on here at James. It's more of an instinct than anything substantive, but I feel there is sufficient evidence on the periphery to warrant a look. I don't know whether someone on Phillip's staff is the source of whatever intrigue there is, or the board, or both. I do know there are enough weak spots in the James' organizational structure that could be exploited by someone bent on damaging this company. By weak spots I mean situations that exist that seem to be open ended. A good example of an open-ended issue is the possible short supply of the raw material for the production of Lifeal.

So, what is your schedule?

I think the first thing we should do is review the Marketing and Finance Departmental plans. Marketing for two reasons. First, because you are familiar with this department. Second, I happen to believe the marketing department is the focal point for all activities that make a product a success. Friday, we can meet with the finance department. There is a board meeting on Thursday and your CFO will be only too happy to take a break from reciting financial reports to the board. Next week I'd like to spend in the production department and the following week with R&D. If you agree with this proposed schedule, I'll call Janet and have her start calling people to firm up the meetings.

Mandi's face suddenly showed concern. J.P. knew she was likely worrying that she would be spending all of her time over the next few weeks, following him around on interviews.

Mandi, you don't have to spend all of your time with me. I realize that a great deal of my work will be covering ground that you are already quite familiar with. I would like you with me when I talk with the department heads. I'll conduct the rest of the employee interviews myself. My main purpose here is to develop a real sense of what is going on in terms of products and projects. I also want to get to know some of the people involved in the critical work. Everyone I talk with will probably peg me as a spy for Phillip so I'll have to win over their confidence before I can get to the real issues that will help us unravel the puzzle. I'll keep you apprised of everything that goes on when I am on my own. Does that sound okay to you?

Fine, J.P., you're off to a good start. I suppose that if we uncover anything we wish to analyze further, we can always change the schedule. She looked at her watch. It's almost time for Phillip's staff meeting. Before we go, I want you to meet Beth, my assistant. She has been with me since I joined James. I have asked her to help you with whatever you require. She's very resourceful. Mandi walked to the door and asked her assistant to step into the office.

Beth, I would like for you to meet Dr. Koenig. As you know, he'll be working with us for a few weeks on a special project for Phillip.

J.P. extended his hand, saying, It's good to meet you, Beth. Please call me, J.P.

J.P. and Mandi took the elevator up to Phillip's floor and then walked to the conference room next to his office.

He was surprised at the reception he got as he walked into the conference room. He knew just about everyone from his previous days as an employee of James. The executives gathered around the table had worked their way up in the James organization, with the exception of Helmut Wahlters. Doc James had hired him specifically for the position of senior vice president of R&D.

Phillip entered the room at precisely 10:00 and took the seat at the end of the table near his office door.

Good morning. I am sure you have all noticed that our friend, J.P. Koenig, is back from the sunny wilds of California. I am also certain that you are all probably wondering just why he is here. Well, to put it bluntly, Lifeal is not setting the world afire. With Mandi's concurrence, I have asked J.P. to work with us on Lifeal for a few months to give us a new perspective on this valuable James product.

He looked around the table, winked at J.P., and said with a smile, It's not that I feel J.P. is altogether brilliant, he just has an uncanny way of looking at things differently than most of us. He wasn't here for the product launch or the marketing that followed the launch, so I'm hoping that he may find something we have missed and am particularly hopeful that he will find some things we're doing correctly.

Mandi will be working with him on this project. I expect each of you to give him your full support. He paused again, looking around the room.

J.P., why don't you give the group an overview of what you have been doing for the past few years and also the tentative plan for your new James project.

J.P. rose from his seat to address the group. Thank you, Phillip. It's good to see everyone again and to be back at James, even if it is only for a short time. First, I would like to comment on the wonderful things you have done for this company. Your outstanding effort is demonstrated in the fact that you are located in this beautiful building and have an exciting product like Lifeal on the market. I have a high confidence level that Lifeal will enjoy the success that was envisioned for it and I hope to help you to achieve that success.

Ms. Hayes and her team have done an excellent job and, let me assure you, there are no shortcomings in your marketing programs. I am here to see if I can lend a hand in identifying other alternative means to success. As those of you who know me can attest, I am a no-nonsense person. If I see that I'm unable to contribute anything, I'll be the first person to say so and exit the scene.

As to what I've been up to lately, I can sum it up by saying that I've been doing some consulting with the federal government, doing some teaching, and writing business strategy books. My last title, The Strategic Continuum, has been well received both in the business world and academia. In between all of that, I ski, hike, and ride mountain bikes. I live in Mammoth Lakes, California at the foot of Mammoth Mountain.

As for my plan for this project, I will be working with Ms. Hayes...Mandi...this week getting familiar with the marketing research studies and the market plans on Lifeal. Brian, if your schedule permits, I would like to talk to you on Friday. Joe, I would like to work with operations next week, and Helmut, R&D the week after that. Janet Williams will confirm my schedule with each of you.

Joe and Helmut, Mandi and I would like to meet with you personally on the Monday afternoon of the week that I have scheduled for your department and discuss Lifeal. The rest of the week I would like to work with people whom you have assigned to Lifeal. This means both the managers and the hourly employees. I don't want to disrupt their working day, but I do want to learn all that I can about Lifeal. Please let me know if I get in the way. I will meet with you personally at the end of the week to debrief you on my findings concerning your respective departments. Finally, if during my discussions anything comes up that you should be aware of, please be assured that I will contact you personally as soon as possible. Any questions?

J.P. knew that his statements had bordered on orders, but he did not want a discussion and he wanted them to know that he meant business. He looked at their faces and was pleased that he didn't have any disagreement. He reminded himself that it was likely that someone at the table had made an extra copy of the 21st Century Plan. For what reason was still a mystery.

Phillip broke the silence by saying, "No questions? Splendid. Okay, let's get on with the agenda. A copy is in front of you." Phillip leaned over to J.P. who was seated on his left and said quietly, "I know of your fondness for gadgets, particularly utilitarian gadgets. Wait until you get a load of this. Welcome to my little command center."

Phillip picked up a remote lying on the table next to him and pressed a button. The paneled wall at the far end of the room split in the middle and separated on tracks that carried the two pieces of wall into unseen spaces on the other side. Three wall mounted video screens were left exposed. Phillip pressed another button and the room began to darken when a set of heavy curtains was automatically drawn across the windows.

He again leaned toward J.P. and said, "The curtains are made of a material that allows enough light into the room to allow people to take notes, yet repels any methods of electronic eavesdropping."

He looked over at Phillip and said, "Very impressive."

Each staff member in the room had prepared their presentations on the computers in their offices and then sent them to the conference computer over the company's intranet. The presentations appeared on the center video screen. If more than one chart was programmed to be up at one time, the first chart was moved to one of the video monitors on either side of the main video. J.P. soon learned that Phillip demanded crisp statistical briefs with specific actions.

Mandi spoke first about sales dollars and units for each of James' major product lines. The actual figures were compared to fiscal year plans and monthly projections. She discussed the product mix changes and product line profit and loss. She next gave a briefing on the current and upcoming sales support programs and ended with the new and refill prescriptions for the previous week. Through various databases and audits, a company could determine how many new and refill prescriptions each product was receiving from physicians.

He noted that even though Lifeal was growing in all prescription categories, it was a very small growth. Certainly not fast enough for what was termed a "hot" product. There was also a large gap between the actual figures and the fiscal year plan. The monthly budget was slightly more accurate, but still too far off to be within business tolerance.

Joe Marshall, the chief operating officer and vice president of operations discussed material availability, capacity, product mix changes, cost of goods changes, efficiency labor issues, and forecast-to-actual ratios for each major James product line.

He never mentioned anything about the possible shortage of Lifeal raw material. Buried in his presentation was a comment that the unit forecast of the higher dosage Lifeal was moving faster than the lower dosage. He concluded that this might be the first sign of a product mix shift. He made a note of the comment to discuss with Joe later.

Helmut was next. He reported on product side effects, regulatory issues, and the status of products yet to be released. He droned on and after his allotted ten minutes, Phillip cut him off. J.P. looked at Helmut and saw a brief sign of anger in his eyes, but he stopped talking.

There was nothing substantive in Helmut's presentation. The expected Lifeal side effects were running at a rate either lower than or at predictable rates. He mentioned that JPC138 was in stage one clinicals, but that there was no clinical information to report.

Brian gave the last presentation. He presented the product P&L's and the expense budgets comparing everything to the fiscal year plan and monthly projections. He knew from his own previous tenure at James that Brian was not a typical finance person for whom numbers ruled the day. He understood what was behind the numbers and tried to intervene on financial situations before they became problems.

Brian was also the largest physical presence at the table. He was 6'7" and had played basketball at Indiana University. He was a good-looking man with an angular face and fine features. J.P. recalled from his reading of the personnel files that Phillip had known Brian from Phillip's days as a James product manager. Then, Brian had shown a lot of promise as an analyst. Phillip had convinced Doc James that Brian should be allowed to attend graduate school for his MBA. After some discussion of Brian's potential long-term contribution to James Pharmaceutical, Doc James agreed to the idea. The company paid for the graduate program at Wharton and Brian repaid the company by finishing first in his class of 180. In subsequent years,

Brian had gone to night school at Columbia and received his Ph.D. in economics.

Brian concluded his financial analysis by saying, "Because Lifeal is not selling up to projections, it is imperative that we tighten up on expenditures and new hires. For four straight months now, we've missed profit plan and monthly projections. The new board directors that Mrs. James brought on board have been on the phone to me asking very detailed questions about the finances. I suspect we're in for a food fight at this week's board meeting. Along with the usual first look at the financial report for year's end, I will have a special financial analysis package on our last six-month expenditures. I'll have a copy of the report on your desk by close of business tomorrow for your review. I would recommend that you and I go over your board presentation on Wednesday. I'll schedule time with Janet. J.P., it's good to see you again and I look forward to talking with you soon."

Phillip wrapped up the staff meeting with a summary of all the presentations and outlined the plans for the week. He reminded everyone that their board meeting briefs were due to him by noon on Wednesday. Everyone left the conference room and returned to their respective departments where they chaired their departmental staff meetings.

J.P. attended Mandi's marketing department staff meeting and met all of the members of her marketing team. He was impressed by her excellent leadership capabilities. She allowed people to present their ideas and observations and then helped them come to conclusions with follow-up actions. She spoke directly to the point without excuses or unnecessary rhetoric.

At noon, Mandi asked J.P. to join her for lunch in the James Executive Dining Room. They took the elevator to the lobby where the kitchen and dining rooms were located. The dining room was spacious with an open area and a number of private booths where business could be discussed privately.

After they were seated, Mandi spoke first, "So how did you like your first morning at James?"

"Very well. I thought you did an excellent job at both staff meetings this morning," he replied. He paused and then said, "Mandi, I would like to make a suggestion." "Please do."

"The first person I want to talk with is Frank Ascot. As the Lifeal product manager, I don't want to put him in a situation where he feels he is on trial. I have to able to ask him anything I want. I don't want him to try to cover up any of his previous actions or alter statistics to make himself look good to you. My suggestion is that you not attend my sessions with your people. I'm hoping that this will make everyone more open...not that they have anything to hide, but I have found in similar situations that conversation is often less strained. When I work with the other department heads, I'll be asking them not to attend the session with their people."

J.P. carefully watched her face for any evidence of how she was taking his suggestion. Seeing nothing, he continued, "How do you feel about that?"

Mandi did not hesitate, "No problem, J.P. I think your suggestion is very good. I have a good group and while I'm certain they will answer your questions the same whether I'm in the room or not, I understand your point."

"Good. With your concurrence I will meet with Frank right after lunch. I want him to show me his Lifeal market plan for this fiscal year. I'm interested in learning how Lifeal is actually performing in relationship to the market plan. After the presentation, I expect to spend the rest of today and probably much of tomorrow discussing Lifeal with him. On Wednesday, I'd like to meet with your sales director and Thursday, with the head of market research. If you want to drop in on any of the meetings to get a feeling on how things are going, be my guest. On Friday, I'd like for you and I to talk to Brian together."

"Sounds great," Mandi said while nodding her head. "I'll have Frank meet you in the marketing conference room at two o'clock."

Their conversation continued through lunch, mostly of the old times at James. Mandi seemed genuinely interested in all of J.P.'s stories and asked many questions about the products and marketing programs that he had been a part of in the past.

After lunch they were drinking coffee when suddenly he said, "I don't know whether you like to work on weekends and I don't want to interfere in your social life, but I would like to go over the results of our first week as soon as possible. If you're not busy this weekend, is there a chance we could meet on Saturday to discuss the results and make plans for next week over dinner?"

Mandi looked up over the rim of the coffee cup as she was drinking. She lowered the cup and smiled. J.P. thought she looked more relaxed than he had seen her since they had met.

"J.P., are you asking me out for a dinner date?"

He felt his face flush. He was almost as surprised as she was that he had even asked. He decided to play it off.

"Eh well, just a test, Mandi. I don't want to mess up your weekend. We can discuss the project on Friday afternoon or Monday morning."

Mandi's smile faded somewhat as she tried to figure out his strategy.

She decided to call his bluff.

"Oh no. You're not getting off the hook that easily. I'd love to go to dinner with you Saturday night."

6:00 P.M., MONDAY, JANUARY 23

BERGEN COUNTY COURT HOUSE WYCKOFF, NEW JERSEY

Ralph Vandermere walked down the stairs of the Bergen County courthouse. He had performed okay in court that day.

He had done everything correctly except for a few episodes when he had to stop and pull himself together. That was the only way he could think to explain it. As he sat listening to the prosecution making their case, he would suddenly become drawn to his own reflection in the acrylic top of his table. He just sat there staring into his eyes seeming to see into the core of his own soul. After the third occurrence, he realized that it had been five days since he had changed his dosage back to the prescribed one tablet every day. He knew the side effect was getting worse. He decided to stop at the pharmacy on his way home and discuss the episodes with his pharmacist.

After court adjourned for the day, Ralph drove the twenty miles from the Bergen County Court House to the small shopping mall off New Jersey Route 208 where the pharmacy was located. Ralph parked his car in the lot and walked into the pharmacy, making his way to the rear of the store where he knew he would find his pharmacist. Somewhere along the way, he thought he heard someone ask "May I help you?" but he didn't pay attention.

When Ralph finally reached the glass enclosed pharmacy department, he saw his pharmacist, Hank Somerset, bent over and thumbing through a large book.

"Hank, hi. How are you doing?"

Somerset looked up briefly from what he was doing and responded, "I'm doing okay, Ralph. How about you? How are you doing on that new medication? You've been using that for a couple of months now haven't you?"

"Actually, Hank, it's been eight months, three days, and I don't know.," he looked at his watch, ".six hours. But that's why I'm here. I'd like to talk with you about some strange side effects I'm beginning to have with that prescription you gave me."

The overweight, balding pharmacist did his best to show concern and moved from behind the glass wall, stepping down the two steps from the raised platform where he filled prescriptions to stand in front of Ralph.

"What's that, Ralph? Are you having problems?" he asked.

"I'm not sure what's happening, Hank. That's what I have you for isn't it?" Ralph said forcing a smile. "I get funny feelings when I take this drug everyday. I tried taking it every other day, but I felt my heart fluttering again. Last Thursday I went back to the original dose of one tablet every day."

Somerset was, at first, stunned by what Ralph had told him. He made an effort to speak without sounding as though he was scolding one of his most loyal customers.

"Ralph, you know better than to change a medication dosage on your own. I instructed you to take the product carefully and exactly as the label stated. Have you spoken with your physician?"

Ralph's gaze shifted slightly to the glass wall where he was again being drawn into his own reflection.

"No, Hank. I don't think it's that bad."

"Well, you should let me decide that. You aren't trained to make those kinds of decisions. What sort of side effects are you experiencing, Ralph? You'll have to be more specific than just saying that you've had funny feelings."

Somerset noticed that Ralph wasn't looking at him, but seemed to be staring at the glass wall behind him. Hank turned slightly to look over his shoulder to see what it was that Ralph was staring at. When he turned back, Ralph was looking directly at him.

"Hank, I know you may think I'm crazy, but I...well...I over think." "What do you mean, over think?"

"When I am actively involved in some mental activity, it seems like I want to perform to higher levels. No, that's not what I mean. I don't want to perform necessarily. It's more like I automatically perform to higher levels. I'm very mentally alert all of the time. The really weird part is that this is especially true when I see a reflection of my pupils. I am able to remember everything I have done and read over my entire life." He paused for a moment and then continued, "I remember things I don't want to remember. It seems like any knowledge I desire is always immediately in my consciousness. I have so much information spinning in my memory that it is even hard to sort out all of the alternatives to answering a question. Sometimes I just sit, mesmerized, as I sort out the information in my mind and then I am.brilliant in its dissemination. I call this my vision." He looked pleadingly at Somerset.

"Just a minute, Ralph, you're getting ahead ofme. Is this information jumbled and confusing?"

"Nope, it's clear as a bell. In fact, if you allowed me to read a package insert, I could remember everything, every word…probably forever."

"I see. Well, speaking of package inserts, let's look at the insert for that drug. Do you have the prescription bottle with you?" he asked.

Up to this point, Somerset didn't know what product Ralph had been talking about. He had been using his standard answers to customer questions hoping to get by without having to answer specific clinical questions.

"Gee, no, Hank. Since I only take it once a day, I always leave the bottle at home. Should I call Joan and get the prescription number or do you have it in your patient records?"

Somerset panicked for a second. His assistant was gone for the afternoon and he didn't understand the record retrieval system well enough to find a customer record, but he wasn't going to admit that to Ralph.

"You better call Joan, Ralph. It'll be easier than going through the new fangled record system that the royal state of New Jersey requires me to keep on all of my customers. I'll even spring for the phone call," he said handing the telephone over to Ralph.

Ralph knew immediately that Somerset didn't know what he was talking about. He toyed with the idea of walking out of the pharmacy to go see Dr. Rosenberg, but that would require more waiting and Ralph felt himself becoming increasingly intolerant of waiting for anything. Ralph took the phone and called his wife. Ralph wrote down the number that she gave him.

Somerset ascended the raised platform behind the glass and typed in Ralph's name. Ralph's entire prescription history appeared on the screen. He found that Ralph was taking the James Pharmaceutical Company product, Lifeal. He walked back into the drug area to retrieve a bottle. The package insert was attached to the bottle. He unfolded the insert and scanned his way to the side effects section. He walked back down to the counter pretending to read as he walked.

"Let's see what we have here."

Hank continued to scan the thousands of words of medical information that the FDA required in a package insert. He knew that whatever else he did, he had to find something that tied in with Ralph's problem. He moved his index finger across the small print until he came across a condition he knew something about, hyperactivity. That could fit Ralph's condition. It wasn't a direct fit, but Somerset knew that Ralph wouldn't understand anyway.

"Ralph, I think I found it," he exclaimed. The package insert states, and I summarize, one of the side effects a patient can experience during treatment is hyperactivity. What you have explained to me seems to fit the definition of this side effect. What do you think?"

Ralph lowered his head slightly, thinking. "Well, I do have more energy. I thought the excess energy was from less strain on my heart and the fact that I've lost weight. I guess you could say that I'm hyperactive. What does it say I should do about my hyperactivity?" Ralph was beginning to feel better about the situation. Hyperactivity did not sound too bad and, in fact, at his age sounded rather good.

Somerset continued, "Since hyperactivity is in the package insert and it says that it's a common side effect during therapy, you should just keep a good watch on the situation. The hyperactivity should go away as your body adjusts itself to the pharmaceutical. When is your next visit with Dr. Rosenberg?"

"In one week. Should I call him before the appointment?"

"Nope." If the situation gets so bad that you're unable to continue your normal daily routine then I would call him. Frankly, the way you've explained this side effect, it sounds like you're benefiting. Maybe we should suggest that James Pharmaceutical bottle the side effect all by itself. Lord knows, I could use a little memory enhancement."

Ralph wasn't so sure. The things he saw in the reflection of his eyes were not the result of hyperactivity, but he could think of no other explanation. He put out his hand to shake and said, "Are you sure, Hank?"

"Sure as I can be, Ralph."

"Okay, Hank. Thanks for your help." Ralph turned to leave the store.

Somerset watched Ralph leave and then moved back behind the safety of his glass wall.

11:20 A.M., WEDNESDAY, JANUARY 25

SPECTRUM OF MEDICINE BUILDING NEW YORK CITY

Yesterday, J.P. had called Phillip's secretary, Janet.

"Hey, how are you doing? I'm sorry I didn't get the chance to talk to you Monday. How about the lunch date I promised you last week? Is Wednesday okay?"

"Sure, J.P., that's great. Is 11:30 okay with you?" Janet had replied in a cheerful voice.

"11:30 is perfect. I'll meet you in the lobby. How about Tavern on the Green in Central Park?"

"Fine! See you Wednesday."

Now as J.P. stood waiting for Janet in the lobby of the Spectrum of Medicine Building, he watched the snow that was beginning to fall in earnest. There was also a strong wind swirling around the tall buildings that caught the snowflakes in hundreds of white whirlpools. He had seen this type of storm before and knew this was the beginning of a heavy snowfall.

He thought back over the last two days of interviewing two members of Mandi's staff. First, he had spent a day and a half with Frank Ascot the Lifeal product manager and this morning he had spent in meetings with the James Director of Sales, Jake Crossman. He thought to himself that he had spent too much time teaching these two managers and not enough time exploring the mystery of the 21ˢᵗ Century Plan. Yet, he had to establish his cover of helping the marketing of Lifeal.

When J.P. had first laid eyes on Frank Ascot sitting at the conference table he looked to be quite tall. When he stood to shake his hand though, he discovered that he was actually about average height. Frank had a medium build and dark hair with sharp facial features. His eyes looked too small for his face and were a dark color that J.P. thought almost perfectly matched his hair. He was wearing a double-breasted charcoal pinstriped suit with a light gray silk handkerchief in the left breast pocket. He smiled as he approached. It was a warm smile, but seemed to J.P. to betray more than a little bit of nervousness.

J.P. knew immediately that Frank likely couldn't figure out whether the meeting would be good or bad for his career. J.P. shook his hand and noticed there was a trace of moisture in his palm and his shirt had French cuffs with gold cuff links. The watch was a Rolex. J.P. had spent his time with Frank going over product management issues.

Then this morning with Jake, this had been frustrating. Jake never gave direct responses to any of his questions. He always countered with a question, which J.P. interpreted as a way to keep the focus off his own performance. When J.P. asked him how he managed his sales force, he responded that he didn't manage the sales reps, rather he directed their every movement. This, he felt, made his sales reps work harder.

He had known sales directors like him before. Jake's personality type usually survived in a corporation when he was responsible for a dramatic product line and fast-growing sales. James had neither.

J.P. had become particularly concerned for Mandi. Her two key Lifeal managers were definitely not the best for this product. A conservative product manager who believed in the uninspiring strategy of maintenance pharmaceuticals was marketing Lifeal and an old-style autocratic sales director was leading the sales force.

His thoughts of the past two days were interrupted when he felt two arms wrap around him from behind.

"Boo!" Janet said. "Have you been waiting long?" "Nope, just a few minutes. You ready to go?"

"You bet. You know it's really kind of a nice day despite the snow, how would you feel about walking to the restaurant?"

"Great idea."

He and Janet stepped out into the snowstorm and began making their way across Central Park to Tavern on the Green. The walk was certainly cold, but the scenery was great. J.P. felt there were few cities as beautiful as New York during and right after a snowfall. The trees in the park were already covered with snow and their was the wonderful sound of snow crunching beneath their boots.

Janet spoke first, "You know, J.P., I'll bet this is going to be a good one. I remember another storm several years ago that had the same size snowflakes and followed the same path up the eastern seaboard. I'll bet most people have already started heading out of the city for home."

He was about to respond when a hard gust of frigid wind hit him in the face and sucked the air right out of him. When he recovered his breath he said, "Yeah, and we should probably be doing the same thing."

"Why, J.P.! Don't tell me you would rather be someplace else other than with me in a snowstorm!"

"Oh no, I can think of no one I would rather be with anywhere, anytime," he answered putting his arm around her shoulders.

It took them forty minutes to get to the restaurant. Once inside they checked their coats and snow boots. The checkroom clerk gave them warm slippers. They walked down the corridor of stained glass to the Crystal Room where the maitre d' ushered them to a table for two. The room was lined with glass windows. Green, red, and blue colored chandeliers hung from a ceiling of pastel plaster. The chandeliers cast shadows on the bright flowered tablecloths. Hundreds of potted flowers were encased in three-foot planter walls, which divided the room like a maze providing a spring retreat in the dead of winter.

They decided to share a bottle of Beaujolais Nouveau and ordered lunch. For a time, their conversation drifted among various subjects. J.P. was happy to be able to spend time in pleasant conversation after his three days of interviews. After a few minutes, the waiter brought out their soups. They had both ordered the soup of the day, carrot and ginger. Their conversation ceased while they ate.

J.P. looked at Janet as she ate and he thought that she looked great. She was wearing a red blazer over a black turtleneck. Her shoulder-length brunette hair streaked slightly with gray was full and shiny. She wore large gold earrings that showed nicely beneath her dark hair. He thought she was a handsome woman and that, Bill; her husband was a very lucky man.

"You know something, Janet. You look great!" he suddenly exclaimed.

His comment had caught her off guard and she nearly dropped her spoon. "Huh? What did you say?"

"I said that you look fabulous," he said with a smile.

Janet blushed slightly, set down her spoon, and looked at him. "Why, thank you."

He was about to say something more when the waiter appeared with their entrees. Janet had a lobster salad and J.P. had the special, Duck Confit with lentils. They ate quietly and sipped the wine.

When they had finished their meal and were waiting for coffee, J.P. decided to broach the subject that had prompted their lunch together.

"Janet, when we last talked you said you wanted to update me about Bill and his new company. Do you want to talk about it?"

She smiled and stared out the window to her right. "It is so relaxing sitting here with you in this wonderful scene and sipping wine. I don't know that I want to discuss work. I haven't felt this relaxed in quite some time. I could sit here forever.

"Uh huh. You can't fool me. I know you too well. You're far from relaxed. I too could sit here with you and cherish this moment, but I would like to know what Bill is up to."

Two years ago, Bill got this opportunity to work with a start-up in clinical chemistry. As you know, he was Phillip's right hand. Bill didn't see himself growing within James nor did he see himself having the opportunity to make big money. He was in his mid-forties, had been with James for twenty years, but he had never been the director of anything."

She paused, her gaze fell back on J.P. "J.P., I know that you've never known how it feels to always be passed over for promotions. You've always been the guy who was offered the really great positions of leadership in companies. At James, Bill never found his own leadership situation. All of a sudden he realized he was growing old and could not handle being in someone else's shadow. When the venture capital guys approached Bill, they gave him the chance to be the boss and make big money. This was an opportunity that James, for whatever reason, did not seem interested in giving him. Bill expressed interest in their proposal. He discussed the position with them for three months. He asked Phillip for advice and tried his best to get Phillip to see his dead-end situation at James. Granted, Phillip has enough worries with James Pharmaceutical, but he never seemed to really listen to what Bill was trying to tell him. When the venture guys made Bill the offer, with a great salary and a 10% stake in the company, Bill felt he had to go for it.

Janet paused and the two of them sat in silence for a moment, just watching the snow falling outside.

J.P. broke the silence, "Janet, what's the project that Bill is working on?"

"Bill's company is in the clinical chemistry business, but not in the general sense. In many respects it is also in the pharmaceutical business. The simplest way to explain what they do is to say that their technology helps to detect disease and titrate patient dosage."

J.P. immediately knew what Janet was talking about and was very interested. Detecting disease was always important and others have been successful in developing chemical analysis instrumentation for detection.

As for the titration, he knew that it has always been difficult to titrate an individual patient's dosage of a pharmaceutical. Each patient has different degrees of tolerance and reaction to a drug. Dosage was usually based on weight and/or metabolism. Most of the time, patient product tolerance was based on subjective criteria such as how does the patient feel or has there been any side effects?

Pharmaceutical companies even established the physicians' sample package to determine a patient's tolerance to their product. The physician is supposed to give the patient one or two days supply of samples and a prescription. He tells the patient to try the drug for two days and then, if tolerated, take the prescription to the pharmacy to be filled. The free product sample also acted as a discount on the price of the pharmaceutical. If the patient had problems with the drug, they were to call their physician who would in turn change the dosage or the product.

"J.P., the company had already worked on some chemotherapy products when Bill arrived as the new president. These tests were very accurate, but the cost-to-benefit ratios were not as good as the physicians and third-party payers expected, so the tests have not sold very well in the marketplace. The volume of tests has to be higher to justify the cost of the instrument so Bill turned research to market segments with a higher number of potential market segments of patients, like tranquilizers, pain, hypertensives, gastric, and hormonal pharmaceuticals.

"The key to developing this test and successful sales is complete cooperation with the pharmaceutical company that manufactures the drug. Bill wanted to talk to Phillip about developing dosage titration tests for some of James products and then work on an enzyme test to determine cardiac arrhythmia. This would help Bill's company and Lifeal.

"He received the cooperation of some hormonal pharmaceutical companies, but he was afraid there would again be a problem with cost-tobenefit ratios. Since Bill has not obtained a test for a high volume product the sales of his company's instruments are not very good and the venture capital companies paying the bills were getting restless and are beginning to tighten the financial screws. To hear Bill tell it, they have screwed things down so tight that he can't move and his efforts to make agreements with pharmaceutical companies is being hampered. Physicians are starting to postpone the purchases of the instrument and the pharmaceutical companies who just a few months ago looked as though they were coming around to an agreement, are now taking a wait and see position. Bill calls it the venture capital whirlpool effect.

"I've been caught in that same venture capital whirlpool a few times and I know it's no fun. There are a few tricks I know that could probably give Bill enough breathing room to operate. I'd be willing to share these with him. Does Phillip know about Bill's company?"

Not really, with all the issues he is handling I don't think he has had time to understand the product.

"Janet, with the next few weeks ask me over for dinner at your home. I'll talk to Bill about some start-up tricks that will at least give him a lifeline in the whirlpool to keep him afloat. I'll also find an opening to discuss Bill's product with Phillip. How's that for a plan?"

Janet's face showed that she was pleased with J.P.'s answer. Now she at least had something to tell Bill. She reached over and placed her hand on top of J.P.'s and gently squeezed.

"You would really do that for me.for us? You're a good friend, J.P. I'll never forget this."

J.P. placed his other hand on top of hers and said in a quiet voice, "I haven't done anything yet, Janet and I don't know how much help I can actually offer, but I'll do as much as I can. You can be assured of that."

J.P. looked at his watch. "Now I think we had better head back. I have an afternoon appointment with Jake Crossman."

Janet's eyes went wide and she raised her hand to her mouth trying to muffle a laugh, "Have you met him yet?"

"I met with him all morning. He's certainly old school. How does he get along with Phillip?"

"Phillip hardly ever sees him. He works through Mandi. I don't know for certain, but I do not think Phillip and Jake are on the same wavelength. Jake seems to do his best to avoid Phillip."

"Between you and I, Jake doesn't seem to fit in with the corporate image at James, but as long as he performs I guess he is okay. I'm not looking forward to the rest of the afternoon with him."

It was two o'clock when the two began their trek back to the Spectrum of Medicine. The wind from the west had picked up considerably in force and was blowing directly into their faces as they walked west on 65^ت Street. The heavy snow made walking difficult. Automobile traffic was beginning to come to a standstill. There were snowplows out on the streets but they were not keeping up with the rate of the snowfall. The only thing moving today would be the subway and the trains. By midnight, the trains would stop and except for walking and the subway, the city would come to a halt.

After they had been walking for a while, J.P. asked Janet about the 21st Century Plan. "Janet, do you trust all of the members of Phillip's staff?"

Janet didn't answer right away. J.P. wasn't sure whether she just didn't hear the question because of the wind or was just forming an answer. He was about to ask her again when she spoke up.

"I have always accepted the staff's loyalty because they are Phillip's team and to think otherwise would complicate my job. Since you've arrived on the scene and I have found out a little about the project you're working on, I have, for the first time actually considered their loyalty. I don't think there is any question about Mandi. I could say the same thing about Brian, especially since Phillip is his mentor... although you never know about financial executives. They're sometimes more loyal to their numbers, but Brian seems very different. So, yes, I would say Brian is loyal and wouldn't do anything to hurt Phillip or James. Joe Marshall is a worker. He does his job. He came up through the ranks and is happy as long as he is allowed to do his job. Helmut, on the other hand, was and is still a Doc James man. He misses Doc because Doc was more of an R&D person than Phillip. There is some strain there, but not enough to purposely subvert James.

"To answer your question, I just don't know. It would seem to me that the board would be more suspect than any of the staff." Janet became silent for the next block. Finally, she said, "J.P., this storm is really bad and I'm beginning to worry about getting home. I think I'll ask Phillip if I can go home early."

"Knowing Phillip, he has already given the employees the option to make their own decision. He doesn't want the employees living outside the city to be stuck in town."

They did not speak again until they arrived in the lobby of the building.

As they came into the building a mass exodus of people leaving met them.

"You know Janet, you should call Phillip from here and see if you can go home now. It's obvious that he has released the employees."

"Good idea. Thanks very much for the lunch and conversation. See you tomorrow, I hope." J.P. entered the elevator for the ride back up to his office. He walked to his office before going to meet Crossman. He wanted to check for messages on his voice mail. He moved around his desk until he could see the voice mail light blinking on his phone. He picked up the handset and dialed the access number for his voice mailbox.

The canned voice greeted him, "Good afternoon. You have three messages in your voice mailbox. First message, received at…1:30 p.m…today."

J.P. immediately recognized Jake's voice, "J.P., Jake here. I am sorry, but I have been called away to a meeting in New Jersey. I'll give you a call in the morning. Sorry about our meeting."

"End of message. Second message, received at…2:10 p.m…today."

It was Phillip, "J.P., it looks like we're in for a big nor'easter, the kind you and I prefer to see atop a ski mountain. I have let the employees who want to go home do so. If you have about thirty minutes before you leave today, I would very much like to go over tomorrow's board meeting presentation with you. I'm going to stay here tonight and not take the risk of going home and becoming snowbound. I somehow doubt that Mrs. James would appreciate my attending a board meeting via telecommute. How about 5:30? Please let me know."

"End of message. Third message, received at…2:15 p.m…today."

J.P. heard Mandi's soft voice, "J.P., how is the day going? Phillip has let everyone go home. I have too much to do here to go home early. I would like an update on the results of your meetings with my people. Would you please give me a call when you get back to your office? Where the hell are you, anyway?" she said half-laughing as she hung up.

He dialed Phillip's number and was not too surprised that Phillip actually answered the phone. He knew that Janet must have gone home.

"Yes?" Phillip sounded testy.

"Phillip, J.P. 5:30 is great. Everything okay?"

"Ah, J.P., it's you. Yes, everything is fine save for the rest of the world not knowing that we have a snow emergency in the making here. I do not have anyone to answer the damn phones and have not had anyone to answer the phones since 11:30, for which you are, by the way, partly responsible. I cannot expect to finish this goddamned board presentation when I have to constantly answer ringing telephones. See you at 5:30," he said as he slammed the phone down.

J.P. called Brian's office and was surprised that he was still there. "Brian, J.P. Listen, Phillip is climbing the walls. Janet has gone home and he is answering his own phone. Can you round up someone who will be here the rest of the day and get he or she up to his office before he goes into sub-space orbit? I have to meet with him at 5:30 and I skipped the part of the MBA program that tells you how to deal with psychotic CEO's, if you know what I mean."

Brian laughed, "I know exactly what you mean, J.P. Not a problem. That's why we've kept a staff pool here. Consider it done even if I have to answer them myself."

"Thanks, Brian." J.P. thought that Brian would do it himself if necessary.

J.P. picked up his phone again and dialed Mandi's number. He spun around in his chair to look out the window. By his estimation, visibility was now probably reduced to about fifteen feet in the wind-driven snow falling outside.

"Mandi, hi. I'm back from my long lunch and I received your message. In answer to your question, I took Janet over to Tavern on the Green. I had a meeting with Jake scheduled for 2:30, but he took off for a meeting in Jersey."

"Yeah, well, Phillip let everyone go who wanted to beat the storm. Jake lives in New Jersey and we all know what it's like over there in a snowstorm."

J.P. thought, "Yeah, right. He probably hit the trail before Phillip ever gave the word."

"Well…so do you want to see me now, Mandi? I can give you an update if you like. I have to see Phillip at 5:30."

"Yes, please, J.P. I'd appreciate knowing how things are going," she said in a very businesslike manner that didn't go unnoticed.

"Okay, I'm on my way over."

He hung up and walked to Mandi's office at the other corner of the building. He wondered what was bothering her.

3:30 P.M., WEDNESDAY, JANUARY 25

SPECTRUM OF MEDICINE BUILDING NEW YORK CITY

As J.P. walked into her office, Mandi got up from her desk, walked to her conference table, and sat down. J.P. took a seat directly across from her as he had before. Mandi smiled at him, but it seemed to J.P. to be a forced smile.

J.P. broke the silence, "I'd forgotten just how bad the weather in New York can get during the winter." They both looked out the window at absolute whiteout conditions.

"Yes. So, J.P., how were your meetings with Frank and Jake?"

J.P. was stunned for a second by what he thought was a very defensive tone in her voice. He decided to proceed cautiously.

"Great, Mandi," he replied with a high level of enthusiasm. "They are both very talented people with a lot of potential. I'm curious, did you handpick them for your marketing team?"

J.P. was probing to find out just how Mandi felt about Frank and Jake before he expressed his full feelings.

"In a way they are my choice," she said.

J.P. noted a softer tone in her voice, "Do you want to tell me about it?" "No, not right now. I would rather hear your thoughts on Lifeal."

J.P. smiled at the way she managed to parry his tactic. He knew she must be a tough manager.

"Okay, straight up. I'm going to present my thoughts about where Lifeal is positioned and then go through why I feel the way I feel. I'll try my best to keep emotion out of my assessments.

"First, Frank is a good short-range planner. You've trained him well. The maintenance dosage market and the Unhappy Patient TMS are good positions for Lifeal. On the surface it seems like this is the most logical and creative TMS for Lifeal, but is it really?"

Mandi leaned back in her chair and crossed her arms across her chest.

She squinted her eyes slightly and pursed her lips as she listened.

J.P. continued, "This is not a direct criticism of the program, but you have to admit that Lifeal does not win the physicians' prescription until another product fails. As you know, it is difficult to wait until a patient fails on another manufacturer's product before you get your product prescribed. An equally difficult sale is to have a product that is only sold for the difficult clinical cases. With that strategy, your sales force has a very tough job selling. They have to get by the physicians' defense mechanism in order to get them to listen to new information. That defense mechanism being a desire to defend their first choice. As you know, the physician feels they make the right choice the first time and never fail in their decisions for their patients. Under the James strategy, they have to admit that they have made a bad decision.

"These defense mechanisms plus the fact that the sales rep has to mention the competitive product which the physician chose as his primary product causes the physician to become very anti-Lifeal. You've chosen a tough TMS for Lifeal, Mandi.

"Frank also told me about the automatic shipment of the higher dosage. I am personally not a big fan of automatic shipments. I realize that they're necessary to fill up the distribution pipeline, which is fine to a point, but the usual reason is to make a short-term sales goal and not achieve product availability. If the reason is to achieve sales, the company will release products that are really not clinically necessary, but give the company a temporary sales hit." J.P. paused to see if she wanted to interject a comment. She made none. He looked out the window and as hard as it was for him to believe, the storm seemed to be getting worse.

"So, I asked Frank where the 50mg tablet was going to be positioned. His response to me was that it would be positioned in the same TMS. I asked him whether the 50mg dosage is a maintenance or therapeutic dosage. He told me that it was therapeutic, which leaves a slight inconsistency in the selected TMS. I didn't discuss this with Frank. My personal assessment of Frank is that he is a very talented person though not terribly creative. Frank would seem to be a good implementation guy as long as he can understand the marketing plan and the program was safe for his career. In other words, if he could achieve the plan without much trouble therefore keeping his job safe from criticism. I would imagine that he becomes very defensive when you stretch his vision much beyond a linear projection within the current year and existing TMS. This is a rough assessment concluded after only two meeting with Frank. Any questions or should I move on to sales and Jake?"

"Please do go on," Mandi replied with a distinct negative edge in her voice.

"My meeting with Jake was to be this morning and continue this afternoon. We had a good meeting this morning and we were to meet again at 2:30. When I returned from lunch, just before 2:00, he had left me a message saying that he had to leave at 1:30 for a meeting in New Jersey. One-thirty was before Phillip's announcement and I doubt that he had originally planned to go to the meeting since we were to meet again at 2:30. He just wanted to go home." J.P. paused and then decided not to pull any punches. "Jake is selling a product by the feature vis-à-vis benefit method. Now, while there is nothing wrong with this sales method, do you really think it is good enough for Lifeal? I detected in Jake a sense of high purpose, but it was what I would call the old fashioned method of sales management. He is placing a great deal of pressure on the sales force to sell, but he is not really helping them to sell. He is demanding that they sell. I was going to discuss this further this afternoon, but the storm prevented the meeting. In summary, I think I received enough information from Frank and Jake to move on to market research tomorrow. Will Carl be in tomorrow?

Carl lives in Manhattan, so yes, he should be in tomorrow. I'll set up a meeting for 9:00. Does that work for you?

That's sounds fine.

Mandi spent the next hour probing his meetings with Frank and Jake.

J.P. began to feel as though he were on the witness stand enduring a crossexamination of his previous testimony. He began to feel uncomfortable and not with her questions. It was her style, which prevented an open and frank exchange between the two of them. Finally, at 5:15, J.P. mentioned that he had a 5:30 meeting with Phillip to go over his board presentation.

Okay, J.P. I guess we've discussed Frank and Jake enough. You can go. I'll see you tomorrow after you meet with Carl.

J.P. felt stung by her curt dismissal of him, but decided not to respond in kind.

Thanks for your time, Mandi. I'll be happy to discuss this further with you as I learn more about Lifeal. Have a safe trip home.

Thanks. I hope I can make it home. I live in New Jersey, she said without looking up from the notes she had been taking during their talk. J.P. closed the door behind him and left for Phillip's office.

J.P. found the door to Phillip's office slightly ajar. He knocked on the door and heard Phillip's voice say, Come on in, J.P. Please take a seat at the table, I'll be with you momentarily.

Phillip was speaking on the phone, Yes, Mrs. James, I did hear you. You want direct answers to the slow growth rate of Lifeal and some specific action plans that will get the product back on track. Otherwise the board will instruct me to start cutting back R&D for JPC138.

J.P. took a seat at the conference table and tried his best not to overhear Phillip's conversation though it was immediately obvious to him that this would be impossible. Phillip was standing behind his desk and looking out the window at the snow as he talked. He was holding the phone about three inches from his ear. J.P. could hear Evelyn Preston-James yelling on the other end. Phillip was speaking in a very respectful albeit strained voice.

After some time, Phillip began to speak again. Damn it, Mrs. James, you know perfectly well that we are doing the very best we can with the resources we have available to us and the regulatory process we have to adhere to by federal regulation. I do not think it is necessary for you to say that we are not trying or that we are just out to spend your money. Doc James would know and understand what we are doing.

He grew quiet as the voice on the other end seemed to increase in both volume and pitch. When Phillip began to speak again his voice was softer, but the tone was very stern.

I will provide my report to you and the other directors tomorrow at the board meeting. I will not provide it for you or any of the other directors one minute before that meeting begins. Now then, I really must get back to work.

I have a meeting this evening. I'll see you tomorrow morning at 10:00. Thank you for calling, Mrs. James and please feel free to call anytime you wish to discuss what we're doing here at James Pharmaceutical Company. Goodbye.

As Phillip was hanging up the phone, J.P. could still hear Mrs. James screaming on the other end. Phillip gently placed the hand piece back onto the cradle. Sat down at his desk and turned towards J.P.

It has been one of those days, J.P. As we get older you would think the frequency of bad days would decrease, but instead they seem to increase in both frequency and intensity. He stopped talking and turned to look out the window. Looking at the snow makes a person long for the slopes. Do you miss Mammoth?

I do. Especially when I'm gone for long periods of time. This storm looks like a dandy.

Yes, I agree. Every time I see snow like this in the city, I always think of a bit from an old Johnny Carson monologue back when the show was based here. He said that the city should park its entire fleet of open dump trucks bumper to bumper on the streets of New York when snow was forecast. After the storm, the trucks would simply drive away with the snow and the streets would be clean.

Phillip smiled which J.P. took to mean that he was lifting himself from his funk.

J.P., I appreciate your being here with me during this stressful time. I also appreciate your help with the board and staying around so late this evening. If you have time I would like to review my thoughts on tomorrow's board meeting.

"Of course I have time."

"As you know, Evelyn.er, Mrs. James as she prefers to be called, has and is stacking the board against my programs. With the annual meeting just four months away, I know she is going to set up situations where board members who have been my allies will be replaced by more of her henchmen. I honestly cannot for the life of me figure out what she's ultimately up to with all of this."

"When does the annual report and 10K come out, Phillip?"

"They are due thirty days ahead of the annual meeting, so let's see...that puts it in the third week of April. The rules of the corporation state that the rough draft has to be in the board members hands sixty days ahead of the annual meeting, which makes that the third week in March. The James staff, especially Brian and myself, always writes the rough draft. Tomorrow I will be presenting some ideas, but I suspect Evelyn will counter whatever I propose."

"Has she actually stated that she wants more input into the annual report?"

"No, it's just a feeling I have about her. Anyway, let me give you my rough ideas about my presentation.

"First, I have to give a situational analysis on the operations of James. Then Brian will present the financial report on the last month and year-todate. I then ask Mandi to give a 30-minute marketing presentation and Helmut a 15-minute research presentation. I ask Mandi and Helmut to be excused and I summarize and present the James planned activities for the next six months. That is followed by a 15-minute discussion of the status of the 21st Century Plan.

"After the James current operational presentation, the other board members give their committee reports. The formal meeting should only take two hours from 10:00 until 12:00. We then have a catered lunch in the boardroom where informal discussions or presentations are conducted. Depending upon the informal discussions this section could take as long as two hours. The informal meeting was old Doc James' favorite time. He always felt the future direction was determined in these informal sessions when the directors were up to date and his advisors could freely discuss the strategies James should pursue. Doc James' board of directors was made of up of healthcare experts, unlike now when accountants and lawyers sit on the board.all of them doing their best to stifle any creative flow of information.

"Before I begin with what I am going to present, I was wondering if you have uncovered anything yet on the missing copy of the 21st Century Plan?"

"No, not yet. I'm still making my way through the organization. So far I've talked to Frank Ascot of market planning and Jake Crossman of sales. I finish the marketing department this week. Next week,

I'll be in Joe's shop and following week with Helmut and R&D. I may take a long weekend after that and head back to Mammoth to write a comprehensive report for your February 6th staff meeting. If I were to give you my gut feeling now I would say the James people I have met with are more concerned with the present than they are about the future. The person or persons who made the copy of the plan have got to be more focused on the future. It's been two months since we know the copy was made and there hasn't been a hint of anything out of the ordinary except for increased pressure on you from the board." J.P. paused and then asked, "Phillip, do you think I could sit in on the informal part of the board meeting? I would like to get some insight into the directors, particularly Mrs. James."

He paused before answering. "Yes, I believe that would be fine, J.P. You are here to help out with Lifeal and this is a positive action on the part of the company. It should also be a favorable sign that I'm being proactive. You are well respected in the industry. Yes, I don't see why not. Come in to the outer office at noon. The board meeting is held in the same conference room where we hold our staff meetings. Now, if I may, I'll quickly run through how I would like the board meeting to go."

Phillip spent the next hour going over the James formal operations presentation. There was nothing new in his proposed presentation. In fact, to

J.P. it seemed that the presentation he was giving was business as usual which didn't seem to him to be a good strategy in situation that calls for dramatic change. J.P. did not comment to Phillip on his concerns. He felt he needed more time to assess the complete picture.

"I will propose that our presentations to the shareholders focus on Lifeal's potential and the strong sales and profit performance of the rest of the James products. We tend to forget that our world is not just made up of Lifeal and JPC138. Our other products, which make up 75% of our sales and 90% of our net profit before taxes are performing better than plan. Last year, we had forecasted a 6% increase in revenues in the product line excluding Lifeal and 8% in total NPBT. Our achievements were actually 10% and 13%

respectively. Mandi's team has established renewed interest in some of the James mature products and achieved higher profitability by raising some of the prices. All of the price increases are holding firm in the marketplace contributing to the 5% improvement in profitability over plan. Joe has also made cost of goods savings by second sourcing some of the raw materials. I'm proud of what they have done to help make up the Lifeal shortfall. Of course, this does not make up for the fact that Lifeal is way below plan and is dragging down the total company revenues. In NPBT we are, in total, slightly above plan. Of course, Wall Street does not recognize our achievement because they say without Lifeal sales, success is short-lived. I agree with this assessment so my argument in support of our non-Lifeal achievements, yearto-date, is not very convincing.

"I intend to give JPC138 limited coverage at the annual meeting. I do not want to have the shareholders expectation outstrip realism especially when the directors might restrict our working capital. I will propose to retain the current board members especially those who support my programs. I'm afraid this will cause a minor fight. Evelyn wants two more cronies on the board who support her views. If my guys hold their seats on the board I will not have a problem. If there is a weakening of my group I could be in trouble. I'll continue to use my argument that we cannot have a board of all lawyers and accounting people. We require a board which helps to create strategy not one that just judges past performance."

"Phillip, I agree with your proposal and have nothing substantive to add right now. I'll be looking forward to the informal session. Is there any presentation scheduled for the lunch period?"

"Oh, yes. I've asked Jack Husted of the Wall Street Journal to talk to us about the global pharmaceutical picture. He should be good. He is a pain in the ass especially when we do not provide information for his advisory point of view in his daily column, but he is honest and very knowledgeable. I usually ask him to give a presentation as we near our annual meting."

"Sounds great, Phillip. If there isn't anything more for me, I think I'll head for my apartment. You are a wise man to stay here tonight. I'll bet the city is paralyzed by morning." J.P. rose from his seat and started for the door.

"See you tomorrow, J.P. Don't forget...noon...here in the conference room. Even with the snowstorm, I'm sure the meeting will not be cancelled. This storm is supposed to blow through sometime late tonight. If anything changes, I'll give you a call."

"Okay, thanks. Have a good nights sleep."

J.P. looked at his watch and saw that it was 7:00. He went back to his office and picked up some reading material, his briefcase, and his coat. He thought about calling Mandi, but decided that she most likely had already gone home. He took the elevator to the lobby and then walked out into the relentless storm.

The building maintenance people had shoveled or blown a two-foot wide path along the sidewalk to West End Avenue. After that, J.P. discovered, he was on his own. It was still snowing heavily, but it felt as though the wind had at least died down a bit since early afternoon. The snow was at least twelve inches deep and beginning to drift.

It was cold and J.P. wished that he had his ski jacket with him rather than an insulted overcoat. He stood for about ten minutes on the corner of 65th Street and West End trying to hail a cab. In the end, he decided to walk.

The snowplows were pushing the snow up onto the sidewalk, making it necessary to walk on the plowed street. The traffic was moderate on the street, so J.P. had to keep a watchful eye out for cars moving quickly along the edge of the curb. Occasionally, he had to scramble up on the pile of plowed snow to escape a certain death by traffic.

After four blocks of walking, a cab with its off-duty light on stopped and offered to drive him to the corner of West End Avenue and Edgar Allan Poe Street. He then had to walk the block to the entrance of the apartment building, but he was grateful for having gotten a ride at all. Charles, the doorman, greeted him.

"Good evening, Dr. Koenig. It's a bad one tonight," he said as he opened the door for him.

J.P. removed his overcoat and boots in the hallway outside of his apartment so that the carpets wouldn't get wet. He felt cold and hungry. He went upstairs and turned on the spa to bring it up to temperature. He looked up and noticed that snow had accumulated on the glass portion of the roof over the bedroom and spa. He hoped the glass was weight tested for wet, heavy snow.

He walked back downstairs and through the hallway to the kitchen. He opened the freezer and removed both food and Stoli. He decided to make fish chowder and began chopping up the ingredients which he dumped into a large crock he found in a cabinet and started cooking. He poured himself a good portion of Stoli and dropped in two olives.

While the chowder was cooking, he went into the living room and searched through the rack of compact discs until he found three CDs of Prokofiev's piano music and symphonies. He placed all three in the CD changer and turned on the stereo. He walked back into the kitchen to stir the chowder when he heard some chimes in the background. He thought perhaps it was part of the music at first, but after hearing the chimes for the third time, it donned on him that it must be the doorbell. He walked towards the door wondering who would be visiting at 8:30 in the evening during a snowstorm.

8:30 P.M., WEDNESDAY, JANUARY 25

EDGAR ALLEN POE STREET NEW YORK CITY

J.P. placed his right eye against the peep hole in the door and saw what appeared to be a woman completely bundled in a coat, scarf, and gloves. She looked as though she had just come inside from the storm. As J.P. watched, she unwrapped the scarf that covered her face and he saw that it was Mandi. He quickly opened the door.

"Mandi?"

"I'm sorry to bother you, J.P. Do you have a guest? If you do, I'll leave. You took a while to answer the door. I know I should have called before coming over, but I was walking on West End Avenue looking for a cab to help me find a hotel. I know it was stupid of me not to have made arrangements for transportation or a hotel reservation, but I simply didn't take the time this afternoon. I kept walking north and the next thing that I knew I was at 84th Street. I knew the apartment was only one block away so I took a chance that you were here alone. May I please come in?"

J.P. realized suddenly that he hadn't moved out of the doorway. The snow on her coat was melting into a puddle at her feet.

"Of course, of course, I'm sorry. Please do come in. I'm just so surprised to see you and I am alone, that is, no guests. You look frozen. Here let me have your coat. Take off those boots."

He hung the coat on the tree just inside the door and set the boots back out into the hallway.

"Look at you, you're shivering. Come in and sit by the fireplace, I'll light a fire. Can I get you a brandy, wine, or something?"

Without waiting for an answer, J.P. led her to the couch in front of the fireplace. He flipped the switch that ignited the gas fireplace.

"I know what you need, it'll only take a second or two."

He left her sitting on the couch in her stocking feet, staring at the fire. She was hunched with her hands clasped together between her knees pushing the black business suit skirt down between her legs. J.P. moved into the kitchen and heated a cup of water in the microwave to make some hot tea. He poured a medium slug of Scotch into the cup. Fumes rose up from the warm liquid and he knew that even if Mandi didn't like Scotch, she would probably like this drink. Before leaving the kitchen he gave the chowder a quick stir and turned the burner beneath the crock down to low.

When he returned to the living room he saw that Mandi hadn't moved from the couch. She was visibly shaking. He gave her the mug of tea and walked to the guest bedroom to retrieve a blanket that he then placed around her shoulders.

"Is there anything else I can get you right now?"

When she didn't respond, he knelt down alongside of the couch. "Mandi, are you okay?"

"Oh, J.P., I feel so stupid. I worked too late and then with this damn storm it became too late to get home to New Jersey. I called a few hotels and everything was booked. I thought I could get a cab to drive me around to a few hotels and see if I could talk some desk clerk out of a room. I'm sorry

J.P. I guess I really don't know you well enough to be taking advantage of your good nature," she said with a smile.

"Mandi, don't worry about it. You can stay here as long as you like. Is there anything else I can get you?"

"No, just let me warm up and I'll use the phone to call a few friends."

"No, no. You can stay here in the guestroom. I'll bet you've even used this apartment to crash when you were in the city."

"No, thanks, I really can't stay here. What would you think of me, especially when I was not the nicest person to you today," she said as she looked up at him. "And, yes, I have used the guestroom a few times after a party here in the city."

"That settles it then. You have the guestroom to yourself. Actually, I have an action-packed evening planned here that you're welcome to participate in as much or as little as you would like. First, there is a large crock of fish chowder simmering that should be done by now. There is warm sourdough bread and Stoli vodka to go with the chowder. When I came in this evening I turned up the temp on the hot tub and I was intending to sit in the tub, drink Stoli, and sop up chowder with the bread while listening to Prokofiev. After all of that, assuming I was still standing, I figured I would find some old movie on television to finish me off. Sounds exciting, huh?"

"Well."

"I know, you're speechless," he said laughing. "You're welcome to join me for all or part of the non-stop fun. I'll tell you what, I'll even wear a swimsuit in the hot tub. I don't do that for just anyone. Well, I'll leave you alone to think about it while I proceed as planned."

As he got up to walk back to the kitchen, he heard her say in a very soft voice, "Thank you, J.P."

When he reached the kitchen he found two large heavy ceramic soup bowls in the cupboard. He ladled out a large portion of chowder into his bowl, took half of the loaf of sourdough bread, and replinished his glass of Stoli. As he walked down the he looked in the living room and saw that Mandi was still sitting in the same position as he had left her.

"Mandi, the fish chowder makings are on the counter, help yourself. If I don't see you before breakfast, I serve at 7:00."

In the bedroom, he removed his sweats and put on a swimsuit, just in case she decided to join him in the hot tub though he figured she would most likely just eat and go to bed.

He set the bowl of chowder on the edge of the tub and slipped his body into the 104 degree water. He reached back and grabbed the bowl bringing it around in front of him. He tore off a large piece of the loaf and proceeded to dip the bread into the chowder. The chowder was good and he finished it in short order. After he finished eating he picked up his glass of Stoli and laid his head back on the edge of the tub.

"Excuse me, J.P. May I join you?"

He was so startled by the sound of her voice that he spilled some of the Stoli into the churning water.

"I'm sorry, I didn't mean to scare you. Guess that's twice tonight that I've surprised you. You looked so peaceful I didn't know how to announce my entrance."

J.P. looked up to see her in the dim light. She was dressed in a short robe that was made of some shiny material that he guessed was probably polyester.

"Well, I'm glad you're here. Jump in. The water's fine."

Mandi slipped into the water with her robe still on. The bottom of the robe flared up as she slid down into the water, but she quickly pulled it back around her legs.

"I couldn't find a bathing suit, but I did find this robe. I don't think my friends will mind. By the way, that chowder was excellent. I wasn't about to try eating in the tub. You Navy guys are used to eating in rolling seas or hot tubs...must be in your blood. I prefer a steady table, thank you. I do enjoy vodka and poured myself a Stoli. Hope that was okay."

"Absolutely. As I told you earlier, make yourself at home. Come to think of it, this place is probably more your home than mine."

Mandi dunked her head under the water and came back up. She pulled her wet hair to one side of her head with her hands and gave the end a twist to ring the excess water out.

She looked over at him and smiled. "You're so tan. How do you keep a tan all winter long? I feel so white."

J.P. laughed and said, "I think it's permanently burned into my skin. I get enough sun year round to keep the tan with skiing and all. Is the water temp okay for you?"

"Just right. Mixes well with the frozen Stoli."

There was no further conversation for about five minutes. He sat with his head back on the edge of the tub, listening to the music. As he looked up at the ceiling, he could see that the heat from the tub had melted the snow away. He could see that it was still snowing.

Mandi broke the silence, "I want to apologize for today. I wasn't a very pleasant person and I'm sorry. You were trying to help me and I was acting like a shithead."

"Don't worry about it. We all have bad days. No need to apologize." "No. My behavior wasn't caused by a bad day, there was, and is, a reason. I realize this isn't the time to talk business, but it's on my mind and I feel badly about the way I acted."

"It's okay. Go ahead."

"Thank you. We can talk about it more at the office." She paused and then continued, "Of course, you were right about Frank and Jake. That is what was making me so angry. They're not the right people for Lifeal. I know this, but I haven't had enough guts to do anything about it."

He was suddenly very interested and sat up. "Why are they where they are then?" he asked, realizing immediately how stupid that must have sounded. He started to phrase the question a bit differently, but Mandi was giggling.

"You don't have to repeat the question, I know what you're asking," she said and started laughing.

The warm water and the Stoli seemed to chase the previous tension of the day away. They began splashing each other and laughing.

"It's too bad the snow is outside. I can throw a pretty mean snowball," she said.

She made a motion as though she were throwing a snowball. When she did, her robe fell open and exposed her right breast. All of the commotion stopped and both of them froze. Mandi quickly pulled her robe back together.

"I'm sorry, J.P."

"This is not a problem, Mandi." They both started laughing again. "Go on with your story."

"Oh, yes...where was I? Oh yes, you wanted to know how those two came to be in positions of authority. The answer is simple. I inherited them. They were there when I took over the job. I took it as a challenge to see if I could bring them around. Guess I've not done such a great job as you so well pointed out to me today. I really wasn't mad at you, J.P. I'm mostly pissed at myself. Thanks for being so open and frank with me today."

"Nothing to thank me for, Mandi. And you shouldn't be mad at yourself. We all stick with people who are in the wrong jobs too long. We always think we can change them but we forget one thing. They feel they have got to where they are on the corporate ladder by being who they presently are, not by being who we want them to be. Did that make sense?" He continued without waiting for her to answer, "I appreciate your being honest with me. I'll help out if you want me to, but as you suggested let's do it at the office. Now then, I have to get out of this tub. You are welcome to remain if you wish."

"No, I think I've had enough." Mandi began to get out of the tub. "I do think I'll take a rain check on the movie. I'm going straight to bed. I'm tired and tomorrow is the board meeting."

Mandi rose from her seat to get out of the tub. Her robe was clinging to her body. J.P. made an effort to avert his eyes by turning to set his glass back on the side of the tub. When he turned back around she was standing on the bathroom floor with her back to him. She picked up a dry full-length terry robe that she had brought in with her and draped it over her shoulders. She began to wiggle out of the wet robe underneath. There was a wet sound as the robe hit the floor at her feet. Her arms pushed into the terry robe and she pulled the robe around her waist and began to leave the room.

She looked back over her shoulder, "Thanks again for everything, J.P. See you in the morning."

He went into his bedroom and looked at the clock on the nightstand. It read 10:30. He decided to forego the movie. He set the timer on the television to go off in two hours and lay down to watch a late night talk show. He was sound asleep in ten minutes.

9:00 A.M., THURSDAY, JANUARY 26

SPECTRUM OF MEDICINE BUILDING NEW YORK CITY

Carl Manningham, Jr., was on time for his meeting with J.P. regarding market research. Carl was a big man. He looked to J.P. as someone who weighed close to 300 pounds. His large baldhead and jowls reminded J.P. of the old Mr. Clean ads.

Mandi had warned J.P. about Carl's dry sense of humor saying that he will try to set you up. She also warned him to not take Carl's observations or comments personally.

After settling themselves into seats at the table, J.P. was about to speak when Carl asked a question.

"Why the hell are you here at James?" he asked in a very matter of fact manner.

J.P. was stunned for a moment. It was the first time since arriving in New York that he had been asked that question. As J.P. formed an answer to the question, he looked closely at Carl. He recalled from the personnel files that Carl was a Ph.D. He replied with what he thought was the classic consultant answer to a question the consultant doesn't want to answer.

"Why the hell do you think I am here at James?"

Carl let out a breath and said, "I was going to give you a wise-guy answer, J.P., but I'll save that for later depending on how this goes. Before I answer, I want you know that I don't appreciate your question as an answer to my question. I would hope after you get to know me you will have a little more respect for me. Since you do not know me I will overlook your lack of respect for, if not me, for my position and knowledge. I hope today's meeting will help you to begin to gain respect for me."

He continued without giving J.P. an opportunity to say anything, "Now as to the answer to your question of why I think you're here? First, I don't think you are here primarily to help us with Lifeal. I realize that we require help with Lifeal and I'm sure your insight into the situation will help, but help with Lifeal is way below the level of expertise for which you are known and for which I am certain you can provide James. There has to be another reason. I have not yet determined the other reason, but if I am right, I want you to know that I am ready to help you in anyway you feel that my talents may be of assistance. If you do not want to share the reason with me, that is fine as well. I do, however, want to make you aware of the fact that I will be watching your actions to see if I can deduce the reason for myself. This, by no means, should be perceived as a threat, just a statement. As you get to know me, which I hope you take the time to do, you will find out that I am very intelligent and very analytical. I am thought of as a funny fat man with a dry sense of humor. I am that, as well, but it is not the true me. I carry this burden of weight. I have, in fact, been likened to a sumo wrestler. I can assure you that in my forty-plus years of living I have tried innumerable means to reduce my weight. Some might feel that I am uncomfortable with my fat. This is not true. Once, a long time ago, I was much thinner. At that time I was uncomfortable with my thinness. Being thinner makes me feel ill. So, now, J.P., I am finished with my discourse. What say ye Mr. Lifeal mystery consultant?"

Throughout Carl's discussion of himself, J.P. had sat staring back him. At one point he realized that his mouth was hanging open and he forced himself to close it. J.P. decided that only time and proof of performance on substantive projects would convince him about Carl's credibility. As to whether Carl could be trusted as to J.P.'s real reason for being at James that too would have to wait.

Carl certainly had access to the data and information that was used for the 21st Century Plan. If he had the cerebral wherewithal that he claimed, he could use a copy of the plan to harm James in any number of ways.

"I say again Mr. Lifeal mystery consultant, what say ye?" Without waiting for J.P.'s answer, he added, "I do not mean to be insubordinate, J.P., but do you have a concentration problem this morning? If so, we can move our meeting to a different day."

"I'm sorry, Carl. No, I do not have a concentration problem," J.P. said as he sat up straighter in his chair. "I have been turning some things over in my head. I considered giving you the full briefing, but I have decided to wait. I respect your comments and insights and will seriously consider the offer of your assistance and talents in my work here. As things are today, let's concentrate on Lifeal.

"I am interested in your thoughts on why Lifeal hasn't achieved its rightful market share or do you think it is just a matter of time before Lifeal takes off?"

"My assessment of the Lifeal situation is that, in my judgment, we have to look back at the original purpose for Lifeal. It was developed as a preventative to ventricular fibrillation or cardiac arrhythmia, not as a treatment. There was good evidence that Lifeal could, in fact, prevent cardiac fibrillation in certain patients, but it was not followed up by James clinical development. Why was it not followed up, you might ask? The answer lies, I believe, though I have never been able to pin down with any certainty, in our availability of working capital.

"The clinical evidence was not as conclusive as James management, that being, Phillip, Helmut, and the board of directors, wanted it to be. They determined that the time and money required to prove the additional clinical indication were simply not available. If they had invested the required funds, the price-to-earnings ratio would have been adversely affected leaving James to face the prospect of losing its rating as a pharmaceutical growth company. I am not making a judgment as to whether this decision was correct. It is a fact that the money was not invested. This decision on Lifeal caused two things to happen.

"First, Lifeal was released without a sustainable competitive advantage and therefore proper product positioning within a very competitive target market segment was very difficult. Second, the expected advantage of a preventative indication has been neither explored nor exploited. In fact, the company has ignored the prospect in order to focus resources on JPC138 and other new products.

"Over the past three years we have been struggling with Lifeal and it's positioning as the product of choice when all other products fail. We constantly over forecast the product sales with an ideology that we can fight the big guys and take away their market share. That is to say, always giving the false hope that we will win market share with poor positioning and no sustainable competitive advantage. I believe we have missed the boat on this product and what we require now is a complete reevaluation into what Lifeal is, what it can be, and what it requires to be a successful product."

"Carl, you have made some excellent points. Have you talked to Mandi about your assessments?" I asked.

"Yes, and I believe she agrees with me but she is caught up in the politics of the day and Phillip's problem with the board of directors' demand of immediate profit returns. I would likely find myself in the same dilemma in her position." He quickly added "Don't get me wrong, J.P., I have no aspiration of being anything but what I am, the director of market research."

"I see." J.P. realized there was nothing he could say at this point until he had an opportunity to meet with R&D to get their perspective.

"Carl, assuming that what you said is true and there is nothing we can do about the situation today, have you done any more thinking about how we can position Lifeal in the maintenance target market segment?"

"As a matter of fact, yes, but my assessment has again fallen on deaf corporate ears. My colleagues, Frank and Jake, certainly don't agree with my point of view." As J.P. waited for him to continue, Carl raised his great hulk out of the chair and walked to the window that looked out over Central Park. It had stopped snowing but the sky was still overcast. The sunlight that made it through the clouds gave Central Park a contrasting look of black and white. Carl stared at the park.

"I love New York City. I grew up over there," he said pointing to the eastern edge of the park.

Carl turned back to face J.P. and smiled. "I had a good childhood, J.P. I was an only child so my parents gave me a great deal of attention. I went to public schools all the way through high school. My folks were Catholic so you can imagine the pressures that were on them to send me to private schools. My dad said the world would be rough and made up of all kinds of people. A New York City public school education would give me a good perspective on life in the next century. He was always pointing me to the future."

Carl paused and bent his head. "My dad was right, you know. I was big in high school. A little fat, but mostly big. I played football, but my knees gave out when I was a senior. Dad was thirty-five when I was born and he's seventy-nine now. He's in the early stages of Alzheimer's. It's not bad yet, but he sometimes forgets little things. We are very close and we both fear the day when he will not able to remember all the evenings we used to spend discussing life. He was a great man in his own right and it's tough for him to know that the great intellectual capacity, which he often took for granted, will someday be gone.

"Both my mom and dad were born in Manchester, England. Their fathers were coal miners. My folks were married in England and then came to the United States to work as a valet and nanny team to a wealthy Brooklyn couple. Dad joined the Army Air Corps and was a W.W.II ace in the South Pacific. He was discharged in 1945 and used the GI Bill to get his bachelors degree in business. He was recalled to active status in 1950 for that Korean exercise in futility. When he returned home after his discharge he went back to school on the Korean GI Bill and received his law degree from St. John's. He became one of the best defense industry corporate lawyers. Most of his years were spent with Grumman in Long Island. He retired in the late seventies just as most of the defense aircraft industry was moving west to California. He remained an active consultant until about four years ago when the Alzheimer's was diagnosed. He now works parttime for the Securities and Exchange Commission as a defense industry analysis expert.

"He is a very positive influence on my life. He did not want me to go into the defense industry and encouraged me to work in the healthcare field." "I can remember his advice. He told me the defense industry had been good to him and our family but one day this earth will get its collective act together and figure out that we will not survive by killing each other. We will survive only by using all of the goodness that each of us possesses to help one another. Dad concluded his advice by saying, Son, what you have to find is an element of goodness and help people to use goodness to work together towards common goals. You should go into healthcare. It is a common ground for all mankind."

J.P. said quietly, "Your father is a very smart man. I would like to meet him someday."

"You would?" Carl paused. "We both would like that very much. I will set up a lunch within the next two weeks. Is that all right with you?"

"Lunch is an excellent idea," he replied.

Carl moved back to the conference table and sat down. "I will finish my life story and then tell you my secret for today's Lifeal.

You might wonder how I got into market research? Well, my father, being a lawyer, was very logical sort of fellow. He felt, and I had to agree with him, that knowing all the facts about the healthcare industry would enable someone like myself to find a position to use my goodness. So I enrolled in the business school at St. John's where I earned both my MBA and Ph.D. I am a true St. John's man. I can do conjoint and cluster analysis with the best of market researchers," he said, smiling. "I do not get much chance at James to display my talents and prove my intelligence, but things have improved decidedly under Mandi's leadership. This is the end of this is your life, Carl Manningham, Jr.

"Now, J.P., on with Lifeal. First, I am a great advocate of your teachings. I am what you might call a closet case J.P. target market segment concept lover. I have read everything you left behind here at James in your formative years and everything you have written on the subject since you left. I am, if you will, sitting here at the same table with my idol."

J.P.'s face flushed. "Please Carl, I appreciate your thoughts, but you are going to make me ill." They both laughed.

"Okay, J.P., with this as background and also the fact that at this point in time we can't promote Lifeal as a clinical preventative to cardiac fibrillation, I have conducted various TMS techniques to try and find a TMS that meets the four elements of a qualified target market segment. First, that the TMS is large enough to generate the volume necessary to be profitable. Secondly, that it is in the growth stage of its life cycle. Third, that it is assessable by existing distribution and sales systems. And finally, fourth, that Lifeal can achieve more than a 20% market share.

"I think I have found a new TMS, J.P. It is not that we are wrong in what we are presently doing, but we have not segmented the maintenance target market segment far enough. When the sales reps explain to the physician that they should use Lifeal when other products fail it seems to set up a textbook win-lose situation with the physician. I have gone one step farther and have found a patient profile that best fits Lifeal as a maintenance product. I call this the Quality of Life TMS.

"Patients who make up this TMS are patients that have cardiac fibrillation problems and have lived a very active life. They desire to continue to live as active a life as possible with their illness. If these patients played tennis or jogged before they became ill, they want, if possible, to return to an active lifestyle. If they skied they want to ski. They also certainly don't want to have the risk of being ill or shortening their life expectancy. I'm certain this story line would have a more powerful impact with physicians than telling them to use Lifeal when everything else fails.

"This Quality of Life TMS makes up $780 million of the $10 billion total market segment. It is not the size of the $2 billion Unhappy Patient TMS, but it is a $780 million TMS nonetheless. I have analyzed our current $100-plus million in Lifeal sales. Eighty percent of the usage of Lifeal today is for patients who fit the Quality of Life TMS."

"Hold on Carl you can stop the explanation. I get it. I like your analysis and I believe you are definitely onto something. Why has this TMS fallen on deaf corporate ears, to use your phraseology?"

"Simple J.P, Frank thinks the present strategy is a good one and manages to convince everyone else that we have not given his strategy enough time to succeed. Jake thinks we will be looking at too narrow of a market for him to expend field sales time and resources to sell into just this TMS. He wants his people to call on as many physicians as possible. He lives by the theory that the more physicians his sales reps call on the more opportunity there is for conversion. These heads are buried in the past and they are ignoring the way the market is going. I, on the other hand, feel it is the quality, not the quantity of physician sales calls. Between the two of them, I get shot down at every staff meeting when I bring it up. They do not want me to rock the Lifeal boat. Status quo is good enough for those two, but not for me. I want James to be a leader, not a follower. Mandi, at present feels she has to back Frank and Jake.

"So I, like all good market research directors who do not agree with market planning and sales, sit back and allow events to take place that will or will not prove my research correct. I love this job J.P., but I have to admit that I hate waiting for a failure and the opportunity to tell management, I told you so." Carl burst into laughter "You know J.P., the sad part about this scenario? I can never say I told you so to Frank and Jake because if it turned out that I was correct and an issue was made of it, they would chalk it up to my arrogance and I would never get anything past those two. It's tough to win in market research. If someone uses your ideas and they turn out to be successful, the idea ends up being their own. If the ideas turn out badly, the fingers always point back to market research."

J.P. had sat listening and was pleased that he had finally found someone on Mandi's marketing team who seemed intelligent and progressive. "Carl I think you may have something. Let me work on your idea with Mandi and then Phillip." He looked at his watch, "It's 11:45 and I have to be upstairs to have lunch with the board. If you have a report on anything we talked about this morning, I would appreciate a copy to study."

Carl looked at him with glint in his eye. "Lunch with the board and you are just supposed to be helping with Lifeal marketing." He put his hand to his multiple chins as if thinking "Hmm. Sorry, J.P., this doesn't seem to compute."

J.P. dodged his question directly by saying, "Hang in there, Carl. Now do you have any reports?"

"Are you kidding, what is market research but a reports factory? The reports will be emailed to you before you return from your board lunch."

J.P. stood up from the table and turned to leave the room. He was smiling to himself as he left the conference room.

He stopped at the door and without looking at Carl said in a joking manner, "I would expect nothing less from a Ph.D. Don't forget about lunch with your dad."

BERGEN COUNTY COURTHOUSE BERGEN, N.J.

One week on the prescribed once-a-day dosage was driving Ralph crazy. No he told himself, not crazy, it was more like frustration. Frustration because others could not keep up with him. It seemed to him that they were all stupid.

Ralph Vandermere had not slept the night before. Everything he was doing at the office and in the courtroom kept running through his mind. If he saw or touched anything his mind seemed to soak it up. His mind continually processed information as though it were in a closed loop. Nothing ever seemed to come to closure, although new information was constantly being fed into the loop.

He looked into the mirror and his eyes just looked back at him questioning his thoughts. Ralph loved the capability of his memory, but he didn't know if he could last until the appointment with his doctor on Monday with his mind turning in a maelstrom whenever he looked into his own eyes. He considered taking two tablets at a time in an effort to quiet his mind and get him through the weekend.

Today was an important day in his court case, but he knew he would be great in court. He had been great every day. His knowledge of law had held the courtroom and even the judge spellbound. He was certain the judge was jealous of his abilities. He shook the second Lifeal tablet from the prescription vial into his left hand and looked at the tablet. It was orange and shaped like a miniature coffin. He placed his right index finger on the tablet and rolled it around in his palm. He suddenly came to a conclusion and placed it in his mouth. He took a swallow of water. He left his bathroom noting the bottle of tablets was getting low.

Ralph drove leisurely to the Bergen Courthouse. No real hurry.

Everyone would be late anyway because of the snowstorm.

The day before, the court had recessed early so that the attorneys could prepare for the final summary. Following the presentation of final arguments the jury would retire to debate the innocence or guilt of Mr. Emmitt in the killing of his partner Mr. Bedlow.

Everyone was properly seated when the judge entered the courtroom with the exception of the defense attorney, Mr. Ralph Vandermere. The judge was just about to ask Dan Patterson, who was seated in the gallery, where his partner was when the double doors at the rear of the courtroom swung open.

It was Ralph, making a grand entrance. He had on a pair of bright green pants, purple polo shirt open at the top, and a white sport coat. A purple silk handkerchief hung out of the right breast pocket of his sports coat. He sauntered down the aisle looking to both sides. He waved at courtroom visitors as they sat stunned by his entrance. Before the judge or anyone could say a word, Ralph spoke.

"Thank you, your honor, I will now begin my summary. The result of this trial is so obvious, my summary will not take very long." He walked up to the jury bar and positioned himself looking at the jury. The judge watched this spectacle with his gravel half raised and his mouth open to speak, but Ralph got the jump on him and started his summary.

"Jason Emmitt has been accused of killing his partner. The prosecuting attorney," Ralph turned and pointed to the prosecuting attorney, "has not proven Mr. Emmitt's guilt beyond a reasonable doubt. Remember my friends on the jury; guilt beyond a reasonable doubt is what you are charged with determining. On the other hand, my defense of Mr. Emmitt was probably the best defense that you will ever hear in a court of law. Even better than you, judge." He glanced to his right at the judge who just sat in his chair, not believing what he was hearing. Ralph turned and again addressed the jury, "Of course, I recognize that none of you has likely ever served on a jury when I was performing. Am I not a better attorney than any you have ever seen on TV.?" He struck a pose that he thought made him look like a movie star. There were hushed whispers and several giggles coming from the gallery.

The presiding judge banged his gavel and looked to the gallery and said sternly, "Silence." He looked back at Ralph and said, "Mr. Vandermere, I don't know what it is that you think you are doing, but I assure that you I am one gavel bang away from finding you in contempt of court."

The courtroom was hushed. The judge, prosecuting attorney, visitors, and press were aghast. The trial had lasted almost two weeks. Ralph Vandermere had started out presenting one of the best defenses most had ever heard from an attorney. During the first week he had presented a case for his client that had every chance of returning a verdict of not guilty.

"Very well, your honor. I am going to cut this summary short because I do not wish to insult the intelligence of the jury. You are intelligent people, are you not?" Ralph pointed to one of the jurors. "You. I am not too sure of your intelligence, but as for the rest of you," he said as he swept his arm in front of the jury box, "with your intelligence you will help this poor juror to see the light and the innocence of my client."

The judge began banging his gavel, "Mr. Vandermere, I warned you. I will not allow you make a mockery of this court or a seated jury panel."

Ralph continued without acknowledging the judge's statements, "So.all of you parasites of Bergen County use your God-given faculties and listen to me. This guy," he said pointing to Jason Emmitt, "is innocent. It is intuitively obvious that he is innocent. If you do not vote for his acquittal, you are, to put it simply, stupid."

The judge now stood up from his seat and raised his gavel to bring the madness to an end. Just as the mallet was about to hit the pad, Ralph turned and walked out of the courtroom. Everyone's eyes followed his walk in a continued silence. No one moved. Once he was through the doors, the room descended into pandemonium.

The judge began banging his gavel and calling for order. Everyone in the room was talking. The judge was yelling at the sheriff's deputy to go after Ralph and bring him back, but the deputy had moved over to the defense table to take control of his prisoner. Dan Patterson rushed out of the courtroom after his law partner.

When he caught up with Ralph, he grabbed his arm. "Ralph, what in the hell is the matter with you? Are you crazy?"

Ralph turned and stared at his partner. His partner could see the anger in Ralph's eyes. "Ralph, you better take it easy. Go home and sleep off whatever has gotten into you." Dan pleaded.

Ralph stared through his partner and began to speak. His voice had a deep resonance snarl. "You ignorant son of a bitch. Do you think I need you or anyone else? You all think you are so smart. You are so ignorant. I know so much more than you do. I can see so much more. I do not need you or anyone else in this half-assed excuse for a town. Now Dan, get the fuck out of my way." Ralph started to move around Dan. His partner moved sideways positioning himself in front of Ralph.

Ralph screamed at Dan, "I said to get the fuck out of my way or I will knock you out of the way."

Ralph folded his hand into a fist and swung at Dan. He hit him square in the face. His partner, not expecting violence, fell backward with the punch. Ralph looked down at him. "You ignorant bastard, stay out of my way and out of my life." He then swung his right foot and kicked his partner in his side and walked off. His partner, bleeding from the mouth and doubled up in pain from the kick, watched his partner walk away.

Ralph got into his car and looked in the rearview mirror at his eyes. It occurred to him that he never knew he was so intelligent. He decided that he really didn't need anyone for anything. He backed out of the space and drove home.

His wife of thirty years met him at the door. "Ralph what has happened to you?" He shoved her out of the way, knocking her down and stormed upstairs to go to bed.

12:00 P.M., THURSDAY, JANUARY 26

SPECTRUM OF MEDICINE BUILDING NEW YORK CITY

"J.P.," Janet greeted him, "Phillip told me you would be joining this auspicious group for lunch. He just called out and told me to tell the caterers that they are running fifteen minutes behind. The meeting started late, the storm you know." J.P. sat down opposite her desk.

"How are things going in there?" he asked pointing towards the boardroom.

"I don't think things are going very well, J.P. I heard a great deal of yelling when the board members were the only people in the room. During Mandi and Helmut's presentations there was a courteous silence but after they left the room you could hear Mrs. James and Phillip yelling at one another. They usually have a few moments of yelling at every board meeting, but this time it sounds much worse."

He decided to change the subject, "So, what's for lunch?" "Sword fish steaks."

"That seems appropriate.. .makes me wonder whose sword is stabbing whom? Good choice, but I am sure the humor will be lost on them.

Phillip stuck his head out of the boardroom. In a very fatigued voice he said, "J.P., come on in. Janet, please inform the caterers that we are ready for lunch. Has Husted arrived?" He looked around and answered his own question. "Looks like he might be late. If he is not here by 12:30 give the Wall Street Journal a call for a status report on his whereabouts. Thanks."

J.P. followed Phillip into the boardroom. Everyone was standing in little groups. He did not recognize any of the board members who had been appointed by Mrs. James. Her supporters were on one side of the conference table while Phillip's remained on the other side.

Everyone had stopped talking when J.P. entered the room and looked in his direction. Evelyn Jones was the first to speak, "J.P., what a lovely surprise. Phillip told us that you would be joining us for lunch. I was shocked, simply shocked. It has been years since you jumped our sinking ship. I assume that Phillip has told you that our ship is sinking. Don't you agree Phillip?"

Phillip's face turned red and though he was visibly angry his voice was steady, "You know damn well Evelyn that I know of no such thing. We are a little behind plan but we are ahead of last year.

Now, please, let's keep our disagreement within the family and not expose our friends to our differences.

J.P. is a good friend of James and will keep our comments to himself. But if you expose our disagreement to Husted then you can be sure that we will be the topic du jour in tomorrow's Wall Street Journal. The prediction of a James decrease in earnings you mentioned this morning that would cause a devaluation of our stock, will in fact happen if you open up to Husted."

Phillip paused and then continued in a mocking voice, "Or, is devaluation what Madam Chairperson desires?"

J.P. watched the blood drain from Evelyn's face. Her right hand came up in a motion that suggested slapping Phillip's face. She replied, "Just what exactly are you implying, Mr. President?"

"You know damn well what I am implying" Phillip replied a little louder.

"Are you seriously implying that I would purposely drive the price of our stock down in order to show up you and the poor leadership and judgment that you have demonstrated as president and CEO of James?" She was yelling now.

"You said it, I didn't," Phillip's voice was quiet but damning.

"You loathsome son of a bitch," she hissed. She raised her hand again, but this time continued the motion towards his face until one of her board appointees caught her hand.

Evelyn turned on the man and it looked as though she would turn her hate on him. He calmly stepped back and said, "Evelyn and Phillip this behavior is not helping anyone, particularly James Pharmaceutical Company. We have one outside guest who must think we are all children in a schoolyard. If you continue we will, as Phillip suggests, expose our disagreement to Mr. Husted. You both owe J.P. an apology for using him as the catalyst to your disagreement."

"No need," J.P. said trying to ease the tension. The room fell silent. He decided to continue as if the nothing had happened. He decided to introduce himself to the board members that he didn't know starting with the man who had stopped the physical confrontation between Phillip and Evelyn.

"My name is Dr. Jean Paul Koenig. I'm a former employee of James, but a good friend of the company. My friends and acquaintances call me J.P.," he said extending his hand.

"J.P., I'm Harman C. Coontz, the fourth. I am very glad to meet you. I have read one of you books on marketing. A very practical treatise, I must say. I have heard many good reports on how you have helped healthcare companies. Welcome to our friendly," Harman stressed the word, friendly with a smile and continued, "informal afterboardmeeting get-together, please don't mind our loud leaders. It must be an after effect of the snowstorm." Everyone laughed and joined in the conversation except Phillip and Evelyn, who were still glaring at each other. Coontz introduced him to the other members of the board.

As he finished the introductions, Janet opened the door and she announced Bill Husted's arrival. J.P. quickly looked over at Phillip and Evelyn who were still standing at opposite ends of the room. They both broke into smiles and walked briskly to greet their guest.

After introductions, everyone, in turn, filed through the buffet and returned with their plates to sit at the conference table. The conversation was amiable.

J.P. had set himself down at the far corner opposite of Jack Husted. When conversation around the table reached a lull, Jack looked over at him and remarked in a vindictive manner, "The almighty J.P. Koenig. What the hell are you doing here? Pray tell us what caused you to descend from your California mountain and visit us poor folks in New York City?"

J.P. didn't reply at first. He continued chewing the food in his mouth and then purposely dropped his fork onto the plate.

"Well, I certainly didn't make the trip to see you, Husted. I also see you've done your best to ruin my visit by arranging a snowstorm. Tell us whose palm you had to grease to make that happen or did you arrange it as you do most of your well-timed stories? Or was it simply a diversion to suspend trading so you could come here for lunch without missing anything?"

The room went silent. Forks were suspended in different positions between plate and mouth. Heads were turning back and forth between the two men who continued to glare at each other for a time. Finally, they both looked at Phillip and the three of them broke out in laughter followed by everyone else in the room.

"Don't let this friendship fool you," Jack finally said. "I don't give preferential treatment to James because I know Phillip. In fact, if anything, I am a little harder on James because I know Phillip and I feel the company can do better than it is presently performing." He looked across the table and said, "Anyway, my good friend, J.P., you can attest to my overwhelming preferential treatment by the review I gave your last marketing book." He finished his remark with a small wink of his left eye.

"Yeah, exactly," J.P. said happily, "His review was so damning I sold an extra million copies to the Husted backlash crowd the day after it was published."

After the brief encounter between the old friends, the mood in the room lifted considerably. Everyone was now enjoying a relaxed lunch with the exception of Evelyn. J.P. kept thinking to himself that she probably didn't know that he, Phillip, and Bill were such close friends from the past and that she was probably trying to reach a conclusion some where in her mind as to whether this was good or bad news.

J.P.'s thoughts were disrupted when Husted announced that he had to get on with his presentation because he had a two o'clock meeting and transportation back to Wall Street was not going to be easy. Evelyn returned to the conference table and took a seat on the side allowing Husted to take the chairperson's position at the head of the table. Husted went through the current problems facing most pharmaceutical companies. J.P. noted that the problems were not any different than they had been for the past twenty-five years. It was what J.P. called the lament of toos. There is too much government involvement in the industry. It takes too long to get a product approved by the FDA. It is too expensive to bring a new product to market. There is too much socialized medicine. And, too much government support of the splinter companies selling generic products against established, wellresearched products.

"I have always been a supporter of James, even though, through some of my columns, you might not believe this statement. I know James is positioned in the middle of the pack of companies that Wall Street analysts like to call corporate pharmaceutical performers. I have personally been disappointed in James because I think of you as a potential bright star. While other companies have been merging and acquiring to strengthen their competitive position, I had thought James would leap the chasm between being a medium company and become a major player on its own merits. This company is different from the other corporations. This can be good and, on the other hand, bad. To this point, you have not used your differences to gain strength. You have used them to create mediocrity. While other Wall Street analysts believed the public relations hype and jumped on the Lifeal bandwagon when it was released, I took a wait and see attitude. I could not see the difference between your product and other products currently on the market. I am sorry to say that time has proven me right.

"You have to believe me, when I say that being correct with my Lifeal assessment does not make me happy. On the other hand, the initial reports that have been leaked," he stressed the word "leaked" knowing that the information leak probably had likely been a plant, "about JPC138 point to potentially good clinical benefits. Please don't screw this one up like you did Lifeal. Tough words I know, but they are from a friend.

"A friend at this board luncheon, but a reporter and analyst after I leave here. I have one thought I want to leave you with today. James still has an opportunity to be the bright star in the pharmaceutical industry. The potential is within yourselves to rise above the pack, but I have to be truthful with you. The indicators on James are flat. They are neither up nor down. Before your annual meeting you will see indications of Wall Street becoming interested in the performance and future of James. Since no analyst knows where you are going and because you don't seem to know where you're going, the market will judge you and grade you on every move you make.

"The choice of whether James is going to descend into a pool of mediocrity or rise as a shining star is yours. Performance can not be measured with false or subjective smoke and mirrors public relations. Performance has to be demonstrated by facts and performance. Mrs. James, Phillip, thank you for inviting me. Good seeing you again, J.P. If you have time during your visit, give me a call. Thank you for the excellent lunch and conversation." Without another word, Husted walked around the table and left the room to applause from the board. Once he had left the room and the doors closed there was silence.

Evelyn was the first to speak, "I guess that's all for today. Thank you for attending the meeting despite the bad weather. We will see you in a month, but I am certain that we will be talking on the telephone. Have a safe trip home or back to your office. Thank you again." She folded her notes, as did the other board members.

She followed her adjournment with, "Phillip, J.P., can you stay for a moment please."

Everyone else left the room saying goodbye to the three of them as they stayed at their places at the table. When the last member had left and closed the door, Evelyn said. "I did not know the three of you were such bosom buddies. If this is the case, how is it that Husted is so hard on us? If he is hard on us because he is your friend Phillip, who needs this kind of friend?"

She continued, "He uses our press releases. He makes a few calls to catch the rumors and then publishes his own slant on what he's able to rake out of the weeds. I do not recall one instance, in the time that I've been the chair of James, that he has printed what we wanted him to print."

"Perhaps you just broken the media code, Evelyn," Phillip said in a very low voice.

"And just what in the hell does that mean, mister?" Her voice was beginning to ratchet up in pitch.

Phil answered in a very quiet and unstrained manner. "It means just what I said. Before you were chairperson, he published the vast majority of our press releases as written. Why? Simply put, it was because he believed us. Since you took over the company, he feels compelled to verify every word and then come to his own conclusion. And from that, Madam Chairwoman, you may draw your own conclusions."

"I am warning you, Dr. Bradsmith, you are skating on thin ice. In this game, I have the best hand and the biggest pot to see it through to the end." She turned to J.P., "What in the hell are you doing here, J.P.? I meant it when I said that you jumped ship. Has our illustrious president provided you with a few crumbs so the deserting rat can come home again and get fatter still?"

Phillip started to speak, but J.P. stopped him, "Thanks Phillip, but I can handle this." He turned back to Evelyn and said, in a condescending voice, "Evelyn….may I call you Evelyn?"

"No," she said shaking her head.

"Fine. Mrs. James. If you look in the list of shareholders you will find my name listed with a reasonable 750,000 shares of stock. As a shareholder with special pharmaceutical and management talents, Phillip has asked me to work with the marketing people on the Lifeal product strategy. Phil is not paying me any wages except covering the expenses I am incurring here at James. In view of my large number of shares, I cancelled all of my other activities and threw my talents to James. I am sure you can not see any harm in all of us trying to make Lifeal a greater success, now can you?" She was about to answer, but J.P. continued. "Now I must get back to work. I've wasted enough time today already. I'm sure that we'll see one another again. Good day, Mrs. James."

J.P. left the boardroom with Phillip following close behind. Evelyn Preston-James remained standing in the middle of the conference table with her back to the windows. Phillip gently closed the door behind him and the two men took the elevator to J.P.'s office.

SPECTRUM OF MEDICINE BUILDING NEW YORK CITY

When J.P. and Phillip were inside J.P.'s office with the door shut, he asked Phillip, "What in the hell went on during the actual board meeting? This was sure some kind of an afternoon."

"J.P., the board meeting was a disaster, anything that was brought up that had any connection to me, she objected to. She accused management of poor judgment, a lack of leadership, and stopped just short of accusing me of outright malfeasance. For instance, when Mandi finished her presentation and left the room, to strong applause from the board, our illustrious chair immediately launched into a tirade about our lack of an aggressive strategy and direction with Lifeal. When I reminded her of our strong performance with the rest of the product line she said, 'So what? We, board members, will not allow these other products to be your performance life rings.'

"She was very pleasant to Helmut. After he left, she warned me that unless Lifeal begins to show some signs of life, I can kiss off the research budget and all of my pet, as she refers to them, bio-herbal projects. With Brian, she tore into him to his face. She and all of her accountant board members picked apart every financial number. They asked him for backup every time he gave an explanation. She finally blew up and demanded an audit thirty days ahead of schedule. With the exception of Brian, she had waited until Mandi and Helmut had left the room before she started in on me. Since Brian was an invited member of the board, she went at me in front of him.

"It seems to me that her next tactic in destroying me is to drive a wedge between me and my staff. She continued objecting to everything even after you arrived. Her last attempt of objection was at the end when she objected to your presence here. By the way, you handled her beautifully. It's probably a good thing that you waved me off. I have to admit that I was looking for any reason to engage her and that wouldn't have contributed anything. I've had quite enough of her for one day. It's funny, she was taken completely aback by your answer."

"Thanks, Phillip.my pleasure."

"Her remarks regarding the company and my leadership, I pretty much took in stride. She did, however, land one decidedly low blow. She has apparently gotten to a board member whom I have always counted on as an ally."

"What do you mean she got to one of the board members? If he was an ally, she couldn't have gotten to him."

"I'm afraid that she got to Dr. David Inglehart on logic. She pointed out that his views were a little out of date and that James needed a fresh look at Pharmacy. As you may remember, Dave Inglehart is the professor of Pharmacology from Rutgers and exDean of Rutgers School of Pharmaceutical Sciences. He was prepared to support my views and to fight Evelyn. He had told me he would remain loyal to my camp.

"During the discussion on the makeup of the James board, she hit Dave's hot button. She announced that she had asked Donald C. Clifton, Ph.D. and just past Dean of the School of Pharmacy of Florida University, if he was interested in being a member of the James Board of Directors. David was not prepared to be replaced by another exdean of pharmacy. He, as well as the rest of my team, had been prepared to fight the addition of more lawyers and accountants.

We had not dreamed that she would propose other healthcare professionals. Her coup de grace with David was her offer to him of 50,000 shares of James stock out of her own portfolio with no strings attached if he understood her viewpoint. I contested her offer, stating that it was tantamount to bribery. She rightly answered that she could give her stock to anyone she chose. She then gave 50,000 shares to the other directors except myself, of course. She then said that she was considering making a proposal to the shareholders to expand the board by adding two additional healthcare executives. She defeated me tactically. The directors that I had considered allies had no other choice but to take the 50,000 shares. If they turned down her offer they knew they would soon be out the door. All of them to a person enjoy their position on the Board of Directors of James Pharmaceutical Company and the $5,000 a month director's fee. I really could not blame them for siding with her. Especially after the board meeting today and Husted's warning. I'm certain that I must seem to them to be a lame duck."

Phillip sat in his chair, head bowed, hands clasped together and held between his knees. His voice lacked the confidence that J.P. knew from the past.

He continued, "There is just so much a person can take, J.P. You work your ass off under the flag of corporate loyalty. Loyalty to the employees, customers, and products. No matter how hard you try to prevent being caught up in corporate politics and greed of power and money, one day they get you.

The greedy grabbers feel they are helping the company, but in my experience, I have yet to tangle with one greedy person that provided one bit of evidence they care about anything else except power." He slowly raised his head and looked at J.P. "I don't think I can fight any more. She has taken away my pride and eroded my power to control the situation."

J.P. felt that Phillip was one of the best pharmaceutical presidents he had known. Phillip truly believed that long-range profitability comes from dedication to the customers, products, and employees, thus enabling the stockholders to achieve a reasonable return on their investment. J.P. knew that Phillip was looking to him to provide an answer.

After what seemed like several minutes of silence, J.P. quietly said, "You can't give up Phillip. You know you are right and they are wrong. This company needs you.

His answer was almost a whisper and lacked any fight. He shook his head back and forth. "You know better than that, J.P. You know as well as I do that no one person in a corporation is so important that they're irreplaceable."

This was not the first time that J.P. had discussed this with Phillip. When Doc James died, Phillip was not the top candidate for the president's spot. The board was planning to use Phillip as a caretaker and find someone outside of James for president. The board felt that James required a fresh perspective. The news had been a personal defeat for Phillip. He felt that he was the top candidate and believed that he would almost certainly be promoted. When he heard of the board's intention, Phillip had taken on a defeatist attitude. He felt that he was the best-qualified person for the position, but no one on the board recognized this fact. J.P. had reassured Phillip that his vision for James was as good as anyone the board could find on the outside, but he was more knowledgeable about the future of pharmaceuticals and the role that James had to play in the future of healthcare.

Phillip knew the weaknesses and strengths of the pharmaceutical industry and how to learn from them and correct them to make James stronger. He knew where James could fit into the global picture. J.P. had encouraged him not to give in to unknown pressures, but to put together a comprehensive plan selling himself and his vision of James and then present his plan to the James Board of Directors.

In the end, when the board had to make a choice, Phillip outshined every outside candidate and the board promoted him to president and Mrs. James to chairperson. Now, Phillip was in another battle and J.P. could see that his self-confidence was again eroding. J.P. knew that this fight was different. Phillip had already won and earned his stripes as a president. He had proven himself, if not to the present board then most certainly to his employees and peers in the industry.

J.P. knew that there was likely something else that was giving Phillip pause to consider whether it was worth it to fight the board to establish his vision for James. His severance and retirement from the company would likely provide

Phillip a comfortable living for the rest of his life. Besides the probability of a golden parachute, J.P. also knew that if he wanted to continue working he would almost certainly be in demand as president or a board member of another company.

J.P. decided that he would take the reverse tactic and encourage him to hang it up and enjoy the rest of his life outside of James. He knew that Phillip would enjoy retirement and the possibility of working as a consultant. J.P. felt that he had to convince him that he had nothing to loose by fighting Mrs. James and everything to gain for the company that he had contributed so much of himself to get it where it was today. J.P. knew that if he could appeal to Phillip's ego that he would hopefully come to a conclusion to stay the course on his own.

J.P. finally spoke, "Phillip, you do know that Evelyn will destroy James, don't you?

Phillip slowly raised his head and looked directly into his friend's eyes.

J.P. could see a deep sadness within his eyes.

His voice was barely audible, "Yes, J.P., but why should I be concerned? I have given all of my energy to James. I don't feel guilty."

J.P. nodded his head in agreement, "You're right Phillip, there is no reason you should feel guilty, but do you want to see James and all the work you have done destroyed with the flick of her pen? Do you want to see everything that this company has accomplished lost to a merger or some other short-term strategy that maximizes her personal financial return and screws the employees and the customers? I don't think Evelyn would even preserve the name James Pharmaceutical Company. James Pharmaceutical Company would disappear like other strong medium-sized pharmaceutical companies have disappeared in recent years. Phillip, think of what Doc James would do if he were in this same situation." Phillip raised himself up. There was the same flash of anger in his eyes that J.P. had seen when they were talking about the board meeting and Evelyn's 50,000 share stock gifts. "Besides, who would Evelyn get to replace you?"

Phillip looked directly at J.P. His hands were now on the arms of his chair. "I don't know J.P. I haven't given any thought to who might replace me."

J.P. decided to push his luck and bait his friend, "I'm betting that she'll put a lawyer or accountant in the president's position and take the chief executive officer position for herself to go along with her chair position. She'll rationalize that she doesn't have to place a healthcare executive at the helm of a global pharmaceutical company that deals with multicountry manufacturing, research, and currency exchange. There would be no reason to know clinical medicine when, in the short-term, the majority of James profits can be made by finance maneuvering prior to the physician writing the prescription."

Phillip stood up. The movement was so sudden that it startled J.P. He walked to the window and then abruptly turned to face J.P. who remained sitting. Phillip's voice was controlled, but anger was bubbling below the surface.

"She wouldn't be that stupid," he paused to reflect and then said, "Yes, I suppose she would."

J.P. saw his opening and moved towards it, "James would begin to fail and then Mrs. Evelyn PrestonJames' team would sell off what was left of James in order to maximize their personal holdings."

"You are right, J.P. That is just exactly what would happen. She is really in a destructive mode. She would tear down James Pharmaceutical Company and indirectly her own financial wealth because her destructive actions against James would be reflected in a reduced value of James stock." Again he reflected, "I wonder what the hell is driving her."

"Phillip, right here, right now, I can't give you any sort of detailed plan on how to win a battle with Evelyn, but there is one forming in my mind. I am sure that by the time the annual meeting rolls around, we'll have something to hang out hats on that will make James the bright star Husted described in his talk today. I will work on the plan and also find out who copied the 21st Century Plan. I'm sure I can do it between now and the annual meeting in May. What you have to do, my friend, is hang in with this company and work with me to develop some sort of strategy to stack the James Board of Directors back in your favor. You can't give in to Evelyn's destructive plans. James, Lifeal, and JPC138 are depending on you and your talents. So, what do you say, Phillip? Are you going to stay in this for the long haul?"

Phillip had turned to look out the window. Small snowflakes were swirling around the corner of the building as the winds began to push the clouds apart. He turned to face J.P. who saw that the sadness in his eyes had been replaced by a look of determined conviction. He was leaning against the window frame when he strongly replied, "Yes.

5:00 P.M., THURSDAY, JANUARY 26
SPECTRUM OF MEDICINE BUILDING NEW YORK CITY

After Phillip left J.P.'s office, he called Mandi to see if she was free to discuss the day's events. Mandi told him that she would welcome the distraction, so he left his office and made his way to the opposite corner of the floor. Judi was not at her desk so he knocked on Mandi's office door. He heard Mandi's voice say, "Come on in, J.P."

As was becoming a habit for their meetings, Mandi got up from her desk and walked around to her conference table. After they had both sat down, J.P. got a sense that things seemed a bit awkward, perhaps from their personal encounter the previous evening. He decided to try and break the ice.

"Good evening, Mandi," he said as he faked a yawn and stretched his arms over his head. "So, do you agree that the past twenty-four hours have set in motion many things moving rapidly along a path of change?" He realized how stupid what he said had sounded, but knew that it was too late to take it back.

Mandi gave him a slightly puzzled look and then said, "It would seem so. I feel change, but except for the snowstorm and my invading your privacy last night, I can't honestly say that I know what that change has in store for James. I don't know whether the change is good or bad. I know it sounds ridiculous, but I feel better about everything at James." She looked directly into his eyes. "My problem is, I don't know precisely how to define the word, things, as it applies here." She smiled at him before continuing. "On a more definitive subject, what were the results of the board meeting?"

"First, everyone said you did a great job today at the board meeting.

Congratulations. Do you feel you achieved your objectives?"

"Yes. I felt I did all right, but I didn't have as much substance as I would have liked. It is obvious that our Lifeal strategy has to change. We can't wait around for the marketplace to dictate what will happen to Lifeal. We have to make change happen. The board is right and, as much as I hate to say it, Mrs. James is right about Lifeal. We have failed. By the way, I appreciated our Lifeal talk last night. It helped me to come to the conclusion that the time for action to cause change is now, not tomorrow. I want you to know that I do want your help. I figured out, with your help, that I now have the best opportunity to change Lifeal and strengthen the marketing organization. I would like you to help me formulate the plan and ultimately sell the plan to Phillip."

"Well, once we agree on the Lifeal strategy the rest of your marketing plan will fall into place. I will certainly help you with your thought process, but you should sell Phillip on the plan yourself. It will be your plan, I will just help you to formulate your thoughts."

"Thank you, J.P."

"Mandi, I just spent the last four and a half hours with the board and with Phillip. What I have to tell you falls within our agreement of secret classification. Okay?" Mandi nodded her head.

"Phillip is in trouble with the board. Mrs. James is making aggressive moves to gain control of the board and with control of the board to move Phillip out and take control of the company. The harmony and good feelings you saw today when you were in the boardroom were a well-orchestrated act.

After you left, Mrs. James went directly at Phillip with every accusation of incompetence she could find in her limited business vocabulary. All the good things you said about products other than Lifeal were rejected with a simple 'who cares.' Mrs. James is buying off the board members who have supported Phillip in the past. She bribed them to come over to her side by giving them each 50,000 shares of her own James stock. I strongly believe that in the long run she will replace them with her own appointees. She says this is not in her plans if the board supports her 100%. With this strategic move she probably now controls the James board. Phillip and I feel that Mrs. James' complete control of the board does not bode well for James Pharmaceutical Company or for Phillip."

J.P. went on to explain the rest of the board meeting and also the challenge Husted placed on James management for this year's annual meeting.

"At a meeting just held in my office prior to my coming to see you, Phillip and I agreed to fight Mrs. James. Mandi, we also agreed that we would need your help." As J.P. told his story of the board meeting, he could see Mandi gradually slip into a slight case of shock. She did not respond immediately to his request for help.

When she finally spoke it was with strong conviction, "You know you both have my total support. When you said things had changed in the last twenty-four hours I thought that you probably meant more than snow and my first visit to your spa."

J.P. smiled and looked down at the table, "I wasn't sure if you caught my complete drift when I mentioned.. .things. Forgive me if what I'm about to say sounds more than little bit presumptuous. I enjoyed our time together last night, but I would like to make sure we keep the project and whatever other relationship may develop on separate paths. I'm definitely a romantic type and the only way I can work with someone I care about and remain sane is to keep business in a business folder and personal in a personal folder. I know I am not saying what I mean very clearly, but do you understand what I mean?"

Mandi smiled and laid her pen back onto the table, "Actually, I kind of like presumption in a man." She giggled slightly. "Yes, I understand and agree. You and I are in 100% agreement on this subject."

J.P. wasn't sure what she meant, so he decided to further test the waters, "I'm certainly looking forward to Saturday night. Are we still on? I thought we could take in a Broadway show and then dinner. How does that sound?"

"J.P., that sounds wonderful. It has been so long since I have had a night out in the City. I am ready to go right now...just kidding. Also can I again impose on you to let me stay at your place Saturday night? I hate to go back to New Jersey late at night."

"The guest room is always available to you whenever you require it. How about coming into the city early on Saturday and we can go for a walk in the park before everything turns to slush."

"Sounds like a wonderful idea. Now that we have our personal issues out of the way, what do we want to do about this board issue?"

"Well, the way I see it, there are really four business issues that have to be handled. First, we have to reposition Lifeal. Second, we have to break the mystery about who made the copy of the 21st Century Plan. Third, we have to seek strategies to ensure the success of JPC138. And fourth, how to help Phillip gain control of James. We only have until the May board meeting to successfully accomplish all of that. At the annual meeting or before the meeting we have to be prepared to wage a fight against Mrs. James. I don't know what form that fight will take, but my guess is that it will be in the form of a proxy fight for control of the board. It is very important you do not mention the possibility of a proxy fight to a single person, not even to Phillip. He has to come to his own conclusion that a proxy fight will be necessary, but eventually he will see it that way. Then it is up to us to be ready with the plan and the ammunition that Phillip will require for implementation."

"I am ready for any kind of fight, J.P. I have never trusted Mrs. James. She has never shown respect for what this company has stood for in the past or what the company could be in the future. She has only wanted money and power. She will destroy James. We do have to stop her." He didn't want their conversation to descend into a prolonged discussion of Evelyn Preston-James so he tried to switch the conversation to Lifeal. "Mandi, what do you think of Carl Manningham?"

"I don't know him very well as a person. As my marketing research director, I think he is one of the best in the pharmaceutical business. He is a little overweight" she paused and smiled, "no, he is a lot overweight. At times he makes me mad because he seems to always be on the opposite side of the issues surrounding Lifeal. I try to listen to him, but I never seem to have time to hear Carl's side completely. I do know that Frank and Jake rarely agree with Carl and usually drown out his ideas before he has had much of a chance to fully explain them to the marketing team. How was your meeting with him this morning? Did he keep you laughing? Sometimes I think he plays the role of the court jester just a little too much. He loses the respect of the team when he turns so many issues into jokes. I don't mind levity, but he uses levity to extremes."

"Actually, my meeting with Carl was one of my best since I've been on the project. I found him intelligent, refreshing, and anything but a court jester." Mandi looked surprised.

"That surprised you? He is, in fact, a very serious manager. I think the humor and what you call playing a court jester is an act he puts on to get attention from your team. He has probably tried to fight Frank and Jake directly and lost. He wants to be heard and he has determined that making things out to be humorous is a way to at least say what he wants to say. In my case, since he had my attention he did not need humor. Anyway, I think Carl is a key element in the repositioning of Lifeal. Let me tell you some of Carl's ideas."

He explained in great detail Carl's idea for the quality of life target market segment. He did not mention the original intended use for Lifeal as a treatment against cardiac arrhythmia. If Carl was right, and he had a feeling that he was, this indication would have to be clinically proven and would not have helped their immediate pre-^annual meeting problem. J.P. was hoping to uncover something new when he talked with the people in production and R&D.

"What do you think about Carl's quality of life TMS?" he asked when he was finished.

Mandi pushed her chair back from the table, leaned back on the back legs of the chair far enough that the chair actually rested against the window frame. She shifted her gaze to stare out the window. The snow flurries with intermittent peeks of sun had ended and the clouds had moved in again. The world outside had returned to its gray condition. Mandi leaned to her right and touched the glass of the window. She suddenly stopped and brought her chair back up to the table.

She was very serious when she spoke. "You know, as I previously said, I always heard Carl's marketing points, but I never really listened to him. I felt I had to listen to Frank and Jake. They were closest to the marketplace. To tell the truth I have never liked the negative sell TMS in which we placed Lifeal, but there was no alternative and so I hesitantly gave into Frank and Jake.

"What it seems to me that Carl has done is provide us with a positive sell TMS. I would like to know more about it, but on first impression I like it.. .I like it a lot. This could pump new life into Lifeal. I know I will have to do a sales job on Frank and Jake." She thought for a second before adding, "You know we could help Carl do some more studies on this TMS and then present it as a package to the marketing sales team. This will give Carl a chance to shine."

"Mandi, that is a very good idea. It will also give him a big psychological lift if you tell him about what you have in mind."

"I will. First thing tomorrow." She sat back in her seat. "So, what is on your schedule for tonight?"

"Nothing special. I have to check in with Mammoth. I have enough leftovers from my fish stew for a second meal. I'll probably watch some television and then hit the rack. Why? You interested in joining me?"

She took his question in a practical manner, "Are you kidding? I have to get home and make sure everything is okay. Hopefully there is no storm damage. I also have to change my clothes. Saturday and Sunday will be fun and I need to clear up a few home chores to clear the decks to borrow a phrase from the Navy's lexicon."

"I understand. Tomorrow is my day in finance. I have always enjoyed working with Brian. On Saturday you can let me know how your meeting with Carl went. I'll see you around noon on Saturday?" He got up to leave.

"I will call you when I leave home. Enjoy your fish stew, it was great." "Good night, Mandi." "Night, J.P."

J.P. returned home to his apartment and called Annie in Mammoth.

Everything was fine with Annie and Mammoth. Her new friend, Skip, called her Wednesday night. He was coming to ski Mammoth again this weekend and wanted to see Annie. It looked like Annie was going to have a new relationship in her life. J.P. liked Skip but something bothered him about this retired Marine colonel. He finally passed it off as his own jealousy for another man with Annie. J.P. told her about his apartment and talked about the storm before hanging up.

He fixed himself dinner and sat down to watch a hockey game, but fell asleep on the couch before the end of the first period.

9:00 A.M., FRIDAY, JANUARY 27

SPECTRUM OF MEDICINE BUILDING NEW YORK CITY

J.P. decided to start his meeting with Brian by going straight to the heart of the matter. "Brian what do you think about all the activity that has been going on with the board?"

Brian thought for a moment before answering, "I would be trying to fool both you and myself if I did not honestly say that the actions of the board haven't left me baffled. It's obvious that they don't want James to succeed. Everything that we do to get ourselves back on track, the board finds some way to thwart. There are too many strings on our working capital. In the past we were a bit more in control of our own destiny. It now seems that Phillip's control has slipped dramatically. It makes corporate life very difficult and causes us to focus too much effort on situations inside the company rather than on the customer and marketplace. If Mrs. James finally has her way with buying off the board and appointing new members with allegiance to her, things will get worse. This is a very precarious situation and we need to be vigilant for the possibility of a start of a downward financial spiral. J.P., I've known you for years and I know how you hate to play the hero, but we really need a hero here. I hope you can help us find a way out of this."

J.P. and Brian were sitting in two large chairs in Brian's office on the 39th floor, located directly below Phillip's office. He had a desk at one end of his rectangular-shaped office. Behind his desk and to his right were floor-toceiling bookcases. The far wall was glass so that Brian could keep an eye on a number of partitioned cubicles that housed the corporation's accounting clerks.

Before he could accept Brian's compliment disguised as a plea for help, he knew that he had to eliminate him as the person who made the copy of the 21st Century Plan. It was hard for him to believe that Brian could be a suspect but he was one of the six who received a copy.

"Brian, Phillip gave me a copy of the 21st Century Plan to read and give my comments. What do you think of the plan?"

Brian's face registered surprise, which J.P. interpreted as surprise that an outsider had access to the plan. J.P. took this as a good sign. Brian's hands started to fidget as he formulated his answer.

"J.P., I know that you and Phillip are good friends and that you are a friend of James, so I will be as truthful as I can regarding the. shall we say, infamous 21st Century Plan. First, and foremost, I was not in favor of writing it. It isn't that I object to forward thinking or long-term strategies. My concerns lie with a plan that is so comprehensive."

He paused to gather his thoughts. His hands were now calm. He picked up his mug from the table and slowly sipped the hot coffee.

"The fact that you are an outsider." J.P. started to interrupt. Brian held up his hand to keep him from interrupting and a smile formed on his face. "Now, now J.P., don't get defensive on me. We both know you are, by every legal definition, an outsider. You are not on the board nor are you an officer of the company. You are an outsider. Friendship is irrelevant to the point I am trying to make. The fact of the matter is, the 21st Century Plan is so comprehensive that, if it got into the wrong hands, it could do irreparable harm to James. We disclosed too much information in the plan. I know we restricted the distribution of the plan, but who knows who may have copies that we don't know about. We're in the pharmaceutical business, not the counter-espionage business."

"I understand, Brian. Let me ask you this, what harm do you think could come to James if someone were to obtain a copy of the plan and who would be a candidate to steal the plan?" J.P. watched his reaction closely.

"J.P., we just talked about someone who might want to harm James. To be specific, the James Board of Directors. Why the board would want to do that is beyond me, but I have seen enough to know that Mrs. James is greedy and has no loyalty to James, to Phillip, or the company short of maintaining her lifestyle. I don't know enough about the new outside members of the board, but I don't think I would be too wrong if I said that they feel the same as Mrs. James.

She would sell us out in a second if it were to her advantage. We are short of cash and she wants cash. How could she sell us out? Well, sorry, but as I said I'm not in the counter-espionage business. I have no idea beyond the traditional merger with another pharmaceutical company or being acquired. There you have my opinion. The plan was too comprehensive and Mrs. James could, I suppose, use the information to some how acquire cash for her own personal gain."

"Brian, the board saw and approved the plan, but as I understand it they never got a copy.

"Yes, I know, but I'm also certain that she could obtain a copy if she wanted."

This statement surprised and angered J.P. "What do you mean, if she wanted? Hell, Phillip made me read the plan in his presence. I thought he placed tight restrictions on the distribution of the plan.

Do you know something about a copy that has gone astray? Is there someone you do not trust?"

Suddenly Brian's mood changed. J.P. saw him tense up and put up his guard. "J.P., why are you asking me questions about the 21st Century Plan? I thought we were going to talk about Lifeal. Instead we are talking about my opinion of the 21st Century Plan. Now you are asking me about people I don't trust. What's going on?"

J.P. considered telling him the whole story, but that would mean removing him as a suspect. As of this point he was still a suspect. In fact, J.P. thought his last statement was a little on the defensive side.

"No special reason Brian. We were talking about the board actions of yesterday and then about Mrs. James possibly wanting to hurt James. We all know she is not a fan of Phillip. We know that if she does want to control Phillip and James, she has to discredit him. To discredit him she has to have a supporter inside James. So, it is only logical that I ask you if there is anyone internal to James, that has access to information that could harm Phillip and James."

Brian again began to fidget. "Boy, J.P., you are taking some small pieces of information and drawing some heavy conclusions." He stared at J.P. for a moment and then said, "J.P., please excuse me."

Abruptly Brian got up from his chair and left the office. He left so quickly that J.P. didn't have a chance to say anything. J.P. sat there running the past several minutes of conversation through his head and trying to determine whether Brian's actions were good or bad. He came to the conclusion that he did not have enough information to make the determination. He just sipped his coffee and waited for Brian to return.

He looked out the window at the gray skies and hoped in his heart that Brian had nothing to do with stealing a copy of the plan. J.P. knew Phillip really trusted Brian. Brian had, in his memory, more information than what was in the 21st Century Plan. Still, if he were aligned with Mrs. James or anyone outside of the corporation the James Pharmaceutical Company was not just in trouble, but also in deep trouble.

Fifteen minutes passed and J.P. decided that perhaps Brian simply wasn't coming back. He was about to get up from his chair and leave when Brian's 6'7" frame appeared in the doorway. He strode into the room closing the door behind him. He actually looked relaxed to J.P.

He plopped himself down into his seat and spoke with a slight smile on his face, "Sorry, J.P., but I had to call Phillip and he was a little hard to find."

He broke out in strong, deep laughter. "J.P., I have a confession to make. I know all about the missing copy of the 21st Century Plan. Phillip told me about the Doylestown incident the Friday that he got the letter before he called you on the telephone. Phillip immediately came to the conclusion that I was not the guilty staff member.a correct assumption I might add." He laughed again. "I know this is not a laughing matter, but I am sorry J.P., I am enjoying the look of surprise on your face. Oh, by the way he would like to see you after we finish today. In fact he wants to see both of us. He will apologize for not telling you when he sees us."

Brian became serious again. "Now then, to actually answer your questions…if you make the assumption that the person who made a copy of the plan is a member of the staff and that it is not Phillip, Mandi, nor I, the only ones left are Joe and Helmut. I have my own opinion, so I would like for you to come to your own conclusion. You have Joe next week and Helmut the week after, right? Let's get back together the week after you work with Helmut's department. Of course, this preliminary conclusion of the guilty party all makes sense unless you are of the opinion that someone got hold of a staff member's copy, made a copy for themselves, and then returned the borrowed copy. I personally think we should concentrate on the party with the most to gain from the information contained in the plan. As far as I am concerned, Mrs. James likely figures prominently in the solution to that equation."

Brian and J.P. went over the board issues again and the history since Phillip took over as president. Brian was able to fill in some of the details that

J.P. was otherwise unaware. They had lunch in the corporate dining room and it was mid-afternoon before the two men began to talk about Lifeal.

"J.P., there is not much I can say about Lifeal. I know we are behind plan and it is hurting our cash flow. Cash flow is necessary for us to continue the aggressive R&D programs we have on herbal pharmaceuticals. We get a nice financial windfall with the new 50mg dosage automatic shipments, but as you know, these are always false highs. I feel the answer is in the marketing of the product and I do not pretend to know anything about marketing. In my opinion, the promotion and sales programs do not have any life at all.. .pardon the pun. I have a hard time staying awake when either Frank or Jake starts talking about Lifeal.

"They are not spending up to the promotional budget so I can't complain about overspending. They believe that I'm impressed with their frugality. Those two have always read me incorrectly. I'm only impressed with success. I wonder if their sales would be higher with better promotional programs that did spend down their allocated budget. I would rather have the sales than the expense savings." Brian smiled at J.P. "I know J.P., this is not the old Brian talking. The traditional financial man has learned a few things in the last few years. The main thing I have learned is the numbers follow the business, they do not cause the business. There is plenty of margin in Lifeal. The gross margin is 80% and the pretax profit is 30%. We could give up a few margin points if the sales volume would increase along with our marketshare. Frank and Jake tell me that the market is not price sensitive and that the cost of goods is relatively steady so I have to come to the conclusion that the solution is in the marketing and promotion of the product. Enter into the equation Jean Paul Koenig, Ph.D. You see J.P.; I believe you are being set up to be the Lifeal hero. Like I said when we began talking this morning. Lifeal needs a hero and you're convenient. There are certainly no heroes here at James. We are all too close to the situation."

"Brian, I appreciate being cast into the role of a hero because it can't hurt future consulting business, but I think the answer is within James. I just have to find the answer, pull it out into the open, have the team massage the key factors, and let good old basic marketing take over. In fact, I have had a very good week with Mandi's people and I already think there is a new slant we can put on Lifeal that will improve its market positioning."

J.P. glanced at the clock on the wall. It was 4:00 p.m. Brian saw his glance and they both got up out of their seats. They knew Phillip worked hard, but they also knew that he liked to leave at 4:30 on Fridays. He liked to beat the Friday weekend exodus out of the city. They walked to the elevator and rode it up one floor.

Brian was the first to speak as they stepped off the elevator. "God, I hate this damn elevator. You should have seen me on my first ride. As you probably noticed, my height places my head close to ceiling. I actually hit my head when we stopped. It almost knocked me out. Did you notice when I rode up even one floor, I bent my knees and held on tight to the rail bar."

"I did notice your odd stance and decided that you were in your protective stance. I fell down on my first trip. Why doesn't Phillip change the programming to a regular elevator service? I can understand Doc James distorted need, but he was weird about things like this."

"I don't know. Maybe, in his own way, Phillip is also weird."

Janet's bright voice interrupted their conversation. "J.P., Brian how are the two James brain trusts this cold and gray winter day?"

"We are both great in our own way." Brian answered.

"Tall man, you sure have a way with words," she exclaimed. We all laughed.

The office door burst open and Phillip was standing in the opening. "What the hell is all this levity? Do I see good friends malingering about? We must not have these happy moments on a Friday afternoon when we are all looking forward to leaving the Spectrum of Medicine for a frolicking weekend outside the Big Apple."

He left his position in the door and walked over to the group and put his arms around the shoulders of J.P. and Brian. "OK, Brian, J.P., let's get to work and leave Janet alone. Besides it is now 4:15 and 4:30 is my slot on the alert-five cat." Phillip announced. J.P. was the only one in the room who understood Phillip's obscure Navy reference to the aircraft that sits on a aircraft carrier's catapult ready to launch immediately when a situation dictated.

When the three men were inside of Phillip's office and seated around his conference table, Phillip's tone turned serious. "J.P., I am sorry I didn't tell you that Brian knew about the extra copy of the 21st Century Plan. I don't know exactly why I kept you in the dark except that I wanted you to look at the total picture instead of going right for Joe and Helmut. I hope everything is all right with my decision."

"Everything is okay, Phillip," J.P. replied. "I was a little surprised at Brian's actions. When he went out to call you and then took fifteen minutes before he came back, I had come to the conclusion that I might not know Brian as well as I thought. His departure produced a feeling that there was a possibility he was a candidate for the bad guy in this scenario. When he came back and told me the real situation, I was so relieved it was impossible to get mad at you or Brian."

"Good, I am glad everything is all right," Phillip concluded.

"Actually, everything is not all right." Brian's voice cut into the other conversation. "Damn it, we had a shitty sales week and a disastrous board meeting. The wolves are dancing at our door. Everything is not all right."

"Ah, leave it to Brian to bring us back to reality," Phillip commented. "I have always wanted to give Brian our 'Back to the Future' award for the person who was best at looking backward while facing the future. But, Brian is so good and conscientious that I feared the tongue in cheek humor would be lost on him. So I gave it instead to Frank Ascot. After your meetings with Frank, I am certain you can appreciate the fact that Frank did not understand why he got the award. You are right, of course, Brian. J.P., did you make any headway this week?" Phillip asked.

"Yes, I believe I have. I feel good about the accomplishments made in the last five days. I am sorry that I haven't made any definitive headway on the 21st Century Plan issue but I feel good about some ideas that have come to light during my Lifeal conversations. I will give you a complete assessment in my Monday morning report. There will be nothing in the report that you should concern yourself with over the weekend. The dramatic issues revolve entirely around the board and you are certainly uptodate on these issues. The Lifeal and 21st Century Plan projects are, at the present, evolving. I have pieces, but still can not make out the total picture."

"I see. Thanks, J.P. And Brian, how was your week?"

"A disaster, thank you, Phillip. We have to do something about the board. We can't let Mrs. James keep undermining us. We've got to come up with a positive plan. I do not have any ideas at this point. I do know that we have to fight or the Mrs. James steamroller will flatten us and James."

"I know, Brian, and I appreciate what you are saying. J.P., do you have any ideas in that regard?"

"As a matter of fact I have a seedling, but not enough to talk about. May I suggest you ask Brian and I to develop a strategy for you? That will then give you something to think over. Maybe give us a deadline of the week before the February board meeting?"

"I agree. Brian, how about you?"

"I'm all for doing something and I would like the opportunity to work with J.P." Brian then turned to J.P. "J.P., let me know when you're ready to talk."

"Let's talk two weeks from next Monday. This will be after I have worked with Joe and Helmut. Does that work for you?" tcp" • "Fine."

"All right, enough chit chat," Phillip announced. "I am now going home to a nice warm fire in the fireplace and spend a quiet weekend with my family. You guys enjoy your weekend."

6:00 A.M., SATURDAY, JANUARY 28
EDGAR ALLAN POE STREET NEW YORK CITY

J.P. had gone to bed early the night before. Although there wasn't anything to which he could attribute his tiredness, he had definitely been feeling fatigued. He had hoped that he would have heard something from Mandi, but he never did. He knew that she would be arriving some time in the next few hours. He lay in his bed for fifteen minutes after waking, planning their day together. He knew that it would be unusual, a combination of private time and public time in the theater district.

Finally, he got out of bed and dressed himself in warm clothing. When he had called Annie on Thursday, he had asked her to express ship two pair of unique thermal full-body underwear that was made in Mammoth Lakes. This particular set of thermals was what J.P. wore when he skied and was the best for pulling moisture away from the skin and keeping a person warm.

He had asked Annie to send a pair for him and a pair of size 6. Annie had been quick to ask for whom the size 6 was intended. J.P. replied that he did not know, but he needed a pair just in case a cold, size 6 person happened through his door. Annie had laughed and warned him to watch out for diseases of the romantic heart.

J.P. ate a good breakfast; put on his boots and light clothes over the twopiece underwear that Annie sent him, and a ski jacket. He rode the ancient elevator down to the front lobby where he talked Charles, the doorman, into loaning out his shovel. J.P. called for a cab and told the driver to take him through Central Park until he said to stop.

The driver turned left on Riverside Drive and drove south to 79th Street turning left so that he could enter the park at the 79th Street traverse. The driving was not easy going since the roads in the park were a low priority for city crews. Fortunately, there were not many cars. Slowly they drove around the park to the side closest to 84th Street. J.P. knew there was a foot entrance to the park at 84th Street. This part of the park was rocky and even with the snow he could make out most of the stone outcroppings. J.P. told the driver to stop at 84th Street. As he exited the cab, he looked to his left and saw a flat area surrounded by trees, which he thought might satisfy his requirements. As he paid the cab driver, J.P. asked him to come back and pick him up at 9:00.

J.P. promised to give him an extra twenty-five dollars if he did as requested.

J.P. stood where the cab had dropped him off and surveyed the surroundings. He knew that it would be easy just to take Mandi to Tavern on the Green where he had lunch with Janet, but he wanted to do something different and special with Mandi. He began walking across a small white field that was surrounded by a number of mature trees.

The snow was more than two feet deep. J.P. walked about fifty yards into the field. The size of the clearing and the trees gave the area an amphitheater feel. Towards the back of the field, he paced off a circle nearly ten feet in diameter. He then dug out the circled area tossing the snow onto the outer edge of the circle, building up the rim to about four feet. It took nearly an hour to accomplish the task. When he finished, J.P. walked back to the road and was pleasantly surprised to find the cab waiting for him. He climbed into the back seat, sat back into the lumpy seat, and gave a deep sigh. The work had been invigorating, but also tiring.

The cab driver looked up into his rearview mirror and caught J.P.'s eye. "What the hell were you doing out there, buddy?" he asked.

"Oh, I was just scouting the area. Essentially, just taking a walk." J.P. replied.

"Takes all kinds. Lived here for fifty years and everyday I find a different New York kook. Someday I am gonna write a book about my passengers. Where to now, buddy, you want I should take you over to the East River so youse can take another walk?"

J.P. laughed. This was one of the things he loved about New York…the taxicab subculture. "Tell you what, how about my hiring you for the day? What would be your charge, say from now until midnight."

He stopped looking at J.P. in his rearview mirror and turned around to look at him directly through that Plexiglas partition between the front and back seat that was intended as a bullet shield between the cabby and the passenger.

"First of all, I am not your friend, buddy. Second, I have to eat and sleep sometime and the Misses…wants me to take her out to dinner tonight. My shift is over at six, see. Youse want I should destroy my love life? Besides, even if youse lives in that big apartment building over on 84th street youse can not afford my palatial limousine for twenty-four hours."

J.P. looked down at his license certificate. The man in the identification picture looked to be about thirty, the man in the front seat was the same man, but he was at least sixty. He was wearing the slouch hat that was the uniform of days past. He had a pleasant and honest looking smile. His name, according to the license, was Roberto Giovanni, license number AA4562.

"Try me on the price, Roberto," J.P. responded knowing full well that he was in for a moving negotiation. J.P. decided that if the driver didn't want the fare he would not have returned to the park to pick him up nor would he have turned around in his seat to address him. Roberto would likely have continued to look at J.P. in his rearview mirror and said something like, "Forget about it, buddy."

"As I said before, youse can't afford me.but for the sake of argument, I'll give you a ball park figure of, oh, say fifty bucks an hour."

J.P. quickly calculated the cost in his head and came up with $600 for 12 hours, noon to midnight. He did his best not to show any expression and turned to look out the side window as he spoke, "Too much for the time I'm going to be actually using you for transportation. Tell you what. How about twenty-five an hour for the time I do not use the cab and thirty-five an hour for when I do?"

"Oh my. Sorry, thirty-five don't cut it, buddy. See dedicated transportation, the type which we are talking about here, doesn't come cheap in this beautiful city." His eyes went from the mirror to the street in front of the cab.

J.P. feigned disinterest and in face turned in his seat to watch a woman walking her dog along a snow-cleared sidewalk. "Okay, tell you what, how about thirty-five an hour for transport around this beautiful city, twenty-five an hour for standby and an additional 150 bucks to take your wife out for dinner?"

Roberto thought for a minute and then said, "Okay, buddy, now youse has my interest. So what's the schedule?"

"I would like for you to pick up a lady friend at Penn Station at about noon, bring her back to the apartment, wait, and then take us back to this place in the park. Pick us up at three and bring us back to the apartment. Pick us up at five and take us to the Broadway theater district. Pick us up at the theater at ten and take us to a restaurant. Pick us up again at 11:30 and bring us back to the apartment. By my calculation that's three hours of driving and nine hours of on call time. $105 for use plus $225 for on call and $150 for dinner totaling $380."

"Make it a minimum of $500 or it ain't worth it."

J.P. sighed, "How about a minimum of $450 and you get paid as we go just in case you get lonesome for your wife?"

"Okay, youse got a deal there, buddy. Of course, this trip before noon is extra."

"Of course, Roberto. Now let's head back to the apartment." "No problem, buddy. Apartment it is, can I call you by a name?" "J.P. and my lady friend is Mandi."

Roberto looked back into the mirror and smiled, "Pleased to meet you, J.P."

The remainder of the trip back to the apartment was in silence. J.P. looked out the cab window. Not much was moving in the city. The commuters were not coming in today and the residents of Manhattan were probably not going to venture out into the cold.

It was going to be a beautiful day. J.P. looked towards the south and saw the Spectrum of Medicine building. It was living up to its name. The morning sun was bouncing off of the grooved aluminum and breaking into its spectrum of light. It looked like a jewel against the blue New York sky. He settled back into his seat telling himself that it was going to be a great day.

Roberto dropped J.P. at the apartment and pulled off to the side to await instructions. When J.P. got back inside his apartment there was a message on the answering machine.

"It is ten o'clock. Where are you, J.P.? I hope that you are there, somewhere. Anyway, I plan on leaving at 10:30. Give me a call before I leave so that I know what to do with myself. Okay?" There was a moment of silence and then a click as Mandi hung up the phone. J.P. looked at his watch and saw that it was 10:15.

He dialed Mandi's number and was relieved when she answered, "Hello?"

"Mandi, sorry I was out doing some errands. What time will you arrive at the station?"

"When you weren't home I was worried you had forgotten our date." "How could I forget our date? It is such a beautiful day I could not think of spending it with anyone but you."

She laughed, "Yeah, yeah, schmooze, schmooze. Well, thanks for the compliment, but I feel anything but beautiful. This snow makes every chore double work. I had to go out this morning and cars were stuck all over the place. I look forward to a calm day. Anyway, I will arrive at Penn Station at 12:05. Will you pick me up or do you want me to come over by cab?"

"Come out the exit for the taxi cab stand. You know the space between the Garden and Penn Station."

"Yes, I know the place."

"There will be a cab at the curb with a sign in the window with your name on it. The driver's name is Roberto Giovanni. He will bring you to the apartment. If he is not there give me a call. Okay?"

"What? Are you spending all of your time making pals with New York cabbies? Sounds different J.P., but okay. Roberto Giovanni, got it. I'm bringing some casual clothes plus evening clothes for the theater and dinner. Is there anything else that I should bring besides myself?"

"You're the most important item and no, you don't need to bring anything else. See you about 12:45."

"OK, bye."

"Bye."

After J.P. hung up the phone, he returned to the lobby to talk to Roberto. Roberto had already found a parking spot and was inside the lobby chatting with Charles.

"Hiya, J.P. So, what is it that I'm to do?"

"Okay, Roberto, I want you to make a couple of errands for me and then pick up Mandi at Penn Station at 12:05. She will meet you at the cab pickup stand inbetween Penn Station and the Garden. I know you have to start before noon when our agreement begins, but I will pay for the errands I'll ask of you at the use fare. Fair enough?"

"Okay, J.P., that's fine. What is it that youse want me to do?"

"Please pick up some flowers and place them on the back seat for Mandi with this note." He handed him a note that he had written before coming downstairs. "Please obtain a piece of cardboard and make a sign with Mandi's name on it to place in your front windshield. By the way, she spells her name, mandi. She'll be looking for the cab with the sign. She is a tall, beautiful redhead, but with the cold she might have her head covered so you may not be able to tell. Any questions?"

"Nope. I have a clear picture and will have the chariot there on time with the flowers and card. Up front money on the flowers and name card?"

J.P. handed him a $50 bill. "Okay, Roberto?" he asked.

"Beautiful. I'm on my way." He drove away from the building spinning his wheels on the snow-covered street, the back end of his cab weaving back and forth. J.P. smiled as he watched him drive off. Suddenly he remembered that he needed to straighten up his apartment for company and pack a lunch. He proceeded back upstairs to get started.

J.P. was just finishing up his chores when doorman's phone began to ring. He looked at his watch and saw that it was 12:45. He picked the phone up on the third ring.

"Yes?"

"Dr. Koenig, Mrs. Hayes is on her way up and Roberto says he will be standing by to take you to the park."

"Thanks, Charles." He hung up the phone and waited for the doorbell to ring. It was nearly three minutes later that the bell finally sounded. He had changed from his shoveling outfit to a more colorful outdoor hiking outfit. He had left his full body thermal underwear and boots on.

He opened the door and there stood Mandi. Her suitcase was on the floor by her side. In her arms was the bouquet of flowers that Roberto had gotten her, a mixed spring bouquet of yellow daisies with tulips, chrysanthemums, and others that he didn't recognize.

She smiled and said. "Hi, J.P. You look ready to weather the great outdoors. Am I a little underdressed?" She took off her coat to reveal that she was wearing jeans and a wool sweater.

"Are you going to let me stand here in the hallway?" she said laughing. "No, no, Mandi please come in. Here let me take your suitcase. I was admiring well, you look fabulous. I was just thinking how lovely your blue eyes and red hair look with you holding the flowers. Sorry."

She laughed again. "Don't be sorry, J.P. I kind of like having that kind of influence on you," she said as she stepped into the apartment and J.P. closed the door behind her.

"Where in the world did you find that beautiful New York cabbie? He entertained me all of the way from the station. He had me in stitches with his stories. And the flowers, they are so beautiful I am afraid to put them down. What a beautiful way to be greeted to the city. Do you have more surprises up your sleeve?"

"I met Roberto this morning and I have contracted him to be our chauffeur for the rest of the day. As for other surprises, you will have to wait and see. We Californians are sly bastards."

"Sly, I will wager, don't forget that I'm a Californian myself, but a bastard I'm not so sure. I will reserve my opinion until tomorrow. Where do you want me to throw my things?"

"Put them in the guest room. We are going out for a walk so I put some special thermal underwear on the bed for you to put on. When you are ready we will have lunch in the park."

"Oh? Do you mean Tavern on the Green?"

"Nope. I mean in the park. As for what in the park means, you'll have to wait for the answer."

"I see, so what's so special about this thermal underwear?"

"It's light and flexible, but very warm. A company in Mammoth makes it for skiers. You'll only need a sweater on top of your shirt. No jacket required."

Fifteen minutes later they were in Roberto's cab on their way to the park. Roberto left them off near the place that J.P. had cleared earlier that morning.

"J.P., this is a beautiful place, but we're in the middle of nowhere and the snow is too deep to walk through."

He led Mandi to the path that he had made. "Follow me, my adventurous friend," he encouraged. They walked to the area he had cleared.

Mandi giggled and asked, "What is this, your special hiding place?" "No, it is our special hiding place."

J.P. set down the canvas bag that contained everything for their afternoon in the park. He spread out a thermal blanket and began to assemble their lunch. He had a bottle of champagne, shrimp cocktail, some warm New England Clam chowder, and fish and chips. The sun was warm and the combination of the thermal blanket keeping the wet earth from them, the four-foot snow banks encircling them keeping their exposure to the wind to a minimum, the food, and the champagne made for a very cozy space.

Mandi looked around at the surroundings and the lunch spread. She looked at J.P. and said, "No, I think I'll give you my opinion now."

"Opinion? Opinion on what?" J.P. asked in surprise.

"On what you are. You are most certainly a sly bastard." She laughed and added; "Now open that bottle of champagne and let's have lunch."

They ate a leisurely lunch and finished the champagne. When J.P. checked his watch it was 2:30. He had instructed Roberto to blow his horn at 3:00 so they would have time to get back to J.P.'s apartment to get ready for the theater. The sky was still blue, but the afternoon light was beginning to dim and it was not as warm as it had been an hour before. J.P. cleared the lunch remains and they lay down on the blanket looking up at the sky.

Mandi broke the silence, "I had forgotten how beautiful New York City could be in the winter. You know we work here and get caught up in the New York City pace and don't take the time to do crazy things like we have this afternoon. Even if you are a sly bastard J.P., thank you very much for a fabulous lunch."

They were using the canvas bag as a headrest. Mandi moved around to that her head rested on his chest. He closed his arm around her shoulder.

"I was thinking of how enjoyable today has been and will be. It is so great to be with someone that I feel so comfortable just being around."

"Today has been filled with simple surprises, J.P. Most of the men I have dated, and there have not been many since John died, try to knock me off my feet. You on the other hand, so far, have taken the simplest of things and made them memorable. Take this little snow room that you've carved out in the park. I know of no other person who would have thought of creating a snow room for lunch. You are a wonder, J.P."

"Not really Mandi. I only thought of doing this when I thought of you. You are a combination of warmth and cold. Do not take this wrong, I meant it as a compliment. You know the difference between these two moods and when it is appropriate to use each of them. Not many people have the talent and the common sense to know the difference." He paused and looked away for a moment.

"Mandi?" he turned his head to look at her, "I don't know much about you. Before I met you I read about your school and work history, but I didn't know much about Mandi. If you do not want to talk about yourself, that's fine, but I would like to know more about who you are. I don't mean the James Vice President of Marketing, but Mandi, the woman. And I might add one of the most beautiful women I have ever met and had lunch with in the middle of a snow drift in Central Park."

She smiled up at him. He could tell that the lunch and champagne had a mellowing effect on her. "I am so content and feel so safe that I don't know if I can talk about myself. I am what I am. I'm not very complex although many think I am because I ask a lot of questions. It is just that I want to learn. I want to learn about everything I can. I don't have enough time in my life to learn all the things I have questions about or the time to experience everything that I want to experience. Part of my past life was structured by the unexpected and devastating loss of John." Mandi stopped talking.

J.P. was afraid he had gotten her to talk about something that she really didn't want to talk about. He remembered Phillip saying that she never discussed her husband's death. J.P. decided to break the silence and give her an out. He didn't want the day to be spoiled for either of them because of an old memory.

"Mandi, you don't have to talk about John. I might not feel your loss, but I do understand."

"No, J.P., it's all right. For a while it wasn't easy, but I finally realized that he was never coming back. It's been nine years. I was quiet because I was thinking about those nine years and how much I have given to James and how little I have given to myself. I haven't talked about John because I haven't had a reason to talk about him or us.

"John was a Navy Lieutenant and a pilot, or a 'Naval Aviator' as he preferred to refer to himself. He was on shore duty at Miramar teaching at the Navy Fighter Weapons School.the old Topgun School. Our romance began soon after I finished my MBA and lasted more than three years. After a year of dating, while he was still at Topgun, he was transferred to the USS Kitty Hawk. After six months of carrier training, his ship was scheduled for a tour to the western pacific. All it took was one seven-month WESTPAC cruise and we were hooked. I visited the ship in Hong Kong where we had six unbelievably wonderful days." She stopped talking again and looked up at the sky.

"I haven't thought of those times for years. They were so much fun. We were young and he knew so much more about life than I did. He had so much that he wanted to show me. We were married soon after he returned from the cruise. At the time, I was a James sales rep in San Diego. He was killed in a carrier training exercise off the coast of California. I don't know many of the details, but I understand that something went terribly wrong during the carrier launch. He tried to bring the plane around and land it on the flight deck instead of just ditching the plane and saving himself. He almost made it, but there wasn't enough power and he crashed into the back end of the ship. He was killed instantly." Mandi fell silent again. J.P. looked down at her and could see tears welling up in her eyes.

She smiled at him and wiped the tears from her eyes. "I guess I haven't gotten it all out of my system and it needs to come out. There is not much more to tell. I was crushed. My life was crushed. I went into a state of depression that you would not believe.

"One day I decided to pull myself out of the dumps and I threw myself into selling for James. Phillip was watching my sales record and soon thereafter I was promoted to district sales manager. In reviewing my records, Phillip discovered that I have an MBA. He asked me if at sometime in the future I might be interested in a marketing position with the home office. I told him I definitely wanted a home office position. So, I moved to New York as a James Product Manager. I bought a little home in Wyckoff, New Jersey. I didn't want to become involved in the singles scene, so I didn't even look into living in the city. I have dated, but not very much. Friends try to fix me up but the relationships never go anywhere. It isn't that I have been pining over John. I just never found anybody that really tripped my trigger. Does that make sense to you, J.P.?"

He replied slowly, "It makes sense if it makes sense to you, Mandi. It is not easy to be alone and hold a top position at James. I would imagine you are just not interested in a long-term relationship. I do understand this because I have felt the same way myself."

"Really J.P.?" She fell silent again.

J.P. was just about to say something when Roberto's horn broke the silence.

"What was that?"

"That's our chauffeur telling us that it's three o'clock and that we have to get back to the apartment and prepare for the theater."

He and Mandi both stood up and gazed into one another's eyes.

"Thank you for lunch, J.P., and thank you for asking me to talk about myself. I feel much closer to you now." She leaned forward and gave him a quick kiss on his left cheek. J.P.'s arms encircled her waist and she put her arms around his neck. They held each other in a tight embrace. After a few seconds, they both turned their heads and their lips met. A long and deep kiss followed, not the kiss of two lonely people, but of two people who had found something in each other. The incessant honking of the cab's horn finally broke their kiss and embrace.

They moved apart and in silence picked up the things that they had brought with them. They were ready to leave when he told her to go ahead to the cab and tell Roberto that he would be along in a minute. As Mandi started up the path towards the waiting car, J.P. began to knock down the walls of the snow room. It took him about five minutes and what was once a place of solitude was reduced to a flat trampled snowfield. J.P. walked slowly back to the cab.

"You were filling in our snow room, weren't you?" Mandi asked softly when he was seated next to her in the back seat.

He took her hand in his and squeezed. "Yes," he said quietly.

9:00 P.M., SATURDAY, JANUARY 28

GLOBAL THEATER NEW YORK CITY

J.P. watched Mandi as they walked back up the aisle following the third curtain call for the actors. Her eyes were moist, not from crying but from laughing so hard at the musical they had just seen. She was wearing a black dress that was cut low in the front and tightly wrapped her slender body to just above her knees. Her bright, silky red shoulder length hair framed her face. The tears of happiness had not affected her makeup; instead it seemed to make here face even brighter. Her full lips were glossy and curled up in a wide smile. Her teeth were sparkling white. J.P. smiled to himself thinking how very lucky he was to have found her and how proud he was to be seen with her.

They held hands as they walked through the cavernous lobby of the theater. Finally she spoke.

"Did you enjoy the play as much as I did, J.P.?" She asked as she turned to look at his face.

"Mandi, I haven't seen a Broadway play for so long I had forgotten how great it is to sit and enjoy a show. That play was one of the best I've ever seen. And sitting next to you added to the enjoyment. I don't recall ever seeing anyone enjoy themselves so much as you did this evening. You really did have fun, didn't you?"

"You bet J.P. I hope I didn't embarrass you by laughing so much." "How could I be embarrassed?

"Well, I was laughing a little loudly at times."

"You helped everyone around us to enjoy it as well. Some people with a hearty laugh, and that is what you have my dear, laugh at the wrong time. Your laugh is always at the right moment and very infectious."

"So, how did you know that I would like this play?"

"Well, with all the seriousness going on at James, I thought we could use a good laugh."

Mandi squeezed his hand and pulled him closer to her, "I loved it. Thank you.

They retrieved their coats and went outside. Roberto was waiting at the curb along with a number of long black limousines. As they approached the cab, Roberto jumped out of his side of the cab and ran around to open the door for them.

As they pulled away from the curb, J.P. asked, "Roberto, how was dinner with your wife?"

"Ah, it was wonderful, J.P. The wife and I ate at Gustov's in Brooklyn. We had the best steak dinner there that we've had in fifteen years. Thank youse very much. Now off we go to your dinner." Roberto drove them to a French restaurant on 56th street.

Dinner was leisurely. They talked about their lives and experiences each wanting to learn more about the other. They had already established a strong working relationship built on trust and mutual respect for one another. Now they were working on building a relationship of a more personal nature.

After their meal, J.P. ordered another bottle of wine and they sat listening to a light-jazz trio that called themselves, "The Legion of Three." The band was set up on the edge of the dining area near their table. The group played a delightful mix of old and new jazz. Mandi reached over and put her hands on top of J.P.'s hands as they listened to the music. At one point, in between songs, one of the musicians announced that they performed three nights a week in the restaurant.

"Hey, we'll have to start coming here regularly. I really like these guys,"

J.P. said as his eyes met Mandi's.

"Perhaps we can become legends in a legion?" She said softly.

"I think I'm already a legend, so why would I want to join a legion," J.P. said laughing. "Are you sure that you want to join the group of legends? You're much too bright, intelligent, and.. .well.. .young."

"Come on J.P., you're the leader, I can feel it when you walk into a room. People look at me and measure me as a female. They look at you and count the money that you will enable them to earn."

"Not true, my love. You just don't see the envy in their eyes at what you have, can, and will be able to bring to any organization. You may not see it, but it's definitely there. One day you'll look in the mirror and realize your full potential."

"Ah, and will you help me get there, J.P.?"

"Hey, baby, anything for you," he said with a smile. "Let's go home before we're tempted to order another bottle of wine. I'm sure Roberto is probably anxious to whisk us back to 84th Street. Ready to go?"

"Ready."

An hour later, they were sitting in the hot tub listening to one of Prokofiev's sympathies. This time there were no swimsuits or robes just Mandi and J.P. and a tub of 104-degree water.

Mandi was the first to speak after they had settled into seats in the churning water, "What are we doing, J.P.? Is it James that is throwing us together or is this for real? It has been a long time.no it has been a very long time.since I have enjoyed being with a man. I was beginning to think something was wrong with me. Do you think that there is something wrong with me?"

"Wow, where did that come from? You're certainly steering the evening towards a definite turn to the serious," J.P. said in a half-laugh, hoping she wouldn't think he was trying to invalidate her concerns. "There is definitely nothing wrong with you, dear. In my humble lay opinion you've just got new relationship jitters. I have to tell you that I am beginning to feel that I'm really falling for you. I know it's probably too early to be using the L-word, but I do think I'm falling in love with you. I think you can probably see that too...perhaps your concerns lie in the fact that it's so early on in this relationship and you feel that things are moving too fast."

She reached over and put her hand on his thigh, "Yes, I do feel the same way. I had considered at some point this evening, probably after the second bottle of wine, that things might be moving a little fast. But that only lasted a short time and then I just decided to roll with it."

J.P. found himself staring at her and she returned his gaze. He was about to lean forward to kiss her when suddenly she said, "J.P., lets get out of this hot water and get ourselves into some hot water. What do you say?"

"I thought you would never ask. Now the question is, should I lift you out of this tub and carry you to the bed. As wet as we are I'd probably slip and break my back. Paramedics would have to come, they wouldn't be able to get the gurney into the elevator, and then some television news crew would be outside taping the action as they lowered me out of a window to the ground below. There I'd be, naked as a jaybird, and tied to a gurney for all of New York City to see. On the other hand, I could show you my Neanderthal side. We could get out of this tub, dry off, and I could throw you over my shoulder and carry to the bed and make primitive love to you, but I don't know how that would play with your feminine sensitivities. Hmmmm, any suggestions?"

Mandi was laughing, "My, my...what an imaginative lover I've found for myself. While I do kind of like the primitive love thing, I would really hate to flip some genetic throwback switch and have you start prowling Central Park for something to hunt down. And, I most certainly don't want to answer some reporter's questions about how it is that you came to break your back, so I have a deal for you. What say, we both climb out of this tub like a normal couple. Then you will dry me off with a towel and I will do the same for you. And then, we will proceed quickly, without running to the bed. How does that sound?"

Without giving him an opportunity to answer, Mandi stood up in the tub and then clambered over the side. J.P. for the first time saw the loveliness of her naked body. He felt himself becoming erect beneath the water and was hesitant at first about standing up in the tub. Finally he decided there was really nothing to be embarrassed about and he stood.

Mandi's gaze shifted down his body when he stood and she said in a voice so low that it was a whisper, "Mmmmm, careful that you don't pass out with all that blood rushing from your head. Now, let's get on with the drying process before we wind up rolling around on the wet tile and catch our death of colds and pneumonia."

Without saying a word, J.P. reached over and flipped a switch on the wall and infrared-heating lamps in the ceiling came on. He walked over to Mandi and began to dry her skin with a large fluffy bath towel.

She said in a soft voice, "Am I too pale J.P.? You are so tan. I look anemic next too you.

"No, you're not too pale. You look great!"

When he had managed to dry most of her skin with the towel, he moved back in front of her and took her in his arms, holding her close.

She giggled and pushed back from him slightly, "J.P., you're still wet!

Here let me dry you off."

Mandi took the towel from him and began to vigorously rub his body.

At times he thought she was going to rub off his skin. "Are you testing my thresh hold of pain?" he asked.

"No, lover, only trying to see if any of this color comes off."

They both laughed. J.P. took the towel from her hands and dropped it onto the floor. Without saying a word, he picked her up in his arms and carried her into the bedroom. He laid her down on the light brown sheets.

Her eyes were closed and she whispered, "Come to bed, J.P. I want your body close to mine. I need your warmth."

When the rays of the morning sun lit up the interior of the apartment, they left the bed and walked to the shower. They washed one another and made love sliding together in the soap lather with J.P. pressing her against the tile wall of the shower. He pulled the drapes over the wall and closed the blinds of ceiling glass. They went back to bed and slept until noon. When they awoke they had lunch and went back to bed and made love again.

At 4:00, J.P. took a chance and called Roberto to ask if he would drive them to Mandi's home in New Jersey and then bring him back to the apartment. He surprised them by agreeing.

On the way to Mandi's house he leaned close to her and asked, "How are we going to act tomorrow and the day I after tomorrow? I'm not sure I'll be able to even look at you unless I'm sitting down."

"You do have a problem with engorgement, don't you?" Mandi responded playfully. "As for tomorrow, You'll just have to show what kind of an actor you can be. I don't expect that we'll be able to hide the fact that we care for each other, but we must not act like a pair of lovebirds. Now we must make some rules or we will never get the James project solved."

J.P. sat back and said, "Okay, we will act like a good friends. At work we should go on as before. I am certain that we can do this because we are both professionals and we don't want to give any impressions that we have any other agenda in mind that would prevent us from devoting our full attention to helping Phillip and James Pharmaceutical. Can you spend Wednesday nights and the weekends in the city? This way I'll have something to look forward to and life will be tolerable."

"I would love to spend Wednesdays and the weekends with you as long as you can stand me." Mandi smiled and gave him a kiss.

After dropping Mandi off at her home the ride back into the city was quiet. J.P.'s thoughts were all of Mandi and what the future might hold for the two of them. Roberto seemed to understand and listened to music on the radio without saying anything.

8:00 P.M., SUNDAY, JANUARY 29
SUTTON PLACE NEW YORK CITY

Sunday evening found Peggy watching television. She thought back over the past week at work. During the week she had concentrated on the increased number of reported routine Lifeal side effects. She felt the increase was due to the simple fact that there were more patients taking maintenance doses of the drug. The routine side effects of sleepiness and slight nausea were increasing in number, but not as a percentage of the total doses being ingested. These routine side effects didn't bother her, they were to be expected. Sleepiness and nausea were common side effects that many patients experienced with many pharmaceuticals. James Pharmaceutical Company, just as any other company, had to keep track of the rate of incidence of all side effects.

A rate of routine side effects below two percent was considered to be within reasonable risk limits. Thus far, Lifeal had a rate of routine side effects of less than one percent.

Peggy had determined that most patients tolerated Lifeal better because it was an herbal-based product rather than chemical. She was slightly concerned over the few reported incidences of, what she could only classify as hypersensitivity. So far, she had received reports of five occurrences. Five cases in five years, this was not a significant number, but the side effect of hypersensitivity had not been reported in any of the pre-FDA approval clinical studies. She decided she would report this new side effect to the FDA as soon as she completed her preliminary report.

She was going to call the physicians that had reported the hypersensitivity side effect and ask them to send her a copy of their patients' records so that she could investigate them for correlation. She would also start animal studies to see if she could reproduce the side effect. Tomorrow, she would call Allen and ask for his advice on this side effect. She did not bother Helmut with side effect results until she had firm data. Helmut always drilled her on her facts to determine if there were any weak points. When she had weak facts, Helmut's demanding management style was not constructive. He would make her feel guilty for bringing the side effect to his attention. Allen gave her advice and helped her to think through situations. She would, of course, give Helmut a complete briefing when she had firm data and conclusions and before she made her report to the FDA.

7:00 A.M., MONDAY, JANUARY 30

SPECTRUM OF MEDICINE BUILDING
NEW YORK CITY

J.P. gave Phillip an oral comprehensive report of his activities of the previous week giving particular attention to the prospects of repositioning of Lifeal.

Phillip waited until he had finished and then remarked, "J.P., I understand your report, but I'm not getting a sense that we're making any headway. I'm actually beginning to wonder if I'm not just tilting at windmills. You saw and heard firsthand what Evelyn James had to say. You, Brian, and I discussed her motives last Friday. She's moving a private agenda along the fast track and I'm not sure that I have the luxury of time to wait while you methodically work through all the Lifeal issues."

J.P. was, at first, stunned by Phillip's words, but then he realized that Phillip was already under a lot of stress and had probably spent the weekend replaying the board meeting in his mind.

"Phillip," he said quietly, "Don't be concerned. And, yes, I know how easy it is for me to sit here and tell you not to be concerned, but believe me, I'm on your side. I am making headway on the 21st Century Plan issue and your overall situation. I realize that I haven't presented anything substantive, but it has only been two weeks." He paused long enough to allow what he had just said to sink in and then continued, "Excuse my bluntness, but there's no delicate way to ask this. If Evelyn were going to dump your programs and you, when would she make her move?"

Phillip shook his head and in a more jovial mood replied "Boy, you sure know how to cheer a guy up on a Monday morning." He thought for a moment and said, "Well, as you so eloquently put it, she would most likely dump me at the annual meeting in May."

"There you go." J.P. said with emphasis. "We have three months until D-Day." J.P. decided to hint at what Brian and he had discussed. "If we were going to prevent DDay in May then we would have to execute a counter plan by the April board meeting. Isn't that correct?"

Phillip sat staring for a moment as he tried to figure out where J.P. was going. "Yes, you're correct. In that case, we only have two months or actually less and by your own report you don't have much in the way of leads. How the hell are we going to prevent what you call, DDay? And, what does the D in DDay stand for? Dump? Devastate?"

J.P. put on his most positive face and acted as enthusiastic as he could under the circumstances. "First of all, Phillip, you have to get your spirits up. You know we can handle this. We've faced bigger challenges in shorter periods of time. We have plenty of time if we work hard together, but you have to want to fight. So the question to you is, do you in fact want to fight? If so, cheer up and make sure your staff meeting has a positive atmosphere. The first time any of your staff gets so much as a whiff of surrender on your part, it's all downhill from there."

Phillip looked down at the floor for some time before turning his attention to the window and the crisp, clear day outside. The morning sun was shining off the Hudson River onto the New Jersey palisades. He got up out of his chair and walked to the window.

"So, tell me, where did you learn cheerleading skills? J.P., come here to the window."

J.P. got up and walked to the large window to stand shoulder to shoulder with Phillip. "Look at the sun's rays.how they skip off the river. I guess I feel like those rays. I have been with James for more than twenty-five years. I have put my life into this company, its products, its customers, and, of course, its people. Ever since old Doc James died, that woman has been bouncing me around like those rays of sun. I get high from achievement and then I hit the water as she comes out of nowhere to knock me back down. I have been knocked around so much I don't know how much longer I can take the ups and downs." He turned towards J.P. and continued with his voice filled with emotion.

"I'm really not sure that I can hold out until DDay, J.P. I certainly don't owe her anything and I am certain that she will destroy James regardless of who is president. No, I'm leaning towards resigning now and walking away from James."

J.P. knew that Phillip was reaching out for help and chose his words carefully. "Phillip, I know you have been knocked around and you feel that it's only getting worse. You have to look at what you've built here at James and what the James potential could be with your continued leadership. You're forgetting your vision of where James can be in the next century. Phillip, look again at the river."

They both looked down at the sparkling Hudson. J.P. could feel himself becoming impatient with Phillip. "You want to talk in parables and metaphors? Here you go. Look, you're looking across the river from east to west. Look again. The river has a finite width, but it also has length. The shimmers you see flow along that length of river to the Atlantic. You have always had a vision of success. You've built upon your daily successes and James has become more successful because of those successes. Mrs. James only sees width, a clear and definable dimension. Your vision takes that in certainly, but also looks out across the continuum. Look at where the East River flows into the Hudson River giving the Hudson that much more strength as it flows beneath the Verrazano Narrows Bridge and to the Atlantic beyond. There's your vision and your answer, Phillip, not to the frigging New Jersey palisades. I'm sorry if I was a bit short with you before, but, frankly unless your thoroughly committed to this, you're doing James Pharmaceutical more harm than good by hanging around. Only you can decide if you have the commitment to see this thing through to the end, whatever that outcome may be. That is the hallmark of great leadership."

J.P. decided to ease up a bit, "This company, its customers, and its people still require your leadership, Phillip. There are millions of patients who benefit from and depend on James products and your leadership. I know it might not seem worth the effort, but it is Phillip. I've never known you to give up anything without a dogfight and I don't think you should give up on this fight without raising some dust.

"Phillip, you have to give your friends here a chance to help you. I'm not saying things will turn around immediately. Nor am I assuring you that things will not get worse before they get better. I do feel and very strongly, that we.. .you.. .will survive and realize your vision. Give us until the annual meeting.

You have nothing to lose. If DDay does in fact happen, then it happens. Financially, a DDay is better than resignation. If you get dumped you get a nice severance package. If you quit, you get nothing and, you know damn well that Evelyn would love for you to quit."

Phillip turned from the window and sat back down at the conference table. "So, J.P.," he said with a smile, "you have convinced me to stay and fight. You believe the payoff is worth the fight. You know, you are really good at what you do…whatever the hell that is," he added with a wry smile. "Now what did you say you're cooking up to prevent a DDay?"

J.P. repeated much of the plan that he and Brian had discussed. They would be repositioning Lifeal to provide Phillip with substance to form a plan for a fight with the James board. He also told him that he would redouble his efforts to solve the 21st Century Plan issue. All of that to be accomplished before the April board meeting.

Phillip's resolve was completely restored when he replied, "You've got it, J.P. I'll see you at 9:00 for the staff meeting."

J.P. turned from where he had been standing at the window and began walking to the door. He was almost to the door when he heard Phillip say, "J.P.!" He turned around. Phillip was standing behind his desk with his hands in his pant pockets. "Thanks, old friend, for everything. Thanks especially for listening to my whining."

"No problem, Phillip. Sometimes a guy needs to whine," he replied and left the office.

He proceeded to Mandi's office for their eight o'clock meeting before Phillip's staff meeting at ten. As he entered her office, he found her at her usual place behind her computer. She got up from her seat and walked over the conference table as she had always done.

"J.P., this is going to be harder than I thought. I missed you last night and want desperately to hug you. I had such a great time Saturday and yesterday that I don't want this feeling to stop even though common sense says slow down Mandi."

J.P. had taken a seat at the conference table. He didn't know what to say, so he remained quiet and just smiled at Mandi.

"For God's sakes, don't let me babble on like a silly college girl. Say something."

J.P. looked down at the table and back to her face, "First, Mandi you could never be a silly college girl. You are most assuredly a woman. I can't begin to describe how very much I enjoyed our weekend together. I don't know where all this will lead us, but I know I will enjoy being with you as much as you and the situation here at James will allow."

He reached over and placed a hand atop her folded hands. The emotions of the hours since they had parted company the night before seemed to well again.

"You know, I don't feel like working, Mandi. I just want to be with you. I don't want my feelings to change, but I…we…have to get them under control while we're here in the office. But after work we will be J.P. and Mandi. How does that sound?"

Mandi gazed longingly at him and said, "Hey! That's no fun! But, I know you're right. It'll be easier this way." She quickly changed the subject, "Now what about this week? What have you laid on for our project? This week is production, right?"

"Right," he replied. "I plan to see Joe this week. Also, before I forget, I made plans last week to have dinner with Janet and her husband, Bill, on Wednesday night."

Mandi's face reflected her surprise and displeasure at his Wednesday night appointment.

"I am sorry, Hon, I know we were saving Wednesday night for us. I made the dinner appointment last week. In the heat of our weekend together, it slipped my mind. Could we make this week a Tuesday visit?"

"Not a big deal, J.P. Tuesday is fine with me." Mandi spoke with excitement. "A day early is just right. If it is all right with you, can we just spend a quiet evening together?"

"I think that's perfect. Going on with the schedule, I have lunch with Carl and his father on Thursday."

"Why the lunch with Carl's father?" Mandi asked with interest.

"I guess it's because I gained a great deal of respect for Carl during our meeting. His father is very important to him and his father is suffering from Alzheimer's disease. He's in the early stages, but as is usually the case, the prognosis isn't good. Carl's father is an excellent lawyer and a good father and there is no better testimonial than for a son to say that he has a good father. Carl wanted me to meet his father and I agreed.

"I think Carl has an excellent start on the answer to the repositioning of Lifeal. I also think he will play an important role in the future of James. Anyway that is my schedule this week. Next weekend is for us. What do you think about a weekend of skiing in New England?"

Mandi replied enthusiastically, "I would love to go skiing." "Great, I'll set it up."

She looked at her watch, "Oops. Time to go to the staff meeting."

1:00 P.M., MONDAY, JANUARY 30

JAMES PHARMACEUTICAL COMPANY MANUFACTURING PLANT BROOKLYN, NY

Phillip's staff meeting was routine. As usual, it ended on time. Joe and J.P. left the meeting together. They went down to the lobby and caught the shuttle van that James sponsored between the Spectrum of Medicine building and the James Brooklyn plant where the major manufacturing complex was located. James had three manufacturing sites one in Brooklyn, one in Sheepshead Bay, and one in Puerto Rico. Sheepshead Bay plant was the original plant. When the business became large, Doc James moved the manufacturing to a plant in Brooklyn. He converted the Sheepshead Bay plant to light manufacturing and pilot plant operations. The Puerto Rico plant took raw material purchased internationally and converted it into finished goods.

The Brooklyn plant was an old building that had been modernized. It was south of the Brooklyn Bridge in the Sunset Park area to the west of the expressway. Most of the buildings in this area were deserted. The days of heavy manufacturing in Brooklyn were over. James Pharmaceutical Company was the only pharmaceutical firm remaining in Brooklyn. When Squibb finally gave up its Brooklyn plant in the late 60's and sold the building to the Jehovah's Witnesses, Doc James remained. He stayed in character. Doc James stayed while others left for the suburbs. He always had to be different. He sunk millions into the old Brooklyn facility and made it a model pharmaceutical plant. The FDA used the James plant as a model good manufacturing practice facility. Joe was very proud of his facility and loved to show off the plant to who ever would visit. He did not have the opportunity to show off the plant very often because visitors never wanted to visit Brooklyn.

When Doc. James was asked why he remained in Brooklyn he would always reply, the labor market was excellent and the people of Brooklyn loved James because it had remained. There was a silent bond between every company with facilities in Brooklyn and New York City. The Boroughs of Brooklyn and Manhattan wanted James to succeed and the people and politicians did the best they could to ensure the company's success. It was family.

The shuttle dropped them off at the front door of the plant. The front lobby was small in size and simple in decor. A reception desk, two elevators, and a door. The door and the entrance door were reinforced. Even though the James employees were family the neighborhood was still not the best and there was a black market for pharmaceuticals. The piers were very convenient for outsiders to smuggle products by boat.

The building was outfitted for maximum security and was built around the employees. There were multiple choices of places to eat as well as recreational facilities all inside the plant grounds. Shuttle buses picked up the workers and took them home or to central drop off points. If an employee drove to work, they parked their car in a maximum security underground garage.

Joe and J.P. took the elevator to the management offices on the fifth floor. Joe's office was filled with a computer, PERT charts, and computer printouts. They sat down at his rectangular conference table. Joe was an excellent VP of Operations. It was hard for J.P. to imagine that he was connected to anything that would harm James. He was a quiet and unassuming person unless it concerned his operations domain. In operations, Joe was the authority and he ran a tight ship. Those that worked hard were rewarded. Those that slacked off, were let go. He worked closely with the Union and very rarely did Joe and the Union disagree. He had worked his way up from the bottom. He had worked part time on the line when he was in high school and college.

After graduation from New York University he was hired as a line supervisor. He then spent the next 30 years climbing to the VP of Operations position. He knew his job very well. On issues not concerning operations Joe was silent. He did what was required of him to ensure the availability of product and he did this very well, but he stayed away from politics.

The two men spent the rest of the afternoon discussing the different product lines and manufacturing processes.

3:00 P.M., TUESDAY, JANUARY 31
WYCKOFF, NJ

Ralph Vandermere walked back to his car from the medical building. He had just left Dr. Rosenberg's office and was thinking back on his conversation with the cardiologist. He concluded that Rosenberg was an asshole and he would start looking for a new physician. Rosenberg just didn't understand what he was going through.

Thinking aloud he muttered to himself, "I really don't require a cardiologist, my heart feels perfect. And, I have never felt more legally capable. Sure, people seem to be getting on my nerves and I have my mood swings, but whose moods don't swing. Things are even better since I increased my own dosage to two tablets of Lifeal everyday. Now, I really am myself. And that damned Rosenberg had the nerve to order me to stop taking Lifeal. Today is the last time I will ever see him again."

Ralph reached into the pocket of his jacket for his prescription vial of Lifeal. He lined up the arrows, pulled the cap off and spilled the last tablet into the palm of his hand.

"Shit," he muttered, "I'd better stop by and see Hank about a refill."

He got into his car and drove to the Somerset Pharmacy. He drove recklessly, weaving in and out of traffic. He laid on his horn at traffic signals. He had to get to the pharmacy to get a refill on his medication. After all, he didn't have his daily allowance, as he had come to call it, of Lifeal in him. He didn't want to take a chance that he would lose the benefits he had gained so far by missing a dose.

Finally, he arrived in the parking lot of Somerset Pharmacy. He virtually abandoned his car in front of store, leaving the door open and the engine running. He walked through the door of the pharmacy and proceeded quickly to the prescription counter in the back. A young pharmacy clerk, who looked to be no more than eighteen, met him at the counter. He looked directly into her eyes without saying a word. He reached into his pocket and pulled out his prescription vial and slapped it down on the counter.

"Where is Hank? I want a refill," he said in a menacing voice.

The young woman was stunned by the venomous tone of Ralph's voice and took a step back from the counter. Hesitantly, she picked up the vial and looked at the label. She surveyed the strangely dressed man who just stood there quietly watching her. He was wearing white slacks that were completely covered with stains of various colors. He was wearing a light blue tee-shirt on top and a large, floor length overcoat that was draped over his shoulders.

She did her best to speak in a confident sounding voice, but the quivering voice that came out betrayed her sudden fear of Ralph.

"I'm sorry, Mr. Vandermere. Mr. Somerset is not here today. It's his day off. Dr. Johnson is the pharmacist today. He will help you."

"Well, sweetheart, move that cute little tail of yours and get this Dr. Johnson off his lazy ass to refill my prescription. I'm a busy man, with lots to do."

Ben Johnson looked up from filling another prescription to see who was using the loud profanity and insulting remarks to his clerk. As he looked up, Ralph spotted him behind the counter and grabbed the prescription vial from the clerk's hand. He moved around to stand in front of Ben who remained behind the glass partition.

Before Ben could say anything, Ralph spun around and threw the vial over the glass partition as though he was shooting a hook shot on a basketball court. The vial bounced on the counter and then fell to the floor. Ben was so busy watching Ralph that didn't really see what came over the partition at him.

"Dr. Johnson, refill this prescription, now!" Ralph demanded. "I'm a busy man who can't doddle in a suburban pharmacy."

Dr. Johnson was only one year out of college, but he knew he had to be careful not to antagonize the strange man in front of him. Ben had recently completed a required continuing education course in patient physiology. The course had really helped out his inter-patient relationships. He knew that this was a patient who had to be humored.

"Do you have the prescription vial?" Ben asked.

"You have it, you dolt. I dropped it over the glass barrier. Now be quick about the refill."

Ben bent down and retrieved the bottle on the floor. As he raised himself he read the patient's name on the label.

"Yes, sir, Mr. Vandermere."

He looked closely at the label and read the prescription number. He then looked up the prescription number in the pharmacy computer database. The prescription was for Lifeal and one refill was left on the original prescription written by Dr. Rosenberg. Mr. Vandermere was acting so strange that Ben decided he had better call Dr. Rosenberg before refilling the prescription.

He looked up and saw that Ralph was wandering away. Dr. Johnson noted that the man's attention span seemed very limited. He spoke to Ralph's back, "Mr. Vandermere, I will be right back."

Ben walked into the back room where there was a private telephone and called Dr. Rosenberg's office. The office receptionist forwarded the call to Dr. Rosenberg. After explaining the situation to Dr. Rosenberg, Johnson was given instructions that under no circumstances was he or anyone else to refill Ralph Vandermere's prescription for Lifeal.

Dr. Rosenberg went on to explain to Ben that Ralph had made a bad scene in the office and wasn't sure that Ralph would be returning to his office for future treatment. Dr. Rosenberg stated that he had been thinking about Mr. Vandermere's case and had an idea. It was obvious that Lifeal was not working for Vandermere. In fact, the drug was apparently having a very bad side effect on him.

He asked the pharmacist to fill the Lifeal prescription with a placebo. After a few days, when the blood levels of Lifeal were diminished and the side effects less, Dr. Rosenberg thought that perhaps Ralph would return to his office for help. Dr. Rosenberg told Ben that he didn't think there would be any withdrawal symptoms from going cold turkey on Lifeal, but he didn't know for sure. At this point, he concluded, anything that would get Ralph under control was a risk worth taking.

"Do you understand Dr. Johnson? Same label, same vial but, with a Lifeal lookalike tablet."

"I understand perfectly, Dr. Rosenberg. Thank you. Goodbye."

Ben Johnson filled the prescription while Ralph unleashed a tirade of verbal abuse about Johnson's lack of intelligence and that Hank Somerset would have filled the prescription much faster and with a much higher level of competency.

After filling the prescription, Ben walked to the counter. He noted that his clerk had completely disappeared. He placed the vial in a small paper bag and asked Mr. Vandermere if he wanted to charge the prescription.

"Of course, you asshole," Ralph growled as he grabbed the bag from the pharmacist's hand and started to walk away. Halfway out of the store he turned back and yelled at Ben, "What manufacturer makes this great stuff? It really works."

Ben almost gave Ralph the name of the placebo manufacturer, but caught himself and replied, "James Pharmaceutical Company of New York City."

"Thank you," Ralph said as he walked out the door.

EDGAR ALLAN POE STREET NEW YORK CITY

Mandi and J.P. moved from the dining room to the living room to watch television after their dinner.

"That meal was great, J.P. Where did you learn to cook?"

"Many years of my life have been spent cooking for myself. I do very well for myself and a reasonable job for two people. Anymore than two and I start dialing for caterers."

Their conversation at dinner had been pleasant and focused on the two of them, both individually and as a couple. A good portion of their conversation was spent recounting their pasts. J.P. soon learned that the past was not as important to him as it was to Mandi. He would have preferred to discuss the future, but he decided that if it was important to Mandi, then it would be important to him as well.

As they settled onto the couch, he reached for the television remote that was lying on the coffee table when Mandi spoke, "Before we watch the movie, how about you tell me about your past two days with Joe?"

He looked over at Mandi and smiled. She had arrived at the apartment after work carrying a small overnight bag and a hanging bag. She had said hello to him and then disappeared upstairs where she changed from her work clothes into a pair of form-fitting sweat pants and a dark colored tank top. Over this she wore a flannel shirt opened down the front.

When she came back down from the bedroom, J.P. was still in the kitchen preparing dinner. He looked up from what he was doing and said, "Well, you look comfortable."

Mandi laughed and opened the flannel shirt. J.P. could see that she wasn't wearing a bra and he could barely tear his eyes from her nipples jutting out from the light material. Mandi turned completely around, modeling her casual ensemble for him.

"You like?" she asked teasingly. "Oh yeah," was his only response as he went back to preparing dinner.

J.P. had been sneaking furtive glances of her throughout dinner. He kept thinking of what the after-dinner activities might bring and it had been all he could do not to shovel his food down to get past the meal, encouraging her to do the same. The last thing he wanted at this point was to discuss business.

"J.P., are you listening to me? Why are you staring at me that way?" Mandi started to laugh. "What are you doing?"

"Oh, nothing. Just thinking about some things. You know I've been really turned on ever since you came down from the bedroom in your health club guerilla outfit. You see what you do to me? I'm fantasizing like some sex-starved pervert. And now you want to discuss business?"

Mandi laughed again, "Oh I'm sorry. If it'll make you feel better, I can go up and change into something more virginal for you. Besides, I can't make love on a full tummy anyway, so let's talk business."

He feigned repugnance over the idea, but then he turned his head and smiled slyly. "Okay, Mandi, let's talk business, but let's make a deal first."

"Uh huh. And what deal would that be, Monty?" She tried to sound as reproachful as possible, but she was having a tough time doing it.

"Well...I was just thinking that since I have information that you probably would like to have, perhaps we can come to some agreement pertaining to the transfer, shall we say, of that information to you."

"J.P., you lecherous bastard! And what sort of twisted circus act will I going have to perform to obtain this information?" Mandi was laughing hard now.

"Oh, I don't know." J.P. said looking up at the ceiling. "What say, you remove one piece of clothing for each bit of substantive information that I give you.

"I knew it! I knew it would somehow involve me getting naked before it was all over. You have some good info, huh?"

"Only the best for you, Petunia," J.P. said laughing.

Mandi picked a pillow from the sofa and hit J.P. with it. "And don't call me, Petunia. All right, you've got yourself a deal. But this had better be good or you'll suffer the consequences later, buddy."

"Oh, I suspect it will be most enlightening for you. A lot of what I'm going to tell you is based on research that I did before I arrived here and some that I've done since I've been here. My meetings with Joe filled in a lot of gaps." His voice had become serious.

"I'm listening. Please go on." Mandi said.

"One of the major issues I've been trying to get my arms around is the supply of the raw material for Lifeal and JPC138. I have a hunch that there might be a problem with the long-term supply. Nothing has been said in any of my meetings nor have I read anything that addresses this potential problem directly. No one in marketing seems to think that there's a problem and the 21st Century Plan certainly never indicates that there might possibly be a problem. As I said, it's a hunch, but it's a hunch based on experience. I've worked with herbs before and they are a great deal different than chemicals. You can increase the production of chemicals faster than you can affect Mother Nature's timing or the politics of another nation."

Mandi's voice was now serious "Politics? When herbs are the primary source of pharmaceuticals, I'll grant you that we're dependent upon Mother Nature. We are also, to some degree, dependent on the countries in which the herbs are grown to allow us to grow and export those herbs. It's always been that way and is really no different today." Then she added, "At least I don't think it's any different today."

J.P. at first didn't respond, he just sat staring at the ceiling and whistling an old Tom Jones song that he had heard earlier on the radio. Mandi immediately knew why he was stalling. She removed a sock and threw it so that it hit his face. He continued.

"I'm afraid things are very different, dear. During the old days the countries were usually dictatorships and not democracies. Landowners were feudal and didn't care much about the people.the peasants, if you will. Today, in most countries, the people who were formerly known as the peasant class now own the land. The best example I can think of to illustrate what I mean by politics is to tell you a story about the rubber plantations. Have you ever heard of the Brazilian town of Manaus?"

"Yeah, it's located at the junction of the Negro and Amazon Rivers. It was supposed to have been a famous and wealthy city in the late 1800's. Today, as I understand, Manaus has suffered the same economic decline as the rest of Brazil. But what's that got to do with."

"You are right on, Mandi. In 1896, the rich European rubber barons built the Manaus Opera House, or Teatro Amazonas, as it was officially known. Teatro Amazonas was built on the same scale as any of the great European opera houses. Even the Great Carrusso once sang at the Manaus opera house. The reason that Manaus was so prosperous was the fact that the extravagant plantation barons around the city had an exclusive lock on the worldwide supply of rubber trees. The greedy plantation owners developed elaborate security plans to protect their monopoly as well as their individual fiefdoms. Manaus was very remote which added to a potential smuggler's burden. It also allowed security police to easily keep track of strangers who visited the city. The goal of course was to ensure that the rubber trees were not stolen and replanted in another country, which would make the rubber market competitive and price sensitive. No one left the Manaus area without being searched.

"The rubber plantation barons had a great deal to lose. They had a monopoly on rubber just when Henry Ford was making the automobile affordable. The rubber was key to a lot of the parts that the automobile needed….hoses, belts, and, of course, tires. The elite in Manaus became extremely wealthy. The wealth initiated the building of Teatro Amazonas and other magnificent buildings right in the middle of the jungle.

"Finally, someone from the outside was able to steal enough rubber tree plants to start a new plantation. With the stolen rubber trees, plantations were planted in India, Burma, and Indonesia where the climate was very similar to that of Manaus. Manaus' worldwide lock on the market was over, competition was established. Suddenly, Manaus' remote geographic location became a burden rather than an asset. The rubber barons were eventually forced out of the market when rubber prices began falling to remarkable lows. Opera was last heard in the Teatro Amazonas in 1907. The sociopolitical scene of Manuas caused the city to fail and its people to lose.

"In 1989, ninety-three years after the first opera, a planned rebirth of Teatro Amazonas based on the growing Manuas tourism and dutyfree port status was launched. $8 million was spent to give Teatro Amazonas a facelift. The exterior of the building was repainted, structural repairs were required due to extensive termite damage, 36,000 specially-made new roof tiles were laid, and thirty-two chandeliers were replaced. Most of the material was imported from Europe where the original materials had been laboriously shipped at the height of the rubber boom. The opera season was to perform thirteen operas, including a performance by tenor, Placido Domingo.

"But, in 1989 another Manuas outsider, Brazilian President Fernando Collor decided overnight to freeze most of Brazil's currency and savings accounts for eighteen months. Consequently, he blocked most of the theater's new funds. The opera season had to be canceled."

"J.P.," Mandi interrupted, "that is a very interesting story. Where did you learn so much about a remote town like Manaus?

"Patience, Mandi, I'm getting there. I've been intrigued by the story of Manaus since I read a novel about the rubber plantations. In fact, I have visited Manaus, but that is another story. Back to the issue at hand, foreign supply of herbs.

"By the way, get ready to lose another piece of clothing. As you know, the basic ingredient for both Lifeal and JPC138 is the bark of particular species of Alstonia scholaris better know as Dita Bark or more commonly, Devil Tree. The tree itself is grown in a remote province in India, in the Philippines, and on a small group of islands in Indonesia known as the Moluccas.

"The genus Alstonia gets its name from a Scottish professor of botany by the name of Alston, who first catalogued it and described its use in treating malaria and various other bowel and digestive complaints. The bark contains a number of strong alkaloids including ditamine and echitanine. All of this I pretty much knew from my previous work in herbal research. What I didn't know until I met with Joe, is that the alkaloids used for Lifeal and JPC138 are derived from a particular species of Devil Tree known as Alstonia spectabilis."

"You know, J.P., I'm not hearing anything here that makes me want to remove clothing," Mandi said with a teasing voice.

"Oh really? Okay try this on.the reason that this particular species of Devil Tree is so critical to James Pharmaceutical and its production of drugs is that the bark of Alstonia spectabilis contains the same alkaloid as Alstonia scholaris with the addition of a crystalline alkaloid known as Alstonamine."

"Yeah, and.?" J.P. once again turned his eyes to the ceiling and began whistling. Another sock hit him in the face.

"Okay, here's the rub. It's apparently the additional alkaloid that gives Lifeal a viable active ingredient...the same for JPC138. But wait, there's more.there is only one place on earth where Alstonia spectabilis is grown. It's a plantation on the Indonesian island of Java. The plantation is owned by a Chinese Malaysian with whom James has made an agreement for the exclusive rights to the bark from his trees."

He paused for affect and Mandi's tank top landed on his shoulder. He looked at her sitting next to him, bare-breasted and then averted his gaze to continue his narrative.

"In fact, James has patents on the bark of the Devil Tree for use in many yettobedeveloped pharmaceutical derivatives. When I determined that there was only a single source of the species required for Lifeal and JPC138, I became concerned. With James' access to all of the scientific and socioeconomic databases, I have become an expert on Devil Tree economics. When I didn't see anyone else becoming concerned, I determined that my fears are either very real or completely unfounded. I'm sorry to say that my fears are very real."

He leaned forward to retrieve his briefcase lying on the floor next to the coffee table. He opened the case and found the accordion folder labeled Devil Tree and removed it from the briefcase. He handed the heavy file to Mandi.

"You're welcome to look through this at your leisure. This file contains a number of articles and point papers that I've been able to locate that address the political, economic, and social issues that could very possibly result in a cutoff of the supply of Alstonia spectabilis. To save time," he said smiling at her, "I'll summarize.

"First thing that has to be considered is that eighty-seven percent of Indonesia's 210,000,000 people are Muslim with the remaining thirteen percent split between Christians and Hindus. That, in and of itself, doesn't mean much. But when you consider that clashes between Muslims and Christians there are on the rise since Suharto left power, you begin to see the makings of a powder keg. Taken with the fact that the Indonesia's population is approaching that of the United States in a country that's less than one-third the size of the United States, it doesn't take much to imagine what sort of internal security issues might arise.

The country's security forces are already stretched to the limit with the guerilla insurgency in the eastern provinces.

"With its roughly 187,000,000 Muslims, Indonesia is the largest single Islamic country in the world. Suppose religious fundamentalism takes root on a scale similar to what we saw in Iran in the late '70's? Do you think we'll be able to sneak our bark out of Java then?" he paused. "Up until the midnineties, Indonesia enjoyed a peaceful religious co-existence. Following Suharto's downfall, it became more and more apparent that he had nearly bankrupted an otherwise prosperous economy in his thirty-some years as leader.

"The overall decline of Asian markets was felt particularly hard in Indonesia who depended heavily on exports to fuel its economy. That and a decided move towards a mostly Muslim government, has caused tempers to flare.

"And then, of course, there's our plantation owner, the Chinese Malaysian gent with whom we have at best, a shaky agreement to keep the bark coming. Indonesia, China, and Malaysia have never been what you might call really close pals. What happens when a strong nationalist movement takes hold? Chances are our friend and his plantation will disappear.

"And then, let's consider this country. Back in the mid-90's an importer who supplies plywood for Hollywood studios tried to bring in plywood from Indonesia for temporary stage sets. A band of environmental activists chained themselves to cranes at the Port of Long Beach, protesting imports of Indonesian plywood with origins in 'unsustainable forestry.' The shipment of plywood was eventually turned away. What happens when the United States government decides to punish Indonesia for human rights abuses by halting all its imports into this country or some group decides to keep the bark out of the United States?

"James Pharmaceutical Company will go dead in the water, as they say. That is, unless, Helmut and his pals in R&D can come up with some method for replicating the additional alkaloid. And that ain't likely to happen."

J.P. was looking down at the coffee table as he spoke. Mandi's sweatpants landed in his lap. He looked up.

"That's a very interesting bit of research you've done there, J.P. I have to be honest with you, I hadn't given much thought to the supply of active ingredient. I see what you mean by socioeconomic and political policies that could effect our production of Lifeal and JPC138. I now see the point in your analogy of Manaus and the rubber barons. Greed caused them to lose their competitive position in the marketplace. What do you think?"

J.P. thought for a moment and then said, "The plantation that James purchases its supply of Alstonia spectabilis is privately owned and the trees do not produce a very good wood for building or furniture. I'm certain the owner keeps the palms of the Indonesian government well greased to ensure that he is able to continue to do business. We just have to watch out for getting caught up in a dynamic situation over which we have little or no control that could cutoff the active ingredient we so desperately need."

Mandi frowned, "Yeah, and we have to watch the cost of the raw material as well. The uncertainty and instability of the government gives the plantation owner a good reason to hike the price for the bark. Where there is corruption, greed is seldom far behind."

"Well obviously James will have exclusivity on the bark of the Devil Tree at least until someone else figures out what James is using it for and wants some of their own. If another company becomes interested in this particular bark of this particular species of Devil Tree, then it's going to become a bidding war on the supply of the bark. So it goes without saying that, at least in this instance, control of the supply far outweighs worries about price.

"I have read the contract that James has with the Chinese Malaysian and it's not a very strong contract. James has a very special price and there are no escalation clauses. In fact, it's an evergreen contract with no expiration date. This, on the surface looks great and it would be, if the supply of Devil Tree bark were in the United States and not in Java. If the James products ever take off and our Chinese Malaysian decides the contract is void, it is my opinion that we wouldn't have a chance of our contract holding up in an Indonesian court. And James could find itself without a supply of its most important ingredient.

"Joe informed me that he has tried to stockpile the bark but there is only a one-year storage period before the bark spoils. As far as I have been able to ascertain, there is no established funding level in James' budget for looking into the supply situation or lengthening the bark storage period. I don't know if spending money on studies is really the answer, at any rate. There is a finite number of Devil Trees and these trees can only supply a specific amount of bark. As far as I know the Devil Tree can't be grown anywhere else in the world. The climate, soil, and altitude of the plantation are perfect for Alstonia spectabilis.

"Joe is moderately concerned about this situation. He knows Mr. Chang, the owner of the Devil Tree plantation and feels that he is an honorable man who will not break the contract. I asked Joe about the age of Mr. Chang. Joe said he did not know his age exactly, but if he were to guess he would say that Mr. Chang is in his seventies. I asked Joe when he last saw Mr. Chang. He told me it was eight years ago when they had signed the current contract.

"Joe wondered why I was concerned. The shipments have always been on time and there was no reason to believe anything would change. He didn't think that I should be concerned."

He was staring at the coffee table as he spoke. He felt Mandi shift her position on the couch.

"J.P., I'm really embarrassed. I knew nothing of this situation and I should have known everything. If our supply of bark were cut off, we would be out of business in less than a year. If the plantation fell into the wrong hands we would be susceptible to industrial blackmail. Now that you have brought this to Joe's attention, what's he planning to do?"

"I got the feeling that he won't do anything. He believes everything is fine. I didn't press the issue with him mostly because I'm not ready to set off the alarm just yet. My main purpose was to determine if there is a potential problem. I accomplished my objective. I have told you because we are a team, but please don't jump on the issue until you and I agree to the disclosure strategy. We can possibly use this information to help James and Phillip. If it gets out in the open and becomes generally known, the information might fall into the wrong hands and we might set off a series of events that could make all of this a self-fulfilling prophecy. Do you see what I mean?"

"Yes, I do and I agree. Two questions." "Fire away, lover."

"First, what did you determine about Joe and the copy of the 21st Century Plan? Second, what are you going to do in the production department for the remainder of this week?"

"I questioned Joe about the 21st Century Plan and came away with the general feeling that he would not steal the plan for himself. Still he could have been an instrument in the theft and stole the plan for someone else. It would be difficult for me to believe that Joe is involved. He is such a straight arrow type. He comes from a very large Italian family of twelve kids. He is the most successful child in the family. Both of his parents are alive, but very elderly. They depend on him for their support. He has five children of his own.

"While it's not impossible to imagine that Joe might be seduced by large sums of cash to commit industrial espionage, it seems improbable that his personal ethics would allow that to happen. That is, unless the person asking Joe to do the job was a James employee. Again, enters the possibility of the involvement of Mrs. James. As

I asked Joe very pointed questions and watched him very closely. I couldn't see any movement in his body or eyes that would indicate that he felt he was doing something wrong. I have left him on our list of suspects but, as yet, I have no motive for Joe stealing the plan except for money for his family.

As for the answer to your second question, I am going to spend the rest of the week learning the extraction process that is used on the Devil Tree bark. Next week, when I am in R&D, I will try to determine if there is any possibility that the alkaloids in the bark can possibly be chemically synthesized. If it turns out that this is a possibility, even theoretically, then in the long-term, James would not be dependent on the Devil Tree.

"Now then, do you have any other questions I can answer?" As he spoke this, J.P. turned his gaze towards Mandi. Her panties hit him in the face.

She moved over on the couch so that she was next to J.P. They kissed deeply and slowly. Finally they rolled off the couch onto the floor in front of the fireplace and made love with deep passion. Afterwards they dozed in front of the fire and later stumbled up the stairs and fell asleep in one another's arms.

7:00 P.M., WEDNESDAY, FEBRUARY 1

ANCHOR STREET PERTH AMBOY, NJ

J.P. spent the majority of the day at the Brooklyn plant going through the Devil Tree bark extraction process. The process was more time consuming than complex. The alkaloid was extracted by a fractionation process. The bark was first scrubbed and sterilized by 300-degree steam heat. The resultant pulp was then distilled and fractionated. The alkaloid was taken off as a liquid and then crystallized. The crystals were crushed into a fine powder. The herb was then combined with a newly synthesized Beta Adrenoceptor antagonist.

The medicinal compound was then stamped into Lifeal tablets. The Devil Tree bark crystals varied in size which indicated to J.P. that there were likely impurities in the compound. He wasn't allowed access to the complete formula for Lifeal, because Joe didn't feel that J.P.'s access to the complete formula fell into the 'need to know' category.

The entire process, from raw bark to Lifeal tablet was four months. Each step of the process took days not minutes or hours. This told J.P. two things. First, there had to be a large amount of product in process and second, the forecast better be as accurate as possible or there would either be a shortage or excess of finished goods. He imagined that the new 50-milligram tablet decision had been made over a year ago for the upcoming automatic shipment. All of these factors made the supply of raw material even more critical, than he had first thought.

He determined that he would have all the needed information he required from production by noon the next day. He could then attend his scheduled lunch with Carl's father. Thursday afternoon he would write his reports and Friday he would start working on the proxy statement that Brian and he were going to put together for Phillip.

After his day at the Brooklyn plant, J.P. took the subway to Penn Station where he caught the six o'clock train to New Jersey. J.P. was looking forward to dinner at Janet and Bill's home.

Later that evening as J.P. sat in his apartment living room he reflected on the dinner at Janet's and Bill's house. As he thought about Bill's new company, Clintec he could see the advantages of James and Clintec working together. With Clintec they would have a great chance of proving Lifeal's prophylactic indication. Even though he had a few glasses of wine and some after dinner drinks, which were always his downfall and usually led to a massive headache he remembered the most important part of Bill's explanation.

As Bill said, "My company Clintec and James should be working together. Working together would help both of our companies."

"What do you mean?" he had said.

"J.P., I know that Lifeal is in trouble and to answer your question before you ask, no, Janet did not tell me about James' problems. All I had to do was to read the pink sheets.

"You know, J.P., I have lived through the total history of Lifeal and, at least up until I left James, I knew the product better than anyone else. I knew what Lifeal was intended to do and understood the marketing strategy.

"As you remember, the original indication for Lifeal was to be a prophylactic against cardiac arrhythmia. The purpose being to prevent the heart from going through the trauma of a cardiac incident. We, excuse me, James could not clinically prove this indication because there was no way to predict the cardiac incident. The FDA disapproval report said that James Pharmaceutical Company did not prove that there was a cardiac incident, so how could James prove Lifeal prevented the unproved incident. James and Phillip gave up on the unique preventative indication and accepted Lifeal's approved indication of maintenance against diagnosed cardiac arrhythmia. Lifeal therefore, moved from being a unique product to a plain old generic product in a crowded marketplace. The rest, as they say, is history. I might add, in my opinion a very short and unprofitable history. I am sure you will agree as you get back up to speed at James and learn more about Lifeal."

He remembered asking the question, "You have summed up the situation quite well, Bill, but what has this to do with Clintec?"

"I'm getting to point, J.P." His voice raised. "Let me ask you a question, what would you say Lifeal's potential would be if I told you I have developed a test that can diagnosis whether a patient is or is not susceptible to a cardiac arrhythmia incident and I...we... Clintec, can do this with a 90% CV?"

He had looked at Bill to see a smiling confident man and asked, "Bill, I find it hard to believe what you have just told me, but if it is true I would say you have made a very significant breakthrough. Have you discussed this with Phillip?"

Bill answered "That is what I have been trying to tell you. I have been trying to talk to Phillip for over six months. Every time I try, he just blows me off. I know it is because I left the James family. I can't go to anyone else at James because I don't trust them. I'm afraid they will steal Clintec knowhow and market the solution to their problem themselves. Phillip is my only hope and he will not talk to me. That is why I need your help."

"Tell me more if you can, Bill."

Bill proceeded to tell him about Clintec's patented diagnostic test. Clintec determined that a patient who is susceptible to a cardiac arrhythmia also carried a very high blood level of a particular enzyme.

The enzyme can be detected in a patient's blood sample and a measurement of the levels obtained by the proprietary Clintec instrument. Bill said that the blood sample can be as small as 1 ml and obtained from a pin prick of a finger. Bill's idea was to market the test as a precursor to the prescribing of Lifeal. The only thing holding him back was the Lifeal formula. If Clintec had access to the Lifeal formula, Clintec could develop the test alone or with the help of James. He had to have the formula to determine the correlation between the diagnostic test, the pharmaceutical, and the disease. He wanted Phillip and James to work with Clintec, but he had been unable to talk with Phillip to explain the benefits to the sales of Lifeal.

A test to diagnose potential cardiac arrhythmia patients was too good to be true. J.P. didn't know for sure if Bill was even giving him the full story.

In J.P.'s business experience, he had found many entrepreneurs, especially in tight situations, practicing a dangerous scheme where they felt that the end would justify whatever means it took to get them there. They expanded the capabilities of their new product or exaggerated the company's sales and profit performance. This was done to obtain additional investment capital or to hold off investors' legal action for nonperformance. The falsely obtained investment capital would be used in an effort to make the lie become the truth. The alternative, of course, was to tell the truth. The truth being, that the product required more testing or more money was required to market the product.

Telling the truth to many investors assured the company or inventor of not receiving the working capital required to bring the potentially beneficial product to market. Or worse, the company actually failed from lack of investment capital and the customer was forever deprived of the company's products.

J.P. had seen that sort of scheme work, but only rarely. Usually telling the truth and working to a better understanding of the business was better than "the ends justifies the means" attitude.

J.P. had done his best to determine whether Bill was stretching Clintec's product capabilities in order to get James' support? He knew that if in fact Bill was telling the full and complete truth that it would potentially be a winwin situation for both parties. On the other hand, J.P. knew he didn't have the luxury of time to pursue this potential solution to the Lifeal problem unless the diagnostic test was as Bill had described it.

He couldn't ignore what Bill was telling him since finding a viable solution to Lifeal's sales woes was one of his objectives. He finally decided that he would have to do more thinking about the test, but it could not be a high priority project. In truth, Bill was asking him to find out if the technology was viable and to resolve the disagreements between he and Phillip.

He had told Bill, "What you have told me is interesting. No, let me raise it to a higher level. It is very interesting. I really have to know more about your product and Lifeal in order to make a recommendation to Phillip. I am this week and next week gathering information that I need on Lifeal. I am working in production this week and research next week. Let me give you a call in two weeks. Meantime, if you can give me some more information on your concept I will study up on your technology. If you need for me to sign a disclosure agreement, I will happily do so. I can coordinate our next meeting with Janet."

11:00 A.M., THURSDAY, FEBRUARY 2

NEW YORK CITY

J.P. had told Carl that he would meet him at the French restaurant on 56th street between 5th and 6th Avenues. He had spent the morning at the Brooklyn plant. Typically, the New York City traffic became gridlock eight blocks from his destination so he paid his fare and jumped out of the cab to walk the rest of the way.

Steam was rising from beneath the sewer covers and mixed with the exhaust from the cars and the respiration vapor of the thousands of people on the sidewalk. The snow from last week's big storm was still piled up more than ten feet high on the corners. The snow had turned black from the soot that was a by-product of the city and ashes that the city crews laid down on the streets. Unlike many midwestern cities, ashes were used in New York City to cover the ice on the streets rather than corrosive salt. The piles of snow restricted the sidewalks so that the pedestrians had even less room to walk. Many pedestrians bumped into one another as J.P. walked along. This was mostly because everyone was bent over from the cold and wind and couldn't see where they were going.

The wind was coming off the park was frigid and J.P. knew from the early morning forecasts that the predictions for that days wind chill was set at 30 degrees below zero.

As he reached the corner of 57th and 6th Avenue the full effect of the wind off the park hit him. The wind seem to channel itself down the park and focus its full force on 6th Avenue or The Avenue of the Americas as the signage in this section of the city called it. The sky was bright blue and the sun's rays uninhibited. J.P. thought that the sun must surely be providing some warmth, but there was certainly none getting through to his body. For the second time in twenty-four hours he longed to be back in Mammoth.

He pulled his coat closer to his body and pulled his collar up around his neck.

J.P. again thought about his previous nights conversation with Bill. He concluded he really didn't have time to devote exclusively to Bill and Clintec. The James board issues and the 21st Century Plan copy were going to take the majority of his time. He decided that he would keep his promise to Bill and contact him after his week in R&D.

J.P. finished his one block walk south on 6th Avenue and was at 56th Street. He waited for the light before crossing the street. He crossed and proceeded east on 56th to the middle of the block where the French restaurant was located.

J.P. entered the restaurant and informed the person at the reservation stand that he was there to meet Mr. Carl Manningham, Jr. The maitre'd told

J.P. that the Manningham party had already arrived and then led him to the table where Carl and his dad were seated. The restaurant was laid out like many old New York City restaurants. Narrow and long with white starch linen draped tables against bench seats, which were built into both walls. The walls were mirrored giving the room the illusion of being larger. In the middle of the room were small tables. J.P. wondered if there was more seating upstairs. He couldn't see the stairs.

Carl and his father occupied one of the tables for four in the middle of the room. The size of the two men prevented the use of a wall table.

As J.P. approached the table, Carl stood to greet him. He was wearing his usual three-piece suit. His vest was a little snug. The buttons actually stretched the buttonholes. He had a gold chain from one of the buttons to the small vest pocket on his right. He had on a starched white shirt. J.P. thought Carl looked dignified.

"J.P., so good of you to have lunch with my father and I. J.P., I would like for you to meet my father Mr. Carl Manningham, Sr. Father, Dr. Koenig."

J.P. looked at the man sitting to his right. Like his son, Carl's father was wearing a three-piece suit with an identical gold chain. On his chain was a small charm that J.P. didn't recognize. The father was larger than his son. He looked up at J.P. and extended his hand.

"I am very happy to meet you Mr. Manningham."

"I am very pleased to make your acquaintance Dr. Koenig. My son has spoken very highly of you. I would ask that you to call me Carl but then you would have to refer to my son as junior and he deplores being called junior.

So we will have to stick with a formal Mr. Manningham or perhaps Ham as my friends and my son's friends prefer to address me." Carl says that everyone calls you J.P. May I call you J.P.?"

"Yes, Ham, you may certainly call me J.P."

Carl's father had a very strong, deep voice to go along with his very dignified look. He looked as healthy as anyone could look at seventy, but looking bad was not one of the symptoms of Alzheimer's disease. J.P. realized that he didn't know much about Alzheimer's disease. He made a mental note to learn as much as he could about the pathology of the disease next week when he was working in R&D.

The waiter with his red vest and traditional white apron wrapped one and one-half times around his waist recited the luncheon specials and waited to take their order. He impatiently stood tapping his pencil on his small white order pad. It was a New York tradition. Restaurants tried to push through as many people as possible for lunch. The waiter took the impatient role with vigor. The customer was intimidated and usually ordered one of the luncheon specials. The waiter spoke to them without any passion, "Take your order folks?" The three men all ordered a luncheon special and ice tea. Within five minutes everything was on the table and they were eating.

Ham's eyes measured J.P. as he spoke honestly about his condition. "J.P., I don't mean to be a bore but I would like to ask you about James' research program. Since I am a Securities and Exchange Commission lawyer I know how I hate people asking me for free legal advice. I also realize you can not tell me anything that has not yet been made public. But I would like to know if there is any chance that this damn disease will be cured in the near future. By near future I mean within the next five years. I want to know because I have to make some personal decisions about my career."

Carl picked up the conversation in order to clarify his father profession. "J.P., I guess you haven't heard of my dad. There is probably no reason for you to know of him because he does most of his work out of the public eye. Dad, is, and has been, for many years, the top lawyer for the Securities and Exchange Commission. You might have noticed the charm on his key chain. This was a special award that was given to him by the American Bar Association. He gained his nickname Ham from two sources. At Yale in law school his last name of Manningham was too long for his fellow law students. The nickname stuck when he went into trial law because he loved to ham it up in the courtroom. His nickname stuck after he joined the SEC. Ham is well known among the ranks of bond dealers, brokerage houses, and the like. He is thought of being a very thorough researcher and when obtaining depositions for congressional hearings he is a very probing, but a fair lawyer. He is able to do this because of his indepth knowledge of his specialty field of law. Six months ago dad was diagnosed with stage one Alzheimer's disease."

Ham picked up the conversation from Carl. "J.P., I am faced with a deteriorating disease that has no timeframe and could, at anytime, seriously affect my work and the people who depend on me. My physician will not, or more likely can not, give me any definitive answers." He broke into a big smile that created wrinkles where there were no visible wrinkles. His wrinkles extended from his eyes almost to his ears. Ham continued, "I accused him of being a lawyer. I think he took my comment as an insult.

"Anyway J.P., I have to make some decisions about my future. Like most people I thought I was going to live forever. Now there is a chance that I may very well live forever, but will not be cognizant of the fact." The smile disappeared from his face at the gravity of his statement.

"J.P.," Carl joined in again, "what my dad requires to know, is if there is any chance there might be a cure within the next five years. If not, he wants to retire. I have tried to get him to retire and enjoy life now and not to wait until the disease gets too serious. He feels he will be letting down the SEC chairman especially now when they are investigating the tax shelters the brokerage houses were selling to investors.

"The SEC, with my father's help, is discovering that the brokerage houses were misleading investors. They hooked the investor on the tax shelter angle and then convinced the investor that the product was a good investment. The only problem was, in most cases there were no plans to make a profit only to pay large salaries and expenses.

"Administering or managing the investment was done by high salaried employees that spent all of the investors' money. Giving them, in return, numerous excuses. Usually there was also a subsequent investment that each investor had to make to stay in the program. Anyway, Dad wants to see this thing through."

J.P. wanted to answer Ham's question on Alzheimer's as best as he could even though he didn't feel qualified to go into specifics. Most importantly, J.P. didn't want the lawyer to make a career decision on his advice alone. Ham had been watching J.P.'s body reactions as Carl had told the story. He turned towards Ham and looked directly into his eyes.

"Ham, I can't give you the answer you want. First, I am not qualified to comment on something as important to you as your career. Alzheimer's is a dreadfully unpredictable disease. Many pharmaceutical companies have been working very hard to find both a cure and a prevention to Alzheimer's. James is working on both, but they will not know the answer in the near future. Are any other companies closer to the answer? I don't think so, at least none that I know of. In pharmaceuticals it is hard to keep secrets once something gets into clinical trial. As of this moment, nothing is in clinical trial.

"My advice to you is to continue to work on your current project, but find yourself a good assistant that could be your replacement. Then phase out of the SEC so you can do some of the things you would like to do before the disease becomes severe."

"Is the James Alzheimer's project moving along as fast as you would like?" Ham asked.

J.P. hesitated before answering, wondering if this was a leading question that Carl had fed his father? He didn't have to wait long for the answer.

"J.P.," Carl spoke up laughing, "I swear that I didn't tell my father to ask that question. I told you he is a probing lawyer."

J.P. looked at Ham. "I'm going to take a risk, Ham. May we speak off the record? What I am going to say is not illegal. It is just a little inside information on James. I don't know how little, maybe nothing at all. I think Jack Husted of the Wall Street Journal has it figured out so it may be public information, at least in the offices of the Wall Street Journal. At any rate, Ham, I must ask you for your confidentiality."

Ham hesitated looking at me with shrewd eyes. "So Husted has his claws in James, eh? He is a smart man. I respect him. Honest, and a proper analyst. Good man for the industry." He paused and then slowly nodded his head. "Yes, you have my confidentiality, but if I think the conversation is going the wrong direction I will ask you to stop. I am sure you understand."

"Absolutely, Ham."

The waiter arrived and took away the plates and asked if they wanted coffee. It was coffee all around. The coffee came faster than dinner. With the coffee came the check. The check was set next to J.P.'s coffee cup. He picked it up, checked the addition, and laid down a credit card on the tray. The waiter picked up the tray immediately and returned the slip promptly. He picked up his card and let the slip lay unsigned. They made small talk during the coffee, waiter, and bill activity.

"Ham, there are some James communication problems that are currently hurting the Alzheimer's project. So far it is nothing too serious, but I am afraid it will become serious if something isn't done about the situation. If you look at the James balance sheet you will see that the company does not have as much cash as is required to correctly complete the Alzheimer's research. Mrs. James has changed the personality of the board of directors. To be quite honest, the board is antagonistic to management and to research.

"The stock dividend has remained high when it probably should have been reduced to provide the financial support required for a brighter future. Mrs. James and her directors have kept the dividend high so that her personal stock dividend income will remain high. I feel that Mrs. James will make a bold move at the upcoming annual meeting in May. Management, Dr. Phillip Bradsmith specifically, is thinking we cannot just sit back and let Mrs. James stop the company's growth. Management feels that the Alzheimer's research product has great future potential but it requires more focus and working capital. Mrs. James will not approve additional funding. We are sure she is planning to establish complete control over the board of directors. If she gets complete control of the board, management will never have a chance to obtain enough working capital to complete the Alzheimer's research."

Ham interrupted him as he was already one step ahead, "So you want to conduct a proxy fight and you would like to know whether I can help you." He held up his hand to stop me from replying. "I can not get too involved in a proxy fight, but I can help you by giving you advice and by reviewing the material you will have to prepare for the shareholders. In this way you can keep the information as confidential as possible and if it is done right you will catch her by surprise. As for payment I want none. I will do this for my son and also for the Alzheimer's project. It will be my indirect donation to Alzheimer's research."

"Dad, that is really great of you."

"Ham, I agree. What you have offered is more than I could reasonably expect. I can see why Carl loves and respects you so much. Here is my card. If you could give me a phone number I can use to contact you I will keep you informed."

Ham took the card and also took out one of his calling cards and wrote a number on the back.

"J.P., you can call me at this number at anytime. I would also appreciate, if you can swing it, using Carl as our liaison between meetings. I would like for him to get the experience, plus I trust him implicitly. Will this be a problem?"

"I'm certain that it will not be a problem, Ham. I will let Carl know this afternoon," J.P. said as he signed the credit card slip.

Ham stood up and brought up his hand for J.P. "Thank you J.P., now I must get back to my office. Thank you for lunch. I look forward to working with you on this project."

"Thank you for your help, Ham. I want you to know that Carl is doing an excellent job at James. He has come up with some new ideas that will help our current product Lifeal. He has a bright future at James." Carl flushed a little.

"Thank you J.P. I appreciate the compliment." Carl commented.

"I am sure you deserve it son." Ham and his son hugged and said their goodbyes.

They all left the restaurant together. Carl and J.P. took a cab back to the Spectrum of Medicine Building.

10:00 A.M., FRIDAY, FEBRUARY 3

WYCKOFF, NJ

It was three days since Ralph had started taking the tablets from his refilled prescription. He was now up to five tablets a day. He was trying to get back to the feeling he had before he had the prescription refilled.

Yesterday, he had tried to go back to his office for the first time since he gave the summary to the jury.

He had driven by the office a number of times, but he couldn't make himself stop. He was for the first time in his life, profoundly depressed. He blamed himself.

Ralph had started to remember how he had been acting the last two weeks. He had lost his partner and his wife had left him and had gone back to her folks' home in southern New Jersey. When they all left he thought being alone was great. He remembered thinking he didn't need a partner or wife anyway. Now he could see just how his life had been ruined by Lifeal. Who was the manufacturer? Who was it that the pharmacist had said manufactured the product? James Pharmaceutical Company? That was the name.

He decided to do something about what James had done to his life. He made a few phone calls to information for the telephone number and one call to James Pharmaceutical Company which got him the address in the city. Ralph showered and dressed in his best pinstriped Brooks Brothers suit. He slipped on his black wing tips,

318

put on a blue button down shirt, and tied a half Windsor knot in his yellow paisley tie.

He went to his safe and punched in the combination on the digital keyboard. When the safe opened, he reached to the rear of the safe and brought out his old Army handgun. He dropped the clip out of the butt and saw that it was loaded. How long had it been since his Colt .45 had been fired? He smiled. All of a sudden now he could not remember things. His memory cells then snapped in and he remembered, 1955, right after the Korean War. Would the gun still work? Were the bullets still good? It doesn't matter, he thought and dismissed the potential problem of a inoperable handgun.

He left a note for his absent wife. Took all but his drivers license and $100 from his wallet. He slipped on his cashmere overcoat, put the .45 in his coat pocket and left the house to make the drive into the city.

12:00 P.M., FRIDAY, FEBRUARY 3
SPECTRUM OF MEDICINE BUILDING
NEW YORK CITY

J.P. looked across the cafeteria table at Mandi. He had just finished briefing her on his week's activities. It was the second time that day that he had made this briefing. He told Mandi about Carl Manningham, Sr., discussing the proxy issue and Carl's dad Ham as well as his evening with Bill. He had spent most of the morning with Brian. Brian had seemed apprehensive at first about having Ham as part of the team. J.P. had reminded him that their team had shortcomings and that their plan could only work if they were able to call on Ham for council when it came to the proxy strategy and the paperwork drill associated with that strategy.

Mandi had listened to every word he said and was more excited about Bill's product than J.P. would have imagined she would be. She was dressed in a navy blue skirt and matching jacket. Her hair was loose and framed her face. It was free flowing with large waves and had a very silky sheen. To J.P. it seemed that the blue of the suit actually intensified her eyes turning them slightly turquoise.

He leaned forward on the table and propped his face against his closed fist, "You know, you look even more beautiful than usual. And I love your hair like that."

Her eyes lit up with the compliment then quickly she turned serious again. "J.P., you have uncovered a great deal of information in a short time. I am impressed. I am also very interested in Bill Williams' cardiac arrhythmia diagnostic instrument. I think we should find out more about his product as soon as possible."

"I will do more work on the possibilities of the product and Lifeal next week when I'm working in R&D.

"Now then, what are we going to do this weekend? If you have no specific ideas, I would like to suggest a ski trip to Stratton, Vermont. I think I can get us a house from a friend of mine. What do you think?"

"I think that would be outstanding. Give me the specifics as soon as you can. We can use my car because I will have to go home to get my gear. Now, I have to excuse myself, I have a full schedule this afternoon. See you later." Her mood had changed from serious to ready for a fun weekend.

She walked rapidly out of the cafeteria. he decided that he would write up a status report for Phillip and set up next week's meetings with R&D. He got up from his seat and went directly to his office.

He sat down at his desk and powered up his computer and reached for the phone to retrieve his messages. There was one message from Annie.

"J.P., hiya. So how is everything in the Big Apple. Haven't heard anything from you. I'm sure everything is fine. Please give me a call when you have the chance. Bye, sweetie."

J.P. picked up the phone and dialed Annie's Bar and Grill in Mammoth. He looked at his watch. It was 11:00 a.m. in Mammoth. Too early for the Mammoth lunch crowd, it would be a good time to talk with her. He felt bad for not having called Anne as he had promised. Annie answered the phone after only two rings.

"Annie's Bar and Grill, Annie here. What can I do for you?" She answered in her slightly western drawl.

"Oh, Annie," J.P. replied half laughing, "what you can do for me, darlin', would be far too expensive, if you get my drift."

"J.P.!" There was real excitement in her voice. "It's snowing tons. You have got to get your ass home. When are you coming home? Have you dropped off the edge of the world?"

"Whoa, Annie, too many questions. I'm very sorry that I didn't call you on Wednesday. I had a dinner date at a friend's house, Bill Williams, an old James business associate, and I talked for a long time about his new start-up company and how James and his company could work together. Sorry, Annie. I'll try harder. What is this about having tons of white stuff?"

"We've accumulated another 100 inches. This storm is about as bad as that storm we had in the seventies. Remember? We had to tunnel into our houses." She paused. "Oh, that's right, you didn't live here then. Anyway it was so much snow we couldn't use some of the ski lifts because they were buried. The one usable lift had walls of snow on each side of the lift chair. It was eerie, but beautiful." Anne went on and he just listened and daydreamed about Mammoth and skiing. She stopped suddenly "So?"

"So....what, Annie?"

"I asked you a question. When are you and Mandi coming to Mammoth?"

"Why would I bring Mandi?"

"Don't try to bullshit me you old desert rat. You and Mandi are probably a major issue back there. Besides, I want you to meet Skip again. Remember you met him in my place last time you were here? He is coming up in two weeks, what do you think?"

"I think you are one smart woman and if it's okay with Mandi, we'll fly up Thursday night the 16th. How's business and, more importantly, how is my house?"

"Both are fine." Annie sounded rushed. "Sorry, J.P. I wish I could talk longer, but I have to hang up the phone. The Mammoth lunch bunch is starting to arrive. Talk to you next week?"

"Yes, I promise. You have a great weekend and I'll call you next week. Bye."

"Bye," Annie answered in a sexy voice and hung up the phone.

He turned to his computer and began typing a status report to Phillip. DATE: February 3, 1995

SECRET Phillip Bradsmith's Eyes Only TO: Phillip FROM: J.P.

SUBJ.: Project Status Report

21st Century Plan: I have not determined who the specific person is that copied the plan or why. I cannot help thinking that the Board of Directors have something to do with the situation. Next week after my week in R&D I will do my best to narrow the field down.

Proxy: I met Carl Manningham's father over lunch on Thursday. He is a highly respected SEC lawyer. He has been diagnosed with Alzheimer's disease. He wants our JPC138 project to be successful. If we have a proxy fight he said he would help you and James at no charge. I have briefed Brian on this issue.

Lifeal: I have uncovered some new ideas about the future of Lifeal. I will keep working on everything and be able to give you a better answer next week I am slightly concerned over the single source supply of the raw material used in both Lifeal and JPC138. Alstonia spectabilis is only grown on the island of Java in Indonesia. There is no other natural source that I know of and it apparently cannot be reproduced synthetically. I know Doc James had a contract with Mr. Chang that is based on honor and loyalty, but Doc James is dead and Mr. Chang is letting his son run the business and plantation. I will do more work with this next week.

Support: Nothing additional required.

Next Week: Working with Helmut and the other R&D personnel.

J.P. pulled up the 21st Century Plan on his computer and began rereading it. He hadn't looked at the report since his first days on the project. He thought that since he knew a great more about James, Lifeal, and the board that perhaps there was something he had missed when he read it the first time.

NEW JERSEY TURNPIKE

There was not a cloud in the sky and the rays of the bright afternoon sun streamed through the back window of Ralph's Lincoln. He had driven south on the Garden State Parkway to the New Jersey Turnpike. He was taking the long way into the city. He had plenty of time before his appointment with Dr. Bradsmith. As he passed the turnpike exit for Newark Airport, Ralph noted that the outside temperature was 20 degrees. In his Lincoln it was close to 100 degrees. The heater was on full fan and at the maximum 90-degree temperature setting. The hot air of the heater added to the sun's heat making the inside of the car extremely hot.

Ralph wanted to change from the left lane to the next lane to the right. His eyes went to the rearview mirror. He had bumped the mirror when backing out of his driveway and the mirror was aimed, not at the rear traffic, but directly back at him. Even though he was not feeling the same as he had before getting his prescription refilled, he still had his vision.

He had done his best to stay away from mirrors and other reflective surfaces which might force him to look deep into his own eyes. Because of the misdirected rearview mirror, he looked into his eyes and again stared into himself. He knew that he had to end these mood swings. He now realized his life, as he once knew life, was ruined. He was not sure how his life had become ruined or for that matter who precisely was responsible, but he did know that Lifeal was at the root of his misery. That morning he had come to the decision that he was going to do one last good thing. Hell, what did he care about life, his body was falling apart. He had to do this one thing before it was too late. It was necessary.

The car next to him was blowing its horn. Ralph snapped back as his eyes left the mirror. He saw, to his horror, he was steadily moving to his right into the other car's lane. He jerked his wheel to the left and almost overcompensated. He looked over at the driver on his right. He was swearing and shaking his fist at Ralph. The man turned his steering wheel to the left to drive into the side of Ralph's Lincoln. Ralph's heart jumped. The other driver then straightened his car, increased his speed to 70 miles per hour, and drove off ahead. Ralph continued his drive to the turn-off for the Lincoln Tunnel.

Thirty minutes later he emerged on the New York City side of the Lincoln Tunnel. He looked at his watch and saw that it was 3:15 p.m. He turned left onto 42nd Street and drove to the Westside Highway. He headed north along the expressway that followed the east bank of the Hudson River. He could see the Westside Corporate Center buildings on his right. What exit did the receptionist say? 78th Street? 66th Street exit passed and he prepared to exit at 78th Street. He looked at his watch again, 3:30.

He would have plenty of time before his 4:00 p.m. appointment with Dr. Bradsmith. That morning he had called James Pharmaceutical Company and found out the name of the President. He then called Dr. Bradsmith for an appointment. He said he was the corporate lawyer for First Boston Investment Bank. He asked Dr. Bradsmith's Assistant, Janet was her name, if Dr. Bradsmith would mind taking five minutes to discuss an issue pertaining to Lifeal. Janet forwarded the call to Dr. Bradsmith. Ralph told Dr. Bradsmith that the First Boston Investment Bank was writing an investors research report on James. He wanted to check out a small point in the patent rights for one of the James products. Dr. Bradsmith asked if he should have the James corporate lawyer present. Ralph assured him that it was not a major issue. Phillip agreed to a five-minute meeting at 4:00 p.m.

Ralph parked the car in the James underground garage and took the elevator to the lobby and checked in with the security guard.

The guard called Janet to confirm Mr. Vandermere's appointment with Dr. Bradsmith. Janet told the guard to send Mr. Vandermere directly up to Dr. Bradsmith's office. The guard pointed to the elevator. He tried to warn Mr. Vandermere about the elevator, but Ralph was not listening. The guard, tired after a long boring day, let Ralph enter into the elevator without warning him of the rapid ascent.

The elevator caught Ralph off guard. By the time the elevator reached the 40th floor, Ralph was dizzy, disoriented, and nauseated.

When the elevator stopped, Ralph fell out of the car and momentarily lay on the carpet.

Janet, on her monitor had watched Mr. Vandermere fall on the floor. She jumped up and ran out into the center lobby.

When she reached Ralph he was sitting. He looked very pale. "Are you all right Mr. Vandermere?" Janet asked trying to show him that she was very calm.

"I am all right." Ralph said. "Just give me a minute." "Didn't the guard warn you about that elevator?"

"No, at least not that I heard," Ralph said as he stood up. "I'm okay.

May I please see Dr. Bradsmith now?"

"Are you sure you would not like to sit down for a minute and maybe have a glass of water?"

"No, I am in a hurry and I'm certain that Dr. Bradsmith has a very busy schedule. I do not want to abuse his kindness in seeing me."

Janet smiled and said, "Fine, Mr. Vandermere, just follow me please." Janet liked this man. He was not mad about the elevator and he was concerned with Phillip's valuable time. He seemed very professional.

Janet had already warned Phillip that Mr. Vandermere was here so she led him right into Phillip's office and introduced Mr. Ralph Vandermere of First Boston and left closing the door behind her.

Phillip shook the distinguished looking gentleman's hand and asked him if he would like to take off his overcoat.

"No, I'm okay and I will not keep you very long, Dr. Bradsmith. Besides for some reason, I'm always cold."

Phillip watched as his guest looked around the office. He wondered what it was that the man wanted.

"What can I do for you and First Boston, Mr. Vandermere?"

Ralph turned to face Phillip. The pleasant expression that had been on Ralph Vandermere's face had changed drastically and his eyes looked cold and hard.

Ralph snarled, "Haven't you done enough for me already, Dr. Bradsmith? What does the doctor stand for Dr. Strangelove or Dr. Death?"

Phillip was visibly shaken. "What? Mr. Vandermere, is this some kind of joke?"

"Joke? You son of a bitch. You, James, and Lifeal are the joke. Your joke has destroyed my body and my life. Because of you and Lifeal, I cannot go on living the life you have forced me to live."

Phillip watched in shock as the stranger pulled a large gun from his overcoat pocket. Phillip thought, "My God, this man is going to commit suicide right here in my office." Then everything began to move in slow motion. Phillip started to plead with Mr. Vandermere not to harm himself when, to his amazement and horror, he saw the well-dressed man in the cashmere overcoat turn the gun, not on himself, but at Phillip.

Phillip watched as Ralph slowly raised the gun. Phillip heard Ralph's voice echoing in his ears. Each word that Ralph spoke was drawn out "You...son...of...a...bitch."

In the background, behind Mr. Vandermere, Phillip saw the door opening and knew it was Janet. He yelled, "No!" to both Ralph Vandermere and Janet. Phillip moved to his right as he heard the snap of the hammer against the bullet. There was no sound of an explosion. Phillip kept trying to move faster, but his feet seemed as if they were in cement and the barrel of the gun kept following him.

Janet was running at Mr. Vandermere. Phillip yelled again, "No!". Janet stopped and turned back towards her office to call security. There was another click as the gun misfired for the second time. Phillip found the strength in his legs then to charge the man with the gun to get it away from him. Then there was an explosion as the gun finally fired. Phillip hypnotically watched the bullet leave the gun barrel and begin its trip towards him. Again in the background, Phillip heard Janet screaming.

Ralph was stunned by the explosion and the dam woman's screaming. He had to end all this noise once and for all. Ralph wanted silence. He stared at the falling Dr. Bradsmith and for a last time, said in a surprisingly strong voice, "Sic semper tyrannis," and then turned the gun on himself putting the barrel into his mouth. Ralph Vandermere, Bergen County criminal lawyer and partner in the Vandermere and Patterson Law firm, pulled the trigger.

Phillip felt the left side of his chest explode. Now, his left side felt very warm. He stopped moving forward as an invisible force pushed him backward towards the windows. He tried to reach back with his left hand to break his fall but found to his amazement that his left arm would not work. He wondered why he was so warm and his arm wasn't working. He started to see flashes of white and felt excruciating shearing pain as he felt himself crash into the windows. He matter of factly concluded, "I have been shot by a stranger in a pinstriped suit and cashmere overcoat. I am dead." Dr. Phillip Bradsmith lapsed into unconsciousness.

Janet saw the hole appear in Phillip's chest as a piece of the back of Ralph Vandermere's skull hit her square in the face. Janet fainted.

When Janet had heard Mr. Vandermere yelling at Phillip she had pushed the security panic button before she rushed into Phillip's office. Now three James security guards emerged from the elevator to hear Janet screaming and the explosion of the first shot. They pulled their weapons from their holsters and rushed to the open door of Phillip's office when they heard the second shot. They stopped outside of the door preparing to rush whatever was going on in Dr. Bradsmith's office. Suddenly the screaming stopped and there was silence. Stan, the senior guard, peered through the door opening.

The carnage that Stan saw shocked him. He saw three bloodied bodies. He motioned to the other guards to follow him into the office. Once the two junior guards saw the bodies, they vomited onto the carpet. As she was closest to the door, Stan rushed first to Janet who was covered with blood. He could see her chest moving as she breathed. His eyes switched to the stranger. He was lying on his back but Stan could see that the top of his head was gone. He then rushed over to Dr. Bradsmith who was slumped on the floor against the window. Blood was streaked down the window where his back had hit and then smeared as he slid to the floor. He was not moving. "Oh my God, I think Dr. Bradsmith is dead or dying, call 911." He reached down and felt Phillip's carotid artery to see if there was a pulse. There was a pulse, but it was very weak. "Hurry up, he's alive but barely."

4:10 P.M., FRIDAY, FEBRUARY 3

SPECTRUM OF MEDICINE BUILDING NEW YORK CITY

As the phone rang, J.P. looked at the clock in the lower corner of his computer's screen. It was 4:10.

It was Mandi her voice was calm but extremely serious. "J.P., please come up to Phillip's office immediately. He's been shot. I'll see you there." She hung up the phone without waiting for any response.

He jumped up from his chair and walked as fast as he could to the elevator. He didn't know how many other James employees had gotten the news or for that matter, knew anything about the situation. Phillip, shot by whom, why, and was he alive? Where was the person who shot Phillip? When he reached the elevator he found Mandi waiting. As he walked up to her, he was about to say something when the elevator light blinked off and the doors opened. They stepped into an empty elevator car. Mandi grabbed his hand and held it tightly, he squeezed back.

"What is the situation?" he asked.

"I don't know anymore than what I told you except that I hear the gunman is dead."

"Who called you?" "Security."

"Who was the gunman?"

"I do not know, J.P.," Mandi paused. "Is the world going mad. What could anyone gain by killing Phillip?" Her voice was choked with emotion.

The elevator reached Phillip's floor and the doors opened to a chaotic scene. The paramedics were standing at the door waiting for the elevator. There were two gurneys. One gurney carried a closed full body bag hiding the identity of its occupant. The other gurney contained Phillip. There was an IV bottle hooked to the vein in his left arm. His face was ashen and an oxygen mask was over his face and attached to the tank beneath the gurney.

His eyes were closed but he could see the rhythmic rising and falling of his chest. A 3-inch diameter spot of blood was soaking through the sheet. The spot was directly over his heart.

Janet was standing on his right side holding his hand. There was blood all over her dress. As they walked out of the elevator into the room, Janet let loose of his hand and the paramedics pushed the gurney into the elevator. They pushed the button for the roof. They were evidently going to transport Phillip to the hospital via helicopter.

"How is he, Janet?" J.P. asked as she followed the gurney into the elevator. He was afraid to ask her about the person in the body bag.

"He is alive. The paramedics do not know how seriously he is wounded. I'm going to go with him to Columbia Presbyterian. I'll call as soon as I know his condition."

Janet looked to be in shock and he wasn't sure if she shouldn't also be hospitalized. He decided to ask about the person in the body bag. "Who shot him?" The doors of the elevator closed on his words. He didn't know if she had heard the question. He turned to look at the second gurney. It was abandoned, pushed against the wall under the picture of Doc James. There were two paramedics waiting for the next elevator. There was no hurry for whoever was in the body bag. He looked around to see if there was anyone who he knew. The security guards were now discussing the scene. No one was paying attention to either Mandi or himself. He walked over to where the security guards were standing.

"No, Dr. Koenig," Stan answered, "can't say that I knew the bastard that shot Dr. Bradsmith. I haven't seen him before. Take a look if you want and see if you know him."

J.P. stepped forward to unzip the body bag. Mandi saw what he was going to do and stepped back away from the gurney. He unzipped the bag and was immediately hit with the odor of rotting human tissue and the site of a face that was not a face. There was no way he could tell who it was. He then began to wonder how this incident was connected with the 21st Century Plan or anything else connected with James.

He called his friend in Vermont and canceled the ski weekend trip. It was going to be a long weekend, but not a skiing weekend with Mandi.

8:00 P.M., SUNDAY, FEBRUARY 5

SUTTON PLACE NEW YORK CITY

Peggy was still in tears. She had just returned from Columbia Presbyterian hospital where she had visited Phillip. Phillip had been released from intensive care on Saturday and was seeing a limited number of visitors for the first time today.

Peggy started to cry as soon as she had left Phillip's room. She had continued to cry during the cab ride home.

"It is all my fault," she said to herself now almost in hysterics. "If I had just moved a little faster on my side-effect research then Phillip wouldn't be lying there in that hospital room half dead."

It was my fault." She mumbled emphasizing the word was. Then out loud, "I should have seen some kind of event coming. Of course there was no way I could have known it would be Phillip who would be a victim, but I should have seen that a patient could go wrong."

The cab driver having had experience in picking up grieving people at hospitals try to console her: "Lady, I am sure it wasn't your fault."

Peggy then realized she had been talking out loud. "I am sorry, please forgive me. I am okay."

"Okay, Lady." He answered.

Once she was home she stopped crying as her professional talents took over from her emotions.

Peggy reflected back on the situation: The animal studies demonstrated that an overdose of Lifeal could cause hyperactivity but she never thought hyperactivity would go to such far reaching actions and she had never considered possible withdrawal effects.

She had methodically followed her experiments on the new reported side effect. Case #6 on hyperactivity had come in last Tuesday by fax from a Dr. Rosenberg in Wyckoff, New Jersey. He had reported that his patient, a Mr. Ralph Vandermere, was taking an overdose and was very hyper. He had alienated all his friends and had been demanding extra refills. Dr. Rosenberg felt that Mr. Vandermere was taking many tablets everyday and that he was addicted to the drug and was experiencing the hyperactive side effect. Dr. Rosenberg had tried to get Mr. Vandermere to stop taking Lifeal, but to no avail.

Mr. Vandermere had gone from Dr. Rosenberg's office directly to the pharmacy and demanded a refill. Luckily the pharmacist was a sharp young man and he had called Dr. Rosenberg on the request for the refill. Dr. Rosenberg had told Mr. Vandermere's pharmacist to substitute a placebo for Lifeal. He had hoped that Mr. Vandermere would come back to his office to see him when his cardiac fibrillation started to bother him. Dr. Rosenberg concluded his report by saying he would write again when he heard from Mr. Vandermere and ended with a question. Had James had any reports of problems like this with any other patients on Lifeal?

Peggy had immediately written Dr. Rosenberg saying that they had five previous cases of mild hyperactivity but nothing so severe as he was reporting. She also admitted that she had not heard of anyone taking a large overdose of Lifeal. She asked Dr. Rosenberg to keep her informed and she, in turn, would keep him informed. She then increased the dosage to her test animals to see if she could duplicate Vandermere's behavior. She also took two of the primates off Lifeal and placed them on a placebo to see if they went through withdrawal.

Friday, a man called Ralph Vandermere had shot Phillip and then committed suicide. This happened the day after she had written her letter to Dr. Rosenberg. When the newspapers released the shooter's name, Peggy knew in her heart that it was the same Ralph Vandermere. As yet, she hadn't mentioned any of this to anybody. She would talk to Allen tomorrow. He would know what to do. Until then, she was left alone with her thoughts. She started to cry again. Quickly getting hysterical. "Oh God, what am I going to do? What is going to happen to me? What is going to happen to Lifeal? What am I going to do?" She could not help blaming herself.

SUTTON PLACE NEW YORK CITY

Peggy woke up feeling terrible. She had cried too much. Although it had given her some relief, it hadn't done anything to solve her problem. She decided to turn to the only person she knew who could help her cope with this feeling of guilt. Peggy had to talk Allen. She did not know if he would be coming into New York City or working at the research labs in Sheepshead Bay. She decided to call his home.

"Hello Pat. It's Peggy McCleary. Has Allen gone to work yet?"

Allen's wife replied, "Yes, he went into the city today. He left about thirty minutes ago, you will be able to catch him at the Spectrum of Medicine."

"Thank you, Pat, have a good day."

Peggy called Allen's voice mail at James. She knew he would check his messages first thing when he arrived at his office.

"Allen, this is Peggy. I have to talk to you as soon as possible. I need your advice. I am pretty sure I know what caused the man to shoot Phillip. I want to talk to you first before I go to the police. It is 7:30 now, I'm leaving my apartment in a few minutes. Leave a message on my voice mail as to when and where we can meet. Thanks. See you soon." Peggy's voice was more chipper than she felt.

Peggy finished dressing, left the apartment, and caught the cross-town bus.

When Peggy arrived at her office, there was a message on her voice mail from Allen. "I am in my office, come on up." Peggy gathered up her Lifeal test results and went to the ninth floor and Allen's office.

Peggy's voice was quivering when she finally spoke, "Oh Allen, I am so afraid. I think I am responsible for having almost killed Phillip and killing that strange man."

Allen's voice was soft and understanding. He placed his arm around Peggy's shoulders and led her to one of the chairs in his office.

"Please take it easy Peggy. How in the world could you be responsible for what happened last Friday? Please start from the beginning."

"Remember we have been working on the hyperactivity side effects of Lifeal? Well, I received a letter from a Dr. Rosenberg in Wyckoff, NJ about a Mr. Ralph Vandermere becoming almost violent from overdosing on Lifeal and that he went through withdrawal after Dr. Rosenberg took him off Lifeal.

Allen, this I am sure, is the same man who shot Phillip last Friday. When I read the name of the shooter in the Sunday Times, I was certain it was the same person. Allen, what am I going to do? If I had just paid closer attention to the side effects this would not have happened." She could not hold it back any longer and began crying again.

When Peggy had settled down, Allen said "Please Peggy, start from the beginning, so I know everything that you know."

Peggy told Allen the complete story and showed him the animal studies. When she had finished, Allen sat back in his chair and just stared at Peggy. His large hands were folded together and the tips of the second finger of each hand rested against his chin. For a few minutes Allen was deep in thought. Just as Peggy was about to interrupt Allen's thoughts, Allen began to speak.

"First Peggy, you have to stop feeling guilty. It wasn't your fault. How were you to know this would happen? You did exactly what you were trained to do. If something is going to happen to Lifeal, then that is too bad. But nothing will happen to you. Now let's figure out what we're going to do to share this monkey we now have on our collective backs."

"Oh, Allen, I'm just really upset at myself, Lifeal, James, and my life." Matter of factly, Allen replied, "Okay, Peggy, now let's fix this thing.

First, we should tell your story to Helmut and then to J.P. If you haven't heard, when Phillip came out of anesthesia from the surgery on Saturday he dictated a memo to the physician placing J.P. in temporary operational command of James. Financial command is still in Brian's hands as the CFO. That move of Phillip's will really piss off Mrs. Evelyn PrestonJames. She was probably in church all day Sunday praying for Phillip to go into a long sleep. I know she is going to get her way if it kills all of us. If I hadn't heard your story, I would have looked to her as an accessory to attempted murder." Allen paused. "Peggy, do you feel that you can tell your story to Helmut and J.P.?"

"I would be lying if said I was feeling in top shape. I would also be lying if I did not say I am 100% better than I was before we had this talk. I'm ready to proceed to the next step, Dr. Allen Stevenson Strong, sir," she answered. She smiled and stood up from her seat.

Peggy and Allen walked to Helmut's office and Peggy told him her story. Allen and Peggy wanted to go up and see J.P. immediately, but Helmut wanted time to think about the situation.

Peggy and Allen stood while Helmut contemplated the situation. After five minutes he spoke, "We must come up with a plan first, so we can present it to J.P. I am not sure if he is up to date on the regulatory issues, so let's make sure we give him a few alternatives from which to choose his course of action.

One hour later the three of them asked to see J.P. on an emergency basis. It was 9:00 a.m. Phillip's staff meeting always started at 10:00 sharp. Allen remarked that they would have an hour with J.P. before his first staff meeting.

They took the elevator to the top floor. The first evident change was Judi, Mandi's secretary, sitting at Janet's desk. "Please go in. Dr. Koenig is expecting you.

Helmut, Allen and Peggy entered Phillip's office.

SPECTRUM OF MEDICINE BUILDING NEW YORK CITY

J.P. was sitting at Phillip's conference table when the R&D group entered the office. J.P. decided to work from the table rather than sit at Phillip's desk. The office had been completely sanitized over the weekend and there remained no evidence of the terror that had taken place in the office only three days before.

The word from the physicians was that Phillip would recover after a week or so in the hospital and then he would spend some time recuperating at home. He had been extremely lucky. The bullet had entered his body above the left auricle just missing his aorta. The round from the ancient Colt .45 did leave a great deal of damage as it exited Phillip's body. He would have a long rehabilitation program to regain full use of his left shoulder.

Janet had asked for the day off. She promised she would be in on Tuesday. She wanted to visit Phillip at the hospital to make sure he was all right psychologically, and then she wanted to rest at home. She wanted Monday to pass without being reminded of the image of Ralph Vandermere's head exploding. J.P. didn't blame her. He also wanted Monday to go by. Why had Phillip given him the reins of the company? J.P. had no idea. He felt that Phillip should have turned the day-to-day operations of James to the CFO, Brian. He was grateful to Mandi for letting him use her secretary, Judi, for the day. He made a mental note to ask Mandi to allow him to keep Judi on a stand-by basis for a couple more days to make sure that Janet made it through the week. J.P. was certain that Janet was probably underestimating the psychological affect the shooting would have on her. He was going to encourage her to undergo counseling when she did return.

"Good morning J.P." the group said collectively as they entered.

Helmut spoke, "Sorry to bother you, J.P., but Peggy thinks she has the answers to a lot of Friday's questions. We feel you have to know about this situation as soon as possible because it could very well result in a recall of Lifeal or at the very least notification to FDA. Sorry to give you such a problem on your first day as interim president, but there it is. Peggy will go through the specifics with you and then Allen and I will go through some alternatives.”

“Okay, sounds like a good agenda to me.” J.P. said. “Go ahead Peggy let’s hear the good news.”

Peggy smiled, “Well J.P., I am sure I know what caused Ralph Vandermere to shoot Phillip.” She then proceeded to tell him about the hyperactivity side effect and her animal studies.

When she concluded, J.P. sat for a moment looking out the window and then said, “Well, Peggy, I don’t see where you did anything that was out of order. How were you to know that this Mr. Vandermere was going to go nuts on us? I have two questions. Were the other five cases as severe as this case? Secondly, wouldn’t you classify Mr. Vandermere’s behavior a little more severe than just hyperactive?”

“The other five cases are classified as no more than restless activity and extra energy. The side effect was red flagged by us only after the five cases because the Lifeal indication of cardiac arrhythmia and hyperactivity are antagonistic. The heart can be racing out of control in cardiac arrhythmia. Hyperactivity could cause cardiac arrhythmia. As you know we always watch for this type of antagonistic situation. The five cases only showed an incidence of less than one hundredth of one percent of the total universe. I started the animal the studies based on the five cases. The differences between my studies and the Mr. Vandermere situation were the high doses and subsequent withdrawal. We think that Mr. Vandermere was taking up to five tablets a day. I was not studying doses that high until last Tuesday when I received Dr. Rosenberg’s notification. I also did not study withdrawal at that high of a dose. I did study withdrawal at twice the normal dose during the original toxicology and pathology studies.

“On your second question, J.P., I would agree that hyperactivity is not a high enough classification. We will have to investigate this further.”

“Thank you, Peggy. Okay, Helmut and Allen, what are our alternatives?”

"J.P.," Helmut spoke first, "we have the following alternatives. Number one, we do nothing now, except accelerate our animal studies and notify the FDA when we know more about the side effect. Number two, notify the FDA that we have a potential problem and that we are investigating the situation and will keep them informed. Number three, pull Lifeal. And, number four; send out a Dear Doctor and Dear Pharmacist letter making them aware of the potential dangers in higher doses of Lifeal.

Allen spoke up, "We think number three is too much action for the total number of incidences. We feel that we have the situation under control. We are concerned over what the press will do when they find out that there is connection between Lifeal and the shooting. The spin that they will put on it to sell more papers could destroy Lifeal. We feel that we should take positive action before we give Peggy's report to the police."

"I agree, Allen. What is the bottom line?"

Allen leaned forward in his seat and spoke, "J.P., I would recommend that we combine our recommendations. We call the FDA and tell them that we have an overdose case and we want to ensure that no other patient overdoses on Lifeal. I don't believe we have to mention withdrawal because Lifeal did not cause the withdrawal or the shooting. Ralph Vandermere got down on himself. We know Lifeal is not addictive or habit forming. Only these two pharmacological actions can result in withdrawal. We don't know exactly why Vandermere did what he did, but it was not directly caused by Lifeal. There is a chance that Ralph Vandermere was an undiagnosed manic-depressive.

"We should write Dear Doctor and Dear Pharmacist letters and send them out as soon as possible. This will ensure that both physicians and pharmacists warn their patients about taking the recommended dosage. We are not the first product to have a bad side effect when a patient overdoses. We expand Peggy's studies and see if they can be accelerated. We go back and review the literature to ensure we know everything about the possibility of a withdrawal. Not to tell you your job, J.P., but I would take the extra step of contacting the

Wall Street investment writer you know. You know, the guy who gives us all the headaches."

"Jack Husted," J.P. said with a frown.

"Yes. He gives us a bad rap sometimes, but for the most part, I think he is fair in his reporting. When he is hard on us, I think we probably deserve the bad press. Anyway, we should be up front with him. It can't hurt. If he finds out on his own, he will be harder on us in the end."

"Yep, I agree. I think you have an excellent plan," J.P. replied. "Peggy and Allen, you work on the investigation of the side effects and the clinicals. Helmut, please contact the FDA and let me know what they say. I will have Mandi draft the letters to physicians and pharmacists and I will call Husted. Peggy, I will also call the police inspector who is handling Phillip's shooting. Helmut will you go over our plan at this morning's staff meeting?"

"Yes, J.P.," Helmut replied.

"Great." J.P. stood up from the table signaling the end of the meeting. "I want to thank all of you for your diligence in this matter. I'm sure Phillip would be very proud of your actions. After the staff meeting, I will be going to the hospital to talk with Phillip. I'll brief him on the situation and any other things that come up at the staff meeting that he should know about." J.P. looked at his watch. "See you in 10 minutes."

"Oh, Helmut," J.P. stopped him just as he was about to go out the door. Helmut stopped and turned back, "Yes, J.P.?"

"My plan, before this shooting incident, was to work in R&D this week. The shooting will cause me to delay my visit to your department until Wednesday. Is this a problem?"

"No, of course not. Whatever you like. I am at your service."

"Please remain flexible, Helmut. I don't yet know what other surprises will be in store for me."

"Again J.P., I am at your service," he said before leaving the office. He silently closed the door behind him.

SPECTRUM OF MEDICINE BUILDING
NEW YORK CITY

After the staff meeting Peggy returned to her office. Even with all of the moral support she had received from Allan, J.P., and Helmut, she was still shaken over Phillip's shooting and the possibility that a Lifeal side effect had helped create the incident. She decided the best thing she could do was to throw herself back into clinical research.

In order to investigate the possibility of withdrawal, she had to look at the basic Lifeal formula. She went to the research department safe, dialed in the combination, and removed the three-inch binder labeled "Master Formula, Lifeal". She had to investigate all of the available information on Lifeal and Dita Bark to ensure there was no chance of addiction or dependence when a patient is taking Lifeal.

SPECTRUM OF MEDICINE BUILDING
NEW YORK CITY

J.P. made two telephone calls immediately after the staff meeting. One to Jack Husted and the other to Inspector O'Brien who was working on the Vandermere case. Inspector O'Brien requested that J.P., Allen, Peggy, and the James corporate lawyer meet with him at 2:30. J.P. readily agreed and set up the meeting to be held in Phillip's conference room.

The morning call to Jack Husted was very rewarding. J.P. hadn't spoken with him since the board meeting so he was very interested in what was happening at James. J.P. brought him up to date and then gave him the exclusive on the Lifeal situation. Husted was very appreciative of the telephone call and was honestly concerned over the trouble James was having.

He told J.P., "I will try and do as much damage control as possible about the shooting and the Lifeal connection. I will use the responsible corporate response scenario. I think the stock will take a small hit, investors are now sophisticated enough to know that humans run corporations and humans err. Just try not to make too many errors."

They ended the conversation with plans to have lunch in the near future.

Later that afternoon, J.P. was seated at the conference table with Inspector O'Brien, Allen, and Peggy. Peggy told the police inspector her story. He confirmed that it was the same Ralph Vandermere. He had questioned Vandermere's wife and his cardiologist. They confirmed that he had not been himself for a number of weeks. Dr. Rosenberg had also told O'Brien that he had sent the customer complaint form to James and to the FDA as directed by the regulations. O'Brien commented that Dr. Rosenberg had stated emphatically that he did not blame James or Lifeal for the shootings. "It was just a regrettable series of events," he said.

The inspector was not too sure how Mrs. Vandermere was going to handle the situation, but the Vandermere's were very well off and even if the insurance company did not pay off on the policy, Mrs. Vandermere was still in great financial shape. He thanked them for their cooperation and as far as he was concerned the case was closed.

After the police inspector left, the remaining James employees and J.P. talked about the potential legal actions that could be taken by any of the parties involved.

After an hour of discussions, Kurt Bershire, the James corporate lawyer, summed up the situation. "I am sure there will be no problem with the police. Dr. Rosenberg and the pharmacist do not think there will be a problem unless Mrs. Vandermere becomes a problem to them. Mrs. Vandermere will not be a problem to James considering that Mr. Vandermere did try to kill Phillip. The FDA should not be a problem if we follow through with the plan that Helmut presented to the staff this morning. I am concerned about what the press will do with this when they find out. I think we should proact with a press release and maybe even a press conference."

J.P. broke in, "I'm going to the hospital to talk to Phillip and will go over our alternatives with him and get back with everyone, except Peggy, tonight at six o'clock. Nothing personal Peggy, there is just no reason for you to stay. You just get the research done on the side effect and then go home and relax. This has taken more out of you than I'm certain you realize. Get a good night's rest."

"Okay, J.P., and thanks" Peggy replied.

The group left the office and J.P. got up from the conference table and went to the chair behind Phillip's desk and sat down. He leaned back as far as the chair could go and closed his eyes. It had been a hectic and chaotic few days and he now realized that he really wasn't ready to come to grips with the problem of what to do with the new Lifeal problem. He swung the chair around so that it was facing the window and opened his eyes. It was a sunny winter day. There were very few clouds and those were moving quickly out to sea. The buildings of the city rose up from Manhattan Island and stood like silent statues against the blue horizon.

What had started as a simple project to find out who stole a strategic plan had now become a full-blown catastrophe and he was right in the middle. He was now in a position to have to make corporate decisions that could make or break a product, company, or a friend. The worst part was that he still had no clue as to who had taken the plan. He longed to just run away and head back to the mountains of Mammoth. He closed his eyes and decided to take a quick nap.

4:00 P.M., MONDAY, FEBRUARY 6

COLUMBIA PRESBYTERIAN HOSPITAL
NEW YORK CITY

J.P. sat in the chair on the left side of Phillip's bed looking at his old friend. J.P. noted that Phillip's normal pallor was even more pronounced than usual and there were dark rings around his eyes. He had an IV tube coming out of his right arm with a 500-ml bottle of Ringers solution gradually dripping into the vein. His left arm was securely wrapped against his chest to keep it immobilized. The bandages went up to his neck.

J.P. had been sitting there for ten minutes. Phillip was asleep. The nurse had said that he would wake in less than fifteen minutes, so J.P. decided to wait. He used the time to think through the various James situations and possible solutions. He felt that he had things under control, but he wanted Phillip's concurrence, that is, if he was capable of giving his concurrence.

J.P. glanced at his motionless friend. He looked at his calm face and, for the first time, noticed the bandages on the back of his head. J.P. didn't realize that his head had been hurt and for the first time, concern regarding Phillip's thinking process crossed his mind. As J.P. sat there thinking that he probably didn't have much business bothering him with James Pharmaceutical business until he was feeling better, Phillip's eyelids moved just a little. Slowly, he opened his eyes. He lay there on his back staring up at the ceiling.

J.P. thought that he was probably trying to figure out where he was. He looked at the ceiling for about fifteen seconds and then began to search the room with his eyes. His head never moved, only his eyes.

Finally, he saw J.P. sitting next to his bed. The expression on his face did not change as he softly said, "J.P., how are you?"

"Fine, how are you?"

"Could be better, but I'm still here among the living and that is something, don't you think?" he continued in a whisper.

"It would take more than a crazy lawyer to do you in, Phillip."

"A crazy lawyer, was it?" a smile came to his face. "I knew those bastards would try and get me one day. Is he in jail?"

"No, he didn't make it. He shot himself after he tried to finish you off.

Are you up to talking about it and about James?"

"Let me think about that question for a moment." He fell into silence for a few minutes and then replied. "I feel good, J.P. A little groggy, but no pain. The local they put in my left shoulder has kept the pain away. The back of my head hurts a little from where I hit the window, but the pain is not too great. Sort of a dull headache, but not thought inhibiting. The real question is whether I want to talk about James. For some strange reason this accident has given me the first peace of mind in years." His smile widened. "I do believe I will stay here for a while and let the great Jean Paul Koenig, Ph.D., play president."

"Oh no, you don't. Not a chance, old friend." J.P. responded with a chuckle emphasizing the words old and friend. "I am not the president of James, you are. To tell you the truth I don't know why I said I would take over for you until you return. You made your request so persuasive it made me feel like I was fulfilling a dying man's final wish."

"It was a good acting job, wasn't it, J.P.?"

In a more serious tone, J.P. said, "From the lightness of this conversation, I believe I will tender my resignation and turn this horror show back over to you. As far as I'm concerned you are ready and able to go back to work. The willing to go back to work is irrelevant to the situation. Now are you ready to talk business or am I resigning?"

Phillip's voice took on a more infirm tone with an accent that sounded to J.P. as being Gabby Hayes, "Oh, no, J.P., don't start threatening a sick and dying man with leaving. I need you to handle the work at hand and to keep the bad guys from taking over the ranch. You must protect our water rights. I have only you I can trust, you can't leave me old friend."

"You missed your calling, Phillip. You should have been in the movies," J.P. said laughing. "Now, whether you like it or not I am going to give you the rundown on today's events and ask your advice and consent. Ready?"

"Ready and able. I'm sorry, but the willing is still absent. Go for it, J.P."

For the next fifteen minutes he went over the day and the Lifeal situation. The questions that Phillip asked demonstrated to J.P. that he was as sharp as ever and he would probably be out of the hospital within the week.

The two men agreed that the staff's plan to keep working on the side effect, inform the FDA of the situation, and write letters to physicians and pharmacists as the best alternative.

SPECTRUM OF MEDICINE BUILDING
NEW YORK CITY

J.P. had set up his first R&D meeting for 2:00 on Wednesday afternoon. He thought it wise to meet initially with Helmut in Phillip's office. Helmut had shown arrogance that he planned to handle by having their meetings in Phillip's office rather than Helmut's office. He figured that Helmut was mostly an administrative leader and was not doing any actual research. One of the main R&D objectives that J.P. had was to learn about Alzheimer's and he thought Allen would be the best person to talk to about that. But first, he had to query Helmut about the 21st Century Plan.

At exactly 2:00 there was a strong knock on the office door. He knew immediately that it had to be Helmut. He was surprised that Janet hadn't warned him of Helmut's arrival, but she still was not herself and Helmut probably intimidated her into taking no action. Whatever the case, it made little difference to him.

"Come in," he said. After Helmut opened the door, he immediately added, "Please Helmut, take a seat at the office conference table. I'll be with you in a minute."

J.P shuffled papers around on the desk and signed a stack of papers that Janet had placed on the desk during lunch. He didn't prolong his action and only made Helmut wait an extra three minutes. J.P. walked around the desk and joined Helmut at the conference table and noted that Helmut didn't appear to be anxious to talk.

"How are you, Helmut?" The two men had known one another when J.P. was at James. In the past, he believed there had been mutual respect between them, but imagined that Helmut had only been tolerating him as Helmut tolerated all marketing businessmen including Phillip. Helmut felt R&D should set the direction a pharmaceutical company. In order to get Helmut to work harder, Doc James encouraged Helmut to continue this philosophy.

"I am well, thank you. That is, considering all the stress that is going around lately," Helmut replied trying to unsuccessfully force a convincing smile. "How are you holding up, filling the man's chair?"

"Just fine, Helmut, just fine. Didn't expect the position when I arrived, but now that I am here, it feels fine."

Silence. They both glanced out the window. The day was cloudy and misty. The sky seemed to be preparing for another snowstorm. They looked out the window for another five minutes before J.P. opened the conversation.

"How is the world of pharmaceutical medicine?" he asked casually. "You know goddamn well the industry is in terrible shape. The changes that have been dictated by federal regulations have damaged our research capabilities almost beyond repair. And, management, ah, now there is one of the many destroyers of our future. Management of pharmaceutical companies is being hired from outside the industry. Executives from aerospace and computers. What do they know about healthcare? Don't ask me why, it is beyond my understanding. Thank God Phillip is an executive who understands why we exist. It is for the patient and not the dollar. The dollar will follow the patients' well being," he jerked his head in J.P.'s direction as if he were Helmut's jury.

J.P. interrupted in a quiet voice, "I didn't know of your passion for the pharmaceutical industry."

Helmut got up from the table and started to pace. He turned suddenly and stood over J.P. and in a firm, but not angry voice he said, "J.P., do you really want to know my views on this subject? It might take up some of your valuable time." The last was said with a slight bitter tone.

J.P. knew he had to find a way to start a conversation about the 21st Century Plan without asking Helmut a direct question.

He knew a direct question would turn him off. Talking about the industry was one way to ease into the subject.

"Yes, as much as this might surprise you, I would like to hear your views. But, please stop pacing and sit down."

"No, J.P.," he paused thinking the tone of his "no" had been too strong. He continued in a softer voice. "Thank you, but I wish to continue to stand. I like pacing you know. I can think better." He turned again and smiled. "Perhaps I require pacing to get my tired blood pumping and nourishing my brain cells before I am able to think correctly."

He turned and walked to the window and stared out at the mist. "I remember when I was behind the research bench and not behind a desk. When I had a research problem, I paced. Sometimes the answer came in minutes, sometimes in hours, but sooner or later a new direction came to my mind and I could go back to my project. So," he turned from the window with a smile, "if you do not mind, I will pace."

J.P. smiled back. This was a side of Helmut he had not seen before. He was almost human. "Of course not, please proceed."

In a very professional tone without too much emotion, but with passion he began, "J.P., research is the backbone of our industry, especially the pharmaceutical industry in this country. During the fifties to the eighties the US pharmaceutical industry led the world in pharmaceutical research. Not to take anything away from American scientists, but much of the research was done by Europeans who immigrated to here. Their native countries did not have the research funds, freedom, or facilities to use their scientific intelligence to develop the new synthetic pharmaceuticals. In the eighties, the foreign companies began to gain a foothold in new pharmaceutical research and the Japanese began their move to gain worldwide pharmaceutical power. In the eighties biogenetics became the future and here it looked as though we would regain our large lead in pharmaceutical research.

"I am not telling you anything that you do not already know, but maybe you do not know the statistics." He stopped his pacing and walked over to a dry eraser board. In his rough handwriting, he drew a wiring diagram.

"On average, it takes twelve years for most experimental pharmaceuticals to go from the laboratory to the patient. This does not include the research time and evaluation of literally thousands of chemical structures and their derivatives before we find a product that is worthy of entering pre-clinical testing. Nor does it include the prior research that was done on a class of pharmaceuticals."

Helmut turned pensive, "All of this time and effort is great and should be done to ensure the safety and efficacy of the product, but at what cost?" He looked directly at J.P. and his tone became more intense. "What of the damn costs?" He proceeded to answer his own question.

"The press and government talk about pharmaceutical profits, but they don't understand how much it costs to bring a single product to market. I know that this is our standard industry argument, but no one talks about what makes up the costs and how the costs are interrelated to the total healthcare sector. As an example, each of the clinical studies listed in phases I to III cost up to $1,000 each or $3,000,000 for 3,000 patients. This money goes to hospitals to keep track of the patient records and to the physicians and staff to pay for their time and expertise in completing the patient evaluation and paperwork. The $3,000,000 helps the hospitals and subsidizes their care of indigent patients. In a Tufts University study, completed in the early 90s, it was determined that it requires more than $231 million for a pharmaceutical company to obtain a new drug approval from the FDA. A great deal of this money goes back into the healthcare industry to pay for services."

Helmut returned to his chair at the conference table. He sat down and looked directly at J.P. "Someone has to pay for this unspecified and uncertain research. Up to this point, in the United States, the companies paid for their own research. Sure the companies made a profit, but, as you know, profits are also taxable by the government and in return are dispersed in federal programs. If we do not protect the industry, we will open the doors to foreign companies to take marketshare away from our companies. With these new profits and government subsidized research programs the foreign companies will gain a research lead that we might never be able to overcome."

Helmut's eyes blazed as he thought of the downside. "Goddamnit, J.P., if there is one truism it is that the best treatment will be used whether the pharmaceutical is researched and manufactured here, in Japan, Germany, or even Iran. The best product will be prescribed for the ill patient and purchased by the US government or third party insurance. It is our makeup to do what is best for the patient. The pharmaceutical industry is not like the automobile industry. If we loose our leading research position we will not be able to regain our lost position for decades. The automobile industry just had to get their quality act together and they regained their lead. They did not have to wait an average of twelve years to obtain FDA approval. The pharmaceutical tax monies, jobs, and knowledge that will be lost to foreign companies and nations are incalculable. I am not an isolationist, but I say let the marketplace seek its own level. Don't let our own government sabotage our efforts and cut off our research capabilities. We here at James are in a free enterprise situation and my research capability has been cut. The government has not cut my research capability, it has been Phillip and the lack of sales of Lifeal that has cut my budget because we have to report growing earnings." He bowed his head, "This is partly my fault," he looked back up, "and the social cost of medicine. Is it our fault that more than 20% of the healthcare dollar is spent on the elderly population in their last months of their lives. Deserted by society, not to die with honor, but to die when Medicare or Medicaid will not pay for their bed and the healthcare system can no longer sustain their life."

J.P. decided to build upon Helmut's statements to show him that he was doing more than listening. He also wanted to draw the conversation to a close. He added, "Is it the pharmaceutical companies' fault that healthcare dollars are spent for sex or drug related diseases. Or the health problems of children born of drug addicts or undernourished mothers. Mothers to be that will not use available prenatal services.

"These problems are being classified as healthcare problems rather than social problems. The burden to the healthcare system is nearly 50% of every healthcare dollar. In the end, nothing is being said or done to change that social situation except establish regulations and government controls that can only hurt the pharmaceutical industry and does nothing in the way of addressing the social problems," J.P. paused. "But what should we, James, do about the situation?" He decided to answer to answer his own question and segue into the 21st Century Plan.

"Helmut, I believe the 21st Century Plan is James' answer to the role we're to play in tomorrow's healthcare marketplace." He closely watched Helmut's face and eyes as he made the statement and waited for his response.

In return, Helmut seemed to search his eyes for any hidden meaning to the statement. J.P. tried his best to remain passive. He seemed satisfied and turned his gaze to the window.

"J.P., look out the window.

"It is cold and wet today. Tomorrow it may be sunny and cold, the next day sunny and warm, and the next day something different. The future is like the weather. There are so many different variables. In science it is the theory of chaos. So is the future, chaos. If we could predict the future we would all be day traders, *ja?*" He laughed. "The 21st Century Plan, J.P. is a plan. Nothing more or less."

J.P. turned back from the window to face him. "But, Helmut, do you believe in the plan?"

"What do you want me to say?" Anger had crept into his voice and his German accent had become more pronounced, "Yes, fine, I believe in this plan."

J.P. pushed, "Will you implement the plan?"

"Why are you asking me this?" he was becoming increasingly hostile.

J.P. backed off, "No real reason, Helmut. I just wanted to know your feelings."

"It is a plan," he responded more calmly. "I believe in the R&D section of the plan. Comments on the other sections will have to be given to you by those who wrote the sections."

"Surely you must have an opinion?" J.P. pushed again.

"I save my opinions for myself. I do not get paid for giving opinions of other people's work."

J.P. decided to take a risk of alienating him and demand an answer. "Okay, Helmut, let's quit this dance. Are you going to follow the 21st Century Plan or fight the strategy and actions that will implement this plan?" He raised his voice as he tried to get a stronger reaction from Helmut. To this point in the conversation he couldn't determine from the researcher's answers whether he knew anything about the extra copy of the 21st Century Plan.

Helmut did not respond any differently than before, "I am not dancing with you, J.P. The 21st Century Plan is just not my top priority at this time." He turned and again looked out the window.

J.P. lowered his voice indicating that he had given up trying to force an answer from him. "Helmut, I want to spend some time discussing JPC138 and, to a minor extent, Lifeal with Dr. Strong. Is this going to be a problem for you?"

"No sir. Certainly not. You are the boss, at least on an interim basis, and you can spend as much time with any of my people as you desire." He turned his gaze back to J.P. and leveled his eyes to meet his and said, "I would appreciate your giving me a report after your visits with my people. Is this possible, J.P.?"

"Of course, Helmut. Is there anything you want to ask me?"

"No, J.P. Now if you will excuse me, I have a great deal of paper work to do for the FDA."

"You are excused, Helmut." I added with a slight hint of sarcasm, "Thank you for your cooperation."

Helmut had gotten up from the table and was almost at the door. He turned and his voice hinted at a slight irritation, "As the kids say, J.P., no problem dude," and he left the office.

J.P. didn't let Helmut's attitude bother him. He had been pleasantly surprised at his depth of knowledge on the politics of the pharmaceutical industry. The Helmut he had known in the past stayed away from politics. He couldn't help but wonder what led him to become a champion of the US pharmaceutical industry.

He picked up the telephone to call Annie and noted that it was almost lunchtime again in Mammoth. Annie again answered on the second ring.

"Annie's Bar and Grill."

"Annie, it's J.P. How are you this fine day."

"You remembered, bless you, J.P. Are you coming home?"

"Sorry, love, I think not." He then told her about all the happenings since last Wednesday. Annie was sympathetic, but disappointed that he was staying so long in New York. He ended their short conversation by saying that he would call her next Wednesday.

He then picked up the telephone to call Mandi.

"Hi," he said when Judi transferred the call to Mandi.

"Hi yourself, lover," Mandi answered with a gentleness in her voice. "How are the physician and pharmacist letters coming along?"

"They have been written and are presently going through our internal regulatory approval. They ought to hit your desk this afternoon. I have everything ready to go. There are about 50,000 pharmacist letters and 300,000 physician letters. The letters are being sent via overnight registered mail at a cost of about $5.00 each or well over $2,000,000 unbudgeted expense. Not counting the overhead. Sorry, J.P., it's the best we could do to honor our commitment to the FDA and ourselves.

"Don't worry J.P. I have my responsibilities under control. How about Jack Husted?"

"He mentioned our quick response to the side effect in his Wall Street Journal column. He built his story around how well we reacted to the situation and downplayed the actual side effect. It's not that he is being nice to us. He wants to give us a chance to research the side effect and then he will make his decision on how to handle the reporting of the hyperactivity side effect.

"In a way this does help James because this strategy will keep the press attention down to a low level. The stock has remained fairly steady. If there were a news media witch hunt on pharmaceutical side effects our stock, plus all of the other pharmaceutical company stocks, would probably have taken a stock traders emotional dip.

Mandi change subjects. "How was your meeting with Helmut?" "What do you think?" he said jokingly.

"I would imagine that he was pompous, only answered questions, and   basically was uncooperative. Correct?"

J.P. decided to keep to himself Helmut's break in character and answer Mandi as she would have expected. "How did you know?"

"That's Dr. Helmut Walthers, J.P." She laughed. "Don't you remember?"

"To be honest, I guess I don't remember him as well as I thought I did.

By the way, are we getting together tonight?"

"Yes, I was planning on staying. Any problem?"

"Nope. I was just doing the courtesy of checking with someone I respect very much."

"Aw, you're such a schmoozer, but thanks. I have some work that will keep me a little late, but I should be home at your apartment by 6:30."

"That's great. See you then. Goodbye"

"Goodbye" He picked up the telephone again and called Allen Strong. "Strong, here." Allen answered.

"Good afternoon, Allen."

"J.P., Helmut told me to expect your call. When do you want to get together?" he asked excitedly.

"How about 8:00 a.m. tomorrow?"

"Sounds like an excellent time of day. Is there anything you want me to prepare for our meeting?"

"Yes, as a matter of fact there is. Please be prepared to give me a 30minute briefing on Alzheimer's disease. Don't get too complex. Just hit the high spots on the physiology of the disease and how you expect JPC138 will help."

"Great J.P., see you at eight." "Thanks, Allen."

"Hi, J.P., I'm home." Mandi slammed the door to make sure he heard her arrival.

"Hey, beautiful, I'm in the kitchen. If you want, get comfortable and then pour us a drink. I'm mighty parched." When Mandi came over he always enjoyed having his first drink of the day with her.

They ate a light dinner in the dining room. Their discussions were of James.

"Did you talk to Phillip today?" she asked.

"I called him this morning and again after I talked to Helmut. He is still in pain, but they are gradually reducing his dosage of painkillers. He thinks they'll send him home on Friday. His left side is still heavily bandaged and he said the physicians are still watching for internal bleeding from both the wound and surgery. So far everything is healing well. I called his physician and confirmed Phillip's assessment of himself."

"Anything about the shooting case from the police lieutenant?"

"No, nothing today. I think as far as the police are concerned it is a closed case. They know who shot Phillip. Phillip will survive with little permanent damage. Ralph did away with himself. Conclusion, case closed. That is according to the police, but not Phillip. He mentioned that he wants to know why Ralph shot him. I have not gone through Peggy's side effect research with him. I figured there was plenty of time to give him a briefing and there was no need to bother him with problems he could not do anything about. And, we have everything under control, right?"

"Right, J.P. I have my responsibilities under control. How about Jack Husted?"

"He mentioned our quick response to the side effect in his Wall Street Journal column. He built his story around how well we reacted to the situation and downplayed the actual side effect. It's not that he is being nice to us. He wants to give us a chance to research the side effect and then he will make his decision on how to handle the reporting of the hyperactivity side effect.

"In a way this does help James because this strategy will keep the press attention down to a low level. The stock has remained fairly steady. If there were a news media witch hunt on pharmaceutical side effects our stock, plus all of the other pharmaceutical company stocks, would probably have taken a stock traders emotional dip."

"Today was your day to call Annie. Did you call?"

"Boy, Mandi, we are full of questions this evening aren't we?"

"Sorry J.P. I haven't seen much of you over the past couple of days and just want to catch up on what you have been doing." she answered with a mock hurt in her voice.

J.P. reached over and placed his hand behind her neck and drew her towards him to kiss. There was a scraping of chairs as they moved their chairs towards each other and then they were out of the chairs and holding each other tightly.

Within five minutes they were upstairs in bed. The dishes were left until morning.

7:00 A.M., THURSDAY, FEBRUARY 9

SPECTRUM OF MEDICINE BUILDING
NEW YORK CITY

J.P. looked at his watch as soon as he arrived at his desk and realized that he had an hour before his meeting with Allen. He swung his chair around to look out the window at the waking day and focus his mind on pharmaceutical research.

Biogenetics was not his major strength because he hadn't personally worked in the field of genetic engineering. He had managed genetic engineering projects, but always worked with the clinical and financial results of the product after it had entered the pre-clinical stage. He was a textbook expert which in the world of biogenetics meant that he was allowed to talk about genetic engineering at cocktail parties, but only after everyone had finished their third drink.

As far as JPC138 was concerned, J.P. wanted an overview of the product and how biogenetics and herbal genetics worked together. Like many pharmaceutical companies, James worked closely with medical research laboratories, universities, and clinics. James was not a leader in biogenetics, but they were a leader in pharmaceutical herbal genetics. The James strategy was to use external and internal centers of knowledge to develop, in the field of Alzheimer's disease, proprietary products with sustainable competitive advantages.

Yesterday, Helmut had stated his views of the pharmaceutical industry situation very clearly, but he did not complete the story. He hadn't mentioned that the pharmaceutical researcher of a new drug entity had to know where every molecule is stored within the body or whether the drug is converted to another chemical, and where, how, and when the drug is disposed as human waste.

All of these drug safety studies are constantly faced with the threat of being attacked by animal rights advocates for using animals for testing, the worry of potential patent infringements because of the complexity of chemical compounds, and the problem of misinformed government intervention by publicity hungry members of congress.

Then there were the lawyers who were always diligently looking for areas they can apply their legal expertise and win major lawsuits from profitable pharmaceutical companies with deep pockets.

Even after a company survived the clinical and political gauntlet and the FDA had given their approval, management still did not know if it had a financial winner. First, the product had to be moved into the distribution system so it would be on the shelves of the pharmacy when prescribed. The product had to be approved by hospital formulary committees to be placed on the hospital formulary and used in hospitals. In today's world a company had to make sure the product was in the mail order house and Internet company pharmacies.

The kiss of death for a new pharmaceutical was to have the physician write a prescription and the pharmacist discover there is no product available to fill the prescription. Or worse, the pharmacist, not having the new product in inventory, calls the prescribing physician and obtains the name of a substitute pharmaceutical to fill the prescription.

After the new product is in the distribution system, the pharmaceutical company has to get the physician's attention and then educate him or her on the products pharmacological actions, approved indications, side effects, bioavailability, drug interaction, dosage titration, chemical reactions, nutritional cautions, storage conditions, and allergic reactions, to mention a few of the pharmaceutical company obligations.

These are reasons pharmaceutical companies, which introduce new products dislike legislation that allows generic companies to duplicate their product. After the pharmaceutical company does all of the work and expense of bringing a clinically successful product to market, generic companies are allowed to walk in and take marketshare without having to do the work or spend the money to have the product clinically established in the marketplace.

Doc James had found his place in this regulatory and political environment by focusing on herbal sciences. In the last fifteen years, James Research, under the direction of Doc James and then Helmut Walthers, concentrated on investigating the bridge between herbal DNA and human DNA.

Dr. Allen Strong was the key person on the research department that Doc James depended upon to come through with a new class of pharmaceuticals. Allen, by his own intelligence, hard laboratory work, the use of medical and agricultural databases, and leased time on a supercomputer for accelerated analyses, had discovered and developed a class of new pharmaceutical compounds, one of which was JPC138.

J.P.'s thoughts were interrupted by a voice from behind his back. He physically jumped and swung the chair around.

"Good morning J.P. Sorry if I startled you. How are you this bright morning?" asked Allen, vice president of Genetic Herbal Sciences.

J.P. looked back out the window at the gray dawning day. "Always the optimist, Allen?"

"Well someone has to maintain the positive spirit around here. If you and I didn't maintain our optimism, everyone might fall into the dumps. That is J.P., if I remember right and you still have your unwavering optimism." He smiled and started to make his way to the door that led to the conference boardroom.

J.P. watched the brilliant researcher as he walked to the door. His walk was full of confidence. He could easily have chosen any pharmaceutical company, but he chose to stay with James and work under Helmut. J.P. wondered why, but, as a shareholder, he was happy that he stayed. He had become world renowned for his work in biogenetics in combination with herbal sciences, but if the truth be known, he was thought of being slightly radical in his pursuit of herbs in medicine. Other companies respected him, but he scared them with his futurist ideas. He was a paradigm shifter. He liked to break tradition and to discover new and better ways of getting to where he wanted to go. This rebel philosophy probably kept the other companies from making him a financial offer that he couldn't refuse. Over the years since J.P. had first worked with Allen, he had maintained a youthful appearance and looked like he worked out regularly.

"No, Allen, I haven't lost my optimism. I still believe you can change negative situations into positive and profitable results. You know, I always look at the bright side of the moon. Especially when others want to go around to the moon's other side into darkness and lost communications," J.P. said as he followed Allen into the boardroom.

"Good analogy, J.P. I've always loved your analogies. Especially the one about the light at the end of the tunnel." He paused and casually asked, "Do you see the light at the end of the James tunnel or is the light, the head light of an oncoming heavy freight train?"

The question had been casual, but the answer was expected to be a true reflection of J.P.'s assessment of the current situation. "To be honest Allen, I haven't traveled far enough into the James tunnel to come to a conclusion, but by the fact that I entered, I am, as you say, optimistic. I don't enter tunnels that I don't expect to exit the far end on my feet." He paused and took a seat at the end of the conference table. "Now let's get to our subject. In terms I can understand, tell me about this mysterious disease called Alzheimer's."

Allen took the seat next to J.P. on the long side of the table. "I hope you don't mind meeting in the conference room. I feel more comfortable here and the audiovisual equipment I want to use in my presentation is available in this room. I hope this is all right with you?"

"No problem."

"My presentation is in three parts. First we'll cover the physiological aspects of the human brain. Next I'll discuss how Alzheimer's Disease affects the brain. And finally, we'll discuss the promise of JPC138 in fighting this terrible condition.

"J.P., would you please push the magic button to draw the curtains to darken the room a little for a computer presentation."

J.P. did as he was asked.

"Thanks. I thought since we are going to be dealing with the functions of the brain, I should first update you on medical studies concerning the brain. As you know, the brain is one the last human organs to be completely researched. With the increased use of Computerized Tomography, or CT, scanning, Magnetic Resonance Imaging...MRI, and Positron Emission Tomography...PET...the pharmaceutical researcher now has a large number of diagnostic aids at his or her disposal. We can now see the brain's physical changes with CT slices and whether a pharmaceutical treatment reverses physical malformations. With MRI, we are able to detect chemical reactions. PET will demonstrate the dynamic chemical functions of the brain. PET will also show us where pharmaceuticals take effect.

"With these sophisticated instruments and our increased understanding of biogenetics we can now do more advanced research. Before these advances in medicine we couldn't break the complexity barrier of the brain. The brain is not an organ we can remove, analyze, and replace in the patient's head. The brain of a cadaver is not a good research tool because of the electrical nature of the brain. A dead brain is shut down and not of much use when the clinical dynamics are what we are trying to study.

"Patients with Parkinson's, depression, schizophrenia, mania, and our specific disease Alzheimer's should see dramatic breakthroughs in diagnostic tests and disease treatments. These listed diseases are threatening the quality of life, which I personally want to see alleviated or at least controlled.

"As you can see this is a medical drawing of the side view of the human brain. The brain is a collection of 100 billion nerve cells or neurons and a trillion support cells. The body of each neuron is 1/100th the size of the period at the end of a printed sentence. Tentacles (dendrites) sprout from the neuron. Some neurons boast a long, wirelike appendage called an axon. Near the end of the dendrite or axon is the end of a dendrite from another neuron. A space of one millionth of an inch separates the two ends. The space is called a synapse.

"Neurons talk to each other by sending down a chemically controlled electrical impulse. Chemicals called neurotransmitters travel across the synapse to trigger chemical activity on the other side. Too much of one transmitter or not enough of another can alter your mood, your thinking, or your muscle strength. Some pharmaceuticals stimulate while others inhibit transmitter output. We have been working on how the chemicals in the brain influence memory and learning.

"Before I discuss Alzheimer's disease let me bridge with human aging. The answer to aging is still something of a mystery, but almost everyone agrees that aging is not caused by a single event or disease. There is a multitude of parallel and often interacting processes, many of them genetically controlled, that combine to ensure eventual aging of the body. As an example it used to be a general belief that, except for the beginning of life, the brain deteriorates. Research has shown that even though we are losing thousands of nerves a day, the brain finds new pathways to carry out the functions of the dying nerves. Evidence even shows that if a brain is exercised, the number of dendrite connections is increased. If you increase the input to the brain like learning new skills, the neural structure is increased. The opposite is also true. If you decrease input, you decrease structure. In the early nineties, Dr. Arnold Scheibel, head of the Brain Research Institute at UCLA stated, "The brain is just like a muscle use it or lose it. As you age, it becomes harder to take on new tasks like learning a language, but you have to do it."

He continued, "The leading causes of death among the elderly are." The screen showed:

LEADING CAUSES OF DEATH AMONG THE ELDERLY

Heart Disease Cerebrovascular Disease

Obstructive Lung Disease Pneumonia/influenza Lung Cancer Colorectal Cancer

"These diseases are the cause of death, but what about the conditions leading up to the cause of death."

J.P. added thoughtfully, "These diseases are terrible, but they are not the diseases that affect the quality of life as we age."

"Exactly, Parkinson's, depression, schizophrenia, mania, and Alzheimer's affect the quality of life and adversely affect the patients family, financial estate, and the cost of healthcare. Medical research can now work on the quality of growing older and hopefully, allow people to die with dignity.

"Genetic engineering has found that human systems do not have an expectancy and then suddenly stop. There is a process involved that can be slowed down and theoretically even reversed. One example is the shortening of life because the process responsible for duplicating DNA during cell division has a strange flaw. The process eliminates a small bit of telomere in every new copy of DNA it makes. All we have to do is repair this flaw. I will come back to genetic engineering in my last section on JPC138.

"Alzheimer's Disease was first recognized early in the 20th Century by Alois Alzheimer. It is most recognized by a progressive decline in memory, cognition, and reasoning. There are a number of behavioral symptoms such as."

BEHAVIORAL SYMPTOMS

Agitation (80%)

Depression (40%)

Delusions (35%)

Aggression (20%)

Hallucinations (16%)

"Studies indicate that Alzheimer's afflicts an estimated 10.3% of the population over the age 65 and half of those age 85 and older. Twothirds of these individuals remain in a home setting and rely on family and community resources for their care. The cost of healthcare for an institutionalized Alzheimer's patient has been estimated at upwards of $2,000 per month. Reports estimate that the number of people in the United States with Alzheimer's is almost 5,000,000 with almost 200,000 dying of the disease annually. Taken with the expectation that the population of those sixty-five and over is expected to grow by 70% over the next twenty-five years, there is good reason to be concerned.

"Treatment of the disease thus far has been limited to supportive care and elimination of the behavioral symptoms. Because there is not a clear definition of the disease there hasn't been any clearly definable headway made in finding a cure.

"As I mentioned earlier there is evidence suggesting that lower levels of neurochemicals result from degenerating neurons. This enzyme deficiency translates into decreased levels of the neurochemical acetylcholine at the nerve synapse. One of the areas that James researched was to treat Alzheimer's by augmenting synaptic acetylcholine.

"Additional work has been done on the oxidation of brain cells. Some believe that, over time, the body's protection against oxidation leads to aging. Researchers at the University of California at Berkeley have estimated that the DNA in each human cell is exposed to some 10,000 oxidative hits every day. This bombardment over time irreversibly damages the cell and interferes with the accuracy or amount of proteins produced by the cell. Cells can also be starved for energy by damaging the mitochondria DNA which is particularly prone to oxidation. Mitochondria are the intracellular power plants that provide cells with critically needed energy.

"According to Douglas C. Wallace of the Emory University School of Medicine, it appears likely that a significant number of mitochondrial DNA molecules may be defective in elderly people. He also speculated the onset of Alzheimer's could be related to mitochondrial failure.

"Much of the research that was accomplished in the early nineties has made great strides in our understanding of Alzheimer's and the total degenerative affect that it has on the brain. Indiana University research in 1992 found that a mutated gene on chromosome 21 causes brain cells to produce an overabundance of part of the amyloid precursor protein, or APP. Too much of the APP component can lead to a buildup of starchy deposits in the brain. These deposits are found in Alzheimer's patients and hamper brain function.

"In 1993, UCLA found that a protein on the surface of key memory cells kills the cells unless a brain hormone called nerve growth factor, or NGF, is locked into the protein through an NGF receptor called p75. They found that p75 is in the exact same cells that are the most severely affected and earliest to die in Alzheimer's disease."

"Allen," J.P. interrupted, "you are getting a little too involved. Let's get into JPC138."

"Your timing is perfect J.P.," Allen said as he pushed a key and the screen dissolved into the title, JPC138.

"JPC138 is unique and we feel it is no less than the beginning of a new class of pharmaceuticals.

"We began to study mitochondria DNA. Mitochondria DNA contains its own snippet of DNA, which bears instructions for the manufacture of thirteen proteins needed for energy generation. If mitochondria DNA slowly became partially defective, the defects could result in production of damaged mitochondria proteins or in the elimination of such proteins. Researchers have identified specific deletions in stretches of mitochondria DNA in aged brains.

"We found that DNA mutations occur within the gene that gives rise to the betaamyloid protein. APP constitutes the plaque that coats memory cells and is thought to be the precursor to Alzheimer's because it causes a degrading of the communication across the synapse. It is our contention that a mutated mitochondria DNA stimulates the formation of APP. The mutation being caused by high levels of oxidation hits.

"JPC138 has two actions. First, it works to repair the mutated mitochondria DNA so that it will cease stimulating the production of APP and secondly it supplies NGF or neurochemicals to help communications over the synapse. This floods of the memory cells with NGF and allows the regeneration of dendrite connections.

"As you know, we are currently in Phase I clinicals with JPC138 to determine safety and dosage. These studies are being carried out at two of the Geriatric Specialty Hospital chain facilities. One such hospital is here in New York near Albany and the second is near Boise, Idaho. The studies have just begun, so we only have preliminary results, which, by the way, are very encouraging."

"Allen, how will the Lifeal side effect of hyperactivity affect the JPC138 studies?

"J.P., you have brought up a very good point. We initially started investigating Alstonia spectabilis or Devil Tree for Alzheimer's because of its expected action on the memory cells of the brain. During toxicology and pathology studies of new compounds we ran the compounds through sophisticated screens to determine if they have pharmacological actions that could be developed for treatments of additional disease entities. During the Alzheimer's screening of Lifeal we caught a mental behavioral change with the

Alstonia spectabilis component when it was injected into rats. This discovery led to further evaluations and resulted in JPC138.

After the Ralph Vandermere incident, it seems that even Lifeal can result in mental stimulation in some overly sensitive patients. After Peggy finishes her studies we will have to examine Lifeal side effects again. I think that Ralph's condition was unique. As we all know, in the chaos theory, there will always be an exception."

"Why haven't I heard much about JPC138 in the press or in scientific publications?"

"J.P., there is no use in fooling ourselves, we have made a mess of Lifeal. Phillip has tried to keep JPC138 a secret for as long as possible in order to keep the hype down. It will be a long time until JPC138 is routinely used in the marketplace, unless the clinicals demonstrate dramatic results. If this happens, JPC138 might fall under the FDA regulations that allow companies to provide experimental drugs to patients enrolled in special treatment programs before the FDA has enough safety and efficacy data to clear the product for marketing. Phillip's strategy is to keep JPC138 under wraps until we are sure of the products pharmacological and clinical efficacy."

"Allen, just what is JPC138?"

"JPC138 is the alkaloid of the bark of the Devil Tree, known most widely as Alstonia scholaris, but in this particular instance, a species known as Alstonia spectabilis. We alter the alkaloid. The DNA string is changed so the pharmacological action is altered from its natural state and the state in which it is used in Lifeal. For a very complex biogenetic reason, the altered DNA product acts on the mitochondria DNA as a repairing mechanism. JPC138 does not prevent oxidation hits on the mitochondria so it does not prevent cells from coming under oxidized attacks. At some point the mitochondria DNA becomes mutated enough through oxidation to increase the protein APP and that's when JPC138 acts.

"Have you had any problems with the development of JPC138?"

"Our major problem is reproducibility. As you can imagine Alstonia spectabilis bark is not a pure compound. Our distillation process does not yield a consistent percentage of purity. It varies by as much as 20% from lot to lot. This is not of concern to us now, but it will be a major financial issue when we have to make large amounts of JPC138. Currently it takes twenty Devil Trees for a years patient supply. Not only is this expensive, but our Alstonia spectabilis plantation in Indonesia has a finite number of the trees. The twenty-to-one patient ratio is entirely related to the yield issue. One thing that we're currently looking at is that the basic difference between Alstonia scholaris and Alstonia spectabilis is an additional crystalline alkaloid called Alstonamine. The fact there is a much larger abundance of the species Alstonia scholaris has us looking into the possibility of somehow replicating Alstonamine in a form as pure or better than what we currently harvest. At any rate, I am certain we will find a way to improve our process. We will have a few years to work on the problem as JPC138 proceeds through its approval process."

J.P. didn't feel it necessary to discuss the potential Devil Tree supply problems with Allen at this point. It would not help his development work. This reproducibility problem did make the Devil Tree supply problem even more urgent to James.

"Allen, your presentation was excellent. At the present time I don't have any other questions, but maybe later. If you receive additional information on the JPC138 clinical studies, please share them with me."

"Thank you, J.P. Yes, most definitely. I will provide you with any additional data that I receive."

"Also, Allen, please keep me informed on Peggy's experiments. Thanks again, Allen. I will tell Helmut of the great job you did in presenting." J.P. then left the conference room and went back into his office to work.

3:00 P.M., THURSDAY, FEBRUARY 9

SPECTRUM OF MEDICINE BUILDING
NEW YORK CITY

Peggy worked hard on Lifeal's new side effect of hyperactivity. She pored over the six complaints at least ten times ensuring that she had gleaned everything she could from the report. She developed a set of specific questions for the physicians who had sent in the complaints. She then had called each of the physicians and talked to them about their complaint and their patient's current status. She learned nothing new.

She was driven to find out what had caused Ralph Vandermere to go to the extreme of trying to kill Phillip. She kept changing the dosages on the research primates, trying to duplicate the side effect. Today she had reached a primate dosage equal to ten tablets per day for a human. The most Ralph Vandermere had taken in a day was five. She was now double the dosage and still no side effect. He must have been overly sensitive she thought to herself. She decided she would keep ten primates on the high dose of 10 tablets a day and five additional primates on a placebo as a control. In two weeks she would take half of the ten off Lifeal and see how they went through withdrawal.

8:00 P.M., THURSDAY, FEBRUARY 9
THE JAMES FARM, GREYSTONE HALL
SEAFORD, NY

"How is the outsider J.P. doing?" she asked.

"He is a crony of Bradsmith. To answer your question, he is harmless," he answered.

"I don't like him hanging around."

"I tell you he is just a marketeer who doesn't matter."

"Perhaps it was lucky that he was here to take over," she mused. "If he is harmless then we might not have to change our plans." She paused and then continued. They were in her large California king-sized bed lying together under a heavy comforter.

"Have they found out any additional information on the nut who shot Bradsmith?" she asked.

"No," he replied.

Her head was on the left side of his chest and her right hand was massaging his overweight stomach. Her hand traced over the ridge of his stomach into his pubic hair where she started scratching the base of his penis. He aroused a little. It was work to get him up, but it had to be done.

"Did Lifeal really destroy this Mr. Vandermere's life?" she asked in a low seductive voice.

"He misused the product, but the publicity could hurt," he answered taking a deep breath as her hand began to massage the length of his growing penis. He continued speaking in short statements as he became more aroused. He continued, "Will this" he paused and took a deep breath, "change our plans? Or shall," breath "we continue?" He roughly yanked her head up to his so that their lips could meet in a very rough, short kiss.

"Have you heard from the NPC?" She had pulled her mouth from his and whispered in his right ear. She noted that her breathing in his ear following the kiss had finally brought him to a full erection, which was not much, but it was enough all things considered. She liked older men. She had always liked older men. Older men allowed her to make love on top. She slid over to straddle his erection. She hardly felt it penetrate her body. The only way she could achieve a climax with him was by rubbing herself. He was so fat she could never feel him inside her unless they were doggy style. But, then again she hated doggy style. She felt that she was placed in a subservient role in that position and she refused to place herself in a subservient role for anyone.

She knew conversation was now hopeless as she rocked back and forth and up and down. His breath was coming out as deep guttural moans. Her breath was steady as she continued to rub herself more aggressively. He reached up and grabbed her breasts. This was telling her he was about to climax. He could not pull her down to him because the size of his stomach would pull her off his erection. He quivered and she felt a slight warming inside her thighs and his hands came off her breasts. She rubbed herself harder and visualized lost lovers and came in a tremendous climax. A smile came to his face as he falsely concluded that it was his lovemaking abilities that had made her climax. She rationalized that the charade was all right as long as he did her bidding outside of the bedroom.

She leaned backwards and his, now limp, stub plopped out. She shuddered again. She was so lucky that she could bring herself to such great orgasms. She looked up his massive hairy body with its shriveled little cock and balls and felt a gag rising in her throat.

"Was it good for you?" He had taken her gag as a sound of affection.

"It was great, lover," she answered hating it when he or anyone asked her whether it was good. She wanted to answer the question a different way. She wanted to say, "Yes, it was good because my hand and imagination made it good you hairy micro-dicked man" She smiled. He took the smile as reward for a good lovemaking session.

She rolled to one side making sure she located the wet spot under his large ass. This was another advantage for being the one on top.

She finally answered the question he had asked before he had become aroused. "No, this will not change our plans." Then she repeated her last question. "Have you heard from the NPC?"

"No" he did not expand on his answer. He was getting sleepy and did not want to talk business.

"Well contact them again," her voice now had a sharp edge. The lovemaking session was over. It was time for business.

"We must have patience. The Japanese do not move very fast." He answered his breathing had returned to normal.

"We don't have time for patience. Do something immediately to get an answer."

"Yes, of course," he replied and then promptly fell asleep.

She knew he would do something about the NPC tomorrow. He was a good puppet. She looked over at his hulk. Again a gag began to rise in her throat. She decided she had to stop him from staying overnight. She turned on to her side facing away from him. In a while he would start to snore. She hoped that she would be asleep before then, but chances were, she would still be awake.

As she lay awake, she listened to the sound of the winter wind blowing off of the Atlantic Ocean and tried to remember happier days. She thought she could hear the sound of the pounding surf on Jones Beach. By the time the wind leaped the sand dunes and traveled across South Oyster Bay it lost most of its ferocity. She could hear the winds musical sound as it pushed its way up the fingers and canals of Oyster Bay and whipped around the new and old homes, piers, and boats which surrounded the low lands. The wind was very cold having lost temperature from blowing over frozen brackish waters. The musical sound was pleasant to her ears. Tears came to her eyes as she remembered Doc and the happy times they had here in their old farmhouse. Tears rolled over and around her nose and down her cheeks onto the blue sheets leaving wet spots that grew as she cried. She was also experiencing anguish when she thought of how she had violated their secret place with this thing that now laid beside her.

She loved the old farm. When she had married Doc she had prejudged his reasons for hanging onto this old Long Island potato farm. She remembered chastising him and, at first, even refusing to visit the farm. It was five years before she made the two-hour trip from their Manhattan apartment to Seaford, Long Island. In the first years of marriage their winter weekends were spent in the city at the theater, Lincoln Center, or Carnegie Hall. If they left the city it was to ski or vacation in the Caribbean. They spent their summers in their Nantucket home. They never went to the old James family home in Seaford, but Doc used to go on his own to think and fish. She knew it was an excuse to be alone and perhaps to get away from her strong and demanding personality. She hadn't cared when he left on his weekend trips. She continued to go to the theater with her social friends.

One day, on a whim, she asked Doc if she could go with him to the farm. Doc had been both pleased and surprised. He had given up asking her to go with him. He did not immediately answer her request. He had looked forward to his time alone and his conversations with the locals. It was his chance to talk to childhood friends and not try to be the young robust husband of the beautiful Evelyn Preston-^James.

She remembered interpreting his pause as a rejection. She had almost burst out in anger and demanded to go with him when he gently replied, "Of course dear, you can go with me. I would like to leave within the hour so we will miss the rush hour traffic. He always left on Thursday afternoon and returned on Monday morning.

When she remembered back to that day long ago, she still did not know why she wanted to go to the farm. In retrospect she surmised the only reason had been her desire to invade Doc's privacy. She had been angry with Doc because she had wanted to go to Florida that weekend and he had turned her down by saying that his work at James prevented him from leaving New York City. She had known that if he had time to go to that damn old farm he had time to take her to Florida.

They made the trip to the farm in the corporate limo. She remembered that time dragged during the drive and the view of the bleak Long Island winter landscape depressed her. More than once she almost asked Doc to drop her off and she would take a cab back to her world in the city, but she was too stubborn. That was eight years ago. Now, just like Doc she looked forward to weekends at the farm. She kept up Doc's practice of making the trip on Thursdays and staying until Monday. When she wanted to go into the city she did not take a limo, she took the corporate helo from Farmingdale's Republic Airport to the top of the Spectrum of Medicine building.

Over the years she had fixed up the inside of the farmhouse and Doc and she had grown to love to be alone together without the hassles of the city. Even though the inside was now a modern country home with all of the modern conveniences, they hadn't touched the outside. The farm still looked like an old weathered house.

Doc's grandfather had built the house in the mid-1800's when he had made enough money to move out of the German section of Brooklyn. He wanted to relive the same feelings he had left behind in Germany. Doc's great grandfather lived near Bremerhaven on the Baltic Sea. He had harvested potatoes and fished for food. The Seaford house was constructed in an Lshape. The long side of the house faced the canal that came off of South Oyster Bay. They had built a deck almost to the edge of the water. Stairs led down to the wooden walls of the pier where Doc's fishing boat was tied up. She now used his boat in the summer, but she never learned how to fish. She just slowly toured the bay, never venturing out into the Atlantic. She did not bother to have the boat removed from the water in winter. The water aroundthe boat was isolated through a series of pumps that kept the water moving so it would not freeze. The back of the house faced away from the ocean. The garage was a converted potato shed. A gravel driveway led to the block long street named John's Court just off Merrick Road in Seaford.

Seaford was one of many small towns which lined the south shore of Long Island. It was famous for the Tackapausha Preserve. A Nassau County tract of land around Seaford Creek that over time had expanded to eighty acres.

The land in this area had been called Arrasquaugh by the Massapequa Indians. The Massapequa Indians inhabited the south shore of Long Island in the 17th Century. When the preserve expanded in 1938 the Tackapausha name was adopted in memory of the chief of the Massapequa Indians.

The receding glacier of the Wisconsin stage of the Pleistocene Epoch over 15,000 years ago had a great affect on what would eventually become the James farm. The receding glacier deposited rock debris on top of the ancient metamorphic bedrock that formed the foundation of Long Island, Manhattan, and the Bronx. This soil combination plus Cretaceous sediments of sand, clay, and gravel made for very good potato crops. Until high-density population destroyed the agriculture of Long Island, the potato crops were one of the major incomes to the residents.

The tears had dried from her face, but not the sheet. Her body and thoughts of Doc gradually succumbed to sleep. Her last thoughts for this evening were troubled. They were a mixture of getting rid of her lover and happier days with Doc, sitting on their deck and sharing a raw potato from the small garden in back of their home.

7:00 A.M., FRIDAY, FEBRUARY 10

THE JAMES FARM, GREYSTONE HALL
SEAFORD, NY

The next morning he wrote a short e-mail to the NPC to be sent from the farmhouse. Before sending the communication, he opened an encryption program that would scramble the message.

He then pressed the send key.

7:00 a.m., February 10 TO: NPC

FROM: James Contact SUBJ.: Business Agreement

I have not heard from you.

I must know immediately whether you are interested in James.

If no answer by February 17, then I must seek an alternative arrangement.

He had to leave immediately. She did not like for him to be in the house when she awoke. He decided there was time for a cup of coffee. He was pouring a cup of coffee when the computer signaled the receipt of an incoming email message.

2400, February 10

TO: JAMES CONTACT FROM: NPC

SUBJ.: BUSINESS AGREEMENT RE: Your e-mail 0700, February 10

NPC interested in hearing proposal.

You will be contacted by a Mr. L. Wolf, please disclose business proposal to him.

"That was a fast response," he commented to himself. Almost too fast considering that it was late Friday night in Japan. He debated whether he should wake her to tell her the new information or just leave her a note.

She had wanted action and he had gotten her action. Perhaps she would grant a little love reward for his efforts. His groin stirred. Yes, he would tell her himself. He printed the email and walked back to her bedroom.

She heard the bedroom door open and looked at the night stand clock 7:10. "What the fuck!" She thought. "He is never to come back in the bedroom after he leaves in the morning. I have warned him."

She bolted up in bed. Her sudden movement scared him and took the breath from his lungs. He stepped back, with a slight case of hyperventilation.

Her voice came to him from the darkness of the room like a verbal bull whip stinging him across his face.

"You asshole. I told you. Never, never are you supposed to creep back into my bedroom once you have left. Who do you think you are, you fat bastard."

"But, but.," he stammered. She was sitting upright, her breasts bouncing as she screamed at him. He was shocked into silence. She had never said words like this to him. His hand reached for the doorknob to steady himself. His right hand surrounded the cold brass surface.

"Don't give me any of your but, buts, old man. Get the fuck out of my house and do it now."

He turned and started to turn to leave. He tried to speak again and managed to mumble in a barely audio level, "But, I have heard from NPC."

The screaming stopped. There was a stillness, broken only by sounds of two people breathing heavily. One in anger and the other in fear. The silence lasted minutes. Finally, from the bed she spoke in a calm, quiet voice.

"What did they say?" she asked.

"They are interested," he answered opening the door and preparing to leave the room.

"What do we do next?" she asked.

"Wait for a Mr. L. Wolf to contact me at the voice mail number."
"Good. When?"

"They did not say," he was now part way out the door.

In almost a whisper she said, "Keep me informed." Then, in a scream "Get out."

He left the room and closed the door softly behind him. He leaned against the doorframe, breathing deeply. He quickly left the farm and drove himself home.

SPECTRUM OF MEDICINE BUILDING
NEW YORK CITY

J.P. picked up the telephone and dialed Mandi's private office extension. "Good morning, beautiful. How are you this morning?" he said as she picked up her phone.

"Oh I'm fine, J.P. and you?"

"Well, I was hoping that we could make up our lost ski weekend this weekend. In fact, I was planning to call north this morning until I saw the stacks of paper on Phillip's desk. Janet had worked late last night and caught up on Phillip's paperwork and piled it high on the desk for my action. Between the paperwork and my continued studies on JPC138, I have decided that probably this weekend is out."

"Out, J.P.?" The disappointment in her voice was very evident.

"Out only in terms of a ski trip to New England. Not out for an evening in the city. Do you have any suggestions?" He asked casually.

"As a matter of fact, I do." Mandi replied with emphasis. "I read the Times last night and saw that the Warsaw Philharmonic Orchestra will be performing at Lincoln Center tomorrow night and playing, guess what my friend?"

"Something by Prokofiev," he replied confidently.

"How did you know?" Disappointment again in her voice.

"Elementary, my dear Watson. You know my favorite composer is Prokofiev. If it were anyone else, you probably wouldn't have asked me to guess. You would likely have just told me. Right?"

"Right you are, Sherlock, but sometimes you should just let me have fun and not be so damned smart," Mandi replied seriously.

He paused, thinking that there was a hidden meaning in her answer. He decided to let it go by, "I am sorry Mandi. What is the program? It sounds like you have a great idea."

"Thank you, sir. I think the concert would be fun if we can get tickets. Witold Rowicki is directing Prokofiev's Piano Concerto

Number 5 and Rachmaniov's Piano Concerto Number 2, both for piano and orchestra."

"Who is the pianist?"

"Sviatoslav Richter. Do you want to go?"

"You bet. As far as the tickets are concerned I'll take care of finding us some good tickets. Do you want to come over tonight?"

"I wish I could J.P., but I have chores to do at home. How about getting Roberto to pick me up at Penn Station at the same time as before? We can take a walk and talk about James." There was a slight humor in the tone of her voice.

"No problem, except for the talking about James bit. I think I can clear my desk by 3:00 today. How about you, Brian, and I getting together for some strategic planning?"

"Great idea, I'll be there. See you at three," Mandi replied happily and hung up the phone.

J.P. replaced the telephone in its cradle and looked at the neatly stacked piles of paper. He leaned back in the chair and raised his arms locking his hands behind his head. He twisted the chair to the left and used his feet to move it towards the window.

At the window he placed his feet on the windowsill and stared out at the murky day. He could barely see the Hudson. The old luxury liner terminal buildings reached out into the river and disappeared into the fog. It occurred to him that Helmut really had the right idea about the future. It is difficult to see the future, but someone had to take a guess. J.P. felt that he was always the person taking the risk and trying to see where events would take the passengers on his ship before it ever left the pier.

He began to reflect on the part of business that he despised, paperwork. Paperwork...now that was the downside of business. For some unexplained reason, paper communications had to keep flowing. It was like a gigantic chain letter. And we were supposed to be in a paperless era. He realized that the paperwork could not be ignored. It never went away. "Oh well," he told himself, "might as well get at it."

He swung the chair back around and scooted to the desk and took the top report off the first pile.

Before he was aware of the passing time, there was a knock at the door and Janet entered the office.

"Did I give you enough work, J.P.?" She asked laughing.

"You know, for an executive assistant you can be awfully sadistic. Can't some of this stuff wait until Phillip returns?" He replied in frustration and got up from behind the desk. "What time is it?"

"What? Are you so buried in paper that you forget how to look at a clock?"

"Yeah, something like that."

"It's almost noon. Are you eating in?" Janet asked.

"Eating in, please. Please order me a corn beef on rye and an ice tea," he answered.

"Do you want me to call Phillip for you?"

"No, I can do it myself. In fact I think I will call him now. He should be awake."

Janet turned to leave the room. "Oh, Janet, I hope this is the last of the paperwork for this week. You haven't generated more, have you?" he pleaded.

"Well," she said smiling. "There was a new supply with the morning mail, but it can wait until Monday."

"Thank you Janet. Another couple of things, I have scheduled a meeting with Mandi and Brian for three this afternoon. Would you please call Brian and ask him to join us. Also would you see if you could purchase two tickets for the Lincoln Center Saturday night concert. Call a ticket agency and pay whatever is necessary to get seats in the middle orchestra section. Thank you again."

Janet left the room and J.P. picked up the telephone and dialed Phillip's hospital room.

A tired and slightly gravelly voice answered, "Hello." "Phillip?" "This is Phillip. J.P.?"

"Yes, Phillip. How are you doing?"

"I am doing better than my voice sounds. Damn oxygen. I breath oxygen for about three hours a day and it makes my mouth very dry and my voice crackle. How are things at James?"

"Phillip, the paperwork is mounting. You have to get back here before I go mad. I now know of another reason why I left the large corporate world. Did the physicians brief you on your injury?"

"Yes J.P. The bullet missed my heart by just a few millimeters. Good old Ralph almost checked me out. Two ribs are broken and my heart cavity is badly bruised. All that said, they said I could be off the disabled list in a few weeks. Can you last that long?" he went on without waiting for an answer. "I can get Brian to stand in if you want to step down."

"Nope. I can handle it for another few weeks. Anything you want me to do or subjects you want to be briefed on?"

"How about Ralph's side effect. Any answers?"

"Nothing so far, Phillip. If anything comes out of Peggy's studies I'll let you know."

"Thank you, J.P. And I do mean thank you. I'm sorry to have gotten you into this mess. I never thought my early morning call to you last month would end up with me in the hospital and you in my chair. Thanks."

"No need to thank me, Phillip. It's my pleasure to help out. I'm sure everything will turn out all right. The good news is that Mrs. Preston^-James has left me alone. Let's hope her silence continues. This afternoon I'm meeting with Mandi and Brian to discuss strategy. If anything significant comes out of that meeting, I'll give you another call. Otherwise, hang in there. I will visit you over the weekend. Now you can get back on your oxygen high."

"Thanks J.P...," and they hung up.

3:00 P.M., FRIDAY, FEBRUARY 10

<h1 style="text-align:center">SPECTRUM OF MEDICINE BUILDING
NEW YORK CITY</h1>

Mandi and Brian were on time for the scheduled 3 PM strategy meeting. Since there was only the three of them, they worked at the smaller conference table in Phillip's office.

"Thanks for joining me this afternoon, guys. I don't think this will be a long meeting, but I thought we should at least touch base before the weekend. Why don't we start with you Brian. Do you have anything to report?"

"Not much J.P. After Phillip's shooting everything else has taken a back seat. I have been watching the stock market and it seems that our proactive strategy with Jack Husted and other public relations contacts has enabled us to prevent a share sell off. Just in case, I was prepared to have the NYSE suspend trading on our stock, but no such action had to be taken.

"Otherwise, I have nothing new to report on the 21st Century Plan or any unusual board activity. Sorry, J.P., there's just not much happening on my front."

J.P. looked away from Brian, "Mandi?"

"Well, we sent out the two letters on Thursday. It is too early for any reaction from the medical community. We, by the way, we do not expect any unusual negative reaction. The marketplace is used to exceptions to package inserts. Physicians pay attention to the warnings, but the profession doesn't generally make radical changes in habits based on a single incident. We expect the new prescriptions to drop slightly, but rebound over time." She paused uncertain whether she should continue.

Mandi decided to continue as Brian and J.P. waited to see what she had to add. Mandi looked at both of them and then spoke in a slightly lower voice. "I don't wish to sound like a cry baby and I don't really even know whether this is important to add, but you are both my friends, so here goes. This situation certainly does not help our already serious Lifeal sales condition. I don't want sympathy, only understanding that the Lifeal forecast from a marketing standpoint is no longer realistic and will have to be reduced again. This will not help our position with the board and Mrs. James. This will probably make our defensive position even harder. I have a question for both of you to consider. Is there anything I should be doing at this point to push Lifeal?"

J.P. knew immediately that Mandi wasn't whining, she was asking for help. He knew this took a great deal of guts, but it really was Mandi's way of conducting business. She was not afraid to ask for help. She knew success came from many directions and if a manager didn't ask for assistance, none would be forthcoming.

"Mandi, of course, I'm not a marketing person," replied Brian, "but I do have a suggestion.

Both Mandi and J.P. looked at Brian and then back at one another.

"I know, I know, you two are the marketing gurus and the silent bean counter should keep his mouth shut and let you two solve all of the world's marketing problems," he said trying to keep his voice light, but his bruised ego came through in the tone of his voice.

"Please, Brian, we're just kidding you. You know I've always appreciated your input. What do you think we should do about Lifeal?" responded Mandi.

"Thanks Mandi. It is probably not important, but as you said Mandi, here goes," Brian paused to gather his thoughts. "I would like to suggest two actions. First, I would delay the introduction of the new 50mg tablet. This is a larger dose and we don't know exactly why Ralph Vandermere did what he did, but we do know that in some way it was dosage related. If we release a higher dosage, it could be interpreted that we are blatantly ignoring a sign that there might be a problem with high dosages of Lifeal."

Mandi jumped in, "That is an excellent observation, Brian. I have to admit my thought process was occupied by the problem and I hadn't even considered the ramifications of the new dosage. On the other hand, we are depending on the automatic shipment sales. What do we do about our budget problem? If we do not release the automatic shipment then we will have to cut our budgets again. It's possible that we may never be able to dig ourselves out of our financial quagmire."

"Mandi, let me give my second point and then I'll address the budget situation." Brian interjected trying not to discount the validity of Mandi's comment.

"My second point is pure marketing. I think we should hold some national seminars on cardiac arrhythmia and Lifeal. We would have a panel of cardiologists, pharmacologists, and pharmacists. It could be billed as a medical team. Not only would they discuss the subject matter, but take questions from patients. Yes, and before you mention it, this will cost us more marketing money and it is not budgeted. But, what do you think about the ideas?"

Mandi's eyes warmed, but she did not immediately answer Brian's question. J.P. thought that she might be trying to find a way to tell Brian his idea was great without losing face. She finally answered. Her voice was sincere. "Brian, I think your idea is brilliant." Mandi turned and looked at J.P. "Don't you, J.P.?"

"Brian, I agree with Mandi. Your ideas are right on. In the future you shouldn't hold back your marketing ideas. I am interested in how we are going to pay for your ideas, but I must say it is refreshing to put the person with the purse strings on the hot seat about where we'll find the money for a marketing program."

"J.P., you have probably hit on the reason financial people do not offer their ideas. They don't want to get caught in the middle. Anyway these two ideas are probably the extent of my marketing creativity."

"Yeah, well, I doubt that. Now, assuming we can implement the program, how about the finances."

"Well, since I'm not a marketing person I don't know how much money you will require, but I do know how we can get started."

Brian got up and walked over to the eraser board and began to write. "Basically we can move to the monies that were allocated to promoting the 50mg tablet into the new program. The following areas have 50mg tablet budget money that can be reallocated." Marketing Budget Promotion Manufacturing Raw Material Glassware & packaging Labor and Distribution Production Overhead

"I know that eventually money will have to be spent on the 50mg tablet release, but not now. Joe works on just-in-time inventory and flex labor. We have not purchased the materials required to make, package, and distribute the 50mg tablet. We will tell our vendors that we have had a delay in the release. They won't like it, but they will understand. What additional funds we will require will have to be taken from other budgets.

"As far as the loss of sales revenue from the delay in the automatic shipment of the 50mg tablet, I don't have a good answer. We'll have to bite the bullet and take the revenue hit. Sales will look bad when compared to last year and to plan, but we all know they aren't sales generated from demand. What do you think, J.P.?"

"I agree, Brian. We take the hit. You know how I hate the automatic shipment trap. If 50mg is a viable dosage we can encourage multiple tablets. I know this is a wild idea, but we could develop a new pricing structure based on the dosage. Since this idea is off the top of my head, I am certain that there are pitfalls. Let's just say that somehow we know the physician wants to prescribe the 50mg dosage. We then provide the current dose tablet at the 50mg price. This will help us in the long run because we don't have to add another product to the line and there is something else." J.P. paused.

"I have discussed this in some detail with Mandi, but I haven't told you, Brian, about a problem area that I've recently uncovered. I have put a number of factors together and come up with this potential problem that could potentially be devastating."

"What problem, J.P.?" asked Brian with concern in his voice.

"I think James, as a company, has not identified the potential raw material supply problem with Lifeal and JPC138. The raw material is from an Indonesian tree commonly called Devil Tree, or Alstonia spectabilis," he said.

Brian responded, "Joe has repeatedly assured me that we do not have a raw material problem."

"I don't think anyone has added together the total quantity of raw material needed for ongoing Lifeal requirements, the now delayed 50mg tablet, and the eventual needs for JPC138. These requirements will not be as bad now, since we have delayed the 50mg tablet, but there are a few other factors that I do not think Joe or James Pharmaceutical are aware of or have considered.

J.P. went into a detailed discussion of the potential problems with obtaining the needed bark from the sole source in Indonesia, covering much of the same ground that he had with Mandi. He ended by outlining his meeting with Allen Strong the day before and Allen's belief that it might be possible to replicate the extra crystalline alkaloid found in the bark of the Devil Trees in Indonesia.

"And beyond the problems that would keep any botanist awake at night, there is our agreement with the plantation owner on the island of Java. The contract is basically a handshake between Doc James and Mr. Chang. Doc is dead and Mr. Chang is very old."

"J.P., please pardon the pun, but I think you have unearthed a devil of a problem," quipped Brian.

"Why is it that I don't feel like laughing?" Mandi dryly remarked with the start of a smile curling the corner of her lips.

"It's okay, Brian. A joke was called for even though we all know the problem could become serious. I say could become serious because we still have time to react now that we have identified the potential problem. Your idea to postpone the 50mg tablet is good for the reason you mentioned, Brian, and also for our supply of Devil Tree bark. Don't ask me why, but for some strategic reason I would like to keep the raw material supply problem just between us for a little while. Is that okay with both of you?"

Both Mandi and Brian nodded their heads in the affirmative.

"Good. Now, my status report. It is not very long and I will go fast by hitting just the high spots. I talked to Phillip and he is better. I think he'll be back in a week or two. I have no new information on the 21st Century Plan. This week in R&D was very rewarding. I think, except for the raw material problem, James possibly has a real winner in JPC138. Allen is a real sharp researcher and I think he has come up with something that will be a major breakthrough in the cure of Alzheimer's Disease.

"Next week we will have to start preparing for the February board meeting and firming up our strategy to help Phillip. That's it, is there anything either of you want to cover that we have not discussed?" Both Mandi and Brian shook their heads no. "Okay, meeting is officially adjourned."

They all got up and walked to the door. Mandi lagged behind and J.P. was able to whisper in her ear that tomorrow Roberto would pick her up at the Penn Station and Janet had purchased great seats for the concert.

9:00 A.M., MONDAY, FEBRUARY 13

SPECTRUM OF MEDICINE BUILDING
NEW YORK CITY

J.P. had spent the morning going through an entirely new stack of paperwork that Janet had placed on his desk. As he worked his way down through the paper, he kept catching himself daydreaming about his weekend with Mandi.

They had a great Saturday and Sunday together. The newness of the relationship didn't seem to be wearing off. J.P. had worried about working so closely together and maintaining a personal relationship. Thus far they had both been able to keep separate their work from their personal lives. The past weekend was no exception. J.P. couldn't recall talking about James once in the thirty-six hours that they had been together. Roberto was, as usual the best chauffeur and made getting from one place to another quick and easy, a difficult thing to achieve on a winter's night in New York City.

He thought about their relationship and what affect it had on the job he had to do for Phillip. The fact that Mandi and he were "good friends" had reached probably every department in the company. He decided that he and Mandi shouldn't try to keep it a secret any longer, but let the situation evolve. Assuming of course that Mandi agreed.

He stood up from the desk and walked to the window and looked east down the Hudson River. It was a clear day and he wished things were as clear at James. He thought to himself, "The president is in the hospital recovering from a bullet wound inflicted by a man gone crazy from an unknown side effect caused by our top product. The major revenue producing product, and the future of the

383

company has had its long range strategic plan stolen by unknown persons and is in jeopardy of going under because of actions caused by a hostile board of directors. Jesus, Phillip, what the hell have you gotten me into? I am sure that when you called me last month you had no idea that things would be as they are today. What you need is the National Guard, not me."

J.P. turned his gaze to the Wachtung Mountains and noted dark clouds building up beyond the rounded peaks of these old mountains. He suddenly wished he were back in Mammoth, sitting in Annie's drinking a beer after a long day on the slopes.

The New York City weather report was not good and J.P. hoped that they weren't in for another big storm. The city was still recovering from the last storm. The countryside was still covered with snow. The temperatures had stayed below freezing most of the time and the snow had been building in depth with small snow showers that blew in off the Great Lakes. He was growing increasingly weary of winter in the East and longed for California and Mammoth. At least when it snowed there it meant skiing and water for Southern California. Snow on New York City had no meaning to J.P. Then he remembered his picnic in Central Park with Mandi and concluded that there was a meaning for him after all.

He turned from the window and walked back to the pile of paperwork Janet had again stacked on Phillip's desk and began to prepare for the staff meeting and the week ahead.

9:00 P.M., MONDAY, FEBRUARY 13

JAL FLIGHT #060 OVER THE WESTERN PACIFIC OCEAN

Nacheda was on his way back to the United States for the February taskforce meeting. He was in high spirits. The time he had spent at Bandai Pharmaceuticals Company had been very invigorating and he hoped that this would be the last team meeting and that he would be able to pursue the ultimate goal that Dr. Nakasone had planned.

Nacheda pushed the seat recliner button and the first class chair reclined. The cabin lights had been turned off so that passengers could either watch the movie or sleep. He watched Reiko talking with passengers about whether they needed a pillow or blanket. He smiled as he watched her and realized that for the first time that he could remember, he was actually looking forward to flying.

Reiko had made an arrangement with one of the other flight attendants. She would have her break just as Nachedasan would be ready to go to sleep. She had also arranged to keep the seat next to him unoccupied so that she could sit next to him.

Nacheda thought back over the last two weeks. He had immersed himself completely in learning the Bandai process for producing a pure active ingredient. Reiko had tried to get him to come down to Tokyo the previous weekend or at least allow her to come up to Bandai. More than anything he had wanted to see her, but he simply couldn't spare the time. He had to understand the Bandai process enough so that, if and when necessary, he could discuss the process with knowledgeable researchers. He felt good about the process and knew that with the right product, it would be invaluable. Now all he had to do was find the right product.

On Friday Dr. Nakasone had invited him into his office. This visit was a great deal different than the one before last month's trip to Los Angeles. Nakasone was very cordial. The rice doors were slid back so that they could gaze out at the garden as they spoke. Nakasone mentioned that he had received favorable reports of Nacheda's progress during his two weeks in Bandai research. This compliment was very unusual and Nacheda was at first flustered, but then accepted his employer's remark with gratitude. Nakasone then abruptly ended the meeting by wishing Nacheda a successful trip to the United States. He added that he expected Nacheda to identify at least one target company though two would be preferable.

Nacheda assured Dr. Nakasone that his trip would be successful. They finished their tea and Nacheda had excused himself.

Nacheda had then taken the afternoon bullet train to Tokyo and by 7:00 he was knocking on Reiko's apartment door. Their evening together was even better than when they had been in Bandai. They had lost their selfconsciousness and loved freely as familiar lovers do. He quickly turned his thoughts to his planned activities after they landed in Los Angeles.

After a quick trip to the Westwood condo to drop off his luggage, he planned to spend some time with Reiko before meeting with Skip for their Monday evening briefing before the task force met on Tuesday morning. He was certain that Skip wouldn't mind his spending time with Reiko. Skip had kept him uptodate with daily emails except for the two weekends when he had been skiing in Mammoth. Nacheda made a mental note to find out why Skip had this sudden urge to be such an avid skier.

Nacheda had closed his eyes and was about to doze off when he felt a blanket being place over his body. He opened his eyes and saw Reiko leaning over him. Very professionally she asked, "Would you like a pillow, Nachedasan?" She smiled and her face lit up. Her white teeth contrasted her complexion. Her breath was as sweet as fresh mint. She leaned close to his ear and he could feel her warmth and smell her perfume. She whispered, "Or a shoulder to rest your head?"

"Yes, I would like a pillow" he replied out loud then whispered "I would prefer a warm body curled up next to mine."

Reiko, blushed as she thought of their lovemaking and anticipating their time together in Los Angeles.

"Stop it," she softly whispered not really wanting him to stop. "You started it," he replied with mock anger.

"I know." Reiko paused continuing her whisper, "In a couple of minutes I will be back for my nap. Then I will help you sleep."

"Your concern for my well being and the well being of your other passengers is very much appreciated," he replied with a smile on his face, but in the same tone as his previous statement.

In the darkness of the plane's cabin, Reiko could not at first see his smile. She hesitated thinking that for some reason he was mad at her. Then she saw his smile and knew he was just kidding.

"You must not kid me so, Nachedasan."

"I am sorry Reiko. I will be waiting for your nap."

Five minutes later Reiko sat in the aisle seat next to Nacheda and wrapped herself with her own blanket to keep warm in the chilly cabin. Their blankets overlapped and their hands clasped in the hidden folds. Both slept peacefully, Reiko for two hours and Nacheda for a comfortable five hours. It was the most comfortable flight he had ever experienced. When they landed, Nacheda was more rested than he had ever been after a trans-Pacific flight.

On the ground in Los Angeles, he said his goodbyes and confirmed that he would call her at the Century City Plaza Hotel. They could then arrange to meet.

Reiko had to take the shuttle bus to the hotel with the rest of the flight crew. JAL really frowned on crewmembers dating passengers especially in foreign countries.

Nacheda followed the same routine that he had followed on each of his trips to Los Angeles. His mind turned from Reiko to the Bandai task at hand. He became excited over the expectations that the task force was about to move from the discovery stage to the implementation stage. The emails from Skip were very encouraging. Skip had been entering the data from the other team members into the computer. Nacheda expected this meeting to be shorter than previous meetings.

"This meeting will be SAM's meeting." He smiled thinking of the computer identity that the unknown team member #8 had created. "Yes, SAM will run tomorrow's meeting," he said out loud as he guided his rental car along the San Diego freeway.

As was the case in the last five trips to Los Angeles, Nacheda did not see the tail that picked him up as he left the airport customs hall. It was odd that he did not see the Asian with the hat because hats, except for ball caps, were not a common sight in Los Angeles. But then, if Nacheda had noticed the person with the hat, he would probably have come to the conclusion that the person was a tourist. Tourists wore hats.

Skip met Nacheda at the door of the condo and they warmly shook hands. Nacheda was shaking hands with a tanner, leaner, and apparently more relaxed Skip.

"Skip, you look great. What have you been up to that has made you look like an American gladiator."

Skip bowed his head just a little in a mock Japanese embarrassment motion and then looked up again. "You should talk Nachedasan you are visibly glowing. I ask you the same question. What have you been up to?"

Both old friends burst into laughter and simultaneously said "Women" and laughed even harder.

"Skip, tell me your story."

"No, Nacheda, you are the guest, you go first." "Guest, hell, this is my condo. You first."

"I live here, you first." "Okay, Skip I give in."

Nacheda told Skip all about Reiko. Skip then told Nacheda about Annie. After they had told their stories they both agreed they would go skiing together as a foursome as soon as possible.

Nacheda then called Reiko and set up a 4:00 pickup time. Skip agreed that Nacheda should spend the time with Reiko. He fully understood. Their briefing could be completed prior to four o'clock and he, Nacheda, needed his rest to ward off jet lag. Nacheda didn't tell Skip that he had slept well on the plane.

Their meeting went well. It was for the most part as Nacheda had expected SAM's meeting. The information from the members had been entered into the computer. All that remained was to update the data with anything new the team would bring with them. Then they would wait for SAM to come to, what he or it, termed a macro conclusion.

At 3:30, Nacheda left to go pick up Reiko and Skip continued to prepare for Tuesday's meeting.

Nacheda's sudden departure from the building caught the man charged with tailing him off guard. This was the first time that Nacheda had left the condo the day before a team meeting. A few times he had left with the American, but never alone. This was most unusual.

The tail followed Nacheda from Westwood to Century City where he picked up a beautiful Japanese woman. The tail concluded that this was something new and should be reported. He noticed that they were very friendly. This was not a new acquaintance. He would have to take a picture of the woman and send it to his supervisor. After watching them kiss a few times in Nacheda's car, the tail also concluded that they acted as though they were lovers. He mentally noted that she might be ofsome help in the future should Nacheda not cooperate when the time came for cooperation.

7:00 A.M., TUESDAY, FEBRUARY 14

WESTWOOD, CALIFORNIA

Captain "Cap" McKennsey was the last member of the team to arrive for breakfast. The rest of the team was laughing and joking while drinking their second and third cups of coffee.

Mary Christian spoke up, "Hey, Cap, how is it that the person who lives the closest is always the last one to arrive?" Cap was about to reply when she waved him off and continued, "And don't give us that crap about LA traffic. That's my excuse."

"My dear, would you believe that I have been in surgery since midnight operating on a patient with a brain tumor?" He replied seriously silencing the group's laughter.

"No," Mary replied. The group broke into laughter again.

"Well now, you win the prize, Mary. I wasn't in surgery. I overslept," Cap replied having been caught in one of his traditional attempts to give himself an excuse.

The group as a whole noticed that Nacheda and Skip were more relaxed than usual. They all sensed that today would be the day that perhaps their work would be completed. This was both sad and fulfilling. At times, in the past, they had felt that this day might never come and that they would fail in achieving their objective. Now, it seemed they had pulled it out in the twelfth hour and snatched success from what most certainly would have been a failure.

At 8:00 they took their seats behind their respective consoles. Skip was the first to speak. There was no laughter now. Everyone was focused on the business at hand and awaited instructions from Skip.

"Okay team," Skip started, "today we have high expectations that this will be the day that, if we are successful, we complete the identification stage of our project." He paused. "Let me restate that if we achieve success we will enter into the implementation stage which may or may not involve all members of the team. We don't know what the future holds, but I for one, want to thank all of you for the cooperation you have given me in the coordination of this project. I realize that, at times, we wondered if we would succeed. Now, before we conclude the day, I want you to know that what we have done hasn't been done before and all of you should be very proud of yourselves. Nacheda, do you have anything to add?"

"Not at this time, Skip. I will give my concluding remarks at the end of the day."

"Okay," Skip announced, "does anyone have any additional information they want to input into the computer?"

All of the team members replied in the negative with the exception of John. He had new information to add. The others had downloaded their information before they had arrived in Westwood.

"John, please type in your new information," Skip instructed.

While John typed in the new information his deep voice filled the room as he summarized what he was typing. "Up to this point I have not been able to contribute very much, but now that we have a great deal of focused material to work with I have come up with some interesting information. I have tried to evaluate where all health-oriented associations have been investing their funds. I have found a young association called the Alzheimer's Foundation. It was founded in 1982, so it is not a very old association, as foundations go. They do not have a celebrity spokesperson, which seems to be what all health-oriented foundations feel they need. "The Alzheimer's

Foundation, or AZ Foundation as they like to be called, has been receiving their funding from the savings of older people plus a few young millionaires who have older parents suffering from Alzheimer's. These young millionaires have helped the AZ Foundation over the financial hump more than a couple of times.

"A few years ago a strategy that the AZ Foundation initiated back in 1982 started to come to fruition. In 1982 and still today, they encouraged wealthy people to provide for the AZ Foundation in their wills. Well, as time has gone by, more than a few of these wealthy folks have died. The AZ Foundation has the potential to be a multi-billion dollar foundation in the next five years.

"I found out that the foundation takes the donated money and invests it into promising research projects on Alzheimer's disease. I looked over the identified corporations from our last meeting and found that there was only one correlation. The Alzheimer's Foundation has invested into James Pharmaceutical Company of New York City. The investment in James was only $20 million, but still it was an investment. I could not find out why they invested, but there it is."

Skip hit the command key on his handset and John's report and data was added to the decision console computer. "Since there is no additional information we will allow SAM to lead us through today's meeting. Before I went to bed last night, I gave the computer instructions to analyze the data at 2200 last night. I think SAM has worked most of the night on the project."

Skip began to type commands into the artificial intelligence program of SAM. It took only one key command to initiate the macro command that would lead to full operation. The screens began to change with various colored designs and then cleared with SAM appearing on the large center video screen.

As the group looked at SAM they could see that he had changed. His alter ego, team member #8, had programmed SAM to look as though he had aged significantly and look very tired. SAM's voice echoed through the room. His computer-generated voice seemed a little lower than usual.

"Well, team you have had me working long and hard on your new material." He paused. His forehead had deep furrows and his hair had grayed just a little around the temples. He had some small crows feet around the corners of his eyes. He was very serious. Then he suddenly brightened. "But, I believe we have a lockin. With John's new material, I am at the 95percentile level. The other five-percent you will have to provide yourself using human judgment. To start with, I would like to summarize the January meeting and then provide you with my lockin conclusion."

The six video screens came alive and the final screens from the last meeting were shown. Terri's screen showed the five compounds highlighting in bright red, JPC138.

John's screen showed his new information on the AZ Foundation and their investment in James Pharmaceutical Company. It was highlighted in red.

Cap's screen showed the five side effects, which had been determined to be significant. Excessive mental alertness was highlighted.

Mary's screen showed the two medical literature search areas of the dormant sperm phenomenon and bone growth stimulant. Neither was highlighted.

Joe's screen highlighted in red the future pharmaceutical area of plant DNA.

Nacheda's screen highlighted pure active ingredient extraction.

The team members looked from screen to screen linking the red highlighted areas. SAM's voice came back on line.

"I asked you to do more investigative research into three areas. First, the subject of herbs as a pharmaceutical class. Second, more information on the dormant sperm phenomenon, bone growth, and excessive mental alertness. And, finally, third, plant DNA bombardment.

"Over the past month you have provided me with more than enough information to make a lockin. First, let me further update your screens."

The team moved restlessly in their chairs. SAM was dragging this out a little longer than necessary.

"Terri did some additional work on all five compounds but what is important to us is JPC138. JPC stands for James Pharmaceutical Company." The words James Pharmaceutical Company printed out on the large wallmounted screen with James highlighted in red. "It also seems that the initial indication for JPC138 is in the Alzheimer's field." Alzheimer's was printed on the screen and highlighted. "Now to John's information. You see his new information, but he also did some patent searches after you had narrowed the field down at our January meeting. He looked into patents on herbs and plant DNA. He entered this information in his remote computer terminal and I have made the following correlation." The large screen refreshed itself. The words AZ Foundation and James Pharmaceutical Company were printed at the top of the screen. Below the names there was a heavy line separating the video screen. Under the line was printed:

Patent 10348765 plant DNA Purdue University licensed to James Pharmaceutical Company

Patent 10267538 Alstonia spectabilis use in Pharmaceuticals James Pharmaceutical Company

Every time James was added to the screen it appeared in red. SAM came back on line. "I am sure the team sees a trend beginning to form."

Nacheda hit the interrupt key on his keyboard to signify that he wanted the sequence to stop. SAM stopped and his head and eyes shifted to his left to look at Nacheda. "It seems that Mr. Nacheda in chair #6 has something to add to this summary. Mr. Nacheda, please begin."

Nacheda turned to the group. "I apologize for not sending this information into you, Skip, for input into the computer, but it slipped my mind. I have been spending my time working in the research department at Bandai Pharmaceutical Company." He looked at Skip who gave him a knowing wink. Nacheda felt a slight embarrassment thinking of Reiko, then went on, "I have found out that Bandai has filed for a process patent on the process that we talked about last month. So please add this information to John's database. Oh, I almost forgot, besides Asia, they have filed for a patent in the US, EEC, and Russia."

"Thank you Nachedasan." Skip then typed in the information.

Everyone watched SAM as he placed his right hand under his chin as if thinking about the information he had just received. He then dropped his hand to his side, looked at Nacheda and said "Thank you Nachedasan. Your information is most useful and correlates nicely." New information relating to Nacheda's information appeared on the large screen.

SAM continued, "Cap has continued his excellent research. Two weeks ago he detected another complaint registered with the FDA by a Dr. Rosenberg on excessive mental alertness. It seems that a lawyer from northern New Jersey went first to his physician and then to his pharmacist and demanded additional refills of a product with the brand name of Lifeal. Lifeal is for arterial fibrillation. The patient had self-overdosed and had gained a tremendous memory boost that enabled him to remember everything he had experienced with tremendous clarity. This is interesting, but what is most interesting is that James Pharmaceutical Company produces Lifeal. And the basic raw material is Alstonia spectabilis."

"We now move to Mary's screen. Although nothing is highlighted we must remember that herbs were part of these product findings thus, giving validation to the use of herbs in pharmaceuticals.

"There is nothing to add to either Joe's or Nacheda screens. So where do we stand?" Jokingly SAM answered his own question. "We do not have to be mental geniuses to see that we have a lockin. I also took it upon myself to look up the financial strength of James. They do not have enough cash to do the clinical trials the way they should be conducted. In conclusion, I would recommend that you look at James Pharmaceutical Company and the product they call JPC138."

Skip began typing a set of commands. SAM looked like he was listening. SAM began to reply to Skip's commands. "Skip has asked me to provide you with a report on James. Please wait ten seconds." There was silence as everyone waited. "Thank you for your patience. You will see on each of your screens a graph and/ or table. These are from their annual report. In my analysis I have concluded that they are short of working capital and that their major new product Lifeal is not living up to its predicted results. There seems to be a difference of opinion between management and the board of directors. I do not see anything here that would change my recommendation. Are there any additional questions?"

"Skip," it was Mary who spoke, "I would like to know more about Alstonia spectabilis."

Skip punched in the question and SAM replied, "Good question. Just give me another ten seconds." After 10 seconds he continued "I have come up with an interesting correlation which I will give you after I explain Alstonia spectabilis."

As SAM began to speak the words were displayed on one side of the large screen. As he described Alstonia spectabilis the tree parts were shown on the other side of the screen. "Alstonia spectabilis grows in only one area of the world, the island of Java in chain of islands that make up the nation of Indonesia."

Alstonia Spectabilis Species *Parts Used: The bark*

Habitat: Java

Synonyms: **Dita Bark, Bitter Bark, Devil Tree**

Description: **The tree grows from 50 to 80 feet high, has a furrowed trunk, oblong stalked leaves up to 6 inches long and 4 inches wide, dispersed in four to six whorls round the stem, their upper running at right angles to the midrib. The bark is almost odorless and very bitter, in commerce it is found in irregular fragments 1/8 to 1/2 inch thick, texture spongy, fracture coarse and short, outside layer rough uneven fissured brownish gray and sometimes blackish spots; inside layer bright buff, transverse section shows a number of small medullary rays in inner layer.**

Constituents: **The basic tree more commonly, Alstonia Scholaris contains three alkaloids, Ditamine, Echitarnine or Ditaine, and Echitenines. The species Alstonia spectabilis, found only in Indonesia has an additional crystalline alkaloid called Alstonamine.**

There are several fatty and resinous substances; the second is the strongest base and resembles ammonia in chemical characteristics.

MedicinalAction and Uses: The basic tree bark is used in homeopathy for its tonic bitter and astringent properties; it is particularly useful for chronic diarrhea and dysentery. Spectabilis species beneficial use is unknown. It has caused dizziness and hypocardia.

Preparations and Dosages: Dita bark: 1 part in 20 for B.P. infusion, to 1 fluid ounce; 1 part in 8 Alcohol Tinc., B.P., to 1 fluid drachm. Dose, 2 to 4 grains.

Other Uses: In India the natives use the bark of the Devil Tree for bowel complaints. In Sri Lanka its light wood is used for coffins. In Borneo the wood close to the root of the same species is very light and white color and is used for net floats, household utensils, trenchers, corks, etc.

"That concludes the official report on Alstonia spectabilis and associated species of what is commonly called Devil Tree.

"Now let me refresh your memory. Last meeting when you were discussing side effects you found excessive mental alertness by reading a report from a hospital in Singapore. The patient had developed the problem while on the island of

Java, which happens to be where the Alstonia spectabilis species of Devil Tree grows. There is a high percentage correlation that the product the patient took was from this particular species of Devil Tree." SAM paused.

"Are there any other questions?" SAM asked.

"If there are no further questions I leave you now awaiting your call. I feel that, with the information you have provided me, you have a company to pursue plus new research technology in which to work with in product development. I wish the team success in the conclusion of your project. Goodnight." The computer shut down and all of the screens went blank.

The team sat silently for a moment and then cheered and clapped. Skip asked Nacheda if he had anything he wanted to say to the group.

"Yes, thank you, Skip. I realize that what we have done has been difficult and at times we could not see the end of the road, but we have succeeded and that is what is most important. Dr. Nakasone will be very pleased.

"Now you must be wondering what we will do next? Well, for the total team I think we should just remain on call just in case we have to go back and find another candidate. As far as Skip is concerned, I will require his help to implement the plan.

"Now for the best part. You have fulfilled your agreement and Dr. Nakasone has authorized me to present to each of you a bonus check of $200,000. He is very appreciative of the work that you have done to provide us with a comprehensive database. He would like to request that you remain on retainer for the next twelve months. He is willing to pay each of you $5,000 per month. All he asks is that you be available for additional projects and you do not tell any person, group, or agency about the SAM process or what we have discussed and identified.

"He also requests that you keep your eyes and ears open in your relative fields to ensure that the database remains current. You can send the information through the same down-link process that you have used over the last year. He again reminds each of you of the secrecy agreement that you signed prior to beginning this project. You are not to discuss anything that concerns the project. He has graciously given you the unexpected $200,000 bonus to confirm the confidence that he has in your integrity.

"If anyone does not want to continue on with the group in the retainer role please let me know and we will work out a way to have you leave the group. Is there anyone who wants to leave?" Nacheda paused and looked at each member of the team. There were no takers. They all wanted to remain on the team.

"Great, I will look forward to working with you in the future. We will not hold regular meetings as we have done over the past twelve months. I will provide you with secret updates on the status of our implementation stage. You will receive an encoded status report once a month from Skip on the same day that we would normally have had our meeting. He will call you and let you know when to expect the report and the password that is required to access it.

"I will be implementing the plan. If I require your assistance, I will let you know. Does anyone have problem with this strategy?"

Again there was no negative response. "Well," Nacheda looked at his watch, "it is 11:30. To use an old Navy term, 'The sun is not yet over the yardarm', so we should not celebrate with drinks here at the condo. Skip has arranged for us to have lunch in Westwood. By the time we get to the restaurant it should be noon, the sun will be over the yardarm and we can celebrate with Champagne. How does that sound?"

"Great," was the resounding answer. "Skip, you have the con," Nacheda announced.

"Okay, team, let's head out to the Renaissance Restaurant on Galey Avenue. We can disband at the restaurant, so if you have anything here at the condo you can either take it with you to lunch or pick it up later. Any questions? No questions, let's go."

The group left the condo and walked their usual route into Westwood Village. After they had traveled about a block the Asian began to follow.

Once inside the restaurant the tail took a position at the bar. The Renaissance Restaurant was not very conducive to eye signals because the bar was in one room and the team was in a separate dining room.

The celebration caused instant enjoyment. It was almost equal to the celebration they had together on the occasion of their farewell from Viet Nam. They were good friends who were glad to be together and relieved that their project had successfully been completed.

The interior design of the restaurant was made to look like an old mansion. Each room was decorated as a dining room from the 1600's. Everyone sat in high-back chairs that were well padded on the seat and back in dark tapestry material. Each seat had cherry armrests set slightly lower than usual to fit beneath the table when pulled close for eating. The walls of the room were dark and covered with tapestries and gloomy renaissance paintings. Chamber music played softly in the background. Drinks were served in silver goblets and the meat was served on giant pewter platters. Light came from two chandeliers hanging over each end of the long table. The lights shaped like candles.

As the meal celebration progressed and the drinking of Champagne continued well into the afternoon, each member of the team in turn went to the restroom. One of the members of the team passed through the bar area and made a quick eye contact with the Asian. As he walked past the Asian he paused an unnoticeable moment and spoke in a whisper, "Successfully completed, I will email report tomorrow, notify NPC." He then proceeded to the men's room and then returned to the celebration. No one seemed to notice his pause at the bar.

The lunch broke up at 3:00. Everyone was slightly inebriated, but they did not care, no one was driving. Even Cap, anticipating the celebration had taken a cab. The group's farewell was more emotional than the previous month's for two reasons. First, because they were mellow from the champagne and second, because they did not know when or if they would ever be back together again as a team.

The last two persons to leave were Skip and Nacheda. They left together and walked back to the condo. The Asian was still following Nacheda. When they were back at the condo they made a decision to wait until the following morning to discuss the plan of action for the implementation. Both felt high on champagne and on success. Nacheda had a plane to catch the next day at 12:30. They would have time in the morning to strategize the implementation plan.

Since it was after 8:00 a.m. in Bandai, Nacheda decided to call Dr. Nakasone and give him a status report. The phone conversation was brief. There was no mention of James or the Devil Tree. A meeting was scheduled for 7:00 a.m. on Friday in Nakasone's office. After concluding the conversation, Nacheda replaced the phone handset and then turned to Skip.

"Everything is set for my meeting with Nakasone on Friday. He wanted me to specifically thank you for your help and untiring work to make all of this happen. He has given me authority to tell you that your bonus would be double that of the other team members. $500,000 will be wire transferred to the bank of your choice. You do not have to tell me now, but as soon as you inform me of the bank, the bonus will be on its way." Skip was visibly moved. The champagne had mellowed him and he could not speak for a moment.

He cleared his throat and said, "That is extremely generous of Dr. Nakasone. It was not necessary, I only did what he asked me to do."

"No, Skip, you did much more. You held the team together and kept it focused on our objective. You were the leader."

"But you are the leader, Nachedasan."

"No, Skip, I was a member of the team and I paid the bills, but I was not the leader. By the way there is also a $200,000 bonus for team member #8."

Nacheda looked down at the floor a little embarrassed to ask the next question. "Skip, I have a personal question to ask."

"No need to ask my friend. Yes it will be all right with me if you spend the remaining hours until tomorrow's morning meeting, with Reiko. I only wish Annie were here so the four of us could go out together. You must promise me that you and Reiko will go skiing with us on your next trip to California."

"Thank you so very much Skip. It is a promise. What will you do tonight?"

"I think I'll curl up with the phone and talk to Annie, then go to bed early. I'm beat. See you in the morning."

Nacheda called Reiko, packed his bag and drove to the Century Plaza with the Asian following closely behind.

6:00 P.M., TUESDAY, FEBRUARY 14

SUTTON PLACE NEW YORK CITY

As Peggy walked through the door of the apartment and walked slowly to the bedroom.

She changed into casual clothes, thinking back on the day. It had been a great day for her. She had a breakthrough on the side effect.

The male primate (they were 60% male and 40% female) named Jake, who was on the 10 tablet a day dosage of Lifeal, began to act differently than the other primates. On Monday he had stopped being hyperactive. Jake just sat and looked at her through knowing eyes. She talked to him and she believed that he was actually able to comprehend what she was saying. He put out his right hand like he wanted her to shake it. She reached through the cage bars and took his small hand in hers. He then put his left hand over her hand. She felt a pressure from his grip.

She knew that she had to be careful. She didn't know what would happen next. These primates could really bite. She had exposed herself to potential danger, but Jake seemed so calm. His grip got tighter and he leaned down his head. Her heart skipped a beat. She thought, he is going to bite me, but the grip was not a force grip. She started to pull away just as Jake's head reached her hand and he kissed the top of her hand and then released his grip. Peggy was so surprised she jerked her hand out of Jake's cage. She then immediately put her hand palm up back into the cage as a sign of trust. Jake just placed his right hand on top of Peggy's and continued to look at her with his knowing eyes. She was very surprised, this species was known to never shown affection.

She looked at the fourteen other primates. Three of the five on placebos were slowly playing in their cages. The other two were sitting in their cages watching Jake. The other nine, on 10 tablets of Lifeal, were very hyperactive. They were moving at a very rapid pace, swinging back and forth and jumping at the barred cage walls.

Jake made a throaty sound, not in his usual high pitch scream, but much lower in scale and softer. His right hand never moved but his left pointed at the two other sitting primates. He made a sequence of sounds. Peggy looked in wonder as the two primates both got up and walked to their feeding platforms and sat down again. Jake made another series of sounds and both started to eat. Sounds again and they stopped and returned to their original starting sitting position. Jake's left hand came to rest under Peggy's hand. She looked into Jake's eyes. She could swear there was a knowing twinkle. His right hand squeezed her finger just as if to say, "Look at what I made them do!"

Peggy could not help but think that Jake had gone through this sequence of events with the two primates to show her that he could communicate with them. Communication between primates was not unusual. What was unusual was that Jake wanted her to know he could get the others to do things for him.

She said, "Jake, are you trying to tell me that you can ask your friends to do things for you?" Jake squeezed her finger and he made a soft noise.

"Jake, do you mind if I leave you now and go back to my office and think about what you have told me?" Jake leaned down and again kissed her hand. His lips were moist and warm. It was just a peck, but there was emotion in the kiss.

Peggy had removed her hand from the cage. She returned to her office and wrote a report on what had happened. She then brought up the statistical information on all fifteen primates and began a methodical analysis of every parameter she could think of to see what made Jake and the two other primates different. She was excited but also a little nervous at what she might discover

8:00 P.M., TUESDAY, FEBRUARY 14

ROOM 212, HYATT LAX HOTEL LOS ANGELES, CALIFORNIA

A member of Nacheda's task force sat in front of his laptop computer typing a report.

TO: Mr. Tanaguchi, Nippon Pharmaceutical Council

FROM: Lonewolf

SUBJ: Project

Subject company identified as James Pharmaceutical Company, Spectrum of Medicine Building, New York City.

Product JPC138

Indication: Alzheimer's Disease

James is short of cash and there is some dissension between management and board.

Await further instructions at (310) 7340123 extension 212./s/ Lonewolf

The team member who referred to himself as Lonewolf removed a black box from his suitcase. He opened up his Japanese daily schedule book. The schedule book had, by each date, a Japanese proverb. The dates were according to the old Buddhist calendar. He calculated the date and time in Tokyo. It was 1300 on Wednesday the 15th of February. The proverb for the day was "One assumes, over time, the personality of the person they pretend to be."

Lonewolf thought that this proverb seemed to be very appropriate for the act he was about to commit. He dialed in the first three letters of the second word ass. He laughed out loud at the ironic code. He then entered the Buddhist date of 3648 and then his symbol for Lonewolf LW.

He plugged his modem into the data connection on the hotel phone. Having completed this task he typed in the NPC secret phone number that would reach the council's communication center on the western coast of Honshu. From there the message would be transmitted to Tanaguchi, wherever he might be. The message would be encrypted by the black box. Decryption could only be accomplished by a similar black box in Tanaguchi's possession. The communications center was located on the western coast because there was less communication traffic on that coast of Japan.

After typing in the secret telephone number, Lonewolf watched the screen as it told him that the computer was dialing, connecting, encrypting, transmitting, and disconnecting.

Lonewolf took out a pack of Marlboro cigarettes and broke off the filter. "Damn California freaks," he grumbled to himself. "They can't stand a little smoke in the air." People at home were civilized and he could smoke when he wanted to smoke. Not in California, they told you where and when to smoke. He figured that they were now probably working on how a smoker should smoke.

He got up from his desk chair where he had typed his short report and sat down in the room's only easy chair. Lonewolf was in full view of the computer screen. An acknowledgment of his coded message would take two minutes. Instructions on what he was to do next would take no less than fifteen minutes. Lonewolf leaned back in his chair and took a long drag on his filterless Marlboro. The smoke burned his throat, his esophagus, and lungs. Ah! The enjoyment of the first good drag of the day. He held the smoke in his lungs as long as he could and slowly let it out through his nasal passage. The yellow smoke swirled around his head.

The notebook computer screen began to blink indicating an incoming message. He leaned forward and read the screen through the haze of smoke. He took a second deep drag and this time he blew the smoke out through his mouth. This was directed at the screen.

On the screen the computer were the words:

TO: Lonewolf

FROM: NPC

SUBJ: Lonewolf communication Acknowledge receipt./s/NPC

The screen then returned to its standby position. Lonewolf leaned back in his chair. He took a third drag on his filterless Marlboro. He switched the finger in which he held his cigarette. He unconsciously switched fingers after every third drag so he did not stain his fingers and give away his heavy smoking habit. Again he held the smoke in his lungs. He had started smoking while in Vietnam. He had been listed as missing in action though he knew where he was, a filthy prison camp. He took another long drag on his cigarette. They had broken him. His body almost convulsed remembering the invisible mental pain. There was not a mark on the outside of his body, but inside. He shook again, but not as intensely as before. After he had been broken he would have done anything they had asked. During his mental torture he had been given Chinese cigarettes whenever he wanted. The Chinese tobacco was so strong with nicotine that he could not smoke the filtered weak cigarettes that Americans now smoked.

No one knew that the Vietnamese had broken him. Sometimes he didn't even realize he had been broken himself. They did not ask anything of him when he was captured and tortured. They explained that when he was free he would be asked to do certain jobs and that he would be paid well for whatever he did for them. They brainwashed him against the democratic free enterprise system and convinced him, beyond any reasonable doubt, that the Communist system was the best. Through the years he had been asked to do various jobs for the Chinese, the Vietnamese, Iran, Iraq, and the old USSR as well as some South American countries. Most of the jobs were either drugoriented or increasingly, corporate espionage. Lonewolf sincerely believed that democracy was corrupt and through its corruptness he would benefit. It never occurred to him that he was one of the causes of corruptness and was becoming rich because of the freedom a democratic system provided.

During the late 1980's and early 90's when communism was being overthrown by the people and replaced by a democratic process, Lonewolf never gave up on his foreign mentors. He was called up by many different people to do special projects. When he was addressed as Lonewolf, he paid close attention to everything the person said following an ever-changing identification code word. The person that talked to him on the telephone was always the same. The contact talked in English, but the accent was Asian. Lonewolf surmised he was Vietnamese.

What Lonewolf did not know was that he was part of a cadre of exprisoners that had been programmed to be industrial spies. The Vietnamese controller contracted the industrial spies to different organizations. When the NPC approached the Vietnam controller and explained NPC's objectives in the United States and formation of the Bandai Pharmaceutical task force, the controller linked all the information in a computer database and determined that Lonewolf was the perfect candidate.

Because of the team make up and the potential commercial value of the outcome, the Vietnamese controller charged NPC a very high price for Lonewolf, more than $2 million dollars. The controller would split the fee 50:50 with Lonewolf, the $200,000 bonus Lonewolf had received from Bandai was peanuts. Lonewolf worked for real money. He was a multimillionaire. His money was in a Freeport, Bahamas secret numbered bank account. He looked forward to many additional contracts now that the Bandai contract was winding down. So far this project had been a way to make an easy couple mil.

The notebook computer screen started to blink. A message was appeared on the screen.

TO: Lonewolf

FROM: Tanaguchi

SUBJ: Project

Excellent work. NPC very pleased.

Coincidence happened to NPC last week. An officer of James Pharmaceutical Company put out feelers to NPC and we assume others. Others being the JPA and other major Japanese pharmaceutical companies. The James officer or officers would not identify themselves. They want to provide the James strategic plan to any Japanese pharmaceutical company that would sign a letter of intent to acquire James at a stock price of 30% above market.

NPC is not interested in dealing with people who will not provide their names. NPC, to this point, has ignored the inquiry.

With Lonewolfs news about James being identified as the company of choice by Bandai project, NPC will now answer last week's inquiry with positive interest.

NPC will require Lonewolf to meet with identified officer to establish parameters of the proposed deal.

For now, return to home base and await further instructions. The screen returned to standby. Lonewolf stubbed out his cigarette.

Lonewolf would wait until told what he was supposed to do for his half of the two million dollars.

4:00 P.M., WEDNESDAY, FEBRUARY 15

SPECTRUM OF MEDICINE BUILDING
NEW YORK CITY

J.P. picked up the phone and dialed Annie's number in Mammoth. As usual, Annie answered after only a couple of rings. This time he had chosen the middle of the afternoon to make his call knowing that she wouldn't be busy with the lunch crowd.

"Annie, hi, it's J.P."

"I know who it is," she replied happily. "How the devil are you and when are you coming home?"

"I'm fine and I don't know when I'll be coming home. Soon I hope, but wanting to come home and being realistic as to when I can actually come home are two different matters entirely."

"Well, how about coming home this weekend and bring Mandi. Skip is coming up for a ski weekend and the four of us can get to know each other. I know you will like Skip."

"I'm sure I'll like Skip. I want you to meet Mandi, but I just don't know if I can. I may have to make a quick trip overseas."

"Where are you going?"

"I'm thinking that I may have to visit the source of raw material for a couple of the James products. I'll probably base myself out of Singapore and then fly to the island of Java in Indonesia." he paused. He wanted to go home to ski. He and Mandi had canceled their trip to New England and they both needed to get away from James, but now was not the time.

"Annie, I'm sorry, but I have to stay here and play president. It pains me, but I'll have to take a rain check."

"I know it's useless to try and change your mind, so I won't bother to try. Skip and I will be disappointed. I have to say though that this is the first time I think I've ever known you to turn down an opportunity to ski."

J.P. moved to change the subject, "Annie, how is my house?" "Everything is in good shape. No real news and no mail of any significance. There was a letter from your editor. I opened it as you instructed. He was just checking to see how your book is coming along. He just asked that you give him a call. Nothing else."

He thought he detected a slight strain in her voice, so he decided to pursue his instincts. "Is anything bothering you?"

"Nothing really, J.P., except that I wanted to talk to you about Skip and myself. Things are moving along and becoming serious.

You are my best friend and I want to talk to you. I also would like to meet Mandi. We have meant a great deal to each other over the years and I feel that because of this New York project we are drifting apart. I'd really like to spend some time talking with you." There was deep emotion in her voice. J.P. realized that he missed her as well.

"Annie, I want to talk to you too and need your advice. Mandi and I are also becoming quite serious and I need to talk this through with my best friend. I will try very hard to come to Mammoth after the trip to Singapore. I'm sure that Mandi is coming with me so we will take a couple of days off on the way back and make the trip to Mammoth. Talk to Skip and see what his schedule is so that we can combine our visits. I'll let you know the exact dates soon. I really do appreciate your feelings and I feel the same way. I'm sorry I can't visit this weekend. Please understand."

"I do, J.P., and I'll talk to Skip. Please call when you have more time to talk." Her voice seemed a little more upbeat.

"I will Annie. Meanwhile have fun with Skip. He seems like a great guy.

I look forward to meeting him again."

8:00 P.M., THURSDAY, FEBRUARY 16

THE JAMES FARM, GREYSTONE HALL
SEAFORD, NY

"Well, have you heard from the NPC?" she asked as she rolled onto her right side to look at him.

"Not yet," was his sleepy reply as he lay on his back and stared at the wood beam ceiling. He shivered a little. He did not know whether it was her sharp question, to which he had no answer, or the strong wind coming off the Atlantic. This old farm, he thought, why did Doc James keep this relic. The wind rattled the windows and the shutters.

"Well?" she insisted.

"Well what?" he didn't feel like bantering with her tonight.

"Well what are you going to do about the NPC? You gave them until the seventeenth and tomorrow's the seventeenth."

"Yes," he said letting out a sigh. "Yes, tomorrow's the seventeenth. That makes tonight the sixteenth, not the seventeenth, so you have answered your own question haven't you?"

"Don't be insolent with me or I'll cut off your nuts. That is if I could find them."

"Look, I don't feel up to fighting with you. I'll take care of it tomorrow.

God, this place is cold. Why in the hell can't you get this place insulated?"

"If I had a decent partner we wouldn't require insulation. Now if you have had all of me you can take for an evening, how about," her voice went up a few decibels, "you getting the fuck out of my house."

He was about to reply when they both heard the alarm on the computer in the study sound, announcing that there was an incoming email.

"Get your fat ass out of bed and see who sent the e-mail!" she yelled.

He slowly rolled to his right and flopped his feet onto the cold floor. Damn he thought, I forgot to put a towel on the floor. A deep shiver went through his body as he turned on the bedside light and reached for his robe. He sat on the edge of the bed for a minute to get used to the cold air as it hit his now limp penis.

"Get your ugly white body out of bed and into the study to see who sent an email. You know it has to be from the NPC. They're the only people who have the address to that account!" she continued to scream. God, this guy is an idiot, she thought, but I need him for a while longer.

He plodded from the bedroom into the study. He opened the message on the computer, saw that it was from Nippon Pharmaceutical and pushed the print button. Before he could grab it the printer discharged the page and it dropped onto the floor. He reached down without bending his knees and felt his back muscles start to tighten.

Oh no, not now, not tonight, not my back. He gingerly reached and picked up the piece of paper and slowly rolled to the floor and straightened out his legs. There was a slight pain in his lower back, but the muscles stretched. He laid there for a few moments to make sure he had stretched the muscles enough and they would not cramp when he stood up.

From the bedroom came, "Well, what is keeping you. I can hear that the printer is turned off. Have you climaxed yourself into a heart attack." The sounds of her strong sadistic laugh echoed off the walls as she responded to her own humor.

When he didn't answer he heard a second, "Well?" much louder than the first. He thought that he might just not answer and she would get worried and think something had happened to him. That would get her out into the cold he thought and a smile crossed his lips then faded. Yeah, and then she would either verbally or physically assault him. She could hit hard.

"I'm coming, which is more than you can do," he replied sitting up and rolling over to be on his hands and knees before standing up straight.

He muttered to himself, "Boy, I hope she never sees me do this. She would kick me in the side and I would be a stretcher case. Why do I put up with this? Only a little while longer, I hope." He answered himself.

He walked into the bedroom. "About time. Don't bother getting back in bed. You are leaving as soon as this is taken care of. Now what does it say?" Her voice was her normal loud.

"It says," and he read it out loud. TO: James Contact FROM: NPC SUBJ.: Business Agreement Meeting

Sorry contact has been delayed. NPC still interested in hearing proposal You will be contacted by a Mr. Smith next week, please meet with him and disclose business proposal to him. If you cannot meet in person, deal is off.

"Satisfied?" he finished.

"Yes," she replied softly. "Now send an acknowledgment of receipt and then leave me alone. Tell me as soon as this Mr. Smith contacts you."

She rolled over onto her stomach and pulled the covers and pillow over her head so she wouldn't hear him leaving. She was quickly asleep.

He picked up his clothes and took them to the study and got dressed. The NPC could wait until he dressed. After dressing he typed out an acknowledgment:

TO: NPC

FROM: James Contact <(215) 8383167>

SUBJ.: Re: Business Agreement Meeting

Looking forward to Mr. Smith's contact.

He then pushed the send key and made sure that it went through before closing the program.

7:00 A.M., FRIDAY, FEBRUARY 17

BANDAI PHARMACEUTICAL COMPANY
BANDAI, JAPAN

Nacheda found his mind wandering back over the past several days as he stood in front of Dr. Nakasone. Nakasone was poring through the report that Nacheda had just handed to him.

The trip back to Bandai was as good as the trip to Los Angeles. Rieko and Nacheda had celebrated the success of the project on Tuesday night. Of course, Rieko did not know exactly what they were celebrating, but she didn't really seem to care.

Skip and Nacheda debriefed the Tuesday meeting on Wednesday morning. They decided that Nacheda would write the report and present it to Dr. Nakasone and await further direction. The one unexpected comment came from Skip.

"Nachedasan," Skip had said pensively, "I think I have an acquaintance at James Pharmaceutical Company."

"What?" Nacheda responded enthusiastically. "This is very good news Skip. Who is the contact?"

"Don't get yourself too excited, Nachedasan, I'm not positive. The night I met Annie in Mammoth, I also met a friend of hers named

J.P. I thought they were more than just friends and it took me a while before I established the fact that Annie was available for dating. J.P. and I talked for awhile, but we seemed to talk around issues. Since I could not be honest with him I didn't take much notice of the fact that I didn't think he was being honest with me. Now that I think back on our conversation we were gambiting back and forth quite a bit. I am almost positive he mentioned that he had, or was currently, working for James Pharmaceutical Company."

"Skip, can you find out more?"

"I don't know old buddy, but I will try. I am going to see when this J.P. guy will be back in town and I'll suggest we get together. Annie did tell me that he has been working in New York City which ties into the location of James."

Nacheda was very interested and had added this information to his report to Dr. Nakasone.

After reading Nacheda's report Nakasone looked up at Nacheda who was still standing in front of his desk. "You have done very well Nachedasan. Not for one moment did I think you would fail."

Nacheda smiled inwardly but kept his head bowed. If what he said was true, Nakasone had been a tremendous actor in the scolding he had given Nachcda before the January task force meeting in Los Angeles.

Dr. Nakasone went on, "I must study the information you have given me over the weekend. Please meet me again in my office Monday morning at seven. Have a pleasant weekend, Nacheda-^san."

"*Doumoarigatou aruji,*" Nacheda spoke as he backed out of the door still bowing.

Nacheda drove back to his apartment, opened the door, and headed straight for the telephone. He dialed Rieko's number. It was picked up after one ring "Moshimoshi, Nachedasan."

"Moshimoshi, Riekosan. How did you know it was me?"

"Who else would it be my love? How did the meeting with Dr. Nakasone go?"

"The meeting went very well. I am a free man this weekend. How would you like to go skiing?"

"I would be very sad if you had not asked me. How about the same train as last time?"

"That would be perfect. I will meet you at the train station at the same time."

9:00 A.M., FRIDAY, FEBRUARY 17

SPECTRUM OF MEDICINE BUILDING
NEW YORK CITY

J.P. spoke in the telephone intercom on his desk, "Janet, please have Mandi join me for a meeting at ten o'clock in the conference room."

"Okay J.P."

Janet paused, "JP?" "Yes."

"Have you given any thought to helping Bill with his new company and blood level test for Lifeal?' she asked in somewhat a timid manner which was completely out of character.

"Yes, I have and thanks for reminding me. Phillip asked Mandi and I over for dinner and I convinced him that it was time to repair the bridge between him and Bill and you are both invited to Phillip's home for dinner tomorrow night. I hope you and Bill can make it."

Janet did not answer but ran over to J.P. and threw her arms around him and gave him a kiss. "Oh J.P. that is so wonderful, of course we will accept. How did you manage to convince Phillip to see Bill?"

"It was not easy but I worked on him while he was sort of doped up on pain killers. I also think the shooting has mellowed him. Anyway we are on our way of solving the situation and helping to solve the long range Lifeal situation. Now please say no more and call Mandi."

Tears were in her eyes as she backed away. "Thank you so much J.P. I will never be able to repay you."

"Just make sure Bill keeps his temper under control and is humble. Let you and I make sure the end result is success."

Janet left the room.

He got up from the table and walked over to the window. New York winters can be very depressing. It was overcast. The weather was still cold and wet. The wind had swung from the west to come out of the northeast, now it came off the cold Atlantic. He visualized the high seas that were smashing up against the hulls of the ships in the Atlantic. The men and women on the open decks would be wrapped in heavy weather clothing to keep the winter seas off their bodies. The long endless nights of steaming at sea. He concluded that his view from the 40th floor of the Spectrum of Medicine Building was not that bad after all. He still ached to get out of town, but he knew that it was not to be. He had finally decided that a first hand trip was the only way to learn about Devil Tree bark, the vendor, and the long-term supply of the valuable raw material so he had to prepare for Singapore. Making the trip was also away to escape New York. He had also decided to ask Mandi to accompany him. There was a knock on the door. He turned around to see Mandi. "Hi let's use the conference table," he said cheerfully.

Mandi caught his up mood. "How come the extraordinary cheerful greeting on such a gloomy day?" she asked smiling.

"I have a proposition." "What's up?"

"You know, I think the supply of Devil Tree bark is essential to the long term success of James."

"Yes."

"Well, I want to visit the plantation and talk to the owner to get a first hand view of the situation."

"Sounds like a good idea to me, but what has this to do with me?" "I thought you might want to go with me?"

Mandi, who had become slightly bored with the way the conversation had developed suddenly, became alert. "Say that again J.P.?"

"I said, I thought you might want to visit Singapore and then the Devil Tree plantation on Java with me."

She did not take a second to answer. "Are you kidding? Of course I would love to go with you. Do you think it is possible for me to go?"

"I am sure you can go. There should be a representative of Phillip's staff and I'm sure I can get Phillip to agree. There is one slight problem."

Her voice reflected her feelings that there was going to be a catch. "I knew there was a catch. It was too good to be true."

"It is not as bad as it seems. The problem is timing. I plan for us to leave next Friday. We will arrive in Singapore on Saturday and visit the plantation the first part of the week. You will not have much time to prepare. Will you be able to leave the office for a week or so? I thought we would be back about March 6th."

"Oh, J.P., I would love to go to Singapore with you. I know you love Singapore and I want to see the city through your eyes. Will we have some free time?"

"I'm sure we'll find some free time."

Mandi surprised him by throwing her arms around his neck and giving him a kiss. His arms quickly went around her waist and they kissed for a long time. They had tried to keep their relationship out of the office, but this time it was not possible.

The next thing they heard was Janet clearing her throat and saying, "Excuse me, J.P. and Mandi."

They quickly broke apart and tried to regain their composure. "Sorry Janet, we forgot where we were."

"No need to apologize, I understand.

"Janet please make reservations on Singapore Airlines for Mandi and myself to fly to Singapore to arrive Saturday the 25th.

The flight should go through Los Angeles because on the way back I want to take Mandi to Mammoth for a weekend of skiing. The return trip should have us in Los Angeles on Friday March 3rd and back here Sunday evening. Please book us in the Raffles Hotel in Singapore. Also check to see what charter air services are available out of Singapore. The ultimate destination is the island of Java in Indonesia. It should be a relatively small plane, capable of landing and taking off on short, remote runways.

"Got it J.P. Sounds like a great trip. I'll get right on it." Janet left the office.

"A minute ago, you didn't say anything about skiing at Mammoth." Mandi said faking an indignant attitude.

"It was to be a surprise, but I knew you would have to pack skis and ski clothes so it was not possible to surprise you. We will leave your ski gear in Los Angles on the way over."

"And what's with the regional security officer?"

"Every embassy overseas has a regional security officer."

He moved towards Mandi and gave her a short kiss and said. "I have to call Phillip and set up the meeting and then I have to get at this paperwork. If I don't see you again today, I will see you at Phillip's tomorrow."

Mandi started towards the door and turned just as she was turning the knob. "J.P."

"Yes, beautiful?" "Thank you."

"Thank you for what?"

"Thank you for allowing Janet to participate in your conversation with Phillip and thank you for our trip to Singapore, Java, and Mammoth."

"You're welcome. See you tomorrow."

He moved around to the back of the desk. As he sat down he noticed the sun was trying to break through the winter overcast.

PHILLIP BRADSMITH'S HOME RIO DEL MAR, NEW JERSEY

"J.P., where do youse suppose people find these New Jersey homes?" remarked Roberto as he drove the cab west on NJ Route 9W towards Phillip's home.

"I don't know Roberto. It just seems that people like to live out in the sticks instead of in view of the beautiful city skyline. They just don't know what is good for them," he answered.

"I think you're right. These people just don't know what's good for them." Roberto looked back at J.P., taking his eyes off the road. "How youse doing, J.P.? Youse is lookin' a little peaked around the gills." He turned back to the road just as his front tires started over the centerline.

"You know Roberto, in the last month you and I have gotten to be good friends, but I have to tell you the truth. When you drive outside the bumper to bumper traffic of midtown Manhattan, you scare me to death."

"Aw! Not to worry. I haven't been in an accident yet." He paused, "Well, least not a serious accident. I don't count the hits in the city. Those are just part of the job. Now tell me how are youse doin'?"

"I'm doing okay, Roberto. I just need to get away from the city for awhile. I need sun and I'm sure not getting any sun here in New York."

"Youse Californians are just spoiled. Life is too easy for youse. Youse don't have to have sun to be healthy. Good clean livin' is what keeps us healthy. Now where did youse say this Rio Del Mar place is located?"

"I believe in your philosophy of the city. I just don't like to live the philosophy. As for Rio Del Mar, it should be up here on the left. Just watch for a stone wall on either side of the side street. The words Rio Del Mar will be on the wall."

They went around two more bends and there on the left side were the two eight foot sandstone looking walls that announced the entrance to Rio Del Mar. Roberto turned left into the long drive. On either side of the road were large homes. Each looked as though it was sitting on at least two acres of land. All of the trees were still barren of leaves.

"Keep going straight Roberto. Dr. Bradsmith's home is at the end on the left."

After a couple of miles they came to Phillip's home. The house sat back from the road about a half-mile. Roberto turned into the driveway. About halfway to the house J.P. saw Phillip walking towards them on the driveway.

"Roberto, stop here. I will get out here." J.P. glanced at the meter, $50.00. He gave him $100.00. "Thanks Roberto. Take the wife out to dinner. I will probably see you next week."

J.P. got out of the cab. Roberto placed the cab in reverse and quickly backed out of the driveway and was on his way back to the city where he felt comfortable.

J.P. glanced at Phillip. His 6'4" frame was now much thinner than before the shooting. His left forearm was bound tightly across his chest. His smile was warm as he strode towards his old friend.

"Hi, J.P., welcome to Rio Del Mar." he reached out his right hand. "Good to see you up and around Phillip. You are looking great considering what you have been through. How do you feel?"

"I feel pretty good. In fact, I want to talk to you about going back to work part time. I thought Wednesday would be a good day to start back to work. What do you think?"

They were now walking towards the house. "I think that would be a good move Phillip as long as you are ready to assume the helm. I sure would appreciate being relieved of the job so I can concentrate on what you hired me to do. I have been here a little over a month and I have done about everything except break the mystery about the 21st Century Plan. I also found out that paperwork is not what I want to do and Janet has sure kept me loaded with paperwork."

"She sure knows how to keep the paper machine moving. Supposedly we are moving towards a paperless society, but all I see are paper reports and demands for new reports. Janet is sure a great trooper. You know she visited me in the hospital more than Sandi."

Phillip seemed to be more relaxed than J.P. had seen him in a long time. He wanted him to be more relaxed, but he didn't want to see Phillip loose his aggressive business drive. He would require that extra drive to lead James through the hard boardroom fights that were bound to take place before the annual meeting. The man walking next to J.P. looked as though he was ready for retirement.

"Why did you ask to come early, J.P.? If it was to talk business, can't it wait until Wednesday?"

"In some respects it is business, but not normal business. It really can't wait and it has to be discussed before the others arrive."

"What is so secretive?"

"I wanted to talk to you about Lifeal and a way to increase the usage."

It was warm for a February day. The sun had warmed things up to about 45 degrees. "Phillip, do you mind sitting in the sun on your porch while I tell you a story about two friends?"

"No, but I am not in the mood for a story." "Indulge me Phillip, please."

"How can I refuse you since you have done so much for James and myself."

They walked up the stairs to the redwood deck and around to the back and sat in two of the summer deck chairs. As they arrived at the chairs the back door opened and Phillip's wife, Sandi stepped out.

"J.P., how good to see you again. It has been such a long time. How have you been? You look wonderful. Nice and tan compared to our wounded New Yorker here. Please sit down. Don't let me keep you to from doing your talking. We can catch up later. Good to see you again J.P." She went back into the house.

J.P. looked at Phillip. "She hasn't changed a bit," he said.

In sequence and triggered by a silent command they both said, "A Midwestern tornado." They laughed as they sat down.

"Phillip, the story is about two friends." He then proceeded to make up a fictional story that was similar to the Phillip and Bill situation.

At the end Phillip turned towards J.P. and said, "Okay, J.P. Enough with the parables already. What are you trying to set up?"

"One of the reasons for Lifeal not realizing its full potential is because of your stubbornness."

"Comeon J.P., cut the crap and get on with it."

"Okay, Phillip." He then told the story about Bill's new company and Bill's attempts to work with Phillip. During his telling, Phillip remained quiet, but his body reflected his distress. When J.P. finished his narrative, there was quiet for a long period of time. The two men sat looking out at the barren trees. It was so quiet that J.P. could hear the water flowing in the creek that ran about 50 feet beyond the redwood deck. As the minutes dragged by he began to have second thoughts about his devious methods. Had he done right by bringing this problem to a head? J.P. had no counter proposal. He silently wished he were back in Mammoth writing his book.

"J.P." Phillip interrupted his thoughts, "J.P., are you asleep?" "No Phillip, just day dreaming."

"Interesting story, J.P. I see what you mean about my stubbornness."

It was difficult to read Phillip's voice. He was not angry which was a good sign. He seemed like he was reminiscing.

"You know J.P., Bill and I were good friends when we were working to make James a leading pharmaceutical company. After becoming president I lost interest in Bill. Maybe it was a defense mechanism because I felt sorry for him, I was still a rising star and Bill was standing still. I don't know the reason. It just happened. When he came to me with his decision to leave, I said to myself, so what? I honestly don't remember his calls for help before he decided to leave James. My ego probably didn't want to accept the fact that he would leave. When he left I was really pissed. You can believe me or not, J.P., but I had plans for Bill. I trusted him and wanted him to be part of the James team. When he said he was going to leave I felt he had deserted James and had let me down. I blanked him out of my mind.

"I can see how things went downhill between us from that point foreword. I don't remember anything about his new company or his requests to work together on Lifeal.

"Now I am trying to figure out my feelings. I can certainly relate to forcing actions. As an example, who of us will be able to predict the results of our up coming board actions? Who will our decisions hurt?"

"I don't know Phillip. All I know is that decisions always cause a sequence of events. Some known, some unknown, some good, and some bad. We only hope that our judgment and experience causes the good to outweigh the bad and we hope when there is a bad event it is relatively minor. We are not geniuses, Phillip. We are just trying to do the very best job we can in positions of power that hard work and fate have placed us."

Phillip turned to the empty forest and again there was silence. This time his reflections did not last as long.

He suddenly stood up and walked to the deck railing. His voice took on the tone of a man that has made a decision. J.P. didn't jump up with him. He wanted to hear what Phillip had to say before showing any physical or verbal response.

He turned around and leaned back against the rail. There was a smile on his face. J.P. knew then that his decision would be good and that he personally would feel good about the decision. "The time for revenge and hurt is over. We must mend this situation. It will be the best for James and Bill's new company. What did you say the name of his new company was?"

"Clintec."

"Yes, a workable solution will be the best for Clintec, Bill, and, yes indeed, the best for James and myself. Do you have a plan?" He added without waiting for the response, "Of course you have a plan. I have never known you to not have a plan. Out with your plan. What do you want us to do to make things right after all of us have screwed things up?"

"Yes, Phillip, I have a plan." J.P. then told him of the plan to confront Bill. Phillip agreed. J.P. looked at his watch and saw that it was close to four o'clock.

"Bill, Janet, and Mandi should be arriving shortly. Does Sandi need any help?"

We both laughed and together we said, "Sandi never needs help."

J.P. had always been fond of Sandi. She had aged faster than Phillip and when you saw them together you would wrongfully conclude that Sandi was years older than Phillip. Reality was, Sandi was five years younger than Phillip. Although after Phillip's shooting he had probably closed the age perception gap. Sandi's hair was gray and pulled back in a bun. Her face was slightly wrinkled from sun vacations. She had not undertaken any cosmetic surgery and probably would not do so as she continued her natural aging process. Her once slim figure had become slightly full from sporadic exercise and regular meals.

Their marriage had been a typical executive marriage. Sandi had her life in supporting Phillip and Phillip lived for James. They went on holidays usually connected with pharmaceutical meetings. When all the pharmaceutical manufacturers met in glamorous watering holes, they went together and stayed a few days after the meeting had ended to play golf, swim, or fish. Sandi was active in their community. Their two kids, Judy and Tim, had completed college, were married, and relocated north of New York City. Phillip and Sandi were grandparents three times over.

From the front of the house there was the sound of a car horn. "If I remember correctly," commented Phillip, "that will be Bill and Janet. They always like to announce their arrival."

"You're memory is correct." J.P. paused before saying, "A word of caution, Phillip. You have not seen Bill for a while and he is not the Bill you remember. He is overweight and when I saw him a few weeks ago, he is bordering on becoming an alcoholic. I don't know what this whole episode has done to his drinking or eating, but I would be prepared to see a Bill you wouldn't recognize if you saw him on the street. Also remember, until today, you wouldn't even talk to him. This afternoon, the conversation will be strained for quite a while.

"I won't have it any other way, J.P. You're plans are always the best way to get started."

They left the back redwood porch and walked around to the front of the house. Not only was the Williams' car parked in the driveway, but also behind their car was Mandi's car. She was just stepping out of the car. J.P. could just see her long legs emerging from behind the car door.

Phillip saw the same scene and felt J.P.'s emotions change. "I told you that you would like your assistant. How are the two of you getting along? I hear through the rumor mill that you and Mandi have a very open and close relationship."

"Before I answer that very personal question, my friend," he answered humorously, "she is one hell of a marketer."

"Don't tell me something I know. Tell me something I don't know." "Yes, Phillip we have a serious relationship. How serious I don't know. Only time will tell."

Mandi was now standing and closing the car door. She moved towards the group that had gathered in front of the house. The wind was blowing her long red hair away from her face. She had minimum makeup and her smile lit up her total face.

Bill and Janet were inbetween Mandi and the two men, so they were going to have to handle this uncomfortable greeting first before they greeted Mandi. Mandi solved part of our problem by walking fast to catch up with Bill and Janet. Mandi shook Bill's hand and gave Janet a hug. They were all laughing as J.P. and Phillip walked into their circle next to Bill's car. Mandi had done her best to break the tension.

As they walked up to the group, Bill and Janet turned to Phillip and J.P.

J.P. walked up to Bill and said, "Good to see you again, Bill," and shook his hand. J.P. smelled alcohol on his breath. He had probably had a few drinks to give himself courage. J.P. moved to give Janet a hug. Bill and Phillip stood uneasily off to the side. Phillip then walked to Janet and Mandi giving each in turn a hug.

Bill was the first to make a move. He walked up to Phillip and put out his hand. Phillip quickly took his hand and the two old friends stood quietly shaking hands. Bill was also the first to talk.

"Phillip it is good to see you again. Thank you for asking us to dinner. I was very sorry to hear about the shooting and your injury. Is everything okay, are there any physical after effects?"

"Thanks Bill. It is good to see you again after such a long time. I am okay. Some healing yet to be done, but from what I understand, no permanent after effects," he paused causing an uncomfortable silence. J.P. was about to break in when Phillip spoke, "I apologize for not seeing you sooner. I miss our conversations."

J.P. noticed that Janet's eyes started to glisten from tears.

"Okay, lets get out of the driveway and into the house," Phillip announced.

The five walked to the front door where Sandi met them.

"Janet, Mandi, and Bill," she exclaimed as if she were surprised that they had come over for dinner, "how good to see you again. It has been such a long time. How have you been? You look wonderful. Please come in and sit down. I must learn what all of you have been up to lately. You go ahead and get started talking. Phillip get our guests a drink. I won't be a minute and then we can catch up on news. Good to see you again." She went back into the kitchen.

Bill, Janet, Phillip, and J.P. looked at each other and together said, "A Midwestern tornado." They all laughed.

Mandi looked perplexed and asked, "What is this, an inside joke?"

"Yes, not to exclude you, but it is a very long and boring story which I will tell you later. Believe me it is not worth the time." J.P. answered.

Mandi announced, "Sounds good to me. I'll be the bartender. Anyone want drinks? I'm having a Stoli on the rocks."

"Ah, a woman after my own heart. Please make mine a Stoli as well, Mandi," J.P. said.

Janet said, "Mandi, a Stoli for you?" Janet looked over at J.P. with a knowing glance. "Sounds to me as though someone may be corrupting someone else," she said with a smile.

"Stoli's are great, Janet. That is if you keep them down to a minimum number. Do you want a Stoli?" Mandi answered in a very happy mood.

"No thank you, Mandi. I'll stick to a gin and tonic. Bill, what will you have?"

"Just a glass of water please," answered Bill.

"I will also have a glass of water," replied Phillip. "The doctor said the drugs and alcohol do not mix. Now where was it that I heard that pharmaceutical warning before?"

They all laughed. Things were relaxing, but J.P. knew that he had to start the action that was hopefully going to lead to a total healing rather than just a social healing. Mandi brought over the drinks and then announced that she was going to help Sandi in the kitchen.

J.P. then suggested the rest of the group adjourn to the porch to catch a few rays from the winter sun. They exited the house through the French doors.

On the redwood deck J.P. walked to the railing and looked out into the empty forest.

Bill again broke the silence, "Phillip, even in the winter your forest is beautiful."

"Bill," J.P. started, "listen to me. Phillip and I have discussed the situation and have come to the conclusion that the pain must stop. We must stop fighting each other. Phillip is prepared to discuss how the two companies can work together to help Lifeal."

"What? What did you say, J.P.?" Bill exclaimed.

"J.P. said that I want to talk to you about how Clintec and James can work together. Are you ready to work things out?"

Bill again jumped out of the chair and stood in front of Phillip. "Are you serious Phillip? You want to work things out?"

"Yes, I do. I know that I am partly to blame and I now know it was selfish and stupid on my part. As soon as you want to work out a solution I'm ready. The sooner the better I think."

"I couldn't ask for more than what you have already given me, Phillip. I will see you this week and give you and anyone you wish a complete presentation on our technology."

"Great, Bill. Thanks," Phillip said with a smile. "Now let's have an evening of fun with a group of good friends that have been battered up a bit, but certainly not knocked down. We still have each other. What do you say, Bill?"

"I say, I couldn't have better friends and let's have a party."

4:00 P.M., SUNDAY, FEBRUARY 19

BANDAI, JAPAN

Nacheda sat down at his computer and started to type his plan of action recommendation for Dr. Nakasone. As he typed, his mind kept drifting to his past few days with Reiko. They had a great time skiing on Bandai Mountain. The snow had been hard packed and was beginning to turn to ice. They were both excellent skiers and approached the icy ski conditions with vigor. Their lovemaking was slow and comfortable, but still with the same intensity as the first weekend in Bandai. Their experiences with one another had grown since they first made love. The hot baths and massages had led to some of the most sensuous lovemaking either had ever experienced.

During a conversation early that morning before Reiko had caught the train back to Tokyo, they had decided that they were truly in love and expressed that love to each other. Reiko had asked Nacheda about his professional life. Due to the secrecy of the project,

Nacheda was still unable to fully answer her questions. He had finally answered that his plan was to continue to work for Bandai Pharmaceutical Company. He said this even though he knew his special project would probably end within a few months. Under the circumstances he felt that it was the best answer he could give. He felt bad about misleading Reiko, but if their romance ever turned to marriage, then he promised himself that he would tell her about his project before they were married. It was only fair that she knew what kind of work he was doing for Bandai. In truth he was working for Bandai. He had not told a lie.

As far as the future was concerned, Reiko had asked a good question. What was he going to do after Bandai? What kind of work could he do to support a wife and a future family? Did he want a wife that was a flight attendant that flew all over the world?

He shook his head. She had asked too many questions and he did not have time to think about the answers, at least not tonight. He would let things evolve for awhile. He missed her already.

He began again to type out his report to Dr. Nakasone and after an hour of typing and editing he printed his report.

TO: President Nakasone

FROM: Mr. Nacheda

SUBJ.: James Project Action Plan

OBJECTIVE: To develop a plan that will lead to a joint venture between James and Bandai that will utilize both companies' technological strengths for the improvement of patients' health while returning a reasonable profit that will be used for future growth to increase the return on investment to the shareholders of both companies.

NEGOTIATING POSITION: Bandai requires a negotiating position. It is recommended that the following action be taken to acquire a negotiating position favorable to Bandai:

Have Colonel Skip Howard meet Dr. J.P. Koenig and determine Dr. Koenig's role with James.

Analyze James Pharmaceutical Company.

Nacheda to visit the Alstonia spectabilis plantation on the island of Java in Indonesia to obtain more knowledge about the tree that is used by James.

Obtain enough of the Alstonia spectabilis tree bark so that experiments can be done to isolate the alkaloids using the Bandai extraction method.

Determine the results of the Bandai extraction process by documenting the purity of the alkaloids as compared to conventional methods of extraction.

Assuming Dr. Koenig is a strong contact executive, approach him with a proposal for James and Bandai to mutually work together on JPC138 leading to a product both companies could market in the global pharmaceutical market.

CONCLUSION:

This action plan will be adjusted to conditions. It is expected that negotiations will begin within four weeks. This timeframe is dependent on the Bandai experiments only taking one week. If this action plan is approved, I will oversee its implementation.

Nacheda placed the report on his desk. It was going to be a rough four weeks. He wondered when he would see Reiko again. If the plan were approved, he would call Reiko and explain that he would be gone for a while.

4:00 P.M., SUNDAY, FEBRUARY 19

LONEWOLF'S APARTMENT ANACORTES, WASHINGTON

The alarm on his computer interrupted his Sunday afternoon of watching the NBA game. Of course it was Monday morning in Japan and they didn't care about who was winning a basketball game. He got up from his recliner chair and went to the computer at his desk. It was an incoming encrypted email from NPC. He waited while the message was received by the computer and then gave his password so that the message could be decrypted. In a minute the message was on the screen:

TO: Lonewolf

FROM: Tanaguchi

SUBJ.: Project

NPC has made contact with James Executive Lonewolf to contact directly and meet executive ASAP. Call (215) 5553167 Immediately to arrange meeting. Provide information to originator immediately after the meeting for next action.

Information Required:

Does he have power to negotiate?

If not conclude contact. We will not waste our time.

Does he have anything of value to provide us? If so we want it immediately in order to establish his good faith to NPC.

What kind of deal does James want to cut?

Determine negotiating edge.

Who is he and who does he represent?

Lonewolf coded an acknowledgment and then went to the phone and dialed the telephone number in Pennsylvania. A woman answered. She sounded very old.

"Yes?" the woman replied.

Lonewolf answered "This is Mr. Smith is anyone there from James Pharmaceutical Company expecting a long distance phone call?"

There was silence on the line.

"Hello, is anyone there?" Lonewolf again spoke, but louder this time. "Yes?" she replied with the same response.

"Is anyone there expecting a phone call?" He was yelling into the phone. Damned old people. They should send them to a home to sleep off their remaining days, he thought.

Finally the old and tired woman's voice came through from Pennsylvania, "I am not expecting a phone call. Do you want me to ask my son if he is expecting a phone call?"

"Yes, please." The 'please' was strained.

Silence. Five minutes went by and Lonewolf was ready to hang up when a man's voice came on the phone.

The man said, "Yes, hello, is anyone there?"

"Yes," replied Lonewolf. "Are you expecting a phone call about James Pharmaceutical Company?"

"Yes, may I ask who is calling?"

"Mr. Smith. Have you requested a phone call," he then tried to trick him into revealing his name, "um, Mr ? May I have your name, please?"

"Yes Mr. Smith, I requested the telephone call and since you are Mr. Smith, I am Mr. Jones."

"Fine Mr. Jones." Lonewolf did not hold back the touch of anger in his voice at the man's response. Who the hell did this sneaky bastard think he was? He was about to sell out his company and he was playing smart-ass. Lonewolf tried to remain calm. He waited until his anger had subsided and then continued in a more controlled voice. "I was asked to contact you and to set up a meeting so that we could discuss the proposition you made to certain Japanese parties. I am available as early as tomorrow."

The response was fast. "No, that would not be good."

"Look Mr. Jones, or whatever your name is, I have other people to meet and I do not have time to mess around. You asked for the meeting not us. How about early Tuesday morning?"

"That would be fine Mr. Smith I apologize for the indecision. I am not very good at this sort of thing. I would like to meet in a small restaurant just north of the Pennsylvania town called New Hope. It is on the Delaware River. It is about 90 miles north of Philadelphia and 90 miles southeast of Newark. Would that restaurant be convenient?"

"Yes, where?"

"The restaurant is located in the Black Bass Hotel. It is on the right hand side of Pennsylvania State Route 32 as you go north. The name of the town is Lumberville. I will be in the restaurant sitting under a painting of King Henry V."

"Fine, I'll be there at 7:30, Tuesday morning. Should I ask for Mr. Jones?"

"Yes," he paused. "Yes, that would be fine. How will I know you Mr. Smith."

"I will have an American flag pin in my lapel," answered Lonewolf. "Goodbye. Mr. Jones."

"Good bye, Mr. Smith."

Lonewolf sent an encrypted message back to NPC telling them that the meeting was set for Tuesday morning.

7:15 A.M., MONDAY, FEBRUARY 20

BANDAI PHARMACEUTICAL COMPANY
BANDAI, JAPAN

Dr. Nakasone set down Nacheda's plan of action report and removed his reading glasses. He picked up his teacup and sipped the hot green tea. They were sitting at Dr. Nakasone's small conference table in front of the entrance to his private garden. The morning sun made the room unusually bright. Nacheda sat quietly with his hands in his lap. His long legs were crossed under the table. His head was bowed as Nakasone read the report and concentrated on its content. Almost five minutes went by before Dr. Nakasone spoke.

"Nachedasan look at me." Nacheda raised his head slightly but did not look into Nakasone's eyes. Nakasone continued "Not just your head, Nachedasan but also your eyes. I want to see your eyes. Please look into my eyes."

He slowly raised his eyes and then looked directly into Nakasone's dark brown eyes. He felt a deep warming in his heart. He saw a caring in Nakasone's eyes that he never realized was there. There was silence between the two as they looked beyond the others eyes and into each other's soul.

Nakasone spoke first.

"I know this is uncomfortable for you Nachedasan, but as you have discovered, I am different from other Japanese executives. It was the teachings of my father. He gave me the skills of both the West and the Samurai. He was not born a Samurai, but of simple farmer stock. When he lived in Japan he sought the teachings of a Samurai. When he lived in the United States he began to understand the teachings of the barbaric westerner. Can you guess what was the first thing my father taught me?"

"I couldn't guess, Dr. Nakasone."

"The first thing he taught me, Nachedasan, was that the west is not barbaric. My mother, being a westerner, also was a good teacher on the ways of the west. One of the things my mother taught me early in my life was, when you want true honesty between two people you must first look through their eyes. If the eyes and the feelings between the souls do not waiver then there is a bonding and a truth. I believe we have this truth bonding Nachedasan."

All during Nakasone's talk neither man blinked nor turned his head away. Nakasone continued, "For what I want to say to you next, it is vitally important that we have this truth bonding between men of spirit, between *shishi*. I know I don't have to ask, but I must, do we Nachedasan?"

"Hai, Shishou!"

"I will not put what I am going to say in writing, it is not necessary. You are not to tell another person what I will now say to you. Do you agree Nachedasan?"

"Hai, Shishou!"

"In my mind I have determined that one day you will occupy my chair. The efforts that you have already accomplished and those that you will accomplish will lead you to this end."

Nacheda started to respond but was stopped with the wave of the old man's arm. The sleeve of his ancient working kimono waving across the table like the flag of a Samurai. "I do not want you to answer me Nachedasan, for I have not asked you a question. Be quiet within yourself and with this knowledge do not change your ways. We will not speak of this conversation again until it is time. Do you understand Nachedasan?"

"Hail"

Nakasone slowly moved his eyes back to the report. His voice changed from teacher to stern businessman "This is a good report Nachedasan. I have thought about both this report and the report about James that you provided me last Friday. I have decided to proceed with this project. Your action plan is acceptable. Please keep me informed." He rose out of his sitting position on the mat.

Nacheda seeing that the meeting was over, unwrapped his legs and tried to get up as fast as he could while the blood rushed back into his legs.

Dr. Nakasone, seeing his displeasure remarked, "The seating pleasures of the western world have made your legs wobbly. Make sure your thoughts stay clear and replenished with fresh blood as you make your way towards the projects end." Nacheda looked once more into Nakasone eyes and he could see the smile that was not on his face, but was in his heart.

Nacheda slowly backed his way out the office door bowing all the way and making sure that he did not hit his head on the low door.

"*Doumoarigatou*, President Nakasone."

Dr. Nakasone sat down behind his desk. The same desk his father before him had sat when he founded Bandai Pharmaceuticals Company. He was very pleased. He turned to face the remembrance of his father and silently said, "Father, Bandai Pharmaceuticals

Company will survive." He turned back to his desk and began the business of the daily operations of his company.

Nacheda proceeded to his Bandai desk. He was bewildered. He sat down and looked at the other managers and employees in the large room. They were all busy at their work. He wanted to put his head down on his desk and think of Nakasone's words. He couldn't do this, as it would be inappropriate. He got up, put on his coat, and walked out of the building. He walked into a nearby park.

The trees were still bare of leaves. Last evening's snow flurries had lightly covered the park's decorative stones. Small green wooden picket fences surrounded each tree. Flakes of snow rested on the wires that held the pickets together. It is like life he thought. Each of us is a picket held together by the wires of communication. When communications are bad and the wires are cold the binding holding us together is cold. When the wires are warm there is love and understanding. We are all form a circle around the tree of life. We depend upon each other. One picket is President Nakasone and another myself. He looked at two of the pickets. The wire between them was covered with snow. As he watched, the morning sunrays hit the wire. The rays bounced off the snow crystals forming many tiny almost invisible rainbows.

As the snow slowly melted drop by drop, he thought of the conversation with Dr. Nakasone and his own future with Bandai. The snow continued to melt. A drop formed on the wire. It hung on to the wire as it gained enough weight to fall. It formed a tear as it hung and then dropped to the next lower wire...the tears of pain and happiness, which are shared between all of us. The drop formed a second time and fell to the next wire down. It was right to know that not one person is alone, but all sharing. Nacheda stared until all the snow on the wires had melted. He felt warm inside, he felt worthy.

Nacheda went back into the building. He drafted and sent an encrypted email to Skip via the computer in the Westwood condo. Skip would probably be back at the condo by 9:00 p.m. Sunday night or 2:00 p.m., Monday, Bandai time. He reread the message:

At 4:00 Nacheda heard the email notification alert sound on his computer.

Suggest you meet with him in Singapore. I can make arrangements.

Annie has nothing but good things to say about Koenig. I have attached a profile on Koenig that SAM provided. Most of the information comes from various Who's Who publications.

SAM alerted to obtaining your requested information and reports. Info should be available for transmission to you by Tuesday LA time. It would be earlier but I have to visit a broker library and get more information and scan it into SAM for analysis.

We are all still looking forward to a possible ski trip with your friend// Regards, Skip

Nacheda sent another message telling Skip to set up a meeting Monday evening, February 27th in Singapore. He also asked Skip to tell Dr. Koenig that he would wait in his room at the Raffles Hotel until Dr. Koenig called him to meet in the Raffles Bar.

Nacheda called the travel agent and made his flight arrangements from Tokyo to Singapore for Thursday returning on Thursday the second. He would have Friday through Monday to investigate the patient with the enhanced memory that was reported at the January task force meeting. He would also be able to track down the information and location of the Alstonia spectabilis tree plantation so he could visit the plantation and see this tree for himself.

Nacheda picked up the phone and called the corporate library and asked if they had any information on the Devil Tree. They informed him that they did not have a specific book on the tree, but there were many references to the tree in botany books. He decided he would read everything he could find on the Devil Tree.

1:00 P.M., MONDAY, FEBRUARY 20

SPECTRUM OF MEDICINE BUILDING
NEW YORK CITY

"Mandi, have you had lunch?" J.P. asked after she had answered his phone call.

"Nope, as a matter of fact, I have not had lunch," she answered softly. "How about lunch up here with me in Phillip' office. I'll update you on our trip to Singapore. Janet will have a sandwich sent up from the cafeteria. What would you like?"

"Corned beef on rye with an ice tea. I will be right up."

"Great. See you soon." J.P. hung up the phone and called Janet over the intercom and ordered lunch.

He got up from his chair, walked over to the window. It was a bright day. The sky was filled with cumulus clouds with large patches of blue sky peeking through. It reminded J.P. of a fall day rather than a late winter day. He could see the USS Intrepid tied up in its berth on the Hudson River. He saw chunks of ice floating down the river from upstream. Spring could not come too early for him. He hoped that by the time he and Mandi returned from their trip, spring would be more evident.

There was a knock on the door and Mandi entered before he could say come in.

"Hi." she said in her happiest voice and closed the door behind her and walked over to where he was standing. "How are you this sunny day?"

He had watched her walk across the room. It occurred to him just how lucky he was to be in love with such a beautiful woman. They kissed lightly. Mandi was wearing a dark coral colored blazer with a matching blouse and a dark skirt with a brown tinge. She wore a short string of cultured pearls with matching earrings.

"I am just great, Mandi. I still have a small tiredness from the party Saturday night." Instead of driving into the city, they had spent Sunday at Mandi's house. They both had massive hangovers and didn't want to do very much.

Mandi and J.P. continued to stand at the window for a while looking over the city.

"It's a beautiful day," Mandi remarked.

"It certainly is. I believe it's what they used to call a false spring."
"Really! A false spring?" she gazed out the window. "Do you like New York?"

"Yes," he replied pensively, "I think this is a great city. It only pains me that the people don't respect what they have. I have tried not to be stuffy and think of New York City as just romantic, financial, and cultural. It is a city of people. It is a shame many of the people that work in New York live outside of the city, but I guess that is a fact that will never change. Wouldn't it be great if everyone could live in the city that works in the city? They would live in beautiful neighborhoods together as one family of cultures, races, and nationalities because they all had pride in where they lived and worked."

She gave him a kiss on the cheek, "J.P., you are an eternal romantic optimist. Now, let's have lunch and talk about our trip to Singapore."

"Okay, I'll stop my day dreaming and come down to reality." They walked over the conference table and sat down.

Janet knocked and then entered. "Perfect timing Janet," J.P. said. "Did you bring your lunch as I suggested?"

"Yes, J.P., I have my lunch," she said with a smile. Mandi said. "Now what about Singapore?"

"Ah! Singapore. Romantic city of Asia. What do you think about Singapore, Janet?"

"I think you both should go to Singapore and enjoy yourselves. I also think you should stop by Mammoth and go skiing. As far as business is concerned, Phillip called this morning and said he would definitely be in the office part time starting Wednesday."

6:30 A.M., TUESDAY, FEBRUARY 21

BLACK BASS HOTEL LUMBERVILLE, PENNSYLVANIA

Lonewolf crossed the Delaware River on US Route 202. He had arrived on the East Coast the night before at Newark Airport and stayed the night at a small truckers' motel on US Route 1. He had left the motel early so he would not be late for his breakfast appointment with Mr. Jones. He glanced down at the map that the rental car agency had provided and noted that Pennsylvania State Route 32 would be the next turn off. He was to turn right on 32 after he crossed the 202 bridge.

He saw the Route 32 sign and made the quick right. The off ramp took him down to Route 32, a small road that ran along the western shore of the Delaware River. His car skidded a little as he made the sharp turn onto the road. There was snow on the sides of the road and a few icy patches. As he had crossed the 202 bridge, he noticed the river steadily flowing towards the Atlantic along with a good number of ice blocks.

He could not help to notice the beauty of the scenery. He felt like he was driving through a Courier and Ives painting. The homes along the Delaware River were built during the Revolutionary War period. They were built of stone and surrounded by farmland. Four-foot stone walls surrounded the fields. Barns were separate buildings. The homes were located close to the river to keep them cool in the summer and out of the westerly winds in the winter.

Some of the homes had been converted into art galleries, but the majority looked like occupied private homes. He wondered if Mr. Jones or whoever he was lived in one of these homes. It sure was a long way from New York City he thought to himself.

He saw the small sign that indicated that he was entering Lumberville, Pennsylvania, population 6,000. The river was about fifty yards to his right. Between the road and the river was the Delaware Canal. The Lumberville General Store appeared on his left. The store was the traditional white color, but was constructed of wood, not stone like the farmhouses. Most of the windows had shutters. In front of the store was one modern gas pump. He imagined how the store must have looked in the 1700's.

It was still relatively dark although the eastern sky was beginning to lighten with the rising sun. It looked as though it would be a clear day.

There were no other cars on the road. Just past the Lumberville General Store he saw on his left a sign for the Black Bass Hotel. It was a wooden sign hanging from a chain mounted on the top of beam attached to a wooden post. At the top of the sign, in black letters, was painted the words Black Bass and underneath the name, in red letters, the word Hotel. The sign was located in the corner of a small parking lot. He looked to his right and saw the old magnificent structure.

There were three other cars in the lot. He wondered if one of the cars might belong to Mr. Jones. He looked at his watch, it was 6:50. He was early so he decided to look around the outside of the hotel.

As he started across Route 32 he looked again at the Black Bass Hotel sign and for the first time that morning he smiled. The bottom of the sign was a checkered red and white tablecloth with two vases with flowers on each side of the sign. In between the two vases was the side profile of a black bass fish. It was standing on its tail and smoking a cigar. Cigar smoke was spiraling upward between the T and E of the word Hotel. Held in the left fin of the fish was a walking stick. Lonewolf actually laughed out loud. Someone had a sense of humor. He looked over at the large two story wooden building built in much the same style as the general store. Each window had two green shutters. It was a long building, perhaps as long as a football field.

Lonewolf walked around to the left of the building where he noticed a footbridge over to a small island located in the middle of the river. He walked to the middle of the footbridge so that he could carefully examine the back of the hotel. He wasn't doing this just to be sightseeing. Whenever he had a meeting with someone he did not know he wanted to know the surrounding area. There was always the chance of a trap or the need for an escape route.

After taking one look at the back of the hotel he saw how just viewing the front could deceive a person. The hotel was on the slope of the riverbank down to the canal. The hotel was actually four stories not two. The two floors below road level were built into the side of the slope. The structure was all wood. There was a sharp drop off from the bottom floor of the hotel to the canal.

He read a sign on the footbridge. The sign reported that the Delaware Canal was built in the early to mid-19th Century and transported millions of tons of anthracite coal and other cargo to Philadelphia. The construction of the canal route made it possible for the canal barges to pull right up to the hotel to offload supplies and take on or leave off guests for the Black Bass.

Lonewolf returned to the front of the hotel and entered the small entrance. To his left was the small reception room where guests registered. At the rear of the reception room was a fireplace. In the fireplace was a roaring fire. He noted that someone had been up and about and had rebuilt the fire with a fresh load of firewood. He walked through the hall and turned right into what seemed to be an area where there were dining tables. Straight ahead was a sun room that overlooked the river. It was empty of furniture. A sign on the doorway indicated that this room was closed for the winter. He continued into the next room. This small room had tables. There was another fireplace, but the fire in here was not roaring but was a gentle, warm fire that had been fueled with only a few logs.

He looked at the walls. There were paintings of British Royalty from the time of the American Revolution. He then saw a table in the right hand corner of the room against a window. Above the table hung a portrait of King Henry V. Next to the painting was the royal shield and another painting. There was no one at the designated meeting table. He walked into the adjacent room where the bar was located and sat at a barstool. Both the dining room and bar were paneled in dark wood with many paintings and photographs of the past. On the far wall of the bar was a glass case with displays of artifacts of the past. Mr. Jones sure knew how to pick an out of way location.

A waiter or bartender emerged from another entrance to the bar. He was a young man. He wore a costume from the revolutionary era and a long white apron tied around the waist.

"Good Morning, sir," the young man greeted him. "Breakfast for one?" "No," replied Lonewolf. "I am waiting for someone to join me. Has anyone else been here this morning?"

"No sir, but the morning crowd will start arriving in the next few minutes. Usually 10 to 15 people stop by for morning scrabble. Would you like to be seated and have a cup of coffee while you wait for your friend?"

"What is scrabble?" asked Lonewolf.

"A Philadelphia breakfast sausage. It is very good and we are famous for it here at the Black Bass."

"Thank you. Yes, I will have a seat and a cup of coffee. I would like to sit at that table over there under the painting of Henry V. My friend wanted to sit at that table. He is scheduled to arrive at 7:30."

"No trouble sir. Please take a seat. I will have your coffee in a second.

Do you want to wait to order breakfast?" "Yes."

Lonewolf look at his watch, 7:15. A few early morning commuters started arriving as the waiter said they would. No one looked like a pharmaceutical executive. At exactly 7:30 he saw the person he believed to be Jones walk in. He looked nervous. Jones looked to the right and saw Lonewolf sitting at the table with his back against the wall. Jones slowly walked over to the table. He nervously looked around the room and at the other people in the small restaurant.

Lonewolf remained seated as Jones walked up to the table. Before Jones spoke Lonewolf said, "Good morning, Mr. Jones." They both took measure of each other. The executive now looked scared as well as nervous. For some reason he kept looking around the room.

"Hello, Mr. Smith," the James executive replied. "Please sit down directly across from me, Mr. Jones."

The heavyset man sat down and they both ordered breakfast. Neither spoke. They ate their breakfast without saying anything to each other. Lonewolf tried the scrabble. It was good.

Lonewolf waited for Jones to speak first. He had all day. He could wait.

He ordered a second helping of scrabble.

Finally Jones, after wiping egg from the corners of his mouth, spoke.

Lonewolf looked at his watch, 8:30.

"Mr. Smith, I represent a member of the James Pharmaceutical Board of Directors." He spoke in a low whisper. His eyes started darting back and forth as if they were a radar scanning for a target. Lonewolf commented to himself that this nervous action was comical because the man was staring at the wall. The occupants of the restaurant were behind him.

"Mr. Jones, stop being so nervous. No one knows who I am and if anyone recognizes you they will stop by and you can introduce me as a business associate. Now first, I want to know the name of who you represent."

"I can't disclose this information, Mr. Smith."

"Mr. Jones, let me be perfectly clear with my intentions and then I will demand that you stop playing games." Lonewolf reached his right hand across the table and placed it on top of Mr. Jones' fisted left hand. Lonewolf started to squeeze the man's fist as he continued his lecture.

"You asked for this meeting we didn't. You are asking for our help. We didn't solicit your help." Lonewolf squeezed until he saw pain on the man's face and then he eased up. "I do not have to tell you anything and you have to tell me whatever I want to know or I leave immediately. Is that clear?" He squeezed harder.

"Yes, Mr. Smith, I understand."

"Now, Mr. Jones, who do you represent?" Lonewolf asked.

Mr. Jones drew extra strength from within himself to gain some measure of confidence and stated, "If you stop squeezing my hand, I will make a phone call and obtain permission to disclose the information that you desire."

Lonewolf released his hand, "Okay, but make it fast and stay within visual sight."

Mr. Jones went to the phone on the bar. It looked like he asked the waiter if he could use the telephone. The waiter must have said yes because he started to dial. Lonewolf watched the number of times that he punched the dialing surface. There was eleven times and then a pause and nine more times. Lonewolf noted that the call was to a long distance number and that he had used a credit card. Mr. Jones came back in about three minutes. He initiated the conversation.

"The person I represent is Mrs. Evelyn PrestonJames, the Chairman of the Board of the James Pharmaceutical Company," he stated confidently.

Lonewolf thought to himself, bingo. He answered in an agitated voice,

"Okay, so go on."

"Mrs. James would like to sell her James Pharmaceutical interests to a qualified buyer. She basically wants to leave the business and she wants to make a great deal of money in the process. There are others who want out and will be willing to sell you their shares. We are working on a major product release and our Lifeal antiarrhythmia product is beginning to show real promise in the cardiac market. James share price was $35 at yesterday's close of the New York Stock Exchange. This represented only a ten times earnings. With what we know about the future, the stock is undervalued. Its market value should be a thirty or more times earnings like the rest of the pharmaceutical stocks. If you paid $70 per share or 20 times earnings the people you represent would be getting an excellent bargain."

Mr. Jones was becoming excited over his dissertation. The room was hot from their nearness to the fireplace. Sweat began to accumulate in little beads on his brow. His sweat beads had not started to run. He was speaking twice as fast as he had when he began the report.

Mentally, Jones began to count the money he would make on the sale of James and what he would do with the money. 100,000 shares at $70 equaled $7,000,000. God, what a win. I could do anything

I wanted. The beads of sweat started to run down his face. A drop rolled over his eyebrow and dripped onto the tablecloth leaving a wet spot next to his plate. The drops of sweat started to fall down his face in a regular stream until he wiped his brow with his napkin.

During this brief pause, Lonewolf stared at Jones. His light blue steel eyes were piercing into Jones' eyes. Jones interpreted the intense stare as sincere interest in what he was saying. He thought to himself 'who said I could not sell?' He rolled on and decided to push Smith.

"Time is important, Mr. Smith. We are at a critical point in our product development and management will be making an announcement that could possibly increase the market value and stock price. This will cause us to reevaluate this proposal upward. So you should tell your people we are ready to negotiate. We would like to close the deal prior to the annual meeting in May. There is a great deal of paper work to be completed before the board meeting in April." In a cavalier manner, he added, "What do you think?"

Jones leaned back in his chair somewhat relaxed for the first time since he had sat down. He had a smirk on his face that said to Lonewolf, 'so there Mr. Smith take it or leave it.' He also made sure his hands were in his lap so that Smith could not hurt him again.

Lonewolf continued his intense stare into Jones' eyes. The flames of the fire had picked up and they reflected the short fifteen feet into Smith's eyes and across his face. There was silence for a long moment. Then, in a low voice that sounded more like a growl he replied to Jones question, "You pompous, sanctimonious, obnoxious, arrogant asshole." Lonewolf had spoken so softly that Jones was sure he did not hear what Lonewolf had said. He leaned forward to hear better. Jones' smirk turned into a smile.

"I'm sorry, Mr. Smith. I did not hear your answer."

Jones made the mistake of again placing his hands on the table. Lonewolf reached across the table and again grabbed Jones left hand and started to squeeze. This time the hand was not in a fist and the pain immediately appeared on Jones' face.

Lonewolf repeated what he had said but in a voice that Jones could not help but hear, "I said you are a pompous, sanctimonious, obnoxious, arrogant asshole." His voice and words shattered Jones face like a hammer hitting a plaster mask. His lips began to quiver and his eyes opened wide. He now saw the look in Smith's eyes and the fire dancing on his face as Smith squeezed harder. Sweat increased again in pools on his brow. This time he did not wipe them away, he couldn't wipe them away.

Jones started to stammer. "But...but...Mr. Smith what do you mean calling me these terrible names. I don't understand."

Lonewolf was silent. He let Jones sweat.

Finally he said, "Look Jones, or whoever the fuck you are, you do not know what the hell you are talking about. Let me give you the facts of life. I am going to be brief and I will say this only once. You had better listen very closely.

"Since you seem to think you have all the facts, Jones and they are, in fact, fucked up you had better take notes." Smith paused and released his grip on Jones hand.

Jones immediately pulled back his hand and started to rub the pain away. He rubbed above the table and then thought better of it and placed his hands in his lap continuing to rub the pain away. He wanted to get his hands away from this mad man.

As calmly as he could, Jones answered Smith's challenge. "I still do not understand your threats nor the reason for you causing me pain. I am not sure whether I should sit here and continue to take this verbal and physical abuse."

A fraction of Jones' confidence came back into his voice. Jones was not a coward, but he had never been faced with the situation he now found himself living. He looked around the room for help. The rest of the room was normal. No one had noticed the exchange of the men sitting beneath the painting of King Henry V.

Lonewolf answered Jones' statement by swiftly pushing the table against Jones and throwing his napkin on to the table. "I will save you the trouble of instructing you in the position your company is in, Jones. I will leave. You requested this meeting and I am ending it." He rose to leave.

Jones face went pale. Oh my God, he thought. I have blown this deal. He panicked and started to beg. "Oh please, Mr. Smith, I am sorry. Please stay. Yes. Yes," he stammered. "Yes.yes, perhaps I do not have my information straight. Please give me your points of negotiation and I will certainly take notes." The sweat was pouring off of his forehead. His underarm sweat had soaked through his suit. The wet stain on his suit coat was two inches over the front of his suit coat and continuing to spread.

Lonewolf stopped his movement to leave. He had this dumb son of a bitch right where he wanted him. He shivered with the pleasure of the thought that he had reduced this bagofshit to a whimpering slave. He stood for a long minute listening to Jones whine.

Lonewolf sat down. Jones immediately pushed the table back to its original position and placed his hands beneath the table. Lonewolf began. Jones took out a small pad of paper and a pen. He was prepared to write, but he would write below the table.

Lonewolf continued "These are the facts, Jones. One, James Pharmaceutical Company is in deep trouble. Your President was shot by someone overdosed on the product you said was beginning to show promise.

Bullshit. Lifeal is in trouble. You have not even come close to your projections and Wall Street is down on the product and the company. Two, your new product, JPC138 is in trouble. James can not successfully complete the clinicals because the compound is not pure. Three, the company does not have enough working capital to have a future. In fact, I would imagine that you are going to have to start cutting expenses because of a lack of cash flow. Four, management and the board are at war. Here you are a member of management, representing the Chairman of the Board. Where is the President? Jones, you gave me a line of bullshit and expected me to believe you. Not only that, which is an insult to my intelligence, but you expected me to make an ass out of myself by giving your story to the investors that I represent. Mister you are not only a jerk, but you are a dumb jerk." Lonewolf paused.

Jones was even paler than when he sat down with his winter pallor, if that was possible. He wondered where Smith had gotten his information. Jones finally found the courage to speak and in a strong confident voice that he certainly did not feel he said, "I am very sorry Mr. Smith. Please forgive my arrogance. What can I do to repair the situation?"

"That is a much better attitude, Mr. Jones." Lonewolf smiled. He had tricked Jones with an effective offense.

Lonewolf continued in a pleasant normal voice. "I don't have the authority to counter your offer, but I can state that we are not prepared to pay any invalid price based on perceived market value. We know Mrs. James' stock options are all below $10 and if we purchase the stock at anything above $10 a share she makes a good profit because of the number of shares she controls. She also doesn't give a damn if the rest of you parasites make any money. So prepare yourself for a price below market value."

Jones again went pale. His options and average share price for holdings were all above $20.00.

Lonewolf went on, "I believe that you were to provide me with a written document. If you are interested in continuing our discussion on a buyout I must have a document to provide proof to the people I represent of your good will. If you do not want to provide the document our conversation is over and I am leaving.

"No, no, Mr. Smith. I, we, are still interested in talking with you. I have the document right here in my suit coat pocket." Jones reached into his inside suit pocket and pulled out a folded copy of the 21st Century Plan. It was visibly wet from Jones' sweat. "Here is a copy of the James strategic plan. We called it the 21st Century Plan." He paused, mustering up the courage for his next request, "I would respectfully request that you keep this plan a secret and not disclose the information to anyone except the potential investors."

"I promise," Lonewolf lied.

"Fine, here is the plan." Jones handed the plan across the table with the left hand that was still deep red from the squeezing.

Lonewolf let the plan hang in the air for a long moment and then gently took the plan from Jones. Jones held the plan tightly for a second and then let it go, his honorable and loyal service to James Pharmaceutical now at an end.

"Thank you Mr. Jones. Please tell Mrs. James that she will hear from us by the end of the week." Lonewolf could barely contain himself. What a bunch of idiots, he thought. With this plan I now have the negotiating ammunition I need to bargain them down in price. What idiots they are. This was too easy. Mr. Tanaguchi will be pleased. He pushed the table back against Jones and got up.

"Thank you Mr. Jones."

"Yes, Mr. Smith. We look forward to your response."

Lonewolf walked out of the restaurant and got into his car. He drove out of the parking lot onto State Route 32, turned left and pulled up to the gas pump in front of the Lumberville General Store as if he were going to purchase gas. It was a self-service pump so he knew no one would bother him, at least for a little while. Now he could watch Jones and see where he drove after he left the Black Bass Hotel.

Meanwhile Jones was still sitting at the table. He began to shake uncontrollably. His hand reached for his cold coffee and the cup chattered against the saucer. The chattering got so loud that the waiter started to come over to offer his assistance. Jones looked as if he were in a catatonic state of shock. He was staring at the door where Smith had made his exit. His hand was completely out of control. The waiter walked over to the side of the table so he could get a full view of his customer. Once he saw his customer's face he stepped back. The customer looked as if he was having a heart attack.

"Sir, is everything all right?" He asked with a mixture of fear and anticipation. "Sir, sir.," he repeated. There was still no answer from Jones' bluish colored lips. "Sir," the waiter said much louder than before. The rest of the customers now turned to look at the man sitting at the table under the portrait of King Henry V. They heard his chattering cup, but could not see his face.

Jones' eyes slowly focused on the waiter. "Sorry, did you say something?" he mumbled.

"I asked if you were all right?"

"No," he replied. He jumped up from the table grabbing his napkin and began vomiting before he reached the door and the fresh winter air of the outside world.

Lonewolf watched Jones as he bent over a snowdrift. It was obvious that Jones was in a convulsive state and was vomiting into the snow.

A smile came to Smith's face. Damn it, he thought. I am good at causing pain and I enjoy it so very much.

It was a good ten minutes before Jones collected himself. The waiter had brought out Jones' coat and came out a second time to ensure that he was all right. Jones walked across 32 and got into his car. He did not look in either direction. Smith could of parked right in front of Jones and he would not have seen him. Jones turned left and drove north on 32. Smith made a tight U-turn and followed Jones.

Jones continued on 32 to Point Pleasant and turned northeast on Tohickon Hill Rd. At the first fork he took a left on to State Park Road. Snow was banked on both sides of the road. If they met a car there would be barely enough room for them to pass without rubbing the snow drifts which were over six foot in height. A sign stating that they were passing the Ralph Stover State Park passed down the right side of the car. He turned left onto Stover Park Road and after a mile, Jones turned right into what looked like a long driveway. It was lined with tall pine trees.

As Jones turned right into the wooded drive, Lonewolf stopped and took note of the names on the mailboxes on the side of the road. There were five metal mailboxes. Only four had names. Smith took out his map and jotted down the route they had taken. He then retraced his drive back to 32 and proceeded to Newark International Airport to catch a plane back to Seattle.

Once home he sent a ten page secret email to NPC describing the day's events. Confirmation of the message came through in the prescribed time. Fifteen minutes later the order from NPC came through to his computer and was decrypted.

His screen read:

TO: Lonewolf

FROM: Tanaguchi

SUBJ: Project

Proceed to NPC via the fastest means available. Tanaguchi

Lonewolf called his travel agent and booked a Wednesday flight to Osaka.

11:00 A.M., WEDNESDAY, FEBRUARY 22
SPECTRUM OF MEDICINE BUILDING
NEW YORK CITY

"Good morning, Annie. Happy George Washington's birthday."

"A good morning to you too, Dr. Koenig. And how is the great east?" Annie responded enthusiastically.

'The great east is just great madam and today even greater. Today I am to be relieved of my president duties."

"What do you mean J.P., to be relieved? You sound like you have found a soul saving religion. I do know you, my love, and a soul saving religion just doesn't fit your psyche."

He laughed, "Only you would associate my happiness with a soul saving religion. I think you have some Freudian belief that my soul requires saving." "Well," Annie replied softly, "you have been in the big city for a very long time."

"Annie, stop with your joking. I am being relieved because Phillip comes back to work this afternoon and will reassume the role of president of James Pharmaceutical Company."

"That's great J.P. Now what about your trip to Singapore and Mammoth?"

'The trip is on Annie. We leave on Friday and plan to be in Mammoth the following Friday. How does that sound?"

"That sounds fine, J.P. I'll tell Skip. Will you be able to fly Skip up with you?"

"No problem. Now how are things in Mammoth?"

"Before I tell you about Mammoth, Skip would like to talk to you about Singapore."

"What does Skip have to do with Singapore?" he asked.

"I really don't know, J.P., but he wants to talk to you about meeting someone in Singapore. Will you call him?"

"Right now. What's his number?"

Annie gave him Skip's number and then proceeded to give him all the news from Mammoth. She informed him that everything was fine with his house and that the skiing was still great and would likely last through Memorial Day. J.P. was only half listening to her. He kept wondering about Skip's connection to Singapore. He sighed, thinking to himself that nothing was ever easy when it came to James Pharmaceutical. At any rate, he would call just has soon as he was done with Annie. After a report on his Great Western Books club, she was finished.

"Annie, I'll see you soon."

"Enjoy your trip, J.P. Call me when you have your final plans." He dialed Skip's number in Los Angeles.

"Howard," came the deep voice after the phone had been answered.

"Colonel Howard, J.P. Koenig here, Annie's friend from Mammoth.

Annie said you wanted to talk to me about Singapore."

"Dr. Koenig, please call me Skip." "And I, J.P., what's up?"

"Well, it's a long story that I will not bore you with unless it is necessary. It's not that I don't want to tell yo u. I have no problem with you knowing, but it is a long story and it deserves sitting over a few beers at Annie's Bar and Grill. Which, by the way, I hear we will be doing very soon."

"We will try Skip. Now give me the short version. Any friend of Annie's can be trusted by me."

"J.P., I wasn't completely honest with you in Mammoth." "I assumed so," he replied.

"Yeah!" he laughed. "We were two middle-aged bulls circling for territory."

"A good analogy," J.P. joined his laughter.

"Well, I have been working on a very secret project for a year with a group of old friends. We are all healthcare experts in one way or another so we undertook a project to find a U.S. company to work with on new products."

"Why would you want a U.S. company?"

"One of our friends represents a company that is looking for a research partner and the name James Pharmaceutical Company came up as a viable candidate."

"That is unusual, Skip. We have nothing to offer."

"You would be surprised, J.P. I believe you have a product in research with a compound name of JPC138?"

A chill ran through J.P., "What? My first instinct here, Skip, is to deny everything and terminate this conversation. You'd better get to what it is exactly that you want and quickly. How did you know this and how did you find out about JPC138?" The missing copy of the 21st Century Plan came quickly to his mind.

"That is part of the long version, J.P. In summary, we put together twelve months of computer research and with the parameters we were seeking, James came out a candidate. If you are thinking corporate espionage, it was not used," Skip came back with concern in his voice.

"You know, Skip, I'm going to be very up front with you. A very valuable piece of information was stolen from the James corporate office last fall. Does this have anything to do with this incident?" J.P.'s voice was slightly threatening.

"J.P., I can tell by your voice this theft is very important to you. I assure you that we received no information directly from James. Believe me, if we had access to this important information last fall, it wouldn't have taken until this month to identify James as a viable candidate. We arrived at James from published information and a very sophisticated artificial intelligence computer that I would be happy to show you when you visit Westwood Village."

"Why do you want a research partner?" he asked, still skeptical.

"We have access to certain research that needs a partner with a specific profile. James has the profile. Believe me it is an honorable project. Everything here is above board," he paused. "I know I have been using the word believe too many times, but it is the only word I can think of to describe the situation."

"Okay, I guess I have to believe you. So what does this have to do with Singapore?"

"Well, the leader of our group will be in Singapore at the same time you are. There he would like to meet with you and explain more about a potential partnership."

"This is real coincidence." Or is it, he thought to himself. "You know, I have no official authority with James."

"We know, but you are well respected by Dr. Bradsmith. We would like your opinion. Mr. Nachedawill explain."

"Mr. who? And who does he represent?" the intrigue was beginning to get to J.P.

"Mr. Nacheda is his name and he represents a Japanese pharmaceutical company. I will give you the name, but it is a secret so I must ask you for secrecy."

"Skip, this is a little too James Bondish for me. Look, you have the blessings of Annie, whom I respect very much. I have listened so far because of her faith in you, but the story is getting a little complex for the telephone."

"I understand. I know I am taking advantage of our mutual friend and this conversation is also making me feel uncomfortable. Please bear with me another moment."

"Okay."

'The name of the company is Bandai Pharmaceuticals Company," Skip replied to his previous question.

"Bandai, as in Bandai, Japan?"

"Yes, you know the company?" asked Skip.

"No. I have never heard of Bandai Pharmaceuticals Company, but I have heard of Bandai. I skied there once. Along time ago."

"Really? I have never been there," replied Skip.

"Well, I have never heard of Bandai Pharmaceuticals Company," he repeated.

"It is a small pharmaceutical company that is outside the usual politics of Japanese pharmaceutical companies."

"I would imagine," J.P. mused. "So this Mr. Nacheda wants to see me in Singapore?"

"Yes, if possible on Monday evening February 27th at the Raffles Bar.

Annie said you would probably be staying at the Raffles."

"I'm beginning to think that Annie knows me too well," J.P. said with a laugh. "Yes, that is where I'll be staying. How do I contact this Mr. Nacheda?"

"Mr. Nacheda is also staying at the Raffles and indicated that he will remain in his room Monday evening until you call and set up a meeting. Is this satisfactory?"

"Agreed, Skip. Is there anything else you want to tell me?"

"No. I look forward to seeing you in Mammoth. I know this conversation has strained our potential friendship, but it is only because I can't explain the situation properly. I am sure that by the time we meet in Mammoth you will understand and any concerns you have, will be alleviated."

"I hope so. I'll see you in a few weeks, oh by the way, I'll give you call again before we land in LA, you're welcome to fly to Mammoth with Mandi and I. Tell Mr. Nacheda, I'll give him a call Monday evening."

"Thanks, J.P. Bye." "Bye."

J.P. leaned back in his chair and placed his hands behind his head. Did this have something to do with the 21st Century Plan? Well, one way or another it is new information. He was worried that he had hit a dead-end after the formula issue. Now at least there is something that could be related to the project. He thought it was a little ironic that he was there at James to find out why someone had made a copy of the plan and in the process there had been an unrelated shooting, a stolen Lifeal formula, and an emerging board of directors battle, all seeming to have nothing to do with the 21st Century Plan.

Maybe Singapore will provide more answers than questions.

8:30 A.M. PST, WEDNESDAY, FEBRUARY 22
WESTWOOD VILLAGE, CA

Skip hung up the telephone and went to his computer to send an encrypted e-mail to Nacheda.

TO: Nacheda

FROM: Skip

Just completed phone conversation with Dr. Koenig. He will contact you in your room the evening of Monday 27 February.

He informed me that last fall a copy of their strategic plan was stolen. He was very suspicious of my connection with you. You will have to win his confidence. He said he has skied Bandai.

Information you requested is on the way./ Regards, Skip

8:00 P.M., THURSDAY, FEBRUARY 23
JAMES FARM, GREYSTONE HALL SEAFORD, NEW YORK

"Well?" she said after he rolled off of her. "Well, what?" he responded.

"Cut the crap, you know damn well what!" she yelled. God, she had to get rid of him. She should bring up business before the sex.

Then she wouldn't have to endure him. Yes, except that she needed sex and he was safe. If she really thought about this situation she would have to admit she looked forward to the sex. That is until the sex was over and then she regretted having even touched him. In a few months it would be over. She would endure.

"As planned, I met with Mr. Smith last Tuesday in Pennsylvania," he replied cautiously.

"Well, what did he say? Why do I have to pull everything out of you?

Why don't you just give me the information?" she said frustrated.

He knew why he was stalling. She was not going to like what Mr. Smith proposed. She was depending on the negotiations to be based on the stock market value, not her average price per share. He remained quiet not knowing how to approach the subject.

"What did he say when you told him that you represented me?" she continued. She had moved to a sitting position with the sheet covering her body to her waist. She knew that her nudity was distracting to him.

She had now asked him a question that gave him a way to explain the deal. "They said I was an acceptable negotiator. I then presented our deal."

"Well, what was his answer? Damn you! Come on, out with it." She started to raise her voice and bounce up and down with excited anticipation.

He watched her breasts bounce up and down. Her body mesmerized him. "You won't like it," he said softly.

"What do you mean, I won't like it?" she took her hand and slapped him across the face. "Wake your brain up and pay attention to this conversation, damn you. Are you brain dead? If you screwed up this deal, after I get through with you, you might truly be brain dead."

He rubbed his face. He was now fully alert and stopped watching her breasts and looked into her eyes. There was definitely evil in those eyes. He sat up in bed. He reached down to where he had thrown his pants when he had climbed in to her bed for their sexual romp. A romp that was becoming more psychologically costly every visit. His thoughts were basically the same as hers. In a few months it would be over. He would endure.

He picked up his pants and searched the pockets to find the piece of paper Mr. Smith made him write at the hotel meeting.

In a very business-like manner he started his report. "After I had given him the terms of the deal at $70 per share, he didn't talk for a few minutes. I thought he was thinking about the terms so I didn't say anything. When he broke the silence, his first words called me a pompous, sanctimonious, obnoxious, and arrogant asshole."

"What? What did you do to deserve him calling you those names?" she asked more calmly. Shocked by the words this man spoke and words that might follow the profanity.

"I told you, I gave him the deal that we had decided upon." He emphasized the 'we'.

"What then?" she ignored his answer.

"He then gave me the facts he had on James. These facts refuted everything I had said. I now quote him because he made me write it down." He read from the piece of paper. "One, James Pharmaceutical Company is in deep trouble. Your president was shot by someone overdosed on the product you said was beginning to show promise. Bullshit. Lifeal is in trouble. You haven't even come close to your projections and Wall Street is down on the product and the company. Two, your new product, JPC138 is in trouble. James can not successfully complete the clinicals because the compound is not pure. Three, the company does not have enough working capital to have a future. In fact I would imagine you are going to have to start cutting expenses because of a lack of cash flow. Four, management and the board are at war." He looked up from the paper.

Then he went on looking at her facial expressions, "Mr. Smith then wondered why the president was not negotiating instead of a representative of the chairman of the board. He said I gave him a line of bullshit when I had presented the status of the company in my explanation of our deal. Then he said I insulted his intelligence by expecting him to make an ass out of himself by giving our story to the investors he represented."

He again looked down at the paper. "He said he didn't have the authority to counter our offer, but he could state that they are not prepared to pay market value. They knew your stock and options were all below $10 and if they purchased the stock at anything above $10 a share you stand to make a good profit because of the number of shares you control. He also said, and I quote again, 'She doesn't give a damn if the rest of you parasites make any money. So prepare yourselves for a price below market value'."

She was shocked. She tried to hide it from him. Her mind was racing ahead. So her deal wasn't going to fly. She wasn't dealing with fools. She had to think. The deal wasn't dead. She would make money even at a deal below what she had offered. She knew it wouldn't be $10.00. They also wanted James and they wouldn't blow the deal with a very low price.

He was sitting quietly waiting for her response when she jumped up from bed and put on her robe. She acted as though he wasn't even in the room. Just has she was about to leave the room she remembered his presence. She opened the bedroom door and pointed at him still sitting on the bed in the nude. "You, out. You can put on your clothes in the car."

He tried to protest, "You can't just kick me out."

"I can't, I can't? I just kicked you out. Now get lost. Call me if anything happens."

He got out of bed holding his clothes in front of him and walked out like a whipped puppy that had just peed the floor.

After he had left she walked to the den and sat down at her desk. She started to calculate a new deal. The wind off the Atlantic made its way up the bay and around the house. It was brisk this evening. The shutters squeaked and there was a low whistling as some of the wind forced its way through the cracks in the walls. The sounds weren't spooky to Mrs. Evelyn PrestonJames. It was music to her ears and reminded her of Doc. What would Doc do in this negotiation? She laughed. He wouldn't be in this kind of negotiation. He would ride his Titanic company to the bottom. Well, not me. She went back to her calculations as the night winds increased.

12:00 P.M., FRIDAY, FEBRUARY 24
NIPPON PHARMACEUTICAL COUNCIL OSAKA, JAPAN

Lonewolf finished briefing Mr. Tanaguchi on his last two months of activities. Tanaguchi had also read through the 21st Century Plan, which Lonewolf had gotten from Mr. Jones. Tanaguchi asked many questions and Lonewolf was becoming impatient. He wanted action. He looked over at his client. Tanaguchi was taller than most Japanese men, at just over six feet tall. He wore a dark business suit, white shirt, and a dark tie with a faint design that Lonewolf could not make out across the distance from where Tanaguchi sat. They were sitting at a large conference table. Tanaguchi looked at Lonewolf and smiled. It was a smile of an actor, it was not sincere.

"Lonewolf-san, we pay you a great deal of money to have you find out simple information. Is this not true?"

Here it comes, Lonewolf thought. The try at renegotiating him down in the middle of the contract. He had been in this situation before. Tanaguchi had to negotiate. He was being set up for a compromise. He had learned to live with Tanaguchi's 'you loose, I win' philosophy. He had learned to live with it, but that did not mean that he had to like it. In fact he hated it.

Lonewolf handled the situation by an offensive countercharge.

He replied, "Yes Tanaguchisan I make good money, but it is not simple information you ask for and it is not easy to obtain. You would not have this information if I did not have special talents. In fact I am thinking I must have more money. You had wanted only information at the beginning of this project but you have me involved in a bigger project and you will make millions off the James potential. I now would like an additional $2,000,000 making the total $4,000,000 US." Tanaguchi did not know that Lonewolf had to split the fee with his agent in Vietnam and besides it was not Tanaguchi's business.

Tanaguchi's face took on a slight red tint. He did not like offensive counteroffers. He was used to people he controlled being submissive. He did not like Lonewolf's challenge.

He countered, "The agreement stands. Our contract was for $2,000,000 when the project is completed and we have a deal with a pharmaceutical company in the United States. This contract is not open for negotiation."

Lonewolf leaned back in his chair. He was pleased with himself that he had managed to outmaneuver Tanaguchi. Not only had he had kept Tanaguchi from negotiating a lower contract, but he had also found out a number of things. First, Tanaguchi knew that what Lonewolf was doing was worth a great deal of money. If he had thought otherwise he would of fought harder to reduce Lonewolfs fee. Second, Tanaguchi needed Lonewolf or he would have ended the contract without paying and gotten someone else to do the remaining work.

Somehow he would get Tanaguchi to pay more for his work, but not today. The gamesmanship was over. All he now wanted was to get going on the next phase of the project.

Tanaguchi continued "After your briefing and reading the 21st Century Plan, I have evaluated that you must leave immediately for Indonesia via Singapore to visit the plantation where they grow this Devil Tree. Here you will meet with a Mr. Chang, Jr. You will negotiate a contract he can not refuse. The contract will be for exclusive worldwide rights to his total production of the Devil Tree bark. You will not fail in re-negotiating the Devil Tree contract. Price is no object. We must gain control of the raw material necessary for James to succeed. With the raw material contract we will name the buy-out price for James stock. Whoever this Mr. Jones is and what he stands for, is irrelevant. From this point forward we will deal only with Mrs. James. As far as we are concerned there is no Mr. Jones." Tanaguchi paused and then shifted subjects.

"Can you leave for Singapore on Monday?" he asked Lonewolf.

"I can leave immediately," replied Lonewolf. The adrenaline starting to pump.

"Good. You have a first class airline reservation on the 6:00 p.m. JAL flight leaving from Tokyo to Singapore on Saturday. You will leave Osaka at 3:00 p.m. on our private jet. The specifics on how to proceed from Singapore to the island of Java will be given to you by one of our people that will meet your flight Sunday morning. I must also warn you that your friend Nachedasan is on his way to Singapore. His objective, we believe, is to locate and tour the plantation although it is not clear as to why he to is en route to Indonesia via Singapore. We also believe it is his objective to acquire the same information we seek, but he is not going to negotiate a contract for Bandai Pharmaceutical Company. Do not worry about Nacheda-san, Lonewolf, but be cautious of a possible contact with him.

"You will stay with our people Sunday night and leave for the plantation on Monday morning for your appointment with Mr. Chang, Jr. at noon. Do not fail, Lonewolf-san. The plans for your success have been laid out very carefully. There should be no, how do you Americans say it.no hitches, I believe. Yes, there should be no hitches."

"I am looking forward to the trip Mr. Tanaguchi. Is it possible to leave earlier?" Lonewolf could not keep the excitement out of his voice.

"No, Lonewolf-san, it is as it is. What we have done so far has been faster than what is considered normal business time. It is also not wise for you to be in Singapore or Indonesia any longer than necessary. An encounter with Nachedasan would be quite unfortunate. To prevent you from becoming bored we will take you to an inn we have rented outside Kyoto on Lake Biwa. We will provide enhancements for all of your senses. I am sure you will be quite pleased. The time before your Saturday flight will go as fast as a bird seeking prey."

"Thank you Mr. Tanaguchi. I sincerely appreciate the extra considerations."

"Fine then, it is settled. My aide will escort you to our inn. Please, as you have previously done, when in Indonesia provide us with daily status reports on your trip to the plantation. Use the usual channels."

"Certainly Mr. Tanaguchi."

"Thank you Lonewolf-san, good luck on your venture."

"Luck has nothing to do with it, Mr. Tanaguchi. I will be successful because I am good. Good^bye, Sir." Lonewolf backed out the door leaving it open.

Another member of the Nippon Pharmaceutical Council closed the door.

Arrogant bastard Tanaguchi thought to himself.

11:00 A.M., SUNDAY, FEBRUARY 26

SINGAPORE

After eating the excellent dinner that JAL Airlines served their First Class passengers, Lonewolf slept during almost the entire flight from Tokyo to Singapore. Usually the beautiful female flight attendants kept his attention. It was frustrating. He usually tried to score with these beautiful Asian women, but he had never been successful. But on this flight, he was not interested in even trying.

Tanaguchi had kept his promise. The inn outside Kyoto had been stocked with liquor, drugs, and beautiful women. After he had finished with one woman another would appear. This would happen whether he was in the hot bath or sleeping. He was exhausted. All he needed, all he wanted, was sleep.

After the dinner he had reclined his chair to a bed position and was immediately sound asleep. The next that he was aware of was the flight attendant waking him to inform him they were landing and that he was required to bring his chair to a full upright position.

The plane's wheels touched down on the long runway of the Singapore Changi International Airport with multiple screeches. The large super-777 settled down as it rolled to the far northern end of the runway. Lonewolf took a deep breath. He was back in Southeast Asia. He was home. He loved this part of the world. He was born American, but he was an Asian at heart.

A young Asian man dressed in perfectly tailored slacks and a Singapore dress shirt met him at the gate. As Lonewolf looked closer at the man's build it was obvious that under his loose shirt, he was very muscular. He looked like a Chinese mob muscle man. Probably not very agile, Lonewolf thought as he sized the man. A habit he always followed when meeting new people whether they were friend or foe. Lonewolf never accepted a person's explanation as to who and what they were and represented. Most people he worked with were playing a role. For his own safety, he had to know the true capabilities of anyone he was working with, for, or against. This person was built of heavy body builder muscle. This type of muscle had its place in hand combat. If not to participate in the combat itself, the muscle was at least used to intimidate potential opponents.

"Mr. Lonewolf, I presume?" the man spoke perfect British English in a bass tone with a very slight Chinese accent. Lonewolf noted the contact had slipped what looked like a photograph into his shirt pocket. So, Lonewolf thought, his photograph had been sent to Singapore in advance of his arrival. Lonewolf did not know whether this was good or bad. He usually did not want his photograph in circulation.

"Yes, I am Lonewolf."

"Fine, please call me Lee. Please follow me to our limo. We must stay in Singapore until tomorrow when we will fly in a private plane to a remote airstrip on the island of Java. We must not be generally seen in Singapore so please try to be as inconspicuous as possible."

"You are the boss, Lee. Lead on," Lonewolf answered in a jovial tone. He was now rested and ready to go. Today he would have a vigorous workout and then a good night's sleep. Tomorrow he would be as good as new and his senses as sharp as the animal from which he took his name.

Lonewolf entered into the limo with Lee. They both sat in the back. "Mr. Lonewolf I have here a complete briefing on the location of the plantation and also a profile of young Mr. Chang, Jr.. I have been instructed to allow you to read this information and then you are to return it to me for destruction. You will have thirty minutes to study the material before we reach our destination. Is this enough time?"

"It is enough time," Lonewolf replied matter of factly.

There were no sounds in the limo as the driver drove out of the airport complex and on to the East Coast Parkway. Lonewolf said a short prayer as he remembered that the airport was built on the location of one of the most ruthless World War II Japanese concentration camps.

Lonewolf read the information Lee had given to him on the plantation and Chang, Jr. In exactly thirty minutes Lonewolf returned the material to Mr. Lee. There was no reason to give Lee an indication of his own capabilities and that he had memorized the information in just eight minutes.

All Lonewolf said as he handed the briefing back was, "You can destroy the report."

Lonewolf sat back in his seat, thinking over what he had read. Chang, Jr. would not be easy to negotiate with, he thought. He is hungry for power and money and to be free of his traditionalist father. This is a dangerous combination. He'll want to have a method of keeping control of the Devil Tree crop even though the NPC will own the rights to the plantation. Chang, Jr. will want part of the action and quite possibly to cut out his father. I had better obtain contingency approval from NPC on whether we cut Chang, Jr. in as a business partner or whether he is to remain just a supplier.

He wrote out a quick email and told Lee to send it to NPC. Lee answered in the affirmative and again there was silence. Lonewolf closed his eyes and walked through the sequence of events he thought would take place tomorrow at the plantation.

Although he did not know where he spent the night in Singapore, he did know the accommodations were first class. He worked out in the fitness room for over an hour, took a hot tub bath, scrubbed by a beautiful Eurasian woman who also massaged out the flight and the workout. He and the woman slept well although she wondered why he rejected her sexual advances. Lonewolf s senses were now well tuned for the work he had before him. Physical lovemaking was not required and he didn't feel the need to explain his actions.

8:00 A.M., MONDAY, FEBRUARY 27

YOGYAKARTA AIRPORT JAVA, INDONESIA

The NPC private Lear jet touched down on the runway at the Yogyakarta Airport. The flight from Singapore to Yogyakarta was just over an hour.

As Lonewolf had taken his seat in the six-passenger section of the plane, the pilot handed him a disk with an encrypted file from Tanaguchi. Lonewolf decoded the message with his laptop computer:

TO: Lonewolf FROM: Tanaguchi

SUBJ.: Current Project REF.: Your email request

NPC does not wish to cut Chang, Jr. in on Devil Tree deal unless absolutely necessary. Chang, Jr. is not to be harmed because of current value to operation. If he will not agree to just being a vendor then negotiate small share. No more than 10%.

Nacheda in Singapore. He still does not know how to find Devil Tree plantation. You have enough time to negotiate deal for NPC exclusive rights to the Devil Tree bark.

If Nacheda leaves Singapore before Wednesday or tries to go somewhere besides returning to Japan our people have been told to eliminate him.

Success on your venture. /s/Tanaguchi

Lonewolf was saddened by the potential elimination of Nacheda. He liked Nacheda, but his friend did not know how to play in this league. Nacheda was in way over his head. He had good business experience, but not very much experience in the international war of business, especially not the way NPC would compete. Nacheda was too nice, Lonewolf concluded.

Lonewolf knew that he would, if necessary, eliminate Nacheda himself. Nothing personal he thought. But, as of this moment, it looked like NPC had the situation in control and Lonewolf would not be called upon to carry out the necessary, but distasteful task of eliminating his friend.

Lonewolf did wonder where Chang, Sr. fit into the picture. NPC was concentrating on Chang, Jr. and not his father. Would the elder Chang play a role in what he was instructed to accomplish? Did the son have the authority or right to negotiate the new contract? He decided that NPC knew what they were doing. He put Chang, Sr. out of his mind until NPC told him to be concerned.

Two NPC men met Lonewolf and Lee at the airport. All four got into a Toyota 4-wheeler. As the Toyota sped out of the airport and the driver took the first curve at almost twice the recommended speed limit, Lonewolf was happy to see that the vehicle was equipped with a steel roll cage.

The maps of south central Java that he had studied prior to landing had told him that the twenty-mile journey from the airport to the plantation on the southwestern slope of the Merapi Volcano would not make for an easy ride. Lonewolf was dressed in rough jungle clothes. The pants and shirt were loose fitting and his boots were high tops. The boots very sturdy and light weight.

The members of the group did not speak unless Lonewolf asked them a question.

The scenery was typical for an island in this part of the world. Mountains, some of which were active volcanoes, would be straight ahead to the left and jungle everywhere else that one looked. According to the map, the plantation was less than ten miles from the ancient Buddhist temple of Borobudur.

Lonewolf had a strong interest in Buddhism and had studied formerly for a time in Japan. He wondered if he might have time during his stay at the plantation to visit Borobudur. The temple was built in the 8ᵗʰ Century and had fallen to ruins until an English explorer in the early 20ᵗʰ Century rediscovered the site and began digging it out.

They reached the turn-off at Blabak in less than forty-five minutes and the Toyota took the sharp turn to the right. They left the smooth modern highway and started their drive on hard packed dirt and gravel. He looked at his watch, 9:45. He had two hours before his noon meeting with Chang, Jr. at the plantation.

Lonewolfwas suddenly jolted out of his private thoughts. He was catapulted a foot straight up off his seat. The Toyota had hit a deep rut in the road caused by the heavy monsoon rains and the large trucks that frequented the secondary roads. He reached up with his right hand and grabbed the roll bar. He looked over at the driver sitting next to him. He was Japanese. He was also very muscular and looked more like a bodyguard than a driver. He turned around to look at Lee who was sitting in the back seat. Lee was wedged into the back seat among the canvas bags of supplies and he had on a seat belt. He had a smile on his face, but said nothing. The other NPC man in the back was also Japanese and was tightly strapped into his seat.

The three other men seemed oblivious to the now continuous jolting from hitting almost every rut that could be seen in the road. In fact it seemed to Lonewolf that the driver was actually speeding up to see if he could find every hole and therefore spring Lonewolf out of his seat. Lonewolf reached down to his right and pulled up the seat and shoulder belts. He then fastened them tightly around his body. Just as he clicked in the belts the driver suddenly slowed down, confirming his suspicions that the driver was having fun at his expense.

Lonewolf turned to the driver and spoke. He had to almost yell to be heard over the roar of the engine, the air rushing through the open windows, and the ramming of the tires through the ruts. After his third yell of, "Driver," the driver turned his head slightly to the right as if he finally had to notice a new sound.

"Yes?" the driver answered.

Lonewolf continued. "Driver, I have two hours before my appointment at the plantation, is it possible for us to visit Borobudur Temple?"

"Temple is behind us. I have orders to take you directly to Chang's plantation. We are not to make any stops."

"Look, driver, I'm in charge here. It would not be good to arrive so early for my appointment. You are to now take orders from me, not some distant boss. Is this going to be a problem? If it is a problem stop the car and we'll deal with this now."

The driver seemed hesitant and turned his head slightly so he could see Lee in the rearview mirror. Lee gave a slight affirmative nod of his head.

"No problem, sir." The driver turned towards Lonewolf and nodded his head and turned the vehicle around. The driver sped up again and the Toyota hit another huge rut which caused Lonewolf's body to try come up out of the seat again. This time the belt kept him from rising, but the belt also caused him pain from the pressure on his lower abdomen.

He gritted his teeth and thought to himself, the son of a bitch did that on purpose. He turned towards the driver, "Look you bastard, stop trying to prove that you're some kind of macho cross-country race driver. I know you did that on purpose."

"Yes, sir. No problem, sir," came the reply.

Fifteen minutes later the driver crossed the highway that connected Yogyakarta to Magelang in the north. The condition of the road here was even worse than what they had experienced when they turned off the highway to go towards the plantation. It was a dirt road barely wide enough for two vehicles to pass when they met. Deep tire ruts on each side were the only indications of lanes.

This was going to be an even rougher ride with this idiot driver he thought to himself. Unconsciously his right hand went up to grasp the roll bar.

About 30 minutes went by on the dual rutted dirt back road. The jolts were still there but they weren't as severe. It seemed that the rainwater used the ruts as stream beds and therefore the ruts were fairly smooth. He also saw evidence that a grader had smoothed the road so that the ruts would not get so deep that a cars chassis would bottom out on the dirt between the ruts.

The jungle almost grew up to the sides of the Toyota as it sped along. At times the banyon trees and the undergrowth would almost cover the road. He had been told this was not the time of year for harvesting, so the road had not been traveled much during the last few months. During the once a year harvest this road was probably widen by the large trucks.

At one blind turn in the road the Toyota suddenly came to a fast halt throwing Lonewolf forward. A tree had fallen across the road and the road was impassable. Lee and the driver got out of the jeep. They went to the storage area in the rear of the Toyota and came away with a gas driven chain saw and a large ax. They then began an orderly process of cutting away the tree in order for them to have room to continue. The event was done with such order that Lonewolf came to the conclusion that this evolution was not unusual, but typical in a semirain forest.

At the one-hour mark, the road split. Lee told the driver to take the fork to the left. He leaned forward Lonewolf and spoke in Lonewolf's left ear. "This is the way to the temple. We will stop for a very short period of time for you to make your inspection."

As Lee spoke, the vehicle traveled deeper into the jungle. There were no road ruts on this road. It seemed as though they were making their own road. The driver brought the jeep to another sudden stop. They were in front of a cleared path leading into the jungle.

"The temple is in there," Lee pointed to the path. "About 100 meters. Watch out for snakes. We will wait here. Please hurry there is a good possibility we will now be late with this unscheduled stop."

Lonewolf started to demand that Lee or the driver accompany him, but then he thought differently and got out of the Toyota. They would not leave him. They knew whom he represented and if any harm came to him they would suffer death.

Lonewolf climbed down and stepped onto the soft jungle floor. He sank about an inch into the plant ground cover. He proceeded down the path. It was quiet except for the distant sounds of animals and birds.

All of the sudden the jungle opened up and the path gave way to the vista of the most architecturally beautiful Buddhist temple is had ever seen. The main structure at the center of the site over 100 feet tall by his estimate.

Lonewolf walked around the perimeter of the structure taking in the beauty of the place. He wished that he had the time to go through it thoroughly and try to locate the 500 statues of Buddha that the temple housed. He glanced at his watch and decided that he had better get back on the road. It wouldn't do to be late for his appointment at the plantation.

The two Japanese NPC men were still in the Toyota. They were napping with cigarettes dangling from their lips. Cigarette smoke hovered in the area to keep away the bugs. Lee was standing at the edge of the jungle. When Lonewolf s foot hit running board the sleeping men woke up.

They had some how turned the Toyota around and were pointed back out to the road to the plantation. Lee silently walked to the Toyota and got into the back seat.

"Thank you," Lonewolf said. No use in being impolite. There was no answer. The rest of the trip to the plantation was completed in silence except for the sounds of the jungle and the vehicle.

It was close to 12:15 p.m. when the Toyota broke out of the jungle into the Devil Tree plantation. The difference was dramatic. One minute they were driving in the jungle and then they were in the middle of orderly rows of trees. It was the Devil Tree. Lonewolf recognized the Alstonia spectabilis or Devil Tree from the briefing materials he had been provided. The trees stood very tall averaging about 75 feet in height and lined both sides of the road as far as the eye could see.

After fifteen minutes of Devil Trees they drove into a large clearing of green lawn. At the far end was a beautiful Batak-style house. With the Merapi volcano as the back drop, the scene looked like a Hollywood movie set for an exotic film set in the South Pacific.

Years before, the first thing that the elder Chang did when he received payment from Doc James for his first shipment of Devil Tree bark was to enclose the old plantation Batak house. He used native mahogany. The traditional shape of the house was evident. It was built at the back of the large circular lawn. A perfect rectangle sitting at the top of the circumference of a perfect circle. The mahogany house had been built about 12 feet off the ground.

There was a staircase, which probably led to the common room. At the bottom of the staircase stood three people. Two men and one woman. Since Lonewolf did not know Chang, he could not tell if these people were Chang or servants or a combination. The driver pulled the Toyota up to the center staircase. One of the plantation men opened Lonewolfs door and the other pulled the suitcases from the rear compartment of the Toyota. The woman gestured that Lonewolf should follow her up the stairs. It was very evident that they knew and expected him. Again evidence that his photograph had proceeded his visit.

The stairs were very steep and the distance between each step was less than the usual western eight inches. These stairs were made for small people. He had learned in Nam to take this type of staircase three steps at a time. He took the first six in two steps. His rate of ascent was so fast that he almost bumped into the small woman. He stopped short of knocking her down and proceeded the rest of the way up the stairs tediously taking each small stair one at a time. As he was plodding up the stairs he looked around. Lee and the two Japanese were nowhere to be seen. He glanced around the yard. It was in the shape of a circle. The radius was 100 meters. It was mostly grass. There was a large palm tree on either side of the stairs. On the outer edge of the lawn the perfect rows of Devil Trees started.

He reached the top step and was jolted hard enough that he almost bit his tongue. He had been so preoccupied with the layout that he had not noticed that he was on the last step. He had tried to take one more step when there was no stair. His foot, expecting another stair, had come down hard on the wooden floor of the central walkway. The loud noise of his boot smacking the floor echoed. The sounds of the jungle went silent as the birds and animals tried to determine whether the sudden noise was good or bad. The woman turned around. If there was a definition for a person who was both old and ancient she was its embodiment.

"Is everything all right, Mr. Smith?" She inquired in broken English with a slight British accent. Probably learned English in Singapore, he concluded.

"Everything is fine. Please go on," he answered.

She turned and started walking down the right-hand side of the long outside central porch walkway. The outside mahogany wood railing had been polished to a bright sheen.

They had passed three doors along the walkway when the old woman turned to her left and opened a door. She motioned for him to enter. He slowly entered the room examining all aspects of the room. The woman remained outside. There wasn't much furniture in the room. A small single bed rigged with mosquito netting. A single five foot high dresser with a small mirror. A table with what appeared to be a water pitcher and a bowl. The only other piece of furniture was a rattan chair. No closet and no toilet.

"Mr. Smith, I am your hostess. Please call me Marisa. My family has lived on this land for more than three centuries. Mr. Chang, Sr., very kindly allows me to believe that I own the land and therefore allows me to live here. I act as hostess to both Mr. Chang and his son when either person is present. I also act as caretaker and manager when they are away. They are away most of the time so it is a good arrangement for all. Mr. Chang, Jr. will meet you for dinner. Mr. Chang Sr. is currently in Jakarta on business.

"At this moment, Mr. Chang, Jr. is inspecting the northeast section of the plantation. Dinner is at 7:00 p.m. Cocktails at six.

Mr. Chang, Jr. is Chinese, but he runs this house like an upper-class British gentleman living in a manor house," a slight smile came to her dark eyes. Lonewolf realized that in her youth she had probably been a very beautiful woman. She also had a sense of humor.

She continued, "Since it is relatively early in the afternoon and you have probably not eaten I have taken the liberty of placing a large fruit basket and some fresh bread in your room. Lonewolf looked at his watch, it was nearly 2:00. He thought the meeting was at noon. Sure, they had been late, but he thought that Chang would wait for his arrival. He rationalized that this was a plantation and nature did not wait when you worked a plantation. Four hours before cocktails. He would eat, take a walk around the immediate grounds, and then take a quick nap before cocktails.

His plan was to conclude business before noon the following day. He wanted to be back in Singapore tomorrow night. He would start the negotiations tonight after dinner. Tomorrow he would see where they prepared the Devil Tree bark for shipment to Jakarta and finish the contract negotiations before noon. It should not be a problem.

He told Marisa what he planned to do and he requested that someone wake him at 5:45 p.m. Marisa advised him not wander into the jungle surrounding the plantation alone because of snakes and other unfriendly animals. She would see to his being awakened at the prescribed time. She then left him alone in his room.

Lonewolf ate the fruit and bread and then went outside. He found a chair on the porch and sat down to mentally go through the material that Lee had given him when he arrived. He wondered where Lee and the two NPC Japanese men had gone. They would come in handy should there be a problem where strength and manpower were required. He decided he would talk to them tomorrow in order to give them instructions about potential problems from Nacheda. He started to get sleepy and decided to go back to his room for the nap.

Once in the room he walked over to the bed and took off his boots, pants, and shirt. He then removed the small pistol from under his left armpit. He went to the edge of the bed, pulled back the netting, and slid the pistol under the pillow. He climbed into bed letting the netting fall back and slid under the cool sheets in his underwear.

He was asleep the minute he closed his eyes. Another trick he learned in Nam. He concluded that at least for today, he was in no physical danger. He again wondered where his three NPC companions had gone. He knew they would be there when he required them. If he required them.

A soft knock on his door woke him up from what had otherwise been an uninterrupted sleep. He looked at his watch and saw that it was 5:45.

"Thank you I will be at cocktails at six." A youthful male voice replied, "Cocktails will be in the common section at the head of the center stairs. If you require the toilet you will find it two doors down on your way to the common section."

Lonewolf got out of bed and walked over to the table where the pitcher of water and bowl were sitting. He poured some water into the bowl. It was cool to the touch. He splashed his face and washed his upper body. He dried off and put on his pants, boots, and a clean shirt and left his room.

He entered the common room after making a short stop at toilet. The common room was very large. He noted a large walkin fireplace on one side of the room with comfortable chairs surrounding a coffee table facing the fireplace. In the far corner of the room was a large circular table. The table had a rotating centerpiece. Lonewolf correctly assumed that this was a Chinese style dining table. Besides himself, there were two other people in the room, Marisa and a man he presumed to be Chang, Jr.. Chang had on an evening jacket and Marisa an evening dress. Lonewolf now understood Marisa's comment about Chang's British style. Lonewolf let a moment of self-conscience at being underdressed go by.

According to the report he had read in the limo, Chang, Jr. was forty years old. He looked younger than his age. He could pass for twenty-five, Lonewolf thought. Chang stood up as Lonewolf moved to the table. Chang had a warm looking smile, but again, the report had stated that inside was a very cold and calculating heart. Lonewolf searched his memory and remembered the exact words in the report:

Do not be placed at ease by Chang, Jr's outward warmth and friendly demur. He has proven to be a formidable negotiator in many business areas other than the James Devil Tree deal which he didn't consummate. The James Devil Tree deal was negotiated between his father, Chang Sr. and Dr. James.

Chang, Jr.'s major motivation is greed. The Chang family is very wealthy. They have over $20 million U.S. dollars in the Bank of Hong Kong not to mention the $5 million U.S. dollar equivalents in Indonesian banks. Chang will be receptive to your offer. He will start very high with the intent to get you to settle on a high number with you feeling that you have won the negotiation. You should settle for no more than a 20% higher price per square meter of bark than what they are currently getting from James.

The bark is sold to James not by weight but by cubic meter. A subjective measurement considering the odd sizes of the pieces of bark, but a measurement that has been honored by both parties since the beginning of the contract. We do not think it is necessary to change the method of measurement. The price James pays is $100 US per cubic meter.

You, therefore, should go no higher than $120 US. If Chang will not accept, after a reasonable term of negotiations, terminate the effort. There are other ways to deal with Chang that will not require your talents.

Adding to the 20% price increase he had, if necessary, the authorization to give a 10% share in a joint venture between Chang and NPC.

As Lonewolf advanced toward the circular table Chang, Jr's coal black eyes took measure of him. Chang's eyes were direct contrast to the smile that was still the dominant feature of his face. Chang's skin tone was darker than most Chinese that he had met. This indicated that he liked the outdoors, but probably more for play than work. Again Lonewolf recalled the intelligence report.

Chang, Jr illustrates no guilt in his ethics, which indicates that he will lie and cheat. This is a dichotomy from Chang, Sr. who is very honorable. Chang, Jr. frequents Macao for enjoyment and manages to have at least one and usually two Thai women as consorts when he lives on the plantation. You will not see them, but they are there in one or two of the rooms. His wife and children (five children) live in Jakarta and never visit the plantation.

Chang was the first to speak. His voice was a low guttural gravel voice with a combination Chinese and British accent. It was the voice of an old wise man coming from the mouth of a young man. The man's personality was full of contrasts. Lonewolf formulated a proverb: What saw or imagined is not alone, necessarily so.

"Good evening, Mr. Smith. I hope you have found my plantation home and accommodations acceptable and comfortable. I apologize in advance for any inconvenience. It is most difficult to have everything one requires or desires here in the middle of the jungle. We do try to do our best." He raised his right arm to shake Lonewolf's hand in greeting.

Lonewolf decided on the strategic tack of being blunt and cold. Americans usually tried to fit into other cultures to illustrate their desire to 'do in Rome as the Roman's do in Rome.'

Lonewolf decided to surprise Chang and take an aggressive strategy. He replied to Chang's courteous opening remarks by not returning his smile. He then drilled his own steel blue eyes into Chang's eyes with a fierce stare. People had told Lonewolf that he had the eyes of a Siberian wolf, a.k.a. Lonewolf. Lonewolf's voice was soft, but direct. He took the posture that he had used with the James executive called Jones. Instead of squeezing Chang's hand he drilled his eyes into Chang. As he spoke he forced the smile from Chang's face and caused him to lower his eyes. The first real negotiating chess move was a win for Lonewolf.

Lonewolf replied, "The accommodations are acceptable, but only barely. With today's access to helicopters and your money, I would have thought your home would be of a higher quality." He had emphasized the words 'your money'.

Chang was silent. He now let his out stretched right arm drop to his side without waiting to see if Lonewolf would or would shake his hand. Lonewolf had not extended his hand so Chang's move was again, a win for Lonewolf.

Chang sat down before he resumed speaking. "So be it, Mr. Smith. As I stated my apologies for the inconveniences."

Marisa remained standing as Lonewolf took his seat. She then acted as the hostess and poured both Chang and Lonewolf a glass of Chinese plum wine. Lonewolf placed a small spoon full of brown sugar crystals into the wine and stirred with his demitasse spoon. Chinese wine is very sweet and viscous and has a very strong fragramce. Lonewolf enjoyed Chinese wine, but in moderation.

Chang spoke again as he raised his wineglass, "To our business negotiations. May they bear fruits to both parties." Both drank. Lonewolf did not answer the toast, which would have been the courteous thing to do. Both men were silent during the serving of the various dishes. Lonewolf did not enjoy small talk so he did not initiate small talk or partake in the gambiting of small talk. He could see that Chang was disappointed in not being able to demonstrate his British dinner formalities. Lonewolf s strategy was to remain quiet until Chang started to talk business. He knew that when he forced Chang to talk business, he would have made another winning move. This strategy would show Chang's eagerness to negotiate which would be a sign of weakness. Lonewolf was prepared to wait all night. Lonewolf was hungry and the food was outstanding, so he ate and the silence continued.

The wills of both men were strong. They ate slowly as if they were carrying on a normal conversation. They would each take a mouthful of food, savor the taste, chew slowly, and swallow. No one was in a hurry. The silence did not worry either of them. It did worry Marisa who interpreted the silence as a reflection on the acceptance of her food. An hour went by in silence.

Finally as a jester of kindness to Marisa, Lonewolf wiped his mouth and looked over at Marisa and spoke. He made sure that he did not look at Chang. "Marisa, your meal has outstripped the capabilities of your environment. It was as good a meal as I would expect in a four-star restaurant in Singapore. You are to be complimented." A large smile came to her ancient face. Her eyes twinkled and the youthful beauty again shown through the years of aging.

Lonewolf assumed that she had probably worked for days on this dinner.

Now all of her work had been rewarded.

Lonewolf noted, from the comer of his peripheral vision, that Chang's dark skin turn a little red. Lonewolf had just delivered another insult. The compliment should have been given to Chang as the master of the house, not to a person that could be considered just slightly above a servant.

Marisa replied, "Thank you very much, Mr. Smith. I will tell my people of your comments." She pushed her chair back and stood announcing to both men, "I will now provide you gentleman with coffee and an after dinner drink and then excuse myself for the rest of the evening. This tired old woman must now go to bed. Mr. Smith, should your require anything to make your stay more comfortable, please push the buzzer on the dresser top. Thank you again kind sir."

She turned towards Chang. The smile was removed from her face. "If there is nothing else sir, I would like permission to retire after my final chores."

"Granted," was the hard and direct answer she received from master Chang.

Both men now sat alone, still in silence. Their eyes slowly came to bear on each other. This time Chang did not lower his eyes. Both men thought to themselves, this was going to be an interesting game.

Another fifteen minutes passed in silence and then Lonewolf changed his strategy and broke the silence. Chang was surprised at Lonewolf's break in strategy. Lonewolf knew that time was against him and in Chang's favor. Lonewolf had to wrap this deal up as soon as possible. Chang already had a deal with James and he could not wait forever. Lonewolf, or rather NPC, could not wait.

Courtesy dictated that business not be discussed until tomorrow. To start discussions tonight instead of waiting would be another winning move for Lonewolf. The key was to get Chang to talk business. Lonewolf continued his visual lock on Chang's eyes as he began to speak.

His voice was cold and direct. "Mr. Chang, as you know, I have come here as a representative of the Nippon Pharmaceutical Council or NPC. We are interested in purchasing exclusive rights to your Devil Tree production. We are developing a new line of pharmaceuticals that will require the particular species of Devil Tree that you grow here. We have an alternative growing plantation site, but as you know, production quantities are eight to nine years away. We have decided to determine if we can work together immediately rather than start our own production in competition with your plantation. Should you decide not to work with us it will be a short-term gain for you and your father. We will, most certainly, put you out of business once we have started. You may be thinking that I am bluffing about a new Devil Tree plantation site. You may be foolish enough to think this, but let me assure you, I speak factually."

He waited a second and then continued before Chang had a chance to respond. "You of course, don't have time to check my statement to determine if it is true or not true so the decision to believe me or not is entirely up to you. We know you have an exclusive agreement with the New York based James Pharmaceutical Company. We ask that you cancel or forfeit that agreement in favor of our offer. Our offer is more than fair and will provide you and your father with a considerable increase in revenue and profit. You will be able to retire and enjoy a life of leisure because we would like to help you run this plantation. We will also make you a contingency offer to purchase the plantation in the future. We offer you $110.00 U.S. per cubic meter. That is 10% above your current contract with James." Lonewolf paused. He knew that he was pushing hard. Perhaps too hard, but he had started on this negotiating tact and he had to proceed and see the strategy through to its conclusion.

He continued, "You should also know that once you have a contract with NPC you will not be able to cancel the contract without drastic damages to your enterprise. We don't carry out our business dealings and breaches of contract in court like many weak American companies including James Pharmaceutical Company." Lonewolf stopped talking and waited for Chang's response. The eyes of both men continued to bore into each other.

Chang's next move surprised Lonewolf and again pointed out his advesary's contrasts. Lonewolf saw in Chang's eyes a look of defeat and yet Chang's next words allowed him to gain back much of the respect that he had lost to Lonewolf during dinner. Chang rose slowly out of his chair forcing Lonewolf to break eye contact.

Chang then spoke in a low voice, "Mr. Smith, you have been a very discourteous guest in my home and you have been extremely blunt. Both are traits that I abhor. Have a pleasant rest. Our meeting begins at 7:00 a.m. in my office at the west end of the house. Good night." He walked out of the room leaving Lonewolf sitting alone.

Shit, Lonewolf thought. The man has a set of balls. He not only returned my insult in spades, but he also got my opening negotiating strategy without giving me his strategy. Tonight he will study my strategy. He can do this from listening to the recording of their conversation that Lonewolf was sure he had taped.

Lonewolf pushed his chair back and decided to take a walk around the house before retiring.

The night air was cool as Lonewolf stepped into the darkness. He stood on the top of the stairs listening to the night sounds. He was startled, but not surprised when a voice came from the shadows at the bottom of the stairs. "Mr. Smith, is everything okay?" Lonewolf recognized the voice of Mr. Lee.

"Yes, everything is okay. I'm about to take a walk around the house.

Would you please accompany me?"

"Yes sir," came the voice from the shadows.

Lonewolf made his way down the small steps to the ground level. The grass was soft. He turned right and decided to walk around the building clockwise. He did not know what he would discover in the dark but he would at least get a general feeling about the grounds.

There was a full moon which gave him enough moonlight to see shapes. Lee joined Lonewolf at his right side, walking between him and the porch that surrounded the house A good man, he noted. Lee was protecting his principal from the side most dangerous to a surprise attack.

As they rounded the first corner of the house, they could see that the circle of grass in front of the house was surrounded by flower gardens. Going around the second corner they saw a second circle of grass. In fact, the house sat in the middle of two circles of lawn. In the back, the lawn did not end in rows of Devil Tree's but with a cliff. At the end of the lawn that were not cliffs were walls of jungle. He couldn't see in the dark whether there were any breaks in the jungle wall, daylight would be required for this detailed information.

As he and Lee walked around the house he did not note any other structures. He wondered where the Devil Tree logging work was accomplished. It was not in the general vicinity of the house and he had not seen anything on the road during the drive this afternoon. There must be a second road he thought. They proceeded back to the front of the house.

"Mr. Lee," Lonewolf spoke for the first time, "I assume that you and the Japanese are, if required, here to assist me. Is that correct?"

"Yes, Mr. Smith. We have been instructed to be at your command. We are trained to carry out any order you feel is necessary to get your mission accomplished. One of us will be here at the bottom of the stairs or under the porch beneath your room all night long. If you require our services, just yell. Have a pleasant rest."

"Thank you," replied Lonewolf. He went up the stairs and to his room. This time he remained dressed as he pushed back the netting. He lay back on the bed. He returned the pistol to its holster and went to sleep. He slept soundly. He felt relatively safe considering he was in the home of a man of contrasts. He did not see any reason to fear being harmed, at least not yet.

RAFFLES HOTEL SINGAPORE

Nacheda was laying on his bed in one of the rooms in the new section of the famous Raffles Hotel. The old section was good enough for the tourists who thought roughing it in a small room was a trip into history, but not for Nacheda. He had enough experience sleeping in the small rooms of Japanese inns. When he got the chance to sleep in a western bed, he took it.

He placed his clasped hands behind his head and closed his eyes. His body was tired from running around Singapore and Jakarta for the last four days.

Before he had left Bandai he had read everything that was available on the Devil Tree. Skip sent him the information that SAM came up with concerning

James. His primary purpose for this trip was to find out who owned the Devil Tree plantation. The report that SAM provided indicated that it was Chang Trading Company in Jakarta, Indonesia. On Friday morning he had taken a flight to Jakarta. After landing it had taken him almost an hour of telephone calls to find Chang Trading Company.

The Chang Trading Company was in an older section of the city and was connected to a medium-sized warehouse.

Mr. Chang, Sr. was an old man and by most appearances, or measures, retired. He told Nacheda that he had turned over the running of the business to his forty-year-old son five years ago. Mr. Chang accepted his son's capability in running the plantation. He added that his son operated the business differently than the way he had run the plantation. He still honored the agreements he had made in the past to Dr. James, but the future was up to his son. The old man smiled as he summarized his son's motivation. Chang told Nacheda that his son was motivated by money and that little else mattered. When Nacheda asked Chang when his son might return to the Jakarta office, he answered that his son would be back in the office on Wednesday. He did not know his location before Wednesday,

Chang then showed Nacheda around the empty warehouse. Chang explained that the bark from the Devil Tree was stripped off at the plantation. The tree was unique because if the bark was properly removed it could be done so without permanent damage to the tree. Within a year, the tree would begin to replenish its bark. Within five years, the bark of the Devil Tree was ready for another harvest. The bark was bundled at the plantation and trucked to the small port at Galur on the Indian Ocean. The bundles of bark were then transferred to small container ships and brought through the straits to Jakarta for further transport to the warehouse. At the warehouse the bark was washed and boxed for export. During Nacheda's visit the warehouse was empty because they had just made a large shipment.

When Nacheda tried to find out the location of the plantation or who was the customer he was met with silence.

While their conversation was taking place in the old man's dark and sparse office, Nacheda had noticed two Chinese characters painted on wooden plaques hanging on the wall. Other than the plaques the walls were empty. He asked the old man what the characters meant.

Chang had replied in broken English. "Tong" which means togetherness and harmony, and "An" which means peace and security. He told Nacheda that these were the symbols that they try to use in our lives which are shared with the Indonesians and in our business shared with our customers.

Mr. Chang impressed Nacheda, but he was worried about the son. Nacheda pressed Mr. Chang about the plantation and meeting his son. Mr. Chang finally suggested that Nacheda phone back on Monday or Tuesday to establish an appointment with his son. He could not guarantee an appointment but he would try as soon as his son contacted the office. Chang would not disclose any additional information. Nacheda left Chang Trading Company, Jakarta and returned to Singapore.

On Saturday he went to the Singapore General Hospital where the patient had died from the hyperactivity side effect. There was only a slim chance that the hospital would still have the records, but he had to give it a try. His accomplishments at the Chang Trading

Company were not very good. He hoped that he would have better results at the hospital.

He visited the pharmacist at the hospital and told him that he was an employee of Bandai Pharmaceuticals Company. The pharmacist was a young and energetic man. Nacheda asked him if he would like to join him for lunch. He replied in the affirmative. They hit it off right away.

Nacheda explained that he was very interested in herbal pharmaceuticals and told the pharmacist about the patient case. The pharmacist's reaction was positive. He said he would try and find out something. Nacheda had told him not to betray any of the policies of the hospital. All he wanted to know is whether the herb the patient had taken was Alstonia spectabilis.

On Sunday, the pharmacist had called him at his room at Raffles to inform him that he had read the records and it was indeed an interesting case. He concluded with the information that the patient had ingested Alstonia spectabilis. It had been written in the patient's record as the Devil Tree.

Nacheda laid on his hotel bed thinking of lay ahead for him in meeting the people from James and hopefully meeting with Mr. Chang's son on Wednesday.

Nacheda had been unaware of the activity that had been going on in the wake of his activities between his personal tail, the NPC, and Lonewolf since he left Japan. Nacheda's tail had been reporting his Singapore activities directly to NPC headquarters and the activities had been very disturbing to Mr. Tanaguchi. Tanaguchi knew Nacheda was in the Singapore area and assumed he was on the same mission as Lonewolf. It would not be good for Nacheda to meet Lonewolf at any time especially before Lonewolf had completed his business with Mr. Chang's son at the plantation.

The tail knew Nacheda did not know the location of the plantation. After Nacheda had visited with Mr. Chang, Sr., the tail had remained behind to question the old man as to what he had told Nacheda. The old man had informed the tail that he hadn't told Mr. Nacheda anything he didn't already know before he had made the visit.

The tail didn't know whether the old man was telling the truth so he had beat the old man until he was certain that he hadn't told Nacheda the location of the plantation. He left the old man sitting in his chair unconscious, but not dead. A few more missing teeth and his Chinese symbols of "Tong" and "An" propped in his lap were a result of the visit. They would also act as a remembrance to keep his mouth shut when he awakened from his unconscious state.

After being informed of Nacheda's trip to Jakarta, Mr. Tanaguchi had instructed the tail to keep Nacheda in Singapore. He was to allow him to leave only to take a flight out of the Singapore and Indonesia area. If he left the hotel again to take any local flights he was to be delayed. If necessary delayed permanently. Nacheda had lost his future importance to the NPC and was now, if he got any closer to the plantation, regrettably, expendable. The NPC mission was now in Lonewolf s hands alone and his identity and mission were to be protected at any cost.

The tail had understood his instructions and for his own information, had asked NPC for the present location of Lonewolf. He had received a twoword answer, "Very close."

After the tail left Jakarta he picked Nacheda up again at Raffles and followed him to and from the hospital. The hospital trip was a mystery to the tail, but seemed irrelevant so further investigation was unnecessary.

As Nacheda lay on his bed waiting for the telephone call from Dr. J.P. Koenig, the tail was stationed in the lobby waiting for further activity or to be relieved by the night watch if no further activity was expected.

Nacheda was putting together all of the pieces of his mission. He had emailed an encrypted status report to SAM via modem. He smiled to himself when he thought that SAM must be up to a 98% correlation by now. In Nacheda's mind he was 100% sure that this plan was going to be successful. He was uncomfortable that he did not know the location of the plantation and did not have a firm meeting date with the old man's son. He understood the ways of Asian businesspeople and knew that meetings were rarely planned and were never a sure thing. Meetings happened when they happened, if they happened.

Nacheda was uncomfortable about a feeling he had about the situation. The feeling rested just under his consciousness. He felt he was not alone and that there was someone watching him. He was almost sure of it, but he had never seen the person. Since he was close to Vietnam and on a special mission his senses were heightened. Which might account for his feelings. He was almost certain he had been followed to Chang, Sr's office. He had tried to spot a tail, but had not recognized anyone in the throngs of people in the streets or sidewalks on which he had been walking. Even though he never saw a tail, the feeling continued to gnaw at his stomach. He would have to be more careful and watchful. He would have to think about taking round about routes to where ever he was going to make sure he had not picked up a tail.

Why would I have a tail? The question emerged in his mind. Who wants to know where I am, what I am doing, and where I am going? He went through the list of the people and organizations involved in the project. Bandai? No, they know where I am and certainly not after Dr. Nakasone's private talk with Nacheda. James? Perhaps they are checking me out, but why? No, I do not think so. Skip? No. Reiko, no. Task-force members? He went through each additional member of the team: Cap, John, Mary, and Joe. No, they had nothing to gain. It must be his imagination and paranoia about Southeast Asia.

9:00 P.M., MONDAY, FEBRUARY 27

RAFFLES HOTEL SINGAPORE

Mandi and J.P. had arrived in Singapore two days before and spent the weekend sightseeing. They had visited every temple, building, and area that had historical significance.

J.P. cut their sightseeing short on Monday afternoon to return to the hotel. He told Mandi that he had to make a phone call as he sorted through papers that he had brought from New York. Finally, he located the slip of paper on which Janet had written the number the American Embassy in Singapore.

"Who are you calling?" Mandi asked.

"A friend of mine lives in Singapore and works at the American Embassy" Mandi and J.P. had gotten as close as two people can get, but not close enough for J.P. to disclose his CMAG network.

"So why are you calling this person? Are you expecting trouble?" "Nope. Technically, because of my work with the Navy and DOD and because I still hold a couple of high-level clearances, I'm required to report my presence in a foreign country. I still have a little concern about meeting Skip's friend later this evening, plus tomorrow we're flying off in a chartered plane to a remote airstrip in Indonesia. It's a good way of letting someone know that we're around." He picked up the phone and dialed the number on the paper.

The phone on the other end rang three times before it was answered. A male voice said, "Hello?"

"Yes, hello. I'm trying to contact a Mr. Stanley. I believe he works somewhere in the embassy."

There was a pause on the other end and then, "I'm sorry I don't know a Mr. Stanley, you should contact the embassy operator."

J.P. breathed a quick sigh of relief, he knew he had gotten it right. "I'm sorry I really must insist."

"Name please."

"Dr. Jean Paul Koenig." "Credentialed?"

"Green 27984," J.P. recited the number on his clearance badge. "You're a contractor? What can I do for you Dr. Koenig?"

"Yes, I am a contractor. There's nothing that you can do for me, I'm simply reporting my presence here in Singapore."

"Are you here on business or pleasure?" "Business."

"I see. How long will you be staying here?"

"I leave for Los Angeles on Wednesday, but there's another side trip before then. I'm leaving for Indonesia tomorrow."

"Oh. Jakarta?"

"No, a remote area near Blabak. Should I contact the RSO in Jakarta too?"

"No, that won't be necessary. Actually, I'm temporarily handling the RSO duties for that Embassy. You're cautioned against discussing any Agency programs that you may or may not be involved in at this or any other time. Further you are not discuss your ties to the Agency as a contractor. Thank you," he said as the phone clicked dead.

With the formalities over J.P. said, "Chuck you old sod. How are you?" "Never better J.P., what brings you to Shangri La?"

"Not a project that you should be concerned with I just wanted you to know I was in town."

"How about a drink, dinner, or whatever. Do you have the time?"

"Fraid not Chuck, maybe next time. I could be coming back soon, then we can get together. FYI I am at the Ruffles."

"Got you, take care shipmate." And the connection was broken.

J.P. smiled to himself. He had achieved what he had set out to do, they now knew he was there.

He turned to Mandi and said, "Well, that's done. What do you say we go shopping and get something to eat?"

"You don't have to ask me twice!"

By Monday evening they were exhausted. They had an early dinner and decided to rest in their room while J.P. considered calling Skip's friend, Nacheda. The ringing of the telephone interrupted his thoughts.

"Yes?" J.P. answered when the phone rang.

"Is this Dr. Koenig of James Pharmaceutical Company?" a voice asked. "Who is speaking please?" J.P. responded. The voice on the other end of the line had an Asian accent. His voice sounded tired and cautious.

"This is Mr. Nacheda of the Bandai Pharmaceuticals Company. I was instructed by a mutual friend to contact you tonight," he answered.

"That's funny, I thought I was supposed to contact you. Who instructed you?

"Skip Howard of Los Angeles. Forgive my impertinence for taking the liberty of contacting you first. I hope I am not interrupting anything." "No not at the moment. Where does this Skip Howard ski?" "Well, currently Mammoth Mountain," he replied.

"You wanted to meet with me?" J.P. asked.

"Yes. I will meet you at the Raffles bar. I am wearing a tan suit with an open white shirt. Please stand near the Bengal tiger until I identify myself to you," the line went dead.

J.P. replaced the phone and thought to himself, "What the hell was that all about? I felt like I was reading from a pocket spy novel."

Mandi asked him if it had been Skip's friend on the phone. Mandi was still wearing the clothes she had worn for the day's sightseeing. She was seated in an overstuffed chair in the corner of the room, reading a magazine.

J.P. looked over to where she was sitting with an obvious look of concern on his face. Mandi commented, "J.P., what is the matter? Was it the person you were expecting to call?"

"I have to admit that I'm a little confused. The person on the phone sounded Asian and seems to know Skip, but he didn't say much. He told me or rather, he ordered me, to meet him in the bar near the Bengal tiger. He talked to me as though we were two spies sniffing one another out. But then again, maybe I contributed to that by making sure he knew who Skip Howard is."

"Maybe he is just an overly cautious guy."

"Maybe, but from what Skip told me about him, this type of behavior would be out of character." J.P. paused. "Tell you what. He doesn't know you are with me. Let's go down to the bar separately. I will meet him while you sit at the bar and play the role of a tourist. You can directly watch what happens. If watching directly is not possible I am sure the bar will have some kind of mirror and you can watch our reflection in the mirror. Also, look around at the other patrons in the bar and see if there is anyone else who appears interested in our conversation. I won't leave the bar without either disclosing your presence to Nacheda or by remaining behind after establishing another meeting with him. Okay?"

"Okay J.P., but I don't understand why all the cloak and dagger stuff is necessary."

J.P. smiled and said, "I don't know either. Just a hunch." Mandi replied, "Okay, Monsieur Bond, I'm on my way."

J.P. waited a full three minutes after Mandi then left the room before heading downstairs.

He entered the bar from the courtyard side of the room and quickly glanced around the room. His visual scan briefly caught sight of Mandi sitting on a stool at the far end of the bar. There was a bar length mirror and she could see the reflection of most of the activities that would go on in the entire room. There was a large glass of red colored Singapore Sling sitting on the bar in front of her. She was sipping the drink through a straw. It occurred to J.P. that anyone in the place could have seen them together in the bar over the last two days, but he decided that it was a risk worth taking.

J.P. spotted the tiger and walked towards it. The local folklore had the original owner meeting a man-eating Bengal tiger on this spot. He killed the tiger and had him stuffed. It was the stuffed tiger that met all visitors to this bar.

J.P. was standing under the left front leg of the tiger. The tiger was standing on its hind legs raised up in a manner that made it look as though it would give the observer a hug.

He had positioned himself so that when he met Nacheda he would still be able to see the bar where Mandi was sitting. He was standing there for only a minute or two when a handsome, tall, middle-aged Japanese man dressed in a tan suit entered the bar. His eyes shifted around the room and lingered for a few extra seconds on Mandi. After he had apparently satisfied himself that there was nothing untoward about the small crowd in the bar, he walked to where J.P. was waiting. He didn't look directly at J.P. as he walked but kept looking around the bar. When he was about two feet away he stopped and his eyes shifted to J.P.'s face. His right hand came from his side to shake.

"Good evening, Dr. Koenig. My name is Mr. Nacheda you may call me Nacheda, to be less formal. Most people do. I apologize for my grade school spy behavior. I will explain the reasons later in our visit. It is nothing serious but I am sensitive to the times." A smile came to his lips.

When J.P. and Mandi dropped off their skis in Los Angeles for storage until their return and ski trip, Skip mentioned, "You will like Nacheda immediately. He is a real person. He acts out the Japanese culture and respects it, but he is western in the way he expresses his feelings." Skip concluded with, "I have no doubts that you will become fast friends. I have known him for more than twenty-five years. He is my friend and I trust him."

J.P. felt some of Nacheda's charisma, but even after the briefexplanation of Skip's friend's overly cautious behavior, he still did not understand the cloak and dagger. J.P. decided to find out now rather than wait until later as Nacheda had suggested.

"Skip speaks very highly of you and tells me I am to trust you. I'm not questioning your judgment for if I am to believe Skip, your judgment is excellent. It is because of this respect that I must insist that you explain the cloak and dagger immediately and not wait until later."

J.P.'s eyes did not leave his and he did not lower his eyes. They were still standing next to the stuffed tiger, staring at each other and shaking hands.

Nacheda released his grip and the two men dropped their arms down to their sides. They stood silently for another minute. Nacheda shifted his eyes to less of a stare and spoke first. J.P. took advantage of the shift in Nacheda's eyes and glanced briefly at Mandi. He noted that she was watching them in the reflection of the mirror. Nacheda saw his glance and looked over at Mandi.

"A beautiful woman, Dr. Koenig." It was a statement, not a question. "Yes, and please call me, J.P."

Nacheda went on with his statement as if he had not heard my comment. "Beauty, many times is in the eyes of the viewer, but then there is true beauty that emanates from both within person and is evident externally. When such a person is in a room there is additional light. It seems that we have both noticed the possibilities of such a person in this bar." He went on obviously trying to place J.P. more at ease and also trying to dodge the direct question that had been put to him. Nacheda continued, "I personally know of such a woman and to tell you the truth, I wish she were here to enjoy our meeting as well. I mention this only to illustrate to you that there is no danger in our meeting, only precaution." The smile again appeared on his lips.

"I understand what you have said, more than you imagine Nacheda."

J.P. returned his smile and continued, "What did you mean by 'being sensitive to the times'?"

"Oh, really nothing, J.P. I was only referring to the fact that we are two corporations and we are meeting in a bar in Singapore by a tiger. If there were a business broker from any industrialized country in the bar tonight observing us, we would start rumors and quite possibly disturb the NYSE and Nikkei averages," he said with a laugh.

"Come," he continued, "let's sit down and make ourselves somewhat less conspicuous." His eyes again swept the room.

J.P. decided that he was not being entirely truthful with him, but he also got the sense that he was not lying. He decided to play along with Nacheda for a while longer and see where the conversation led. He glanced at Mandi as they moved to the nearest table and sat down. She was not watching the two men, but was ordering what J.P. figured was her second Singapore Sling.

"Nachedasan, as I am sure Skip informed you, I am a consultant to James Pharmaceutical Company. He told me that you are a consultant of Bandai Pharmaceuticals Company and you wanted to talk to me as soon as possible. I realize that most Japanese businessmen do not like to jump into a heavy business conversations immediately after being introduced and I do not wish to be discourteous, but I am tired from a strenuous weekend of sightseeing which is of little consequence to you, but there it is. I am also on a very tight schedule. So I apologize for being blunt, but perhaps you can enlighten me as to why we should be having this conversation?"

"I appreciate your frankness," Nacheda explained, "but I do not think I can fully explain my reasons for the conversation in one short meeting. In this first meeting I will try to give you a good reason to squeeze me into your tight schedule and meet with me again while you are in Singapore. I'll give you a synopsis of my situation and then you make the decision as to our next move. Is this acceptable to you?"

"Sounds fair to me. Please go ahead," he replied.

He leaned forward over the small table that they shared. J.P. felt somewhat compelled to also lean forward, but resisted. Nacheda began, "I know a great deal about James. I cannot disclose my sources, but I assure you that they are honorable. You will immediately have to trust me on this matter."

"I understand, please go on."

"I know that James is going through a very tough period. There are problems with the Lifeal sales performance and with some of Lifeal's undesirable side effects."

"This is true Nachedasan, but that's common knowledge."

"Yes J.P., but there is more. I know there is trouble brewing between the James management and the James board of directors. I also know there is a short supply of working capital and because of this shortage, your research programs may be in jeopardy."

J.P. was momentarily stunned by the amount of knowledge that Nacheda possessed regarding closely held information about James. He decided to play it off. "I am impressed Nachedasan, but you could have deduced this information from published reports."

"You are correct, but I do not think I could use deductive analysis to conclude that you are here in Singapore to investigate a potential problem with your supply of the raw material Alstonia spectabilis that is used for Lifeal."

J.P. froze, unsure now how to proceed. As far as he was concerned, there was no legal way that Nacheda could have obtained this information.

"Hold on Nachedasan." He broke in doing his best to keep the creeping anger out of his voice. "Where in the hell did you get this information? Trust can only go so far and you have surpassed the level of trust that we have established here this evening. If I were to tie this information together with your strange behavior you can easily see why I am now suspicious. You will have to do some fast explaining or I am going to get up from this table and leave. At this point, I only remain at this table because Skip and is presently dating my best friend, Annie."

All during J.P.'s outburst Nacheda kept lowering his eyes and head. J.P. glanced over Nacheda's shoulder and saw Mandi looking directly at them. His voice had not been loud, but Mandi had heard the change in tone. She had turned her barstool and was staring at the two men. She looked like she was waiting for orders. J.P. looked at Nacheda^ who was now slumped in his chair. Mandi pointed to herself and then at the table where he was seated. J.P. shook his head. He waited.

After a short silence Nacheda began to speak, but in a less confident voice.

"Dr. Koenig, I am a strong and honorable man, but I am not good at playing the role of a politician. I have not been able to command the art of indirectly approaching a sensitive subject. I sincerely apologize, but I ask you to hold your judgment of me and listen to my story a little longer. You must believe me that neither Bandai nor myself are your enemies and we want to be your friend. Please honor Skip's judgment of me for just a little longer. I promise you that neither you nor the company you represent will be disappointed. I should not have been blunt, but I provided you with this information in good faith and not as a threat." He stopped waiting for a response and was again looking into J.P.'s eyes.

J.P. softened, slightly. "Nachedasan you say you are not a politician, but I beg to differ with you. You just talked yourself into more conversation, but my friend, the explanation better be good or I am out of here."

"Thank you J.P. Perhaps we should ask Ms. Hayes to join us. I understand that she is an officer in your company, perhaps she would like to hear this as well.

J.P. flushed red, embarrassed that he had been caught in his own attempt at counterespionage. "How did you know?"

Nacheda smiled, "J.P. it wasn't difficult. Skip told me that Mandi was traveling with you. When I walked into the bar this evening, it was apparent that it was she from the photo I saw in the James annual report."

J.P. waved to Mandi to join them at the table, "Mr. Nacheda, I would like for you to meet Amanda Hayes. She is Vice President of Marketing at James Pharmaceutical Company."

"I am very pleased to meet you, Ms. Hayes." "Please call me Mandi, "she replied with a smile.

The three chatted informally for nearly thirty minutes before J.P. decided it was time to get back to business. He asked Nacheda to continue his original discussion.

"It is true that I work for Bandai Pharmaceuticals Company but not in a traditional capacity. For the last year, I have been conducting a special Bandai project. The project is to find a pharmaceutical company that would be compatible with Bandai technology. The purpose would be to sign an agreement to work together on a mutually advantageous project." He paused waiting for a response.

J.P. replied, "Please go on, we're listening."

"As I said before, at this point in time, I am not at liberty to disclose how we came to know about the James situation, but it was done legally and by a method I believe you would find very interesting. Let me give you a hint, it is a database management system that uses an artificial intelligence platform. That is all I am at liberty to say, but if we end up working together, I will disclose everything to you.

"Thank you, I understand. Please continue."

"Bandai has developed a patented process of isolating pure active ingredients from herbs and we have a great deal of cash that would help in funding a cooperative project. Unlike many Japanese companies, we do not wish to make an acquisition, rather a joint venture. I realize what I am providing you is a great deal of new information and is probably a surprise, but I think it is worth a second meeting. Wouldn't you agree?"

His knowledge of James and the possibility of an agreement surprised

J.P. Still, things were going a little too fast and he hoped that Nacheda was not going to ask for some kind of commitment. "I agree Nachedasan and I appreciate your being persistent with me. Tell me, what brings you to Singapore at the same time that we are here?" he asked in, what he hoped was a very friendly voice.

Nacheda did not answer the question right away, but thought through his answer. "To tell you the truth, J.P., I am here to meet you. Skip informed me that you were a straight shooter and I, we, did not know how to reach out to James," Nacheda replied a little uncomfortably.

J.P. interpreted this admission and his obvious discomfort as an indication that he was still hiding something. He spoke, "Nacheda that is very fortunate, perhaps a little too fortunate, for both of us. Tell me again who is we and why do you want to reach out to James?"

"We, is Bandai Pharmaceuticals, Dr. Nakasone, the president and founder, and I. Why is because we believe that we have technology that would greatly benefit James and in return, benefit Bandai."

"I'm sorry to be asking so many questions Nachedasan, but I must have a clearer picture. How did you find out that you had a technology that would benefit both companies?"

Nacheda answered. "We...Bandai and I.... did some investigation into U.S. pharmaceutical companies with a knowledge of herbal medicine. James

Pharmaceutical Company surfaced and we began to investigate James as a potential research partner. We are very interested in herbal medicine, as is your company. Therefore we thought there might be something that we could do together."

Mandi joined the discussion. "Why do you want a partner? I would imagine that you can get all the Japanese investment dollars and partners you require to do all the herbal research your company desires." J.P. noted that there was a slight edge to Mandi's voice.

Nacheda answered in a very respectful tone, "Bandai Pharmaceuticals Corporation_Dr. Nakasone to be specific_is different than most other Japanese pharmaceutical companies, particularly in terms of corporate leadership. A dramatic example of this difference is our location in Bandai. As you know, the majority of the pharmaceutical companies in my country are located in Tokyo, Osaka, or Kyoto_not hundreds of miles north of Tokyo. Please believe me when I say that Dr. Nakasone is not one of the members of the, as you would call it, good old boys club. The club consists of members of the Japan Pharmaceutical Association or Nippon Pharmaceutical Council. These pharmaceutical executives do not respect Bandai or Dr. Nakasone's strategies or tactics. They outwardly view Dr.

Nakasone as a rebel and not very important to the future of the pharmaceuticals industry in Japan. Inwardly, they also do not like the fact that Dr. Nakasone lived overseas for many years. They consider him a pseudo westerner. Being thought of as western is not a compliment in Japan.

"So you see Mandi, the vast Japanese investment coffers or partnerships are not readily available to Bandai Pharmaceuticals Company."

He went on, "Bandai has a global vision just like most other growing worldwide companies, but Dr. Nakasone does not want pursue his vision alone. He would like to find a partner who shares the same vision. Other Japanese pharmaceutical companies want to acquire U.S. pharmaceutical companies and are very control oriented. This is not Bandai's vision." He paused again trying to collect his thoughts and then continued, "A year ago we established a task force to investigate U.S. pharmaceutical companies. We wanted to find a company that would fit the model we had established for the perfect Bandai partner."

Mandi finished the thought "And you came up with James as the perfect partner." She turned to me and in a laughing tone said "There are some New York Wall Street analysts who would argue with you and state that we are not perfect for anyone, much less a Japanese partner."

J.P. agreed, nodding his head. Nacheda looked bewildered.

"Sorry, Nacheda. An inside joke. As you know Nachedasan, and if you do not know you could easily find out, we are not being romanced by the U.S. investment community. They are having trouble with our short term financial projections and our performance to plan."

Nacheda replied, "Ah, thank you." He then turned to Mandi, "Did I answer your question Mandi?"

"Yes, but I have another question." Her tone had eased quite a bit. Nacheda's charm was winning her over. "What kind of model were you using to determine a perfect partner?"

Nacheda said without hesitation, "We want a partner that does basic research in herbs, has demonstrated they can produce and market an herbal product, and perhaps was looking for, or could benefit from, a partner with excess cash and new herbal technology."

"That was….is….a very impressive model."

The conversation had come to logical stopping point, so J.P. gave it a push to see how Nacheda would answer. "So where do we go from here?"

His answer was very perceptive. "Bandai, through myself, has approached you, James, with interest in talking about how the two companies we represent can work together. I believe, J.P. that the proverbial ball is in your court. I await your expression of interest." He stopped, but added before

J.P. could respond, "I might add, to show you that there is more to this than a casual interest that we have a patented process that would be of tremendous value to James. What if I told you that this process is capable of isolating the pure alkaloid that you will require to successfully produce the product presently known as JPC138?" He paused to allow his statement to sink in.

He smiled at the surprised expressions on the faces of Mandi and J.P. Mandi's mouth had dropped open and she was staring at Nacheda. She turned to look to J.P., expecting some sort of explanation as to Nacheda's insider knowledge. J.P. did not have an answer.

Her voice again took on a slight edge, but it was respectful. "Nachedasan, I would say that your research into James has been quite thorough. There are aspects of our business that we feel you should not know unless you have some insider information. We're playing games with each other and we should either get down to serious business and you should place all of your cards on the table or let's just have another Singapore Sling and call it a night. I say your cards because it seems like the topic of conversation is about James proprietary information and not about Bandai. I know that we may have of caused you some discomfort at the onset when J.P. and I played our little cat and mouse game with you, but you're continuing to play with us. Although I respect you, Nacheda-san, I am becoming increasingly uncomfortable about how much you know about James and how little we know about Bandai or its real motives. It is just a little too convenient that all three of us met here in Singapore. I, for one, would like to know what other reasons you have for being here in Singapore, besides drinking Slings with Skip's new acquaintances.

Nacheda was stunned by the directness of Mandi's verbal attack. Nacheda again paused to think over the situation and how he would answer Mandi's question. He suddenly relaxed as if he had made a very important decision. "You are right Mandi and I apologize to both of you for being overly careful or, what you might interpret as being coy. I will tell you more about Bandai and our research. As for my reasons for being here in addition to meeting friends of Skip, I would like to hold that answer until tomorrow. Is this acceptable to both of you?"

Mandi answered for both she and J.P., "Yes. We can wait until tomorrow, but we want an answer and, of course, we can give no assurances that there is a possibility of working together unless we have the complete story. Is this acceptable to you?

"Yes, of course."

Nacheda used the next hour telling them about Dr. Nakasone and the exciting research into isolating pure active ingredients from herbs. J.P. determined that from what he now knew about JPC138, Nacheda had been right about the clinical and production importance of isolating the pure alkaloid. In several glances at Mandi, he was sure that they were both gradually coming to the same conclusion. Bandai with their research and cash resources could make for a win-win situation for both companies.

Nacheda ended his story with another of his surprise questions. "And now, do you want to tell me more about why you are in Singapore?"

It was now J.P. who hesitated before answering a pointed question. Mandi also waited for him to answer the question. J.P. ran all the possible answers through his mind. If he told him the total story, would he be telling him too much? Could he tell him without loosing a future negotiating advantage? He quickly thought back over his conversations of the evening. If he confirmed Nacheda's suspicions about the Devil Tree supply situation, the potential deal might be blown because the risk would be too high. On the other hand, there was nothing wrong with saying that they were going to visit the supplier of herbal raw material. If Nacheda's task force had done as much research as it seemed they had done on James, Nacheda already knew about the Devil Tree supply. J.P. decided there was no harm in telling that him they were on their way to visit the plantation.

"Nachedasan, Mandi and I are going to visit the plantation where they grow the Alstonia spectabilis that is used in both Lifeal and JPC138. We are supposed to visit the plantation once a year to satisfy good manufacturing practices, or GMP, regulations. Mandi is the official James corporate officer for the visit and I wanted to learn more about using herbs in pharmaceuticals."

Nacheda again lapsed into silence. He seemed to be absorbing what J.P. had said. His expression changed as if he had arrived at a conclusion.

"That sounds very interesting, J.P.," he replied. "What time are you leaving?"

J.P. looked at Mandi. "Mandi has the agenda because it is her meeting," he answered.

Mandi gave J.P. a quick look and then said, "We are leaving on a 9:00 a.m. chartered flight from Singapore tomorrow morning. Our visit starts with lunch on Tuesday. We plan to return Wednesday morning. We are guests of the plantation owner, Mr. Chang, Jr., Tuesday night."

"Mandi, J.P. if I may, I know this is very presumptuous of me, but I would consider it a privilege if I could accompany you on your visit to the plantation. Do you think this is possible? In return, I would like to invite you to visit Bandai before you return to the United States. The trip would give us time to get to know each other better and perhaps see if there is the possibility for our two companies to work together. What do you think?"

Mandi looked at J.P., who nodded yes. "Nacheda-san, that would be acceptable to us, but I'm concerned that the host will mind."

"I do not think that he will mind my accompanying you if you say that I am also working with James. If he does mind, then I will find accommodations nearby until you are ready to leave."

"I think this would be acceptable to everyone concerned," J.P. replied. "Then it is settled." Nacheda said with finality in his voice. I look forward to enjoying the trip with you and hearing more about Annie as well as your company. Skip is a dear friend and I know he is very taken with Annie." He pushed back his chair and as he was rising he said, "I must get some rest and call Bandai."

"We also look forward to tomorrow. Shall we meet at 6:00 a.m. for breakfast in the coffee shop?"

"Sounds good to me," Nacheda said. "Have a good rest. I will see you tomorrow morning."

"Good night Nachedasan," the two Americans said in unison. Nacheda left the bar.

J.P. and Mandi ordered one last round of drinks despite J.P.'s concern that any more alcohol would not help them to be at a 6:00 a.m. breakfast meeting. They still talked about how Bandai and James might work together and concluded that although it sounded exciting, it was probably too good to be true and they would have to find out more about Bandai Pharmaceuticals Company before making any conclusions.

When they had finished their drinks, J.P. signed the bill and they went back to their room overlooking the city. The Raffles tower was one of the tallest buildings in that section of Singapore. The view was tremendous. They were on a corner with a balcony. J.P. slid back the door and they walked out onto the balcony. There was a light warm sea breeze that felt good on their faces and ruffled Mandi's hair. They stood for a moment looking out over the Singapore Strait in the direction of the northern shore of Sumatra in Indonesia. Merchant ships dotted the horizon like little fireflies. J.P. placed his left arm around Mandi's slim waist. She folded her arms across her chest moving her right hand to cover his hand.

Mandi gently squeezed his hand and said, "It is beautiful here, isn't it J.P.?"

"Yes, it is. Singapore is one of my favorite cities," he answered. "It is as beautiful in the sun as it is in darkness. You can't say that about a lot of places. The city is even more beautiful for me now because you are here and we're together."

J.P. turned her around to face him and their lips met in a kiss. They pressed their bodies together as they kissed. The on-shore breeze picked up and Mandi's red hair and blew it around their faces. Her body shivered and he could feel small goose bumps forming on her arms.

"You're cold?" he asked in a whisper. "Only, where you are not touching me." "Let's go to bed," he whispered.

Mandi answered by kissing his ear and saying, "We still have to make up for the day we lost when we crossed the International Date Line." With a smile she said formally, "If you will excuse me I will retire to our dressing room and prepare myself."

Mandi grabbed her small suitcase and went into the dressing room leaving me standing just inside the sliding door that led to the balcony. He undressed and opened a bottle of Champagne. He removed the bedspread and neatly folded it and placed it on the luggage rack. He then put on a silk robe that hotel provided with the room and then lay down on top of the sheets. It was a full ten minutes before Mandi came into the room.

Mandi emerged leaving the light on in the dressing room, which silhouetted her body. She wore a new lavender gown that clung to her body. Her red hair gently fell and rested just below her shoulders. J.P. rose to hand her a glass of Champagne. As she took it, the scent of her perfume flooded over him.

"You look magnificent, Mandi. I don't think I have ever seen you look so beautiful and radiant."

She raised up and kissed him. "Thank you, my love. It is you that brings out what you see in me." She started to move to her side of the bed.

"No, wait a minute please," he said softly. "Let's turn on some soft music and dance for a little while."

"That's a great idea J.P., I would love to dance."

He walked over the audio unit that was part of the room's entertainment system. J.P. located a station that played soft Jazz. She came to him and they began dancing slowly, relishing the music and the feel of their bodies moving against one another.

"I love you," he whispered in her ear.

"I love you with all my heart," Mandi whispered back.

They danced for a long time, kissing and whispering. Finally their bodies couldn't take anymore and they found their way to the bed.

RAFFLES HOTEL SINGAPORE

Nacheda was right on time for breakfast, as were J.P. and Mandi much to their own surprise. They were seated at a large table for four in the coffee shop of the hotel. Each of them had, in turn, ordered a large breakfast.

They spent most of their time over the morning meal discussing the possibilities of James and Bandai working together.

After the plates had been cleared from the table and another round of coffee was poured, Nacheda disclosed that his secondary reason for his coming to Singapore was to learn more about the Devil Tree.

"I was able to reach Dr. Nakasone last night. He has given me permission to be absolutely frank with you. Dr. Nakasone's vision for a partnership is based on an open dialogue and complete cooperation. In this way he expects the relationship between Bandai Pharmaceuticals and James Pharmaceutical Company to be that of a true partnership.

"If this is to be the case, then there is something else that I must tell you. My trip to Singapore was intended not only to meet you, but also to visit the plantation in order to find out more about the Devil Tree. I was also instructed to obtain sample quantities of the bark in order to test the Bandai alkaloid isolation process specifically on the Devil Tree bark. Please forgive me for not explaining this last night, but I felt that is was better to be overly cautious because you were the first contacts that my company had made at James. We were afraid that you might be scared away by being contacted by a Japanese company because most contacts by Japanese firms are generally thought of as being hostile. Further, I did not have the authority to disclose everything because Dr. Nakasone had instructed me not to disclose everything at the first meeting. I knew, after our meeting last night that I could trust your judgment and would have disclosed everything, but I wanted to obtain Dr. Nakasone's permission first. I hope you understand."

It seemed to J.P. that Nacheda was being sincere and that he wanted their approval and understanding.

"Nachedasan," J.P. replied, "Mandi and I both understand large corporation policies and chain of command. We accept your apology and we understand. We have both been in the same position that you found yourself in last night."

"Thank you," Nacheda replied in a cheerful tone. He then discussed his abortive attempt to visit Mr. Chang's son and how the father had told him that the son would be back in Jakarta on Wednesday. After a discussion J.P. and Mandi were encouraged that the elder Chang had not disclosed the location of the plantation to someone outside of the James organization.

8:00 A.M., TUESDAY, FEBRUARY 28
RAFFLES HOTEL SINGAPORE

When they had finished their breakfast the three went back to their rooms and agreed to meet in the lobby at 8:00 to catch a cab to the airport. They changed into casual clothes for the trip to the plantation. J.P. had been warned, during his time with Joe in the production division, that the road to the plantation would be rough and if it rained the road was virtually impassable.

They were standing in the lobby and about to walk outside to have the doorman hail a cab when a fourth person, an Asian, joined their group. J.P., Mandi, and Nacheda paid little attention to the man and turned to walk away. The Asian put his hand on Nacheda's arm and gently tugged. Nacheda turned to him and the man spoke to him in Japanese. J.P. and Mandi had stopped and turned around to watch Nacheda and the other man converse. The conversation seemed to J.P. to be very serious. He had initially thought that this person must be a friend of Nacheda's even though he was fairly certain that Nacheda was in Singapore alone. J.P. became a little more concerned when the stranger's tone turned somewhat menacing.

Nacheda tried to back away from the man who then tightened his grip on Nacheda's right arm to prevent him from moving. The stranger then said something else in Japanese, which sounded like an order. J.P. started to move forward to see if Nacheda required any help and to determine whether the man was a friend or a threat. As he got closer, Nacheda put up his left hand to stop him. The Asian barked another order at Nacheda and started to pull him away.

"Nacheda is something wrong?" J.P. asked. He felt Mandi at his side.

She had stayed close to him and now slipped her arm through his.

"I am afraid so, J.P.," replied Nacheda. "This person has informed me that I am not to leave the hotel. He has a very tight grip on my arm and he says the object that is sticking in my back is a gun. He has informed me that there are three additional people somewhere in the lobby who have their weapons trained on us. He recommends that we cooperate with he and his associates."

"Is there anything we can do?" J.P. asked.

The Asian spoke again in a very stern manner, but in a voice low enough so that others standing in the lobby wouldn't hear. The other people in the lobby were oblivious to the activity that was going on with Nacheda.

The man spoke again, this time in English and directly to J.P., "Dr. Koenig, that is your name, is it not?" He did not wait for a reply. "I would suggest that you remain silent and follow instructions and you and the lady will not be harmed."

J.P. glared at him trying to decide what he should do. He looked around the lobby that was becoming increasingly crowded and was able to pick out three additional Japanese men who seemed to be watching them with interest. All of the men had draped jackets over the right forearms covering their hand. Nacheda and the man were speaking again in Japanese. There was anger in both of their voices, but the volume was kept low.

After a lengthy exchange, Nacheda turned to Mandi and J.P. and said. "Mandi, J.P., it seems we are to be taken to an unknown location and detained for an unspecified amount of time. If we do not come along in complete cooperation they will drag me off after silencing me with a pistol. I have tried to negotiate with them so that you might be left behind because this is between them and I, but they will hear of no such thing. You are now part of this situation and are expected to cooperate or there is a very good possibility that we all might be harmed. If we jump the man behind me the others will finish whatever he is unable to complete."

"So," the man said in English, "now that Mr. Nacheda has explained the situation, we would like for all of you to move to the side door on my left. After we exit the hotel you will turn left and proceed to a white stretch limousine. A man will be standing at the rear door and will assist you into the backseat. Please do not try and escape. My associates are now positioned on the street and they will prevent you from ever leaving here alive. So now please, very slowly, turn and walk towards the door on your left. All of your lives depend on your following my orders."

Mandi and J.P. turned towards the door that he had indicated. Mandi had not taken her arm from J.P. and her grip had gotten tighter as the tension had increased. The lobby had become increasingly crowded in the time since they had come down from their rooms. There were about fifty people milling about, waiting for tourist buses or for the rest of their party to join them. There wasn't very much open room so the group of four had to walk in a tight group. Mandi and J.P. led the way followed by Nacheda and the stranger with a gun.

He noticed that the door that they were walking towards opened inward. He quickly whispered to Mandi, "After going through the door turn right, drop to your knees, and crawl like hell."

She squeezed his arm in acknowledgment.

They reached the glass doors and Mandi released her grip on his arm. Being the first to reach the door, she reached out to grasp the handle and started to pull the door open. There was a rush of warm, humid air as the door moved from its frame. Since the door had to be pulled the group bunched up. Nacheda was now slightly behind J.P. and crowded against his left side. The man with the gun was almost on top of them so he couldn't tell Nacheda of his plan. Because the man wasn't wearing a suit or sports coat, it was very difficult for him to hide the gun without remaining right up against Nacheda.

J.P. had formed a plan but it depended on the man not being able to hold the muzzle of the gun directly against Nacheda's back for fear of being noticed. He assumed that the gun would be parallel to Nacheda's back and if discharged would fire to the side. It was a risky proposition either way, but he felt that he had to take the chance. He had already decided that there was no way that he was going to allow Mandi or himself to be taken to a location that was controlled by kidnappers.

As Mandi stepped around the door and over the threshold she turned to her right. She immediately dropped to her knees on the pavement and began crawling away. J.P. slipped through the partially opened door and as he did, he spun around and grabbed Nacheda pulling him forward through the opening with his right hand. His left reached for the door handle as the gunman, caught off guard by Nacheda's sudden move, now tried to come through the doorway himself. Nacheda caught on to J.P.'s plan and also grabbed at the handle. They both gave the door a yank.

The clearance between Nacheda and the man had not been enough and the man's left foot was caught in the threshold. The gun discharged. It did not make a load sound because it was fitted with a silencer, but J.P. heard the pop. At the time he heard the muffled pop he was dropping down to the right to crawl off in the direction that Mandi had gone. His right knee hit the pavement hard sending a sharp pain up his thigh and into his spine. He fell to the right against the building and then proceeded forward after Mandi. Another silencer pop reached his ears. He glanced over his shoulder and saw Nacheda just a foot behind crawling on his hands and knees.

By this time all the bystanders in front of the hotel knew something was going on. They could see men running around with guns drawn and three people crawling along the side the building. Most of the bystanders were just staring with their mouths hanging open. One woman began to scream.

Mandi took a sharp right turn through another door and went back into the hotel lobby and stood up. Nacheda and J.P. followed. Nacheda now took the lead and said out loud, "Follow me." The three of them moved quickly through the lobby and down the hallway into the coffee shop kitchen area.

J.P. noticed that the back of Nacheda's pant leg in the area of his calf was turning red with blood. He had been hit. J.P. assumed that it was not as bad as it looked because he seemed to be moving without any physical problem although the loss of blood looked to be at a rate that would soon be a problem. He took a turn into a staircase and began climbing the stairs two at a time. Mandi followed with J.P. bringing up the rear. He stopped for a moment to listen for sounds of people following, but heard nothing.

J.P. focused his thoughts on who might yet be in front of them. He yelled to Nacheda, "No one is following. Stop!"

He stopped, as did Mandi. They were all breathing hard and no one spoke until they had each taken a number of deep breaths. They listened in silence. In the background there were only the normal sounds of a kitchen.

"Nacheda, you're hit!" Mandi exclaimed in a concerned voice.

"It is not bad," Nacheda answered. "I will tend to it later. There might be someone following us. We should wait and surprise them."

"I don't agree. What is in front of us is more important to our survival than what has passed," J.P. stated.

"You are correct, J.P. Now we must get to my room and figure out what has happened."

"No, I disagree again," J.P. said. "Whomever is behind this attempted kidnapping was after you not Mandi or I. They likely have been watching you and will know your room number. There may be someone waiting there for you to return."

"I agree," Mandi said. "Let's go to our room, look at that wound and then get out of the hotel as fast as possible."

"Agreed" said Nacheda. "What is the room number?"

"636," she answered.

J.P. looked at the stairway door and the floor number where we had stopped. The numeral 4 was painted in bright red in the middle of the door.

"Two more floors, but be careful stepping out into the hall," he instructed.

"Right," Nacheda answered.

They continued their climb to the sixth floor. They had no further incidents and in a few minutes were in the room. Once inside, J.P. bolted the door and moved a small table with a marble top against the door as a barrier. He went into the bathroom and came out with a large towel.

"Nacheda, take off your trousers and let's see how bad your wound is. You can wrap this towel around your waist. And while we are looking at your leg how about telling us what the hell is going on. Is there something else you have forgotten to tell us?" J.P. was having a hard time keeping the anger out of his voice. "Whatever is going on has placed us all in grave danger and most importantly, we were unprepared for this kind of danger. Now let's have the full story, Nacheda or Mandi and I are splitting company with you right now."

"J.P., based on everything that has transpired since we met, you have every right to be mad at me. But I swear to you. I am in the dark about this kidnapping. I do not know why anyone would want to have me kidnapped or why it was today and in Singapore. If someone wanted to kidnap or kill me they have had numerous chances here, in Japan, and in the United States. It doesn't make sense. The only thing that is different about today is our planned trip to the Devil Tree plantation and I'm with the two of you. I agree with you though, it was me that they were after, not you or Mandi.

"Since my arrival, I have had no warning or indication that someone was after me. I have, though, had a general feeling that someone has been following me. This feeling was especially strong when I went to see the elder Chang in Jakarta. At one point, I tried to trick my invisible follower by changing patterns and looking behind me unexpectedly, but this was to no avail. I finally decided that it was just my imagination. The bottom line is, whatever triggered this kidnap attempt is most probably connected to our trip to the plantation."

"Why would anyone be so interested in your trip to the plantation that they would try to kidnap and kill you?" Mandi asked.

Nacheda answered "As I am sure you both know, although you have not acknowledged the fact to me, the Alstonia spectabilis tree is known only to exist, in quantities large enough for commercial harvesting on the Chang plantation. I know, and because I know, it is possible that others have this knowledge. With this and the knowledge that the plantation supplies James with the necessary raw material for Lifeal it is just possible that someone besides James and Bandai are interested in either acquiring the supply of the Devil Tree or want the James supply to be shut off. Since you and James have every right to be at the plantation then I must conclude that it is Bandai that someone wants to prevent from visiting the plantation. Your next question will be who is this someone? I am sorry, but I can not answer that question. I have no idea who would not want us to be working together."

J.P. looked over at Mandi. Almost simultaneously they said, "The 21st Century Plan."

Nacheda was startled at their strange response. "What in the hell is the 21st Century Plan?"

Mandi and J.P. laughed at his use of the word hell. It relieved some of the tension between them that had been building ever since the episode in the lobby. After a second Nacheda joined in laughing.

"Nacheda, your surprise at our mentioning of the 21st Century Plan is understandable and also a relief to Mandi and I. Let me look at your wound and Mandi will explain the 21st Century Plan. Okay, Mandi?"

"Fine, J.P." Looking at J.P., she remarked, "If Nachedasan knew anything about the theft of the 21st Century Plan he would have reacted differently." Mandi then turned to face Nacheda. They were in the living room of the suite. Mandi was seated on the couch and Nacheda who had been sitting on the marble coffee table facing Mandi now stretched out on the floor so that J.P. could examine his wound.

Mandi continued addressing herself to Nacheda. "I would like a little more explanation on how you know so much about the Devil Tree before I do my explanation about the 21st Century Plan."

Nacheda was quiet again. He was going through the same thought process he had used previously when to answering some of their questions. "I told you about our task force, but I did not tell you about our computer system. I am not at liberty to go through the entire system in detail because it is highly secret to Bandai and it is not germane to our working together. Please do not get me wrong. If it were germane then I would tell you everything about SAM. SAM is what we call the computer system. SAM stands for strategic analysis manager. Let me just say that SAM is a very comprehensive information gathering system connected with an artificial intelligence platform. These two interactive systems came up with the conclusion that the supply of Alstonia spectabilis or Devil Tree was critical to James immediate success and to survival as a viable pharmaceutical corporation. My mission, as I have told you was to verify the importance of Devil Tree. I have studied all the books I could find on the subject and SAM has researched the literature. There hasn't been much written on the Devil Tree, but what has been written, I have read. Is this a satisfactory answer?"

"For now, yes. In the future, if we are going to work together we would like to know what other little tidbits of information SAM has come up with in regards to James. I guess, since you were surprised at the mention of the 21st Century Plan, that this plan was not one of the areas about James that SAM uncovered." Mandi then began the story of the 21st Century Plan and the extra copy. The two James employees both knew that they were violating some of Phillip's trust, but they had shared the threat of death with Nacheda and saw no reason not to let him in on the existence of the 21st Century Plan.

During Mandi's story, J.P. was examining the wound on the back of Nacheda's calf. There was a long shallow groove cut across the top of the calf muscle where the bullet had grazed him. There was no harm to a vein or artery, but it was bleeding fairly heavily. J.P. determined that all he would likely need were a few butterfly strips to pull the skin together and hold it until the wound healed. He had a first aid kit that he had brought along and he went to get it from his suitcase.

While they were talking in the hotel room, they heard the sound of several sirens down on the street. They all assumed that three things had or were happening. First, that the kidnappers had most likely gotten away. Second, there was a good possibility that the hotel and police did not know who the attempted kidnapping had focused on. And third, there was probably still confusion in the lobby. Now they saw the task ahead was to fix Nacheda's wound and then get themselves safely out of the hotel without any further delay.

Mandi continued her explanation as J.P. applied an anti-biotic ointment to the wound, used the butterfly strips to hold the skin together, and then wrapped the wound with adhesive gauze. Nacheda winced a few times, but said nothing. The wound was not as bad as it looked. J.P. knew there would be a scar since the wound wasn't stitched shut, but it would not be an unsightly scar. As he was dressing the wound, he noticed other scars along the backs of both of his legs. He didn't ask Nacheda how he had received the other scars.

Mandi finished her explanation. "So Nacheda-san, does this help in determining who else is involved in our present situation?"

"Mandi, all it does is confirm that there is another player. Who and why I still do not know. I do believe that they do not play by our ethical rules so we must be prepared for further problems. How does my wound look, J.P.?"

He explained what he saw and then gave them his proposed plan of action. "I figure we must leave the hotel as soon as possible and to do so without alarming the hotel or our pursuers. If we hurry we can still get to the plantation this afternoon.

"Nacheda-san is there anything in your room that could be used to protect us?" he asked.

"Nothing, J.P." answered Nacheda. "Firearms are not allowed in Singapore. If the police catch the kidnappers they will be severely punished. It is even a good possibility they will be executed. When I come to Singapore, I do not even tempt this possibility. I do have some small oxygen canisters that I have altered. One is filled with mace and the other tear gas. Either canister can be sprayed and the tear gas can be thrown. I have four of each." Nacheda noticed the questioning looks on our faces "You are surprised? Well, we Japanese are freaks for fresh oxygen. In Japan it is the 'in' thing to periodically fill your lungs with pure oxygen. Everyone accepts the fact that Japanese businessmen travel with small oxygen canisters so officials inspect them and the airport scanners are programmed to highlight them, but then pass them through as safe. Business in this part of the world can get kind of rough and tumble sometimes, so it pays to be prepared. I am quite good at the martial arts but every once in a while I require some help to keep the odds even or slanted my way. A small dose of mace or a cloud of tear gas in the right place, at the right time can do more damage than a gun. I have these items with me in my briefcase, so the only items we have available for protection are already with us. There is no need to go back to my room."

"Well, there is a small tear in your pant leg and some blood that stained the fabric. I have a pair of trousers that will probably fit you. Hang on and I'll get them from my bag."

"Thank you. I know a side entrance to the hotel. We can leave that way and very few, if any hotel staff will see us leave. We can catch a cab on Victoria Street. I suggest we call the air service that you've chartered your plane through and change our flight departure. Let's shoot for a 10:00 departure. J.P., why don't you call Mr. Chang, Jr. at the plantation and tell him that you've been delayed, and you will be late. Do not mention me. I think my attendance should not be announced."

"I agree, Nacheda-san. Mandi what do you think?"

"Whatever. Let's get on with it," Mandi answered with stress in her voice.

J.P. put the call through to Chang and told him that they would be late. Chang told him that it would not be a problem.

They called the air charter service to move the departure to 10:00. They cautiously stepped out into the hallway and closed the door. Nacheda then led them down the stairs and through empty hallways that appeared to be used for temporary storage. Before long they were at the end of a hallway in front of a fire door. They had managed to reach the exit without meeting one other person. J.P. pushed the crossbar and they all stepped out onto the street. They walked to the corner and looked left to the main entrance of the hotel along Beach Road. There were many people and police cars in front of Raffles. They walked right and started looking for a taxi.

After a block of walking they found a taxi and soon were on their way to the Airport. They kept looking for the limo that the kidnappers had been using, but saw nothing. If there was another attempt they figured it would be at the airport.

J.P. had the cab driver stop at a pharmacy so that he could purchase a few more supplies for Nacheda's wound. Nacheda said the pain was minimal. There was some pulling of the skin as the wound dried. He told them that he had learned in Vietnam that he was a fast healer. J.P. decided not to follow up on the admission that a Japanese soldier had been wounded in Vietnam.

At just past ten o'clock, their plane lifted off for Java.

9:00 A.M., TUESDAY, FEBRUARY 28

KATONG DISTRICT SINGAPORE

As Mandi, JP, and Nacheda were making their way to the airport, the kidnappers were apprehended by the Singapore police. Witnesses to the incident at Raffles had described the limousine and one person had actually written down the license plate. When the Raffles doorman called the police to report the trouble he was able to give them all the information that they required in order to make a quick apprehension. The kidnappers had not gotten more than a mile from Raffles on the East Coast Parkway before the police forced the limousine off of the road. There was a short skirmish between police and the three occupants of the limousine. During the fight the occupants of the limousine were killed.

The NPC backup car to the limousine witnessed the police forcing the limousine off of the road and turned off into the Katong District and onto Mountbatten Road where they were able to watch the ensuing gun battle. The Japanese man in the passenger seat picked up his digital phone and dialed a number in Japan.

After two rings the phone at the NPC headquarters in Japan was answered. "Tanaguchi here."

"Mr. Tanaguchi, Singapore here. I am sorry to report that the Bandai man was not stopped in Singapore. He has joined the James people and I am sure they are now all on a flight to Java and then to the plantation. They escaped the trap we had set for them at Raffles. We did not anticipate the capabilities of the James people. The man known as Koenig aborted the attempt to kidnap the Bandai man. Our three associates here in Singapore were forced off of the road by the Singapore police and from what we have seen, we must assume they were killed by the police. There are no other witnesses to the attempted kidnap and I was not identified. I await further instructions."

"Fools, fools," Tanaguchi said loudly. Then he paused. His Singapore associate waited patiently for instructions.

"Your instructions are to go to the Singapore airport and wait for the return of the Bandai and James party. Obtain additional help and apprehend if they succeed in eluding the plantation trap. Is this clear?"

"*Hai. Wakarikiru, Tanaguchisan*," and the connection was disconnected.

9:00 A.M., TUESDAY, FEBRUARY 28

NIPPON PHARMACEUTICAL COUNCIL HEADQUARTERS OSAKA, JAPAN

Tanaguchi hung up the phone. "Fools!," he said out loud. It was a good thing that they had all died. It saved him the problem of having contracts eliminated before they could talk to the police. Tanaguchi trusted no person's loyalty. It was safer to eliminate them before testing loyalty. The problem now was that Nacheda had been alerted to danger. This made him a very dangerous man. Tanaguchi felt that he must warn Lonewolf.

He wrote an encrypted email to send to the plantation that he hoped Lonewolf would receive prior to Nacheda's arrival.

TO: Lonewolf

FROM: Tanaguchi

SUBJ: FLASH COMMUNIQUE

Lonewolf via corporate communications FLASH priority Nacheda escaped Singapore trap.

Believed to be en route your location accompanied by Koenig and Hayes of James Pharmaceutical Company.

Terminate Nacheda's ability to interfere with our plan.

We believe that Koenig and Hayes don't know of NPC involvement. Ensure they do not find out, terminate with prejudice if necessary.

Report actions ASAP. /s/ Tanaguchi

Tanaguchi could only hope that Lonewolf would receive the email in time.

8:00 A.M. LOCAL, TUESDAY, FEBRUARY 28

CHANG'S PLANTATION OFFICE JAVA, INDONESIA

Lonewolf awoke at 8:00 and went to the common room for breakfast.

Only Marisa was there to greet him.

"Good morning Mr. Smith. Mr. Chang is outside somewhere on the plantation. He said for you to enjoy your breakfast and he will meet you in his office at nine o'clock. Breakfast buffet is on the table. I am sure you will find an assortment of various foods that will satisfy your tastes. I will leave you to eat in solitude. Mr. Chang's office is to the right after you leave this room. Is there anything else I can do for you, Mr. Smith?"

"No thank you, Marisa, everything is fine."

Lonewolf ate his breakfast in silence. Everything was not fine. Chang's snub began to eat into Lonewolf's psyche. He was well on his way to being really pissed with Chang Junior. He knew it would not do any good to get angry. Getting angry hampered his negotiating skills. He sat back in his chair and forced himself to calm down.

After he had finished his breakfast, he rose from the table and went outside. Again he walked around the house committing every angle and stairway down to the ground to memory. He surveyed his surroundings looking for openings into the dense jungle. Finally, he returned to this room and lay down for fifteen minutes.

At just before 9:00 he walked the length of the porch to Chang's office.

He knocked and entered after he heard Chang beckon him inside.

"Good morning, Mr. Smith," Chang said as he jumped up from his chair.

The two men shook hands across the desk. Chang's office was all natural wood with the walls made of mahogany. Somewhere in the room camphor wood had been used because there was a very strong and distinct odor of camphor. The walls were empty of any decorations. Except for a lamp on the desk and one chair in front of the desk, there was no other furniture in the office. Even though it was a bright day outside, the wood made the room very dark. The lamp had a bark opaque shade. Light only shown through the top and onto the ceiling and downward onto the desk. It was difficult for the men to see on another's faces. The room had an eerie glow. Lonewolf assumed that Chang was used to the conditions and had created them to give himself some sort of edge.

Chang motioned to Lonewolf to sit in the chair. "I trust you slept well and had a satisfactory breakfast. I again apologize for not having the best menu, but we do what we can." Chang's words dripped with honey.

"The sleep was great and so was the breakfast. You do not have to apologize. Marisa prepares an excellent meal and should be complimented." Lonewolf replied doing his best to maintain a civil tone in his words.

The animosity that had built up during dinner the night before had disappeared. It was difficult to see in the dim light, but Chang appeared well rested.

"If you do not mind, Mr. Smith I would like to get right to business." Chang's voice had taken on a serious tone. "I am very sorry that I can't accept the kind offer that you made me last night to acquire the exclusive rights to the Alstonia spectabilis tree. It was a very generous offer, but I am afraid my father and I know the Devil Tree is worth more than the value you have placed on the bark. If you have no counteroffer then I think our business discussions are completed. You are welcome to stay through lunch, but after lunch I have new guests coming to the plantation."

As Lonewolf sat outwardly quiet, listening to Chang's eloquent speech inside he was fighting the urge to reach across the desk and grab Chang by the throat. He remained cool because he knew Chang was not through negotiating. Lonewolf would try to exercise patience.

"Mr. Chang," Lonewolf said trying to be as polite as possible, "did you speak to your father about my proposition?"

"Yes, Mr. Smith. He was in total agreement with my decision."

"Mr. Chang.," Lonewolf remained polite hoping the impact of his next words would knock Chang down a few pegs. He was careful that his voice did not indicate anger or threat.

"You are a lying snake in the grass." Lonewolf was smiling as he talked. "I know for a fact that your father is in the intensive care unit of Cipto Mangunkusumo General Hospital in Jakarta. He had an accident recently. So I know that you could not have talked with him yesterday or today. If you do not show some sign of cooperation with me and the people that I represent.," he paused to ensure Chang heard him, and then continued, ".I understand there is an empty bed next to your father's bed."

Chang was silent, but his face and eyes showed terror, anger, pain, and sorrow. Even in the dim light, his face had taken on a red tinge. Tears formed in Chang's eyes from anger and sorrow. Anger began to dominate his face pushing back the other emotions. He spoke, but his voice did not reflect his feelings. Chang was thinking he would show this arrogant American that he was strong.

"I am not frighten by your threats, Mr. Smith. You're in my county now, as your television actors say. You might think you are safe, but you are far from safe. I can eliminate your three friends that came with you the second I choose to do so. I can then make the remaining hours of your stay here on earth very painful, but since I haven't given the order and we are still sitting here, I have chosen not to take these aggressive actions. The accident to my father is very unfortunate, but he is a strong old man. He is what you Americans call a survivor." He paused. "Very much like you and I, Mr. Smith. We too are survivors. So I choose to negotiate. I still cannot accept your offer, but what do you think about $130.00 per cubic meter and 10% of the gross sales from any product derived from the bark?"

Still in an outwardly calm voice Lonewolf answered Chang. "I appreciate your strong willpower but I do not believe you heard what I said last night. Allow me try to explain our position a little more clearly. No fucking way!" The last three words were said loudly and with venom.

Chang sat coolly and took Lonewolf's insult. He then spoke again in a very calm manner. "Mr. Smith, I can see that the plantation and the groves of Devil Trees are very important to you and those whom you represent. I must assure you that, since we are the only plantation of this particular species of Devil Tree sufficient to provide production quantities of raw material, you would be lost without our plantation." He held up his hand stopping Lonewolf from answering "No, please Mr. Smith let me finish. I do not care what you think about me because it is irrelevant to our negotiations." Lonewolf closed his mouth.

"Good, Mr. Smith. It is a pleasure to know that your mouth is not always open and spewing foul words. To go on, I had determined, without my father's immediate permission, that in the event that we are unable to reach an agreement and you threaten or harm me in anyway, I would systematically blow up and burn the plantation. What you will be left with is a burned and useless field of dead trees. Since you know so much about the Devil Tree, I am certain that you also know that it takes fifteen years for the tree to reach maturity. Therefore, sir, you and the people you represent will be out of business, at least as far the Devil Tree is concerned."

The information sank into Lonewolf's mind and negotiating stance. So this is Chang's hidden card. It is a good card. Lonewolf was quiet. He had to think this one out. He had to have the trees. The entire project would be blown without the trees. This was a formidable card. Was he bluffing? He could not take the chance that Chang was bluffing. Lonewolf had to come off his position, but first he required time to think about this new information.

"Mr. Chang," Lonewolf began, "I believe we have reached a standoff position in our negotiations. May I suggest that perhaps we should take a walk and visit some of your plantation facilities that process the Devil Tree bark. During this walk we can discuss different alternatives. I am sure that we can reach an agreement that would be satisfactory to both of us. First, I must state that I am just a representative and only have certain negotiating parameters. Once outside my approved parameters I must go back to my clients for approval. I am sure you will see my point."

"Your suggestion is well timed, Mr. Smith. I accept your suggestion."

Both men got up from their chairs and proceeded outside. At the threshold of the door Chang stopped and turned to Lonewolf. His black eyes now bore into Lonewolfs blue eyes. "Mr. Smith, even if you have threatened me many times yesterday and today, I know that you are an honorable man and a man of your word. But, I must inform you, if I have any kind of fatal accident or for some reason I am not back here at twelve o'clock my people have been instructed to ignite the plantation. There is no way that you or any of your friends can prevent this from happening. You must believe me, Mr. Smith, I am not bluffing. I have too much to lose."

"I believe you Mr. Chang. As I stated before, we have a standoff. You and I both need each other and we need the trees. Please be comfortable and let's enjoy our walk." This creep would make a good poker player Lonewolf thought to himself. They started off across the lawn.

12:00 P.M. LOCAL, TUESDAY, FEBRUARY 28
CHANG'S PLANTATION OFFICE JAVA, INDONESIA

Chang and Lonewolf finished their tour of the plantation and its facilities and returned to Chang's office at the plantation house. During their walk they had come to an agreement $118.00 U.S. per cubic meter and 5% of the venture.

Lonewolf knew the NPC would be very happy with the deal. He had kept the terms under what the NPC was willing to pay. He felt that he should receive a bonus. If not, then he might be able to cut himself a side deal with Chang and have him charge the NPC at a rate of $120.00 U.S. and 10%.

As they were walking, Chang had shown Lonewolf land mines in the groves. Chang explained that the mines were placed throughout the plantation. They were safe unless a major switch was thrown to activate the mines. There were two modes. One mode was for single detonation when triggered by something coming within the proximity of the mine. The other mode was set for complete destruction. Complete destruction was initiated at a number of key locations around the plantation and required the input of a digital pass code. Lonewolf now believed that Chang genuinely had the capability to blow up the plantation. He also concluded that this minefield security system would come in handy for the future management of the plantation.

Chang suggested that they have lunch to celebrate the agreement. "My visitors have been delayed and we may therefore have lunch together."

"Sounds like a good idea to me," replied Lonewolf. He did not want to hang around any longer than necessary. He believed that when a deal is cut, it is time to cut out. They entered the common room. Marisa was at her normal place at the table. The table was set for Chinese food. Chang and Lonewolf sat down to eat and to enjoy a newfound mutual relationship.

1:00 P.M. LOCAL, TUESDAY, FEBRUARY 28
DEVIL TREE PLANTATION JAVA, INDONESIA

The vehicle that had been sent for them at the airstrip left the road to Yogyakarta and made its way up a road that pointed to the summit of Mt. Merapi. Mandi and J.P. were in the backseat of the Toyota four-wheeler, hanging on to the passenger handles above the doors as the vehicle bounced over the ruts in the road. Nacheda, in the front seat, looked to J.P. as though he was having a similar experience. The Indonesian driver, who had been sent by Mr. Chang, Jr. from the plantation, seemed to be enjoying himself as he piloted the Toyota along the road. He told his passengers to imagine that they were on an amusement park ride and not be worried. He was a small man who had given his name as Luther when he picked them up. He spoke English very well and kept the group of visitors entertained during the drive.

The day was beautiful. There were small white cumulus clouds floating in the blue sky. While they drove along the smooth highway Luther had kept up a continuous chatter about the sights along the way and sights that they were going to see.

The vehicle had turned off the access road and was halfway through the Devil Tree plantation when Nacheda saw the first Japanese guard. Using his head instead of his hand, he pointed out a man standing next to a tree in the second row of trees.

"Do you see that guy standing part way in the trees?" He asked to no one in particular.

Mandi and J.P. looked in the direction that Nacheda had indicated. "Is he a worker?" J.P. asked.

Luther answered, "No, doctor. I do not know him and he doesn't have the clothes of a worker." The man in the trees wore tropical slacks, a Philippine dress shirt, and a pith helmet.

"He looks Japanese and appears to be guarding something. Luther, do you have an explanation?" Nacheda asked.

Luther suddenly became serious, "No, Nachedasan. I do not know the man. I left the plantation Monday morning to visit family and pick up supplies in Magelang. The man must have come to the plantation yesterday or today. I believe that Mr. Chang said that he was going to have visitors, but I thought he meant you. I am sorry, I did not pay any attention to what he was saying."

"Do not worry about it, Luther. He doesn't look like he is threatening." Nacheda assured Luther.

"Nacheda-san are you sure you aren't seeing ghosts from Singapore?" Mandi asked in a sincere manner.

"Maybe so Mandi, but keep your eyes open for other indications of strangers."

Nacheda asked the driver to go slower so they could have more time to react to potential problems. As they drove along they saw more men in the Devil Tree groves, but they were definitely workers. Luther knew these men and hailed each of them as he drove.

The Toyota finally broke out of the trees and entered the plantation house grounds. J.P. quickly surveyed the situation. A large typical Sabat-style house was sitting in a clearing of grass. The area of grass looked to measure fifty meters in radius. He mentally noted that there was a great deal of open space before a person had the cover of the trees.

J.P. told the driver to stop. They were halfway up the drive when he spotted what looked like another guard standing on the stairs between two large trees that straddled the stairs. At that point another Toyota pulled up behind theirs. Nacheda turned around and quietly announced that the man he had seen in the trees a few miles back was driving.

"He is definitely Japanese. If there is something funny going on, I am sure when he saw us on the road he telephoned ahead to have his partner waiting at the house."

"I don't know these men," Luther announced in a soft voice.

J.P. looked at the posture and position of each of the guards. The one on the stairs stood with his legs apart and arms folded in a stance of defiance. He could not see the man's hands so he didn't know if he was hiding any firearms.

The man in the stopped vehicle had not moved from behind the steering wheel. His arms were also folded across his chest. J.P. thought to himself that if they had guns they would be caught in crossfire. He recalled Nacheda's words on the flight from Singapore about the morning's events, "If one Japanese was involved in this intrigue then the person or persons behind this would also be Japanese." These Japanese guards seemed to indicate a definite Japanese connection.

"Luther, pull off to the left and let the Toyota drive past," he ordered.

J.P. was hoping to get them out of the potential crossfire. He wanted both men in front of us so we could see them and watch their actions.

Luther moved the vehicle to the left and onto the grass. The other Toyota did not move.

"Shit. Okay, proceed to the front of the house very slowly and stay to the left," J.P. instructed. "If something potentially happens as we are driving to the front of the house, Luther, you make a hard right and drive back out the driveway and then into the trees."

Luther said, "Sorry Dr. Koenig, I cannot drive into the woods. The groves are mined against intruders."

"Okay, back out to the road then as fast as you can. Mines? Did you say mines, Luther? Why mines?"

"I don't know," he replied. Luther drove slowly up to the front of the house and stopped. J.P. looked over his shoulder and saw that the Toyota had proceeded up the driveway and was stopped about twenty-five feet behind them.

"What the hell do you think is going on Nacheda-san?" he asked.

"I'm not sure. They are expecting you, Mandi, and Luther. With these dark windows they likely haven't spotted me yet. Of course, if they are associated with our unknown Singapore kidnappers and knew that I was in the car then I think we would have had some hostile activity before we reached this point. I believe they are waiting to see what we do and for orders from someone in the house. There is a good possibility that whoever is with Chang could be the key to our discovering the identity of the mystery group who wants to prevent me from visiting the plantation. What do you think Luther?"

Luther was startled by the question. He wasn't used to being asked for an opinion. He simply remarked, "I don't know who these men are. We don't usually have guards here at the plantation. There is no reason for guards. I think there is someone in the house that is a stranger and could also be a problem for Mr. Chang. Do you want me to go into the house to see what these men do?"

J.P. answered quickly, taking control of the situation. "No, Luther. I have another suggestion. Since the guards are not expecting Nacheda-san and might think he is part of our Chang escort, let's play along. These windows are dark, but I'm certain that they can make out four persons in the vehicle. We have acted suspicious and they're probably wondering why. Let's try to act normal and see what happens.

"Mandi and I should go up to the house as if everything is as it should be. Nacheda-san, you stay back and watch the two Japanese guards. Perhaps you could strike up a conversation with them. Position yourself so you can neutralize the guards should you recognize the person in the house and determine them all hostile. Luther this is not your business. You should disappear.

"Once we are inside, if we can identify the person and we determine everything is okay, we'll call you inside. If we don't recognize the person we will lure both Chang and the person outside for your identification. When you see the person you will have to find a way to tell us if you know them and if they're hostile. If we determine that the situation is hostile, when we are inside, we will use one of your tear gas canisters. At that point everyone will have to fend for themselves as best they can. What do you think?" J.P. wanted their opinion, but with every passing minute, he knew their lack of action was causing the guards to become increasingly suspicious.

"Great plan, J.P.," responded Nacheda. "If I figure the third person is bad then I will mace the guard on the stairs as well as the other if he is close. You will have to take care of Chang and the unknown person. That might leave a few loose ends so everyone will have to be alert to other danger. If the guards have guns I will try and get their guns while one or both of them are reacting from the mace. Mandi you take one each of the canisters. Nacheda slipped Mandi the two canisters. "I am ready, are both of you?"

"Ready" replied Mandi as she opened the door and began to walk around the back of the vehicle. As she came alongside J.P.'s door he got out and they walked together up to the stairs.

As they approached the first step, the guard asked, "Who may I say is calling?"

J.P. could now see that one of his hands was inside his shirt. There was an excellent chance he had a gun. He formed his right hand like a pistol and waved it against his side hoping that Nacheda would catch on to the rough hand signal.

Mandi answered the guard's question, "We are Ms. Hayes and Dr. Koenig of James Pharmaceutical Company. We have an appointment to see Mr. Chang."

"Yes," the guard answered. "Mr. Chang told us to expect your arrival. Please proceed to the common room directly at the top of the stairs." He unfolded his left arm and pointed to the door with his left hand while keeping his right hand inside of his shirt.

J.P. and Mandi began to climb the small stairs to the porch. J.P. looked back at the Toyota and saw that Nacheda had gotten out and was slowly walking towards the stairs. The driver of the other Toyota had also gotten out and was coming up behind Nacheda. Good, J.P. thought, both guards would be close to Nacheda.

Mandi and J.P. reached the top of the stairs and walked across a wooden porch that stretched the length of the house. He opened the door to what he believed was the common room and preceded Mandi. He didn't want Mandi to be on the receiving end of any surprises. As he entered the room, he quickly determined that things looked peaceful. He held the door for Mandi to enter. The room was sparsely filled with furniture. In the far right-hand corner was a dining table where three people sat eating lunch. One man had his back to them, there was a Chinese man that J.P. assumed would be Chang, and an older woman. As they entered the room, the Chinese man jumped up and walked rapidly around the table towards his visitors.

"Mrs. Hayes and Dr. Koenig, what a pleasure to meet you. After your phone call, I did not expect you for hours. Please, please come in. I want you to meet my new partner.

He moved quickly back to his place by the table and prepared to introduce the other two people. The man with his back to them had not moved. He wore a tight fitting safari shirt. J.P. noted that his shoulders did not look Japanese and he had blond hair. He could feel his tension begin to ebb. Then it occurred to him that Chang had referred to him as his new partner.

Mandi and he walked towards the table. J.P. noticed that Mandi's purse was hanging from her left shoulder and that she had her left hand inside the purse. She probably had her hand on the tear gas canister. She had not relaxed.

Chang began the introductions "Mrs. Hayes and Dr. Koenig, I first want you to meet Marisa, she runs the house. This is the home of her ancestors and I honor her right to live here and help me manage the plantation." Marisa rose and bowed.

Chang went on with the introductions, "And this is my new partner, Mr. Smith." He paused and then added as an afterthought, "Mr. Smith is from America also."

Smith raised up from his seat. He wiped the corners of his mouth with his napkin and turned around while tossing his napkin on the table. He reached out to shake J.P.'s hand.

"Welcome to the plantation we are honored to have representatives of our best customer visit. Dr. Koenig and Mrs. Hayes," he shook Mandi's outstretched hand, "I look forward to working with you on the supply of Devil Tree bark." He looked to be just less than six feet tall and had a very muscular build. He was a handsome man in his late-forties. The shirt was so tight across his chest that J.P. could see the outline of a holster strap that seemed to end in his left armpit. He held his left arm normally indicating the pistol was probably not in the holster.

J.P. decided to immediately go into a discussion on business. He addressed Chang. "There has been no previous mention of a partner, Mr. Chang. How does this affect the James agreement?"

Mr. Chang started to answer, but was silenced by a look from Smith. Smith answered his question, "Here in Asia it is usually impolite to enter into a business discussion immediately upon introduction, Dr. Koenig, but since we are both Americans and you did ask the question, I will answer. This new arrangement will mean the rewriting of your contract. We...Mr. Chang, Jr. and myself," he gestured to Chang, "feel the price that James Pharmaceutical Company pays for the bark of the Devil Tree is too low for the value of the products that they are ultimately producing."

Chang started to enter the conversation, "No wait."

"Mr. Chang," Smith silenced him, "I will handle Dr. Koenig's inquiry." "I don't understand, Mr. Chang." Mandi said. "The James agreement was with your father. You have no right to change the contract without mutual agreement between James and your father. What does your father have to say about your new partner?"

Chang did not immediately answer Mandi, so again Mr. Smith answered for him. "Mr. Chang's father was in an accident recently and will not be able to carry on as an active partner. Mr. Chang, Jr. has his father's power of attorney, so there will be no argument. We have not had an opportunity to discuss the terms of the new contract so you will have to be patient."

J.P. decided that Smith's announcement of the partnership, his tone of voice, and arrogant attitude were all very bad signs for James.

Where had this American come from and what were his real motives for entering into the bark business?

Smith continued, "We will have a new contract prepared for you this afternoon."

"Wait just a minute, Mr. Smith," J.P. said. "This is going a little too fast and I don't want to be run over by a runaway train with a new deal that you are trying to push through. James doesn't agree to this or any other change in the current contract. We are the major contractor for the Devil Tree bark and contractually we have a say-so in what goes on with the plantation."

"I'm sorry Dr. Koenig, didn't I tell you? You are no longer the major contractor. My company is now the major contractor and under Indonesian law."

"I don't give a fuck what law we are under. Who the hell are you, Mr. Smith and what rock did you crawl out from under?"

"Dr. Koenig, I am surprised at your locker room language. We are trying to be civil here," Smith replied. He folded his arms across his chest in a manner that accentuated his biceps.

Mandi spoke up with venom in her voice, "Smith, we are in the jungle and you're taking the role of a cannibal. There is no civil language here. You're bringing a new dimension to a very important aspect of our business and we aren't going to stand by and be intimidated by your words, your phony contract, or your repulsive rippling muscles."

"Lady. If I may call you lady," Smith countered, "we. I. don't have to take this shit from you or James Pharmaceutical or your friend Koenig. It is what it is, take it or leave it. Look, face it, you and James are out of luck. Now I am going to have to break up this small cluster fuck before I come to the conclusion that this situation should become physical in order to arrive at a satisfactory conclusion." He took out a package of filterless Japanese cigarettes and lit one. He inhaled deeply and blew the smoke back out through his nose.

Both J.P. and Mandi saw the cigarettes. Mandi's eyes looked to his. She was silently asking permission to release the tear gas bomb. J.P. answered by shaking his head no.

Chang, trying to break the tension, moved quickly around the table, almost knocking over Marisa who had been sitting quietly with her head bowed.

Chang said anxiously, "Yes, please let us all leave and go outside into the fine air. I am sure things will work out to everyone's benefit. Yes, please out to the sunshine. My home is no place for anger. It is a lovely place."

He began to nudge Mandi towards the door. Mandi and J.P. turned towards the door. Smith preceded them. J.P. noticed the butt of a gun sticking out above his belt and covered by his shirt.

J.P. allowed Chang to get ahead of him. He didn't want anyone at his back. He looked quickly over his shoulder at the table and saw that Marisa had disappeared. The room had double French doors. Smith chose the door on the left and Mandi the door on the right. She was a full step behind Smith.

J.P. was still positioned behind Smith and Chang behind Mandi. J.P. kept his eyes on the gun butt. He figured that if Nacheda knew Smith, then Smith would know Nacheda and how quickly he went for the gun would be the first indication of whether he was a friend or a foe. Smith and Mandi had moved through the threshold of the doors and were silhouetted against the bright sunlight. The sudden brightness made J.P. blink and he did not see the initial movement of Smith's right hand going to his back and the gun. The scene had been quiet as they were leaving the common room. Even the sounds of the jungle had been silenced. The only sound came from an audible squeak from the opening of the left door.

The silence was broken by Nacheda's voice screaming, "Joe!" and Smith yelling, "Nacheda!" Smith's hand was fast. He had gotten the gun out of his belt and was almost to a firing position when J.P. sprang at his legs to tackle him and interfere with the shot. In Smith's sudden recognition of Nacheda he had forgotten that anyone was behind him. A gunshot rang out.

Just as J.P.'s shoulders hit the man's knees, Mandi pushed him to the side with her shoulder. She then brought her left hand out of her purse and was holding the tear gas canister. Smith fell and

Mandi released the tear gas and stepped back to keep clear of the mist. Smith's knees buckled and the two men landed in a heap at the edge of the porch. The tear gas was above them as J.P. reached for Smith's gun hand. He was pointing in the direction where Nacheda had been standing. J.P. brought his right fist down on Smith's right forearm. It was extended half the way over the first step and the force of the blow and the porch step broke his arm. The gun sprang free from his hand, but not after firing a round. Smith screamed in pain.

J.P. knew that Smith was temporarily out of action and turned to help Mandi. Chang was coming at her with his arms raised in a position to give her a chop to her neck. J.P. saw her fall back to place her weight on her bent left leg while she brought up her right leg landing her kick directly in Chang's crotch. His forward movement stopped as he was literally lifted off the porch by the force of Mandi's kick. His face became contorted in a pain and he fell to the porch wretching.

From somewhere below the stairs J.P. heard Nacheda's voice yell, "Three points!" J.P. smiled, knowing that we were all unharmed, so far. He turned his attention back to Smith who had crawled to where the gun lay. He was reaching for it with his left hand. J.P. bent over to pull him backwards by his belt when he saw Nacheda's foot come down on Smith's hand with such force that J.P. actually heard bones crack. Smith's second scream was louder than the first.

The tear gas had drifted to J.P. and his eyes and throat began to burn. Nacheda reached down, pulled him to his feet, and walked him down the stairs. J.P. raised his hands to his eyes and started to rub, but Nacheda pulled his hands away.

"Don't rub them J.P., it will only make it worse. Get some water and splash your eyes to dilute the chemicals. I do not think you received a heavy dose."

The stinging was easing now that he was away from the cloud. "You're right Nacheda-san, but look at Smith or Joe or whoever."

The man was lying with his legs on the porch and his upper body hung over the first four steps in a spread eagle position. His left arm was outstretched with his left hand looking swollen. His right arm was stretched out with the lower forearm dangling off a step. His face was contorted in pain and he was whimpering either from pain or the tear gas. Tears were streaming down his face. His broken right arm was bleeding. The blood was mixing with his tears and saliva in large pools on the stairs. The liquid was being absorbed into the wood leaving dark stains.

J.P. looked around at the results of their short visit. Chang was lying on the porch in a fetal position, both hands cupping his crotch. He was also was whimpering. Mandi was standing over him close enough to guard him, but out of the tear gas cloud. She was holding Smith's gun on him in case Chang decided to move. On the front lawn were the two guards, unconscious.

Nacheda said angrily, "J.P., this man is Joe Berger, a member of the task force that had identified the James Pharmaceutical Company. Until a few minutes ago he was a trusted friend. Now I know he was never a friend and he was just using Skip, our other friends, and me. We will now find out who sent Joe and why he is here. You take Chang back into the common room. I will take Berger into the woods." There was anger in Nacheda's voice that scared J.P. He turned to Mandi, "Mandi-san, may I please have Berger's gun."

Mandi reluctantly handed Berger's gun to Nacheda.

"Nacheda-san," J.P. said with concern in his voice, "are you sure you want to do this? I can interrogate Berger."

"J.P., it has to be done and I am the person who will take care of the situation."

J.P. nodded and went back up the stairs to where Mandi was still standing over the moaning Chang. "Mandi, let's take this bag of manure back into the room and see what he knows about this situation."

They lifted Chang to his feet, Mandi on one side and J.P. on the other. They dragged him by the armpits with his feet dragging the floor. Marisa opened the door. They entered the room and literally threw him into a chair.

"Okay Chang, let's have the complete story," J.P. demanded.

"Dr. Koenig," he whined, "I don't know anything about this Mr. Smith. He came to my home with his guards and made me an offer that I was unable to refuse. He threatened me and said that if I didn't make a deal with him, he would hurt me as his people had hurt my father. I was forced to make a new contract with him even though my heart was not in the negotiations or the resulting contract."

"Chang, you tell a good story, but it isn't good enough. You are now trying to convince us that the happy scene we saw when we arrived was not a celebration? That you were, in fact, under duress? Please, you insult us with your bullshit."

Mandi spoke up, "Admit it, Chang. You are a greedy bastard who is in this only for yourself. You violated a contract that was made between your father and Doc James."

"Chang, who was Smith working for?" J.P. asked.

"I do not know Dr. Koenig. He would not tell me," he softly replied. "Where is the new contract?"

"It was to be written this afternoon. We made the contract on a handshake."

"You mean to tell me that you would break an honorable contract with a handshake between yourself and man you did not know nor the people he represented?" Mandi asked incredulously.

"I know it sounds bad, but the situation called for me to make the decision." Chang replied.

"What was the contract?" J.P. asked.

"He would pay $118.00 per cubic meter of bark and I would receive 5% of a joint venture between his company and mine." He paused and then continued. "We would still sell the Devil Tree to James. You wouldn't be out of raw material. It might cost a little more, but you would still be in business." As an after thought he added, "Your American business can afford the extra cost."

Again Mandi spoke to Chang. This time there was more venom in her voice than J.P. had ever heard. "You are lower than anyone I have ever known. How can we ever trust you again?" He was watching

Chang's reaction to Mandi's statement and did not see her hand extracting the second canister from her purse. She brought out the canister and sprayed mace directly into Chang's face. It was not a direct stream into his eyes, but it was close enough. Chang screamed and brought both hands up to cover his face. Mandi stopped and coolly replaced the canister in her purse.

"Nice move Mandi," J.P. said. "Wish I had thought of it myself." Chang was writhing in pain and his screams seemed to be getting louder. Marisa was at J.P.'s shoulder with the ice bucket that had held the Champagne that he and Berger had been drinking when they arrived. He smiled at her and took it from her hands. J.P. upended the ice bucket over Chang's head. For whatever reason, when the ice water hit Chang's face, he passed out.

Suddenly, they heard a shot. All three of them ran to the door. J.P. reached the door first and stopped. Mandi and Marisa stopped behind him.

"Let's not rush outside, we must be sure the shot was not aimed at us." They waited for a few moments and then J.P. eased out the door. All he saw was Nacheda walking slowly across the lawn on his way back to the house.

He opened the door fully so that Mandi and Marisa could come out. They stood on the porch until Nacheda had climbed the stairs. Nacheda's face was drawn and in obvious mental pain. He reached the porch and stopped.

"Where is Chang?" he asked.

"He is sleeping in a chair. He said he knew nothing about Berger, but he did give us the provisions of the contract. How about Berger?" J.P. asked.

"Berger is no longer among the living," Nacheda stated in a matter of fact manner. "He did not tell me anything. I knew he wouldn't. His kind never do."

Mandi and J.P. were shocked and silent. Killing Berger in cold blood did not fit the Nacheda they thought they knew.

"Nacheda, you shouldn't have killed him," Mandi said. "We could have turned him over to the authorities."

"I understand what you are saying Mandi, but this isn't the way of the Bergers of the world. He had been turned while he was in Vietnam. He was a for-hire business espionage thief, a new breed of crook. He was here on a contract from his current employer. He had been on this contract the entire duration of my task force. He only told me this much and no more because a long time ago we had been friends. I do not know whom he was working for except that, as we ourselves have deduced, they must be Japanese. The guards maybe, could have given us some information, but I doubt it." He then turned to face the lawn "As you can see they have also departed."

"Okay, Nacheda-san, but to kill Berger!" Mandi reiterated.

"Mandi, I did not kill Berger. He killed himself. I did supply him with his own weapon. It was his wish. He knew he was finished. Even his powerful arms would not have repaired to their original strength. He was through and wanted to make an exit. All I did was provide the means." He paused and looked down at the porch. "It did not make me happy, Mandi. Even though he cheated all of us... our friends, James, Bandai, and me, he was a comrade in arms and a very intelligent biogenetic engineer. Greed and whatever happened in the Vietnam jungle many years ago managed Joe's life. Too bad, he could have been an asset to humanity, but instead he chose to be a poison. In the end, humanity and the world will be a better place without Berger."

Mandi broke the solemn silence that followed. "What now, J.P.?"

"Well I suggest, that while our host sleeps, we find his office and draft a new contract for his signature. When wakes up we'll have him sign it."

"Sounds fine, J.P. Perhaps we can make the contract a little better so he can never claim we took advantage of him. Perhaps a slightly higher price but a ten-year contract renewable every subsequent year unless both parties agree to cancellation."

"That sounds like a great idea, Mandi. Let's do it."

They found Chang's office and typed out the agreement. Chang was coming around as they brought him the new contract to sign. Marisa witnessed the signatures. Chang's eyes could not focus and he could not read very well so Marisa read to him. He readily agreed to the terms and signed the document.

JAMES FARM, GREYSTONE HALL SEAFORD, NEW YORK

She had made her decision. She would only see him if he had new information on the deal with NPC. Even though she physically desired the sex, she was growing very tired of him.

She picked up the phone in her office in the farmhouse and dialed his number

"Yes?" he answered. "It's Evelyn."

"I know. What do you want?" he replied somewhat irritated that she had called him at the office.

"Have you heard anything?" she asked trying to keep the growing anger out of her voice.

"Nothing," he replied.

"Fine!" she answered, the anger coming through. "Since it is nothing, you get nothing. Please refrain from visiting my home or bed until the nothing is a satisfactory something. Do you get my point?"

"Evelyn," his voice was now a pleading whisper so no one could hear him say her name. "Please. I need you. Please just tonight. I will try and find out what is happening. Please?"

"No. Not unless you have substantive new information and even then I'm not sure I want to see you."

"I will call them and then call you back. Okay?" his voice was begging. "If you obtain new information, call me and leave a message on my machine stating the new information. If I deem it important enough then maybe I'll call you back. If I don't call you back, stay away from here. In fact, stay away from me until you have a definite answer. If your ego can't handle this rejection, rationalize that I have a perpetual headache. Now stop your begging. Do you get the message?" she commanded.

"Yes, but.," he begged.

"No yes, buts," and she hung up.

He immediately called NPC, but no one answered. He called her back, but, again no one answered.

AMERICAN AIRLINES FLIGHT 298 OVER THE EASTERN PACIFIC OCEAN

J.P. and Mandi finished their dinner in the first-class section as they were flying over the Pacific on their way back to Los Angeles and Mammoth following a short holiday in Hawaii. After dinner and the beginning of the movie Mandi had gotten drowsy and wanted to try and get some sleep. She had been asleep in less than five minutes. As she stirred in the seat next to J.P., he looked over at her and smiled, thinking to himself how beautiful she was. She slowly opened her eyes and saw him looking at her. She smiled and fell back into a deep sleep.

The last eight days since they had left the Devil Tree plantation had been an exhilarating whirlwind for the two of them. After they finished their business at the plantation on Tuesday, they flew back to Singapore and were relieved to discover that there were no personal repercussions from the attempted kidnapping. No one had identified them as the intended victims. They were particularly vigilant in their activities and always watched for strangers. They had figured that whoever was managing Joe Berger had arranged the kidnapping as a means to ensure that Nacheda didn't identify Joe.

The next day J.P., Mandi, and Nacheda made another trip to Indonesia, this time to Jakarta to visit Chang's father in the hospital. They told him the full story of his son's activities and of Berger's tragedy. He was very embarrassed for his son and the shame that he had brought on the family. He agreed with the terms of the new contract and summoned his personal attorney to the hospital to formally witness his signing the document. He wanted to keep the agreement with James because the agreement had been good to his family and he hoped that the same was true for James. He surprised them by informing them that he had another son who had been in training with another trade company. His other son would now take over the running of the plantation. They told him of Marisa's loyalty and he said that she would be rewarded.

J.P. was impressed with the old man's inner and outer strength. His face did not look particularly battered from his beating, but his chest was heavily bandaged. The physician later told them that he had four broken ribs and a broken leg.

Nacheda asked Chang if he had any idea who Berger might have been working for. Chang told them that he had no idea except that he was certain that the man who had beaten him was Japanese. Before ending their visit with Mr. Chang, Sr., J.P. explained the potential for a new joint venture with Bandai Pharmaceuticals and asked if it might be possible to obtain a small sample of Devil Tree bark from his warehouse to take back to Bandai for tests. Chang was only too happy to oblige and contacted the foreman at his warehouse operation and instructed him to package a small amount of bark and deliver it to the hospital. Chang also agreed to increase the size of the plantation in view of the potential use with JPC138.

Nacheda had invited J.P. and Mandi to return with him to Bandai before they flew back to the United States. J.P. was anxious for he and Mandi to meet Dr. Nakasone and determine the scope of a possible agreement between Bandai and James firsthand before returning to New York. He also wanted to study the research on the pure alkaloid isolation process. So after some coaxing by Nacheda, they finally agreed to make the trip.

The three of them arrived at Narita Airport early Thursday morning and took the train into the city. Nacheda had called ahead and made arrangements for Reiko to meet them at the Tokyo Central Train Station in downtown Tokyo. The four of them then boarded the train to Bandai where they arrived Thursday evening.

Friday was filled with lectures, demonstrations, and negotiations. J.P. and Mandi found Dr. Nakasone to be a tough, but fair negotiator. He was honest and wanted Bandai Pharmaceuticals Company to be successful by working together with an American company. He didn't agree with the traditional Japanese strategy of gradually taking over the U.S. company. Dr. Nakasone felt that the true global company would be successful only if they learned to work together as a team. Each side had to respect the capabilities and culture of the other. One member could not rule the other and there had to be a fair distribution of the profits based on agreed performance.

J.P. stated to Dr. Nakasone that James Pharmaceutical also wanted to work together but the key to success was to take the final result of the team effort as the measure of success. In their mutual situation it would be the development of JPC138. He believed that every aspect of a products development and commercialization was equally important. If each step was not accomplished on time, within budget, and with expected clinical results, then there was a possibility of a team failure. The team as a whole, not any one corporate partner or individual, had to make adjustments. R&D cannot overpower the development program as finance and marketing cannot overpower the program. If they could share in the final success and not be greedy in the steps leading to that success then they could truly form a team.

Nakasone agreed with J.P.'s philosophy and they were finally able to work out the basic parameters of a James/Bandai agreement.

Dr. Nakasone suggested that Bandai would provide the technology to isolate the pure alkaloid and invest a substantial amount of cash into the project. The total amount of the investment would be determined after both companies reviewed the research protocols. James would provide the DNA bombardment technology and share the R&D and toxicology/pathology work accomplished to date. Both companies would share herbal technology on a continual basis. The companies would form a joint venture on the JPC138 product. The headquarters for the joint venture would be set up in a location agreeable to both parties. Nacheda would head up the Bandai share of the joint venture.

During the afternoon they reviewed the Bandai pure active ingredient technology. Mandi and J.P. were not engineers or pharmaceutical researchers, but this didn't prevent them from realizing the full value of what Bandai Pharmaceuticals had developed.

They watched as Dr. Noguchi, the Ph.D. who had made and refined the discovery, took a three-inch square piece of the Devil Tree bark and placed it in a vacuum chamber. It was then bombarded with electrons breaking down its molecular structure and therefore changing its chemical structure. The resultant sludge was then analyzed and transferred to a second vacuum chamber that was made up of a number of magnets. The sludge was literally pulled apart by varying the power of the different magnetic fields. While in the chamber, a spectra analysis profile was made of the sludge and plotted using a computer algorithm.

The computer plot provided the necessary information to isolate the selected active ingredient. The active ingredient was then recovered in an almost pure state. The remaining sludge was reconstituted and discarded. One of the most important advantages of the process was the fact that no chemicals were used. Since the raw material was actually plant life, the disposal of the sludge was no problem to the environment.

The pure active ingredient was then collected as a coarse white powder and pressed together in one-inch cubes. This would be shipped by special plane to the James facility for DNA bombardment. The current shipment route of the Devil Tree bark from Indonesia to James would be changed by adding a stop in Bandai. The rerouting of the bark was one of the first tasks that Nacheda had to do as president of the Bandai half of the joint venture. Mandi and J.P. agreed that there was a better than 75% chance that Nacheda could find a location closer to Tokyo to build a dedicated processing plant. Nacheda told them that he loved the Bandai area, but he was more of a city person and Bandai was too quiet for year round living. They felt that Reiko might have had some influence on his decision.

They spent Saturday in Bandai skiing and looking around town. J.P. had skied in Bandai years before. Although things had changed in and around the village, he was pleased to see that it had not become overdeveloped.

Mandi, Reiko, and J.P. took the train to Tokyo on Sunday morning so they could catch the Sunday evening flight to Hawaii.

On their second Sunday morning after crossing the dateline, they landed in Honolulu. They rented a car and drove away from the overcrowded area around Waikiki Beach. J.P. knew of a hotel on the windward side of Oahu that most visitors didn't even know existed. It was quiet and they were able to enjoy themselves.

Before leaving Singapore, they had spoken to Phillip by phone about their itinerary and he had agreed to the side trips. Phillip remarked that as time for the March board meeting approached, things were heating up once again between himself and the board. Mandi and J.P. decided to begin to develop the strategy for the proxy fight during their holiday.

Monday evening they had dinner served on the porch of their villa. The ocean was relatively calm so sound of the surf sliding onto the beach was not too loud. The soft continual rhythm of the waves provided a relaxing and romantic background.

Mandi, as usual, looked as beautiful that night as J.P. could ever recall seeing her. Her hair was long and had flowed down over her shoulders. The flame's reflection from the table candle bounced off that wall as it danced in the breeze. Mandi's blue-green eyes sparkled with moisture. Her teeth were pearls against her tanned face.

"J.P., this is so fabulous," she said as she looked out towards the sea. "Where do we go from here?"

They were holding hands and drinking Champagne. It was not a direct question, but kind of a general reflection.

"Where do you want the relationship to go?" He squeezed her hand and took another sip of Champagne.

She looked at him and laughed. "You weren't supposed to answer my question with a question."

"I know, it was not fair, but still this is a we thing. I don't know if your question can be answered separately. We have to find our way together in making the decision of whether we go together through a part of our lives or separately. Today, I don't think we know the direction this relationship will take. Do you?"

"I guess I feel like you do J.P., but I do wish things were a little more certain."

He reached over and took both of her hands in his. "Well, as far as I am concerned, there is only one thing for certain and that is that I love you very much and I feel very lucky to be with you." He leaned across the small table and kissed her.

After their lips had parted she said, "I love you Jean Paul, with all my heart.

"Not to break our romantic spell, but why don't we just see where things take us. When we get back we are going to have a rough time pulling off the proxy fight. Mrs. James now has a good head start in the implementation of her plan. We haven't even formulated our plan."

"That's one of the things I really love about you, J.P., you always know how pull things back down to business." She giggled and then added, "But, you know

Mrs. James doesn't have you and I or Nacheda. We will pull it off. If we don't win we will surely give her a rough fight and, if she wins, we won't leave her anything of value."

As she finished her comments about James, she surprised him by standing up and letting her wraparound dress slowly unwrap and fall to the porch. To his further delight, he discovered that she wasn't wearing anything underneath. The candlelight danced across her sun-bronzed body.

"Well, I know where I now want to go," she said in a seductive whisper.

J.P. leaped up from the table without pushing back his chair and nearly tipped the table onto is side. Only Mandi's quick action kept their wineglasses from falling.

She laughed, "Easy there, boy."

J.P. walked around the table and they embraced, enjoying mutual warmth of their bodies as they touched. They were bound in candle and moonlight. After a long and very passionate kiss he lifted Mandi in his arms and carried her into the villa.

Tuesday evening, as they sat together in the Admiral's Club at the airport waiting for their flight's departure to Los Angeles, J.P. brought out his laptop and began writing a status report that he would email to Phillip and Brian.

TO: Phillip Bradsmith

FROM: J.P./Mandi

CC: Brian Smith

SUBJ: Status Report

21st Century Plan Status. I feel the solving of this puzzle is still a few weeks away. We think the primary suspect is Mrs. James, but I have not yet determined her accomplice or exactly why she would want a second copy. Believe the end objective was for this person to provide her with continuous information to help move you out of the way enabling her to take complete control of James. You must be prepared to go to war with Mrs. James and we are prepared to assist you in this regard. Who ended up with the copy of the 21st Century Plan? See paragraph 2.

Devil Tree Supply. Briefly, the supply of the Devil Tree bark had been in serious trouble. The question we have is why this wasn't identified earlier? It was fortuitous that Mandi and I showed up at the plantation when we did. If we had arrived only minutes later, James would have quite possibly lost the supply of Devil Tree bark altogether. As it turns out, Mandi and I have secured a steady supply under the provisions of a new contract with Chang Trading Company. I will provide you the new contract for your review, approval, and signature. The complete report on our visit to the plantation will be verbal. Two items of note. One, we found another company in negotiations with Chang, Jr. for the rights of the Devil Tree in violation of our contract. This was successfully handled, but we don't know the name of the other company or why. We believe the other company has had access to the 21st Century Plan. They determined the Devil Tree was important to James and wanted to gain control of the bark before James woke up to the fact that the supply was vulnerable. Second, as we mentioned in a previous conversation, we made a connection with a Mr. Nacheda representing Bandai Pharmaceutical Company. See paragraph 3.

Bandai Pharmaceuticals Company. The visit with Dr. Nakasone, President/CEO of Bandai Pharmaceuticals was excellent. I have, in my possession, a draft of an agreement between the two companies that I will review with you. Nothing has been committed, only preliminary discussions.

March Board Meeting. I would recommend that you proceed with the March board meeting with no changes in our previously agreed strategy. We should learn and observe whether Mrs. James plays any additional cards in the game she is playing. After this trip we believe your team will have more trump cards than Mrs. James. I don't want to expose our hand until we know we can win. I know you are not in full agreement with a war with Mrs. James, but after you hear our report I think you will be convinced that you have no choice, but to go to war. We recommend we start to play her game by our rules starting at the April board meeting. Until then we keep our plan to ourselves. I think only you, Brian, Mandi, and myself should be involved in the fight. As for outsiders I have two recommendations. I will discuss these with you in person.

Conclusion. We are entering into a period where James is threatened. I believe we should act accordingly. In this regard we should now keep all correspondence to a minimum and destroy past memos and electronic storage media. We will explain more upon our return next Monday.

Warmest, etc. //s//J.P.

The email was sent on Tuesday afternoon.

J.P.'s reflections of the past week stopped when he realized that he was about to fall asleep. He pushed the button to raise the leg rest on his seat and pushed a second button to lower his seat to the recline position. He unfolded the blanket that was next to him in the seat and pulled it over him. He turned onto his left side to face Mandi and placed the pillow under his head. He watched Mandi sleeping as he closed his eyes. Her faced remained fixed in his mind as he drifted into sleep.

The next thing he knew, the flight attendant was asking if they wanted coffee and juice. He nodded in the affirmative raised himself back to a sitting position. He began to become accustomed to the bright sunlight that was now streaming through the windows. Mandi was already awake and sitting up. The attendant informed them that they were one hour from LAX and that a light breakfast would be served in a few moments.

"Good morning, J.P.," Mandi said with a smile.

"I better hit the head before they make us strap in. Be right back." He looked back at Mandi staring out the window at the early morning sun bouncing off the clouds beneath the plane.

3:00 P.M., THURSDAY, MARCH 9

JAMES FARM, GREYSTONE HALL SEAFORD, NEW YORK

"Hello?" he answered. "Well?"

"No. Nothing yet." "Do something." CCTJ.... _ •

I m trying. "Try harder." CCT

I am.

"The hell you are!" she screamed as she hung up the telephone.

7:00 P.M., THURSDAY, MARCH 9

ANNIE'S BAR AND GRILL
MAMMOTH LAKES, CA

"Mandi, Annie, Skip, and J.P. were seated at the table closest to the roaring fire at Annie's. They had just introduced Mandi to her first kangaroo steak. She took the joke like a good sport, but J.P. didn't think she was enchanted with the idea of eating kangaroo.

"Skip, I don't think we've made a convert," he said.

"J.P., I just can't think of eating a steady diet of kangaroo. I also don't think I could eat a steady diet of bear or bison. I am a domestic person and I think we should only eat animals bred for meat. I'm sorry to disappoint guys," Mandi replied.

"You see," Annie said in her best business voice, "Mandi has the attitude that most people have about kangaroo steak. It will never catch on. I think I'll stop trying to be a culinary pioneer and take it off the menu."

"Annie, you never had it on the menu. You only served roo steak to those of us you want to trick. Perhaps you should place it on the menu before giving up and see what happens. You never know, you might have a winner,"

J.P. advised.

"Yeah, well, maybe you're right. I'll give it some thought." Annie turned her attention to Mandi. "How was your first day on Mammoth Mountain?" she asked.

"The mountain lived up to everyone's billing. I have never had such an exhilarating day. There were very few people on the mountain and the conditions were outstanding. The only disconcerting factor was all the snow bunnies know J.P. and kept telling him how much they've missed him this winter. J.P. has refused to talk about why these nymphets missed him. Now, J.P., in front of your friends would you like to explain yourself?" Mandi asked faking a stern look.

"Hey, you guys know I love to ski. I am just a lonely bachelor up here on the mountain. All the nice young ladies just look to me as a father figure. Do you actually feel I can compete for their charms when there are hundreds of young ski studs from LA. No way. I'm just a friendly old man that they like to tease," he replied humbly as he bowed his head.

With perfect timing, the lift operator from chair lift #9 walked by the table and said to him, "J.P.! How's it going? I have missed seeing you. When are you gonna come up so we can go down together," she threw her head back and laughed.

"Soon," he called after her as she walked away.

"There, you see?" Mandi said to the group. "You all are witnesses. This guy is a dirty old man."

"Let's change the subject. I'm getting myself into deep shit." He looked at Skip, "How are things in Westwood Village?"

9:00 A.M., MONDAY, MARCH 13

SPECTRUM OF MEDICINE BUILDING NEW YORK CITY

"Good morning Janet."

"Good morning J.P., I hear from Phillip that you had a rough trip, but by the look of that beautiful tan I'm a little suspicious."

"I guarantee it was rough, it's just that most of our business activities took place outside in the sunshine of Southeast Asia," he answered seriously.

Janet smiled and looked up and over her desk. A slight chuckle was in her voice when she commented "Uh huh. You know, J.P., I never realized that Hawaii and Mammoth had relocated to Southeast Asia? A person learns something new each day."

"You caught me there Janet, but a guy and a girl have to have some fun sometime don't they? Is Phillip available?"

"Go right in, the man is waiting for you," she replied going back to her business voice.

"Thank you Janet. By the way, you look great. I hope everything is going well with Bill and Clintec?"

"Everything is working out. Thanks to you, he's like the old Bill that we both knew. He's lost twenty-five pounds and he's stopped smoking and drinking. He has thrown himself into making Lifeal and his company a success. Thank you for asking.

"That's great Janet. Give him my regards. How is Phillip?"

"I will, thanks and Phillip seems just.," she paused, "okay. I really can't read him anymore. It seems like the fight has gone out of him. Now that you are back I hope he will show some life. If there is anything I can do, please ask."

"Thanks Janet. See you later." J.P. walked past Janet's desk. He knocked and then opened the door to Phillip's office and walked in. Phillip was sitting behind his desk. His head was resting in his hands with his elbows propped on the desk. He looked up without lifting his head off of his hands.

"Ah, J.P. Good to have you back." His voice was low and had no enthusiasm. He wore his traditional dark pinstriped suit, but it was wrinkled under the armpits and what was most unusual to J.P. was that his shirt was unbuttoned at the collar and his striped tie was pulled down an inch. His skin color was that of the winter New York pallor. This was not unusual to many New Yorkers but by mid-March it wasn't normal for Phillip. Normally he would have taken a trip to Florida and somehow acquired a tan. J.P. didn't know whether it had been the gunshot wound, the problems at James, or his fight with the board that was the cause of his apparent depression. "Good morning Phillip," J.P. said cheerfully "You look great."

"Bullshit," was all he said. His eyes returned to a spot in the middle of the desk where he probably had been staring for a long period of time.

"Come on, Phillip, get your butt from behind the desk and let's go to war."

He raised his head this time and let his arms fall from his chin to the desk. He looked directly at J.P. "Don't try to rile me. I have had about enough of this pharmaceutical business and the corporate politics bull crap that comes with the job. Who needs this stress? All I want to do is grow James and help physicians to provide better medicine. The situation with Lifeal and Bill is good and I have to admit I was wrong to have shut Bill out for so long, but I'm afraid it is too late to save Lifeal. By the time we get the FDA to approve the new test and allow us to promote it, I will be long since retired."

"Hey Phillip, stop looking at the glass half empty. You know the trend is up. Things are getting better. We have a better plan for Lifeal and the 21st Century Plan mystery is beginning to unravel. I know things don't look that good, but from my perspective things are looking up. I hate to repeat a bad quip, but things always get worse before they get better. Usually the reason for the downswing is that we know more about the situation so it just seems to get worse. What we need is a great action plan for your leadership of the proxy fight."

"Bullshit," he said again with more conviction.

J.P. persisted in his attempt to pull his friend out of his depression, "Phillip, you're a great leader, don't give up now. I feel good about things. You have to have an open and positive outlook about the future of James. The employees and the board have to see you as the fighter not the shot-up has-been."

His eyes shot an angry look at J.P. He waited a second to see if Phillip would respond any further before he continued antagonizing him.

"Well Phillip, I'm really surprised that you are going to let the scheming Mrs. James beat you. And beat you without a fight. How could you throw away all these years with James just to make that woman richer? There's a person without any operating experience whatsoever and she's going to make a mint of money off of Phillip T. Bradsmith, Ph.D."

Phillip was becoming increasingly angry. J.P. could see that his hands were balled into fists. His eyes were staring directly ahead and his face was reddening. J.P. decided to take the intensity of his prodding up another step and possibly risk their friendship.

"You know something, Phillip? With your current attitude, you're a hasbeen and a loser. She deserves to win. All in all, I'd say she's damned lucky to have you as her ally."

Phillip jumped up from his desk. His chair shot back on it's caster wheels and smashed against the window. He smashed his fists on the desk. His face was red as he spoke through gritted teeth.

"Get the fuck out of my office, you ungrateful bastard. Give me your written report. I don't know if I want to ever see you again. I do know that I don't want to see you at today's staff meeting." His voice had risen in volume with every syllable. "Now get out of my sight."

He turned to find his chair. As he turned J.P. walked forward and laid a copy of the report that he had emailed from Hawaii on his desk. J.P. knew that in his present mood he likely hadn't read the email. J.P. turned and walked to the door. As he opened the door, Janet was standing on the other side looking as though she was deciding whether or not to open the door. J.P. nearly bumped into her. He closed the door softly and turned to Janet. She looked terrified. She had obviously heard Phillip's shouting and wondered what had happened in the office. J.P. was smiling as he turned to her. The smile really threw Janet off guard.

"Wha…wha…what happened, J.P.?" she stammered.

His smile got bigger, "Janet, you are a stut…stut…stuttering." "Stop joking and tell me what was all the shouting about!"

"Phillip was the only one shouting. I was, speaking to him very slowly and softly. I was prodding the lion with his ego. What you heard was the roar of a lion in pain before he starts to fight back and let me help him to take the thorn, namely, Mrs. James, out of his paw. If the man needs me I'll be in my office."

He walked to the elevator and pressed the down button. His smile to Janet did not reflect the acid feeling in the pit of his stomach. Had he gone too far? Had Phillip reached a point where he would just yell and not fight? Would he read the report and reconsider his remarks to give up? He thought he knew Phillip, but he began to realize that he really didn't know the man now sitting in the president's office. J.P. began to worry that he had underestimated just how much of a toll the last three months had exacted from his friend. The elevator arrived and he push the eight button and prepared for descent.

Seconds later when he stepped off at the eighth floor he had made a decision to wait through that day. If nothing changed during the business day, he would see Mandi that night and fly back to LA the next day. He looked at the clock on his desk. It was 9:30. He thought of calling Mandi, but decided to just wait things out. He pushed his chair back away from the desk and turned towards the window. He leaned back in the chair and placed his feet up on the window ledge. A bright, sunny day was emerging across the city.

His daydreaming was interrupted by a knock on his door. He answered the knock with a lazy "come in" and continued his gazing out the window.

"J.P., is something wrong? You didn't call my office after you saw Phillip. I thought we were going to give our report to him together before the staff meeting? You wanted to spend a few minutes with him alone and then you would send for me." Mandi was indignant.

He still hadn't turned from the window when he answered her. "I never had a chance to give our report, Mandi. Phillip has asked that I leave James."

"What? What do you mean he asked you to leave?" She lost her indignant tone and spoke with concern in her voice.

He turned around and faced the woman that he was in love with. She was wearing a traditional business suit with a mint green blouse. Her tan complexion and the green made an excellent combination. J.P.'s mood began to fall at the thought that he would have to leave New York and Mandi. Beyond their new personal relationship, he was concerned about her having to finish their project by herself. It wasn't that he felt that she couldn't do a great job, but it was not a one-person project and it was still potentially dangerous. They still didn't know who had been running Berger and why. They knew the situation could be dangerous, they had seen just how far someone was willing to go in order to gain control over James and Bandai. Nakasone had told them that he would not work with Mrs. James or a weak Phillip Bradsmith. If this were to happen, the BandaiJames deal would end and with it JPC138.

"Well, he didn't exactly ask me to leave. He kicked me out of his office and said that he didn't want to see me. He especially didn't want to see me at the staff meeting."

"What's wrong? What happened in there?" Mandi asked again since he hadn't answered her question. She began to move around to his side of the desk. He got up slowly from his seat and took her in his arms. "Everything is all right, I think. I just stirred up Phillip's ego this morning and he kicked me out of his office."

"Why did you do that, J.P.?"

"Phillip was acting like a beaten man. Janet told me that since we left town, he had lost all signs of fight. I decided I had to rattle his cage. I went pretty far, Mandi. Maybe too far. Only time will tell whether we have a leader or a beaten, defeated man. I am hopeful that he'll pull himself out of his defeatist attitude and start to fight Mrs. James. I only hope the situation is not out of control when he wakes up to his responsibilities to himself and to this company."

"What are we going to do?" Mandi asked and then added, "What can I do?"

"I honestly don't know Mandi, wait and see, I suppose," he mused. "I have decided to give him today to straighten himself out. If he doesn't come around by this evening, I'll do as he requested and leave tomorrow."

"Oh, J.P., surely you don't believe that he is going to let you go, do you?" Slight panic edged into Mandi's voice.

"I don't think either one of us knows the man that is presently sitting in the president's office. The shooting incident may have taken more out of him than we had first thought. Let's just wait and see."

He paused. "You had better go to the staff meeting. You don't want to be late."

There was a slight moistening in Mandi's eyes but her mouth was set in a determined expression. "I'll go on up to the staff meeting." She turned to leave.

"Dinner tonight, at our place?" he asked.

Mandi turned and she was smiling again. "Our place," she replied and left the office.

He sat down again and looked out the window. Some clouds were forming in the south. He looked at his watch, it was 9:45. He wondered what Phillip would do at the staff meeting. Would he show his defeatist attitude? Would he button his shirt and straighten his tie? Too many questions and not enough answers.

The sharp ring of the phone brought J.P. back from his thoughts. He glanced at his watch, 10:35. He wondered who was calling. Most of the people he knew were in Phillip's conference room. He hit the speakerphone button.

"Yes? J.P. here,"

"J.P..," it was Mandi. All kinds of conclusions jumped to his mind. Did Phillip not show? Did he just cancel the meeting?

"Yes, Mandi," he replied, turning to face the phone.

"Phillip wants to know where the hell you are." There was excitement in her voice. "J.P., he is back. We have our fighter."

1:00 P.M., MONDAY, MARCH 13
SPECTRUM OF MEDICINE BUILDING
NEW YORK CITY

The staff meeting earlier that morning was for the most part routine except for the electricity in the air. Phillip looked great. J.P. even noticed that he seemed to have managed to have some color in his face. He was in a jovial mood. When J.P. arrived, he kidded him about being a hypocrite by always demanding punctuality, but not living up to his own standards. He never mentioned the trip status report in the meeting, but asked that Mandi and J.P. give him a briefing after lunch.

The man that was now sitting across the table from Mandi and J.P. was the old Phillip. "First, J.P., I want to apologize for being such an insipid fool this morning and for being such a disappointment to you. I have no excuses nor do I wish to hide behind personal reasons. I want to say to you in the presence of Mandi that I apologize and I am ready to fight."

"Apology accepted." he replied. There was nothing more to be said. It was now time to develop the battle plan.

"Okay, where do we go from here?" Phillip asked. "The March board meeting is a week from Thursday and the annual meeting is only two months away. Not to over dramatize the issue, especially when I have been asleep at the switch for a few months, but the future of James is in our hands. What is the plan?"

"Phillip, the specifics of the plan are being developed but the general idea is that we….you….have to get the shareholders to elect a set of board directors that reflect your vision of the James future. To be specific, you are going to have to wage a proxy fight with Mrs. James and her cronies."

"Can we win?" Phillip asked.

"We have some really good ammunition, but we also have some problems. The largest problem being product sales. No matter what we can produce as an argument against Mrs. James, she still has a large hammer. The hammer being our lack of sales performance vis-a-vis our budget plan. Shareholders want performance and you are the president/CEO and, truthfully, at least in the independent and institutional shareholders mind, your team has failed."

"Yes, but can we win?" Frustration began to creep into his voice.

J.P. answered with one word, "Yes." Phillip responded with one word, "How?"

"We will win with surprise, intellect, and information. Mrs. James is dealing with corruptness and emotion. It will be hard, but if we do what we are capable of doing we will win." J.P. stopped for a second and almost sounding as though he was trying to convince himself, he added, "Yes, we will win."

He waited for his answer to sink in. Phillip remained motionless and without expression. Finally, he turned towards Mandi and asked her the same question.

"Mandi, will we win?" There was more confidence in his voice, but there was still some doubt. Mandi caught the doubt and immediately responded. "Yes, Phillip we can win, but we will require you to be our leader and be as strong in your commitment as we are." She then went out on a limb. "We don't need you to be wishy-washy or show us any indecision. We can and will win but only with you. I think I am speaking for the majority of the staff and employees. We realize that you have been through a lot during the last few months and we appreciate this fact, but we need your commitment. A commitment to your employees and to James. Phillip, are you committed to this fight or are you just putting on a show?"

There was a long silence. J.P. wondered if Phillip would understand their position or just lash out at Mandi as he had done with him.

Phillip was staring at Mandi thinking of how best to answer her question. After what seemed to be almost too long of a pause, he answered.

"Mandi, I appreciate what you have said and what you are asking. I apologize for taking so long in answering your question. I assure you that it was out of respect not indecision."

His voice was strong and confident. J.P. realized that his staff meeting earlier that morning had been a stepping stone in the rebuilding of his will to fight. Mandi, had really touched the major issue. It wasn't about whether Phillip himself was going to fight, but whether or not Phillip would lead the fight for James and the James team. A team he had built now looked to him for leadership and was dedicated to providing as good a pharmaceutical product as humanly possible.

Phillip continued, "I had to be absolutely sure of my answer to you and to the James team. It is one thing to put on an acting job for the staff. It is something else entirely to search deep down within myself and make the true commitment to myself, you two, and to this company. I have worked hard for James and I would be lying if I said I was not tired. There are things I want to do in my own life that James and a proxy fight will either postpone or cancel. I want to make sure that when I," he looked at J.P. and smiled, "sign up for J.P.'s war, I am in it for the duration.

"I know one thing for sure, if I sign up for a proxy fight and I do not really fight, that you," he pointed a finger a J.P., "my friend, will have nothing to do with me in the future. After my outburst this morning, you can either believe this next statement or choose not to believe it. Your friendship and counsel, J.P., are very important to me. So, Mandi, my wise and lovely VP of Marketing, I have come to the conclusion to fight that woman back through perdition's gates." He laughed. "Win we will and it will be an uncompromising win. From your report, and by the way, I did read your report, there is more conspiracy to this situation than meets the eye. As you wrote in your report and as you both experienced on your trip, Mrs. James is apparently playing with a marked deck. It is incumbent upon me then to use any means necessary to take back James and to build our company to its full potential."

J.P. sat back in his seat and smiled. "Great speech, Phillip. I hope you have it imprinted in your head. We will need some great speeches at the annual meeting to ensure a win for James."

Mandi spoke up with sincerity. "Phillip, thank you very much for your commitment, it will be a great fight and I know that 99% of us are behind you. We still haven't found the one rotten apple in the James barrel, but we have a good idea who it is and I think we will be able to isolate the person."

"Okay, now let's have the full report on your trip," Phillip requested.

J.P. and Mandi gave him a complete rundown of everything through their time with Dr. Nakasone. Phillip interrupted the narration a few times with questions, but mostly he listened.

When they had finished, Phillip said, "Great! That was some story, but if my dates are correct, that leaves one week unaccounted for and the plane trip from Japan does not take a week."

"Phillip, we informed you that we wanted to take a weeks vacation," Mandi replied defensively.

"I know, I was just joking. Mandi, don't always take me seriously. I hope you had a great time. By evidence of your tans I assume that you enjoyed the surf and slope. Now," he shifted gears, "what is your battle plan?"

"Well Phillip, as I said earlier, we have to win a proxy fight. We have one chance to prevent a fight, but I think Mrs. James is committed to her plan and will conduct a counteroffensive to a proxy fight."

"What is the one chance?" Phillip responded.

"We have two board meetings before the annual meeting. The March meeting is next week. This is too early to spring a surprise counterattack. I have not analyzed her complete situation, but after our experience at the plantation, I'm beginning to think she has more business savvy than we have given her credit.

"Somehow she has launched a very good conspiracy plan. If we think back on the moves she has made with the board directors, her strategies are very good and illustrate that she has been preparing for this event for a long time. I would say for at least a year. You, Phillip, have been, to some degree playing into her hands by allowing the conflict with the board to be based on emotions rather than issues. All along she has been slowly replacing board members, giving them stock options to increase her controlling percentage when the members exercise their options. She implemented her planning process by possibly copying the 21st Century Plan and who knows what her role was with the Japanese connection at the plantation.

"You know Phillip, one of the mysteries of the missing 21st Century Plan is if Mrs. James had access to the plan why would she have made a copy. What would she have to gain? I still don't know her exact role, but I think I know what she would do with an extra copy."

"What J.P.?" both Phillip and Mandi asked in harmony.

"I never thought you would ask," he replied. "Two reasons for an extra copy. First, to recruit someone on your staff, Phillip. She needs someone close to you to be in her camp as a source of inside information. Someone she could use and depend on to be loyal to her over everything else. She would seal the loyalty by asking him to go against your strict orders. You ordered no copies to be made of the 21st Century Plan. She ordered him to make a copy."

Mandi said, "You keep using the term him. Do you know who made the copy?

"I think so, but I have to check out a few more leads. One is to make a trip to Doylestown where the copy was made. I am sure there are some answers at the pharmacy, I know both of you have your own ideas, but let's keep them to ourselves until I return."

"When are you going?" Phillip asked.

"In two weeks. The week after the board meeting," he replied. "What was the second reason?" Phillip asked.

"The second reason was right before our eyes, but we couldn't see it before our trip to Indonesia. Mrs. James needed a product to sell."

"What do you mean a product to sell?" Mandi asked.

"Again, we have underestimated Mrs. James. We thought she was a stupid emotional chairperson who only wanted power and money. Well, we aren't wrong about the power and the money, but we are wrong about stupid and emotional. I would now judge her as very intelligent, calculating, and a very capable adversary."

Unconvinced, Phillip asked, "What has made you come to this conclusion?"

Mandi jumped in with the answer, "Excuse me J.P., can I answer Phillip?"

"My pleasure madam," he replied bowing slightly at the neck and gesturing with his hand as to give her front stage.

"Thank you, sir," she replied sitting up straighter in her chair. "Phillip, we forgot a number of things. First, she is an adversary to what we stand for in terms of ethical pharmaceuticals. We thought we had to tolerate her and learn to live with her tantrums against you. We didn't see that she was throwing up a smoke screen so that she had time to execute her strategic plan. Second, this lady is not a dumb person. Remember, she has a Masters from Wellsley, magna cum laude. This is no easy accomplishment to begin with and she did it in economics."

"What?" Phillip almost shouted.

"Yes, Phillip, economics. This explains a few things, doesn't it? Lastly, we underestimated Doc James."

This time J.P. was surprised. "You have me there, Mandi, what does Doc James have to do with this except she was his wife and now his widow."

"Exactly right, J.P. We have underestimated Doc James' choice in women. He wasn't a dirty old man. Men his age aren't looking solely for someone to bed, they're looking for someone to share the remainder of their life. He was looking for a soulmate who shared his passion for business, among other things."

Mandi went on "You can bet that they talked business.. James business. She was probably mentally working on the plan to take complete control of James from the day he died. You, Phillip, and the rest of us have gotten caught up in what is probably a very carefully laid out plan. Now, and I agree with J.P., we have to turn the tables and the board meeting next week does not give us enough time."

"Mandi, that was very good," Phillip said and turned to J.P., "You didn't explain your statement that she needed a product to sell. Also, earlier you said that there was one chance to stop a proxy fight, but you never said what that chance is or, at least, I did not hear you say what it."

"Yeah, sorry I got caught up in Mandi's analysis of Mrs. James. Mandi, I agree with Phillip, you've given us an interesting perspective on her." He paused. "The product to sell is the 21st Century Plan. To whom is not definite, but there sure are a number of Japanese business interests coming in and out of this mystery. Now, as to the one chance to stop the fight at the April board meeting. To date I'm not too sure what Evelyn knows that we know. I would imagine that once last week's events get back to her she will begin to wonder what is going on with all of us. Until now she has been hiding behind the diversionary tactics we just talked about and the fortuitous shooting of Phillip. I am sure the shooting and the theft of the Lifeal formula and Bill's company were not in her plans. On the other hand, they did not hurt her cause. The plantation event, again, has caused a diversion. The plantation incident is a positive link to the possibility of a James conspiracy. I don't think she is aware of us knowing some of her plan, so a surprise from us just might throw her off guard and give us an advantage.

"In April we will know a lot more about the potential conspiracy and we could present this information to her and to her cronies at the board meeting and then ask for their resignation."

"That sounds viable J.P., but why don't you think it will work?" Phillip asked.

"First, as I said before, I don't think she will quit without a fight. She has worked long and hard on her plan and if she causes a proxy fight she knows she has the votes. So why should she stop? In addition, Phillip, with all due respect, she probably thinks from the way you have been sucked into her plan, that you're a pussycat and will not fight because you have lost your spirit. She will figure that you won't fight because it will hurt the reputation of James and yourself when you lose.

"Second, at this time, we only have circumstantial evidence of a conspiracy. I think we will be able to obtain firm material evidence in the next sixty days but certainly not before the March Meeting and possibly not before the April meeting. I can't guarantee enough material evidence by the April board meeting. I don't think we should make our counter bid for control at the April meeting. We will ask for their resignation, but we must also be prepared for a full proxy fight in May at the annual meeting."

"J.P., all of this sounds reasonable, but I know that I don't know a damn thing about proxy fights. Unless you or Mandi have gained some recent experience, I don't think you have much experience in these matters."

"You're right Phillip, but we have two additional members of our proxy team that are not in this room. Onc you know, namely Brian your CFO and the other is Carl Manningham's father Carl Manningham, Sr."

"Carl's father, J.P.? Who the hell is he?" Phillip asked.

J.P. went on to explain Carl Sr.'s involvement with the SEC and also his recently diagnosed Alzheimer's disease. He concluded, "He can't take an active role in the proxy fight, but he can give us good sound advice. Probably better advice than what is being given to Evelyn. I feel that with the three of us, plus Brian and Carl, we can do whatever is necessary to set up our slate of candidates for the board. Once we expose her plan at the April board meeting I am sure we will have plenty of volunteers to help us to win the proxy fight."

"J.P., what about the rest of the board?" Mandi interjected. "I haven't had much personal involvement with the board, but as I understand things, Evelyn has stacked the deck with lawyers and finance experts. What role will they play in a proxy fight?"

"Good question Mandi," J.P. replied. "Phillip, do you have an opinion? I will have to research their backgrounds before I can answer that question."

Phillip did not answer immediately and when he did speak it was cautiously. "I am sorry but as we pointed out earlier I was focused on the emotional issues and not the actual actions she was making in changing the personality of the board. J.P. is right, we will have to research her appointments to the board. Mainly, we must find out what they have to gain. I would assume that the most obvious is money, but maybe there are other gains that are not as obvious."

"Good point, Phillip. I have one question to ask and one suggestion, then I would recommend we adjourn and meet later this week with Brian and Carl Sr. joining the group. My suggestion is that we continue to play possum at the March board meeting. They will be looking for some indication as to our knowledge of the conspiracy. We should do our best to show that nothing has changed in our complacency towards what Mrs. James is doing to James. Phillip you will have to be more passionate showing Evelyn that you are still wrapped up in her charade and that you will not fight her plan to control the board. This will not be easy. You will have to be a good actor. Do you agree?"

Mandi and Phillip agreed.

J.P. continued, "Second is my question. Phillip, do you have a general idea of the number of shares you could count on for support, how many she has, and how many are not committed to Evelyn? We must realize votes are the bottom line in a proxy fight. Who has the most shareholder votes? We must also assume that the stock options she has given to her board members will be exercised by the time of the annual meeting election. Can you give us a rough idea?"

Phillip paused and thought through his answer. "Again, I must apologize for not having a more accurate answer, but I depend on Brian to keep track of the shareholders and I never expected a proxy fight. That having been said here are my estimates."

"I would say that she locks up 30% and we have 20%. That leaves 50% that we will have to fight over."

NIPPON PHARMACEUTICAL COUNCIL HEADQUARTERS KANAZAWA, JAPAN

"Please forgive me, Mr. Tanaguchi, everything went wrong. I have no excuse for my failures," apologized the Lonewolf associate who was responsible for the recent Singapore NPC operations including the kidnapping and plantation failures.

He was kneeling on a tatami mat in front of Tanaguchi. His head bowed so his forehead rested a quarter of an inch above the mat. The associate spoke in a voice that was barely audible. Tanaguchi sat cross-legged behind a low cherry wood Japanese desk. He wore the clothes of a modem samurai warrior businessman. His outer robe was black silk, the inner robe silver silk, and the sash crimson silk. The room was bare of furniture except for the desk and dual crossed samurai swords that hung from wires attached to the ceiling beams in front of the shoji behind the executive.

The room was part of the west coast headquarters of the NPC. This was different in every way from the offices in Osaka. The rooms of the traditional Japanese mountain inn had been converted to offices. Everyone associated with these NPC offices wore traditional dress not the western style dress of the Osaka offices. It was a one-story building built in the 1600's and located next to a mountain stream. Each office had a balcony built over the mountain stream. When meditation was necessary, the modern samurai would sit on the balcony within the serenity of the surroundings of water, tree, and nature. No outsiders were ever permitted to visit the inn.

It was here, in these serene surroundings that the NPC ran its clandestine activities. It was here that the NPC associate had voluntarily come after the bungled mission in Singapore and Indonesia. He had to come here voluntarily. If he hadn't come voluntarily or if he had resisted being brought there against his will, he would have been eliminated.

"I do not care about the apology for your failure," replied Tanaguchi. "You have completed your contract as an NPC employee. You will never be trusted again and you will never have a second chance, is this clear? In past history you would be expected to take your own life. Today, we do not expect this from you."

The associate, still kneeling and with head bowed let out the breath he had been holding for almost a minute. Except for the sound of air escaping from his lungs, he remained silent. Tanaguchi continued in a tone of voice that had a very strong guttural accent. "You are banished to Fukuro Island with only the material items you can hold in a small suitcase. Your financial worth has been confiscated and you are as worthless in wealth as you are in spirit. You may never leave the island or you will be accident prone."

"*Hai,*" escaped the associate's lips.

The associate knew that his punishment would be severe. Although he would live he would live as a dead person. He had acquired great wealth working for the NPC and now it was gone, confiscated all because of one mistake. Thoughts of failure raced through his mind. Not just one mistake, but many. He had been in charge of the Singapore/Indonesian mission. He had failed with the old man Chang when he should have had him killed. He had failed in trying to have Nacheda kidnapped and he had failed at the plantation. Through his failures Lonewolf, two NPC guards from the plantation, and three kidnappers from the limo were dead, six in total. All that remained alive were himself and Lee.

Tanaguchi now asked one question of the associate. Since the associate was now banished he was referred to as a foreigner, a gaijin. "Gaijin, where is the man called Lee?" Tanaguchi commanded.

"Forgive me, I don't know from my own eyes, but I was informed that he joined Chang's employ after Lonewolf's demise. My intelligence sources say Lee remains at the plantation a self-inflicted prisoner."

"Are you certain?" commanded Tanaguchi.

"It is the truth as far as I know," replied the associate.

What did the associate care about Lee when his life, which had been rich in wealth and power was now over. Banished. He thought of his one alternative. He had hidden a quantity of money and pictures of NPC activities in a box buried near the Bandai railway station. He knew that if things went wrong in Singapore he would either be dead or banished and sent north by train. Before turning himself in to the NPC, he had made the train trip to Bandai and placed three million-yen in a plastic bag and buried it in a park near the Bandai train station. It could give him a chance to escape and begin life again elsewhere.

His head wavered above the tatami. He couldn't relax because if his head touched the mat, Tanaguchi would send a message by first kicking him in his ribs and then in his head. Tanaguchi continued his ravings about his failure and how he would find Lee.

The associate's thoughts continued to form a plan for his escape from NPC control. Where would he go? The NPC would find him wherever he went. His passport would be useless. He was a prisoner in this island nation. Once he arrived on Fukuro Island, he would never be able to leave. He would be a beggar in a cold, barren, and inhuman environment. He and Tanaguchi knew that he wouldn't last though the next winter and possibly not through the remainder of this winter. He had grown soft in spirit. His body was strong but required nourishment to retain his strength. The only solution was to join NPC's competition. He had to find Nacheda and convince him that he could help Bandai and James. It was a slim chance because in Japan a traitor is not even respected by those he joins on the other side. He struggled to think of what his worth would be to Nacheda. Would Nacheda shelter him? Would Bandai Pharmaceutical Company shelter him? He had no choice, but to take his only option and try to win over Nacheda, it was better than banishment. He began to plot how he would retrieve his money and meet Nacheda.

Tanaguchi was concluding the last sentence he would ever direct to the associate, "Now get out of my sight and may your life be as miserable as you have made my life."

The associate backed up by scooting on his knees. He had never once raised his head to look at Tanaguchi. If he had, he would have been terminated. His eyes focused on the tiny squares of the mat. Now the tiny squares began to blur as he rapidly backed out of the room. His knees reached the sharp metal edge of the doortatami mat molding. He slowly turned with his forehead gradually raising off the mat as he turned away from Tanaguchi. He reached behind and slid the shoji to the closed position.

Two men, his same size, appeared. One on his right and the other on his left. They did not touch him. They did not have to. There was no way for him to escape, at least not here in the NPC western headquarters. He would have to wait until he reached the train station at Bandai. Until then submission was his only role. Later today he would again become strong. One more time he would be a samurai he thought as he was ushered into another room.

This room was on the other side of the inn and was bare except for a pile of clothing in the center of the floor. The clothing was peasant clothing and it was soiled. NPC had soaked the clothes in a cesspool so he would repel the people around him.

He slowly removed his expensive tailored clothes and neatly piled the silk suit, shirt, tie, socks, and shoes in the far corner of the room. He placed his 24k gold cuff links and diamond tie tack on his silk handkerchief and laid it next to his alligator shoes. He slowly put on his used and foul smelling wool undergarments and torn kimono robe. He then put on a wool quilted jacket over the kimono. Next he pulled on dirty white socks with the single large toe for the sandal strap.

He stood and walked to the door of the room. The two men had stood silently at the entrance and watched him change. The exchange room, as it was called by the associates and guards, was bugged and surveyed with video cameras.

He knew the ritual. He had stood where they stood a few times in the past. He reached down and visibly removed his wallet from the folded suit pants. He removed about 100,000 yen from the wallet in full sight of the two men. They watched as he slid the yen into the inner side pocket of his quilted jacket. He had watched other gaijin do this when he had been an escort. It was an unwritten courtesy that the survivors allowed the condemned. They watched, but never spoke. The taking of the money was done in full view not in secret. It was a silent but open gift. The condemned person was silently asking for one last favor. The favor of survival money. The escorts had given their silent permission by watching his actions. He had silently and openly begged for one last gift from his previous comrades and it had been granted.

If he had taken the money in secret or with his back turned to the escorts, the money would have been physically removed from his person as he left the room and he would have been severally beaten. Silent begging now provided him with all the money he would have to exist on or so his two escorts thought.

The associate, now a peasant, and two escorts left the inn and proceeded by taxi to the train station. At the station, one escort left and the remaining escort and the new peasant climbed on board the train to Tokyo where they would change trains. A different train would take them to the port where they would take the boat to the island of his exile.

Eight hours later his train arrived at Tokyo station. During the trip no one bothered the two travelers. When other travelers came near, the peasant's stench was overwhelming and they would move as far away as possible within the confines of the train or station.

Walking from the train from the west to the train to the north, they passed one of the many construction sites around Tokyo Station.

The peasant noticed a pile of construction debris as they had come around the corner of the passageway between train tracks. He had been walking in a clumsy manner trying to get used to his sandals. He had faked a stumble and fell hard to his knees. The pain of his knee caps hitting the cement passageway floor was excruciating. He did not make an audible sound, but the escort knew it had hurt. The peasant knew the escort would not bend down to help him back up on his feet. He depended on the escort not providing any assistance. As he fell he made sure that his kimono had flowed around his legs over a pile of debris. In one swift motion he found a spike. As he painfully started to rise from his fallen position he hid the sharp 9" spike in the folds of his quilted jacket. Once he was on his feet, the now armed peasant continued his clumsy and painful walk to the train platform to catch the train that would take them north.

The northern train was now two minutes from Bandai station and the peasant was ready to implement his escape plan. The escort was in the aisle seat guarding the peasant's exit from his window seat. He had been watching out the window and studying the reflection of the escort. The escort had slowly fallen asleep from boredom and the rhythm of the train's motion.

The peasant continued to gaze dreamily out the window at the passing forests of pines, but his mind was plotting his escape.

He saw the sign for Bandai station and knew that he had to make his move before the station announcement awoke the sleeping escort.

He slowly slid the spike from its hiding place in his quilted coat. His hands were steady and dry. It was certainly not his first kill, but the escort was a former comrade, a fellow Japanese. He paused as if trying to determine if what he was doing was morally right. In the eyes of the brotherhood of guards, escorts, and associates he was wrong. He was supposed to accept his exile with honor. His escort had assumed that he was an honorable man and had allowed himself to fall easily to sleep.

The escort did not expect any trickery only submission from the peasant, but the peasant had broken the code of conduct when he had hidden the money and again when he had picked up the spike. Maybe his lack of feelings of guilt about the breaking of Japanese honor was the reason that caused him to fail in his mission. He again paused. This was no time for reflection. It was time for action. The spike was now firmly gripped in his right hand. He looked around the train car. There were only a few passengers and because of his odor, they were not within five rows of his seat. They had watched the peasant and well-dressed man get on the train but over the miles, the curiosity of the fellow passengers had been replaced by boredom and the two large men had just become two more travelers.

The bulk of the escort and the closeness of the seats in front of them prevented the peasant from making a frontal thrust of the spike into the escort's body. The peasant was also on the wrong side for a sideward thrust into the escort's heart.

He had to kill the escort with one quick silent thrust. He could not miss. He only had one chance. He also knew the escort was not in a deep sleep. He would awaken easily. He knew, because he had been in this situation himself.

He had to make his move now. The spike was in his right hand. He gripped it tighter as he pulled his arm out of his quilted jacket so that the bulky material would not impede his arm. With one fluid movement he brought his right arm across his own body and past the right arm of the escort. The spike was now turned toward and perpendicular to the escorts body. The peasant's body rolled to the left as his right arm had moved with the thrust. He had to get his full weight into the thrust. It entered into the left rib cage just under the heart. The peasant's body now was over the right side of the escort. To an observer he looked like he was climbing over the large man to get into the aisle. With all his strength he gave the spike a final thrust into the escorts body. He heard a rib crack as the thick spike cleared the rib cage. He then turned his hand from a stabbing grip into a position where the blunt end of the spike was against his palm. He thrust upward steering the spike into the escort's heart. The escort's eyes snapped open and his left hand strongly gripped the peasant's right biceps. He looked into the escort's eyes and was amazed at how much white was showing.

The peasant, now free, placed his right foot in the aisle and dragged his left leg across the dead escort. The escort's left hand dropped from the peasant's right arm. His hand felt a small warmth as the first blood from the ruptured heart began to ooze around the spike. He quickly released the spike. The other passengers noted the escort seemly went back to sleep after his peasant seat partner had safely navigated his way to the aisle.

The peasant whispered, "Sorry my friend." Then in a voice that could be heard throughout the car he said, "Enjoy the remainder of your trip, kind sir. I enjoyed being your companion. He bowed slightly and while in the bowed position he pulled the escort's overcoat closed over the spike and the reddening white shirt. He took a chance and quickly unbuttoned the coat and swiftly reached in and stole the man's wallet from his inner suit pocket. He would not need these worldly items he thought.

He straightened and began his slightly bent peasant walk up the aisle just as the loud speaker announced the train's arrival at Bandai station. He did not look back. He was certain the escort looked as if he were asleep. It might be a few hours before he was discovered. The passengers will remember that the peasant got off the train in Bandai. And the Bandai police would be looking for a smelly peasant. He had, at most, two hours of freedom. He had the 100,000 yen in his pocket plus whatever the dead escort had in his wallet. He also probably had the escort's passport. This he had not planned on. The passport would only be good for a short time. Only until the NPC learned of the murder. The NPC would know something had gone wrong when the escort failed to check in by telephone at the port. They would learn of his death when they read about it in the next day's newspaper.

Then they would place all their resources to the task of finding the peasant. He had, at the most twenty-four hours before he was hunted.

Now he had to retrieve his buried money.

As he stepped safely off the train at the Bandai train station, he thought, so far so good.

11:00 P.M., TUESDAY, MARCH 14

BANDAI, JAPAN

Nacheda stirred in his sleep and then quickly awoke though he didn't move. His eyes searched the darkness of his apartment bedroom. He slowly reached down along the right side of his bed, which was against the wall, and felt for the pistol. Ever since the Singapore/Indonesia trip he had kept a pistol at his side. He felt the cold steel as his right hand closed around the grip of the weapon. To an observer's eye there had not been any outward sign that Nacheda was awake.

He heard the noise again. It was coming from direction of the entry door. Someone or something was scratching the surface of the wooden door, which was only about twenty feet from where he lay.

He rolled to his left as if he were turning in his sleep. The scratching continued. He was now certain it was from the front door. He got to his feet and slowly walked to the front door in a zig^zag pattern. He took a crouched position on the hinge side of the door. If someone shot through the door he would be off to the side. If they shot as he opened the door he would be under the normal height of a person opening the door. An assassin's bullet would be fired above his head. In his crouch he would be in a position to spring upon the intruder and disarm or kill him.

The scratching continued. "Who is there?" Nacheda asked in a voice loud enough to be heard outside the door. The scratching stopped.

"A friend," came the soft reply of male voice.

"I have no friends that scrape my door this late at night."

"I know, but I am a new friend and I am unarmed. I come about the American in Indonesia known to you as Mr. Smith and to me as Lonewolf."

Nacheda was startled. Only enemies knew of Mr. Smith, not friends. He told his visitor as much.

"Those who knew Lonewolf are not friends of mine. I have information you would want to acquire. I am not armed. I come as a friend," he said for the second time.

Nacheda reached over to the door lock and turned it to the open position. He then backed off into the shadows. This time Nacheda spoke in a louder voice, "Open the door very slowly and enter the room on your knees. Do not make a sudden move. I have a gun pointed at you and I won't hesitate one second to shoot a new friend from Indonesia."

The door began to open very slowly. An empty left hand appeared then an empty right hand. A peasant gradually appeared in the doorway and slowly raised both of his hands above his head. "I am unarmed and have only come to talk."

"You look like a peasant and you smell like a shit truck driver. You don't look or smell like a person with knowledge about Mr. Smith. Besides, who is Lonewolf?" Nacheda announced.

"Please hear me out, Nacheda-san. I am sure you will be very happy with the knowledge I am prepared to provide you at relatively no cost."

"Continue into the room on your knees and take a seat on the couch facing the front door."

Nacheda remained in he shadows with his pistol aimed at the intruder. "Speak, and make your story fast and clear. I have no time for you, Mr. Smith, or your Lonewolf. My trigger finger grows tired from the tension of the moment."

"I will be only but a moment. Please put down your pistol, you will not need it tonight. I would have nothing to gain by either hurting you or by getting myself killed. I will be short and then if you do not value my input or presence I will be gone as silently as I arrived."

"Speak!"

The exNPC associate explained that Mr. Smith and Lonewolf were the same person. He did not know Lonewolf's real name. Nacheda felt there was no need to tell this intruder that Lonewolf's real name was Joe Berger. The intruder then told Nacheda his story. He spoke of his times as Nacheda's shadow in Westwood Village, Singapore, Tokyo, and Bandai. He explained his work with the NPC and how he came to know Lonewolf. He finally told of his failure and how he came to be a midnight visitor. When he explained the killing of his escort, Nacheda's hand tightened around the pistol grip. In a quick ten minutes, Nacheda had learned all he wanted to know. He now knew how Berger had gotten the job and who he had been working for. He still did not know what the NPC wanted from him, Bandai, and/or James. He also knew that this traitor would not have the answers.

"I am tired of you, traitor," Nacheda said in an authoritative voice. "What is it that you want of me?"

"I am now a fugitive and my chances of leaving Japan are very slim. I beg of you to give me guidance. I have a small quantity of money and also some pictures of NPC activities.

Nacheda was silent as he thought through the situation. First, he could not trust this traitor, but he did need physical evidence on NPC activities. He decided he would require time to think. He would shelter the traitor until morning or until he had a plan for this unexpected situation.

"First you are going to wash yourself and then I am going to tie your hands and legs so you can not move. The bonds will not hurt, but believe me you will be immobilized. I want to think this situation through and I also require sleep. If you try to escape I will interpret the attempt as a hostile action and a breach of trust. I will kill you or turn you over to the police which ever is most convenient to me. I do not trust you and there is nothing you can do or say that will change my opinion. Is this clear?" *"Hai."*

After the visitor had taken his bath and Nacheda provided him with a different set of clothes and threw the old into the trash, he bound the man. Nacheda used strong shipping tape and bound his visitor in a kneeling position. His hands were behind him and attached by tape to his feet. The tape was not tight, but he would not be able to break loose. In a show of sympathy he helped the visitor to lay on his side so as not to be left kneeling all night.

"Doumoarigatou," was all that the visitor said.

Nacheda went back to his bed and replaced the gun under the bed pad.

He had first thought to keep the gun in his hand but had second thoughts when he envisioned the possibility of a nervous twitch in his hand accidentally causing him to shoot himself in his sleep.

He slept more soundly than he thought was possible considering a stranger was in his home.

Morning arrived as a crisp late winter day in the mountains. The temperature was three degrees Celsius and the wind had a cutting edge. Nacheda woke with the first rays of the morning sun. He slowly rolled from his bed and looked into the living room at the visitor. He was still on his side and sleeping. Nacheda got dressed and went outside. He decided he could think better in the fresh air. He walked to a small park and sat down on the trunk of fallen tree.

How could he get the information without committing himself to help this traitor? After an hour he had devised a plan. He then returned to his apartment and his visitor.

8:00 A.M., WEDNESDAY, MARCH 15

BANDAI, JAPAN

"Okay, whatever your name is, I have a plan that should benefit both of us. I cannot guarantee your success, but there is a good chance you will get away."

"Please tell me your plan," the traitor replied.

"We must get you to Hong Kong where I have some friends that will provide you with false papers. You can then disappear into the millions of people coming and going from Hong Kong. This is especially true now that the PRC has taken control of Hong Kong and its territories."

"This sounds too good to be true. What is the price?" he replied suspiciously.

"The price is the pictures of the NPC activities. Of course, the price depends on how good the pictures are and how I can use them in the future. You must show them to me immediately so that I can determine their value. If they have no value to me, you are on your own. I won't help you in any way and you must leave immediately. You must show me all of the pictures." Nacheda paused. The man's face expressed fear. Nacheda continued, "I know you will want some of the pictures for your own protection, but that is not possible. I want control of the pictures and I don't want the possibility of you telling the NPC that the photographs exist. That is my offer, take it or leave it."

The traitor searched Nacheda's face for any sign of weakness. He knew he wouldn't be able to find a better deal, but he must try to keep a few pictures. He will sneak them from the package when Nacheda is not looking. His plan for keeping some of the pictures was destroyed with Nacheda's next words.

"I don't want you handing me the pictures while you are unbound. I want you to tell me where they are and I will retrieve them myself. Don't worry about the money I will not take any of the money. You will need it to obtain new papers. Now where are the pictures?" His voice became a command so there was no question as to who was giving the orders. The traitor was quiet too long for Nacheda's patience, which was growing short.

"I wouldn't advise that you wait too long, you are in no position to bargain. Where are the pictures?"

"They are in a belt around my waist."

Nacheda reached down and parted the folds of new clothing he had supplied the night before. He felt the large belt at the man's waist. He uncovered the belt and untied it. He took one end in his hands and yanked it from the traitor's waist. The force spun the man as the belt came free.

Nacheda opened the belt and removed its contents. There was a large stack of 1,000-yen notes and seven photographs. He inspected the belt to ensure there were no additional contents. He put back the money and threw the belt down in front of the man.

Nacheda then inspected the photographs. The first one was of Berger and some Japanese executives. They were sitting around a table talking. "Who are these people?" Nacheda asked showing the traitor the picture.

"These are the executives of the NPC and Lonewolf discussing the James project. This is the name the NPC gave the project concerning you, Bandai, and the James Company. When you take off the tape around my hands I will write down their names for you.

Nacheda uncovered the second photograph. It was a picture of Berger and some men emerging from a large office building. There were other people in the same scene. There was a newspaper stand in the picture. "What is the value of this picture?" Nacheda asked.

"There are two. First, it shows the NPC executives and Lonewolf at the NPC building. Second, if you enlarge the picture you will be able to read the date on the newspaper posted on the wall of the newspaper stand. This places the date the group was meeting at the NPC Osaka headquarters. You will find that it is a date in mid-October of last year.

Nacheda said to himself, the bastard was working for them as far back as last October and probably from the beginning of his task force. He felt a deep since of regret that a man he called friend had betrayed him and the rest of their friends in the group.

The third photograph showed Berger and the rest of Nacheda's task force coming out of the Westwood Village condominium.

The fourth and fifth pictures were of the attempted kidnapping in Singapore. The last five were photographs of the plantation on Java. Three of them were of Lonewolf and Chang and the last two were of the front of the plantation house with Nacheda at the bottom of the stairs, Berger (Lonewolf) lying on the stairs with J.P. lying on top of his legs. Mandi was standing on the deck holding a pistol on Chang who was doubled up lying on his side.

"Since you were present at the plantation and I wasn't, you might wonder how these pictures came to be in my possession?" asked the traitor.

"It did cross my mind," remarked Nacheda.

"I had many spies. A plantation worker took these. After witnessing the tragedy at the plantation he drove to the Yogoyakarta airport where the NPC private jet was waiting. He told the pilot about the deaths and told him to carryout his orders. He gave the roll of film to the pilot to deliver to me. The pilot gave me the film when he reported back to me in Singapore. It was then that I decided that I was most certainly a dead man unless I had a good contingency plan. You are now part of my contingency plan. Are the photographs satisfactory?"

"First, answer one question. These photographs have large periods of time between events. I am sure they weren't on one roll of film. There must be additional photographs. Where are they?" Nacheda's question was more of an order.

"You are very observant, but since you haven't lived the life of an NPC associate you wouldn't know the answer. There were other photographs, but they were destroyed. Like you I didn't want many copies available for others to use. Many copies would diminish the value. I can assure you that I destroyed all of the other photographs and all of the negatives. The pictures you have in your hand are the only photographs I have or were taken of these events with my knowledge. Are these photographs satisfactory for our deal?' he asked again with anxiety.

"These photographs are satisfactory," Nacheda replied. "I will cut your tapes and you will cook us both a morning meal. You will be under my guard and I will kill you if you decide to make a sudden move. I have no reason to keep you alive except that I gave my word that I would help you. If you do anything stupid, I will consider my promise invalid."

"I assure you, I have no reason to be difficult. You have promised me more than I would have expected under the circumstances. You will have no trouble from me. How will you get me to Hong Kong?"

"That's my problem. Now I will cut the tape and you will cook while I make a phone call." Nacheda called a friend from his Vietnam intelligence days who worked for Japanese intelligence. He promised he would fill him in on the illegal activities of one of Japan's most respected associations. The friend would have to wait until June to receive the material evidence. He would also have to do a favor for Nacheda by exporting a Japanese man to Hong Kong. No questions asked.

The friend knew and trusted Nacheda. He would do as Nacheda requested. A private plane would pick up the passenger this evening and be on the way to Hong Kong before midnight. Have the passenger at the Bandai airstrip at 4:00 p.m. Nacheda thanked his friend and hung up the telephone.

Nacheda wrote down two Hong Kong names and their phone numbers. The traitor would obtain new identity papers from one and transportation papers from the other. He told the traitor to memorize them and then Nacheda burned the paper.

By midnight the traitor was on the way to Hong Kong and Nacheda was on a flight to New York City with the material evidence to tie Berger to the NPC and James. He did not stop to see Rieko in Tokyo. After the traitors report, he did not know if anyone was following him. All he knew was that he had to get this information to J.P. as soon as possible and it had to be hand delivered.

2:00 P.M., THURSDAY, MARCH 16

EDGAR ALLAN POE STREET NEW YORK CITY

J.P. looked around his living room. Present were Mandi, Phillip, Brian, Carl Sr., and Nacheda. He had received an e-mail early Wednesday morning from Nacheda saying he was on his way to New York to see him and to meet Phillip.

Nacheda arrived the night before and was picked up at the airport by Roberto. J.P. had brought him up to^ date on their proxy strategy. Nacheda showed J.P. the photographs and went through the traitor's story. They now had proof that the Nippon Pharmaceutical Council was spying on the Bandai Pharmaceutical Company task force through Joe Berger and ultimately trying to harm the James Pharmaceutical Company through control of the Devil Tree plantation. They discussed the reasons for the NPC activity late into the night and could only come to one conclusion, the NPC was interested in James, and they wanted to keep Bandai out of the picture. Why and to what extent they were interested in James had yet to be determined, hopefully very soon. It seemed only logical that a move would be made either before or during the annual shareholders meeting in May.

Early that morning Phillip, accompanied by Mandi, had arrived at J.P.'s apartment to meet with Nacheda. They had determined that there was a good chance Nacheda was still being followed by the NPC and they wanted to keep him away from the Spectrum of Medicine Building. They went through the BandaiJames proposed agreement. Phillip and Nacheda hit it off right away. Things were looking up as the team and the proxy fight were beginning to take shape. At the morning meeting they decided to have a proxy team meeting in the afternoon at J.P.'s apartment.

Carl, Sr., began by summing up the situation. "I have a good news and bad news story. First, the good news, this is St., Patrick's Day weekend. Now for the bad news, you have a less than a fifty percent chance of winning your proxy fight," the lawyer matter of factly announced. He waited for the significance of his statement to sink into the minds of the team. Just as they were all about to ask why, he continued with his summary. "The patient is dying, but not dead. Let me explain. It is very hard to undo what has already done. Mrs. James has you on the defensive because she has more shares under her control. A share is a vote, as you all well know, and she has shares...lots of them. She doesn't have to work very hard to win over additional shareholder votes because of her status within the organization. The fact is, she is the chairwoman of the board and the founder's widow. Many people will vote with her because they will rightly assume that she holds the power.

"In order for you to win, you will have to win over shareholders and also convert some of the shareholder votes that she is counting on for her win. As you can imagine, this will be very difficult. The idea of a joint venture with Bandai is great, but you have to win the proxy fight in order to implement the plan. So, Bandai, the cash infusion, and their potential role as a shareholder are somewhat irrelevant as far as the proxy fight is concerned.

"Bandai is a solution for the future. I'm not saying that the Bandai alliance isn't important, it is, but it is the future, not today's proxy fight. The alliance with Bandai provides Phillip, with a strategic platform, but no firm votes. If there is already an alliance between Mrs. James and the NPC, which, by the way we have no real proof of, then they might also have as good a future platform as the BandaiJames platform. It could even be better because the NPC has more money and power. The biggest advantage to Mrs. James and her side is the real and perceived failure of James under Phillip's leadership. I know this hurts Phillip, but the fact is, you have not achieved plan and you have lost some of your credibility. Since this is historical fact it can't be undone. This will hurt you in the voting. Shareholders want change when performance has been poor. Mrs. James offers them change. The U.S. shareholder is fickle. They think they know everything about business, but really don't know anything except how to be a Monday morning quarterback. The shareholder will vote against the past before they will vote for the future."

Phillip interrupted. Frustration was in his voice, "But Carl, what of the possible illegalities that surround her activities?"

"You said the important swing words, Phillip, 'possible illegalities'. Do you have positive proof of illegal activities. No, you have circumstantial evidence, not proof. The shooting can't be tied to Mrs. James or the NPC. Nor can the Devil Tree plantation incident be tied directly to her. I'm sorry, but so far she is clean. You might say she plays dirty, but some would also say she plays smart. It all depends on your perspective and who is going to get the shareholders the best return on their investment. I say again, Phillip, whether you like it or not, to date, you have failed in the eyes of the shareholders. She has not had a chance to fail. Will the shareholders give her a chance to fail? The next two months will provide the answer to this question."

"Carl," J.P. interrupted, "this is all gloom and doom, but you said there was a chance to win. What is the chance and what is it that we have to do to take the chance?"

"You are right, I did say there was a chance." He paused to get their full attention and to reverse the feeling of impending failure. "First, there is the possibility of getting the current board to resign based on the circumstantial evidence you now have from Nacheda.

They might be scared off because of the slanderous publicity that disclosure might bring to them and their respective companies. I agree with previous statements by J.P. that they won't actually resign. They have gone too far with Evelyn's plan and they have too much money to lose. So resignation is remote, but it should be tried. The second choice is to risk the outcome of the vote by relying on the good judgment of the shareholders. This, again is a shot in the dark and, I am sorry to say, history tells us that we will not win. The third choice is to commence a class action suit against the board of directors for actions detrimental to the survival of the corporation."

This was a new choice to the team that none of them had ever considered. They listened to Carl, Sr. with more interest as he continued.

"This choice has its downside as well as its upside. The most obvious downside is that Phillip and the board members that support Phillip are also part of the board and will also be named in the suit. Therefore, we will have to place into the proxy a totally new slate of directors. We will not be able to include Phillip or the other board member supporters of Phillip. It is not as bleak a picture as you might imagine. The new board will choose the new president and CEO as well as the other officers of the corporation. If this is done right then nothing will change except the makeup of the board. The new board will then hire Phillip as president and CEO as well as elect him to the board. If you had planned to have Phillip assume the position of chairman of the board by replacing Mrs. James you wouldn't be able to carry out this strategy, at least not in the short term."

"Carl," Phillip replied seriously, "I want you and the rest of the team to know that my goal is to protect James and the principles on which it was built. I'm not after personal gain. In fact I would welcome a new chairperson as long as they were helping to build James and not tear it down as Evelyn is trying to accomplish. I have plenty to do in successfully implementing the James 21st Century Plan. I don't need the chairmanship."

The mention of the 21st Century Plan reminded J.P. of something. The latest developments concerning Bill Williams' company Clintec, the newly reported side effects of Lifeal, and the Bandai connection had rendered the 21st Century Plan written last fall as, for the most part, obsolescent.

"Not to drift off the subject," J.P. commented, "but, we must rewrite the 21st Century Plan. With everything that has happened in the last few months, I'm sure you will all agree that the 21st Century Plan, as we know it, is obsolescent. We can undertake the rewrite effort along with formulating the strategies we will use to win the proxy fight. We will need to define our new objectives so when asked, we can inform the shareholders what plan will be followed under the new James board."

"Exactly right, J.P.," Carl chimed in "What you are pointing out isn't that irrelevant. We will have to develop a new strategic platform for the new board. I would expect the following sequence of events to take place in order for us to win our fight for control. And make no mistake about it we are in a fight for the control of James. If you think these words are too harsh then we shouldn't even start to fight. I remember a quotation by General MacArthur after the Korean War. 'We should not enter a war without the will to win'."

Carl continued his schedule of events, "First, at the upcoming April board meeting, we will ask the current board to resign based on the circumstantial evidence that we have gathered. If we have hard evidence of wrong doing and we are almost assured of getting them to resign, then we most certainly will consider using this evidence for its value of encouraging the directors to resign. If we are not certain, then we should hold the evidence for the annual meeting. I will jump to a conclusion. I think Mrs. James and the board will refuse to resign and will submit to the shareholders the plan they have developed in likely cooperation with the NPC.

"This will cause us to file a shareholders class action suit that will have to be based on hard evidence. This will surprise them and force them into an aggressive action. I would imagine that a public relations campaign would be launched against the present officers of James. Phillip, you must be prepared, psychologically, to handle a negative PR campaign. There is also a possibility that your reputation could be permanently damaged. I don't think this will happen once the facts are known, but it is a possibility and you must be prepared." Carl paused for effect. "I don't think the shareholders class action suit will actually take place. No one will want to go through this type of legal case, especially the Japanese. If we present the BandaiJames plan, the shareholders will hopefully see the light and force the issue against Mrs. James and her selected board members. Mrs. James is not stupid and she wants money. Her James stock will be devalued in a proxy fight. At what share price will she agree to quit so it won't go any lower? I don't know the answer, but I do know that her kind will, at some point, quit. They won't ride the corporation train into failure."

Phillip jumped to the heart of the issue. "I again state my objective to see James grow. If this growth takes place without my active participation then so be it. I will be disappointed but not devastated. I have enough shares that, with a healthy James, the money gained from their eventual sale will enable me to retire and live quite nicely."

Carl continued without addressing Phillip's input, "Well, that is the way I see the next two months. It's up to this group to decide what to do and how to implement your decision. I will advise you, but as I have previously informed J.P., I can't be an active participant."

Brian spoke up for the first time, "Carl, we certainly appreciate your counsel, but why are you doing this and what do you expect in return?"

"Good question Brian. I assume by 'return' you mean monetary gain?" Carl replied.

"Well I did not mean the question to be as direct as you have interpreted it, but yes, what monetary gain will you get from this situation."

Seeing that Carl was going to be placed in something of an embarrassing situation, J.P. spoke up to answer the question for Carl. "I would like to comment on your question, Brian. Only Carl can specifically answer the question, but I can shed some light on the situation in which Carl finds himself. Carl is helping James and us for his own personal reasons and for this assistance he is not receiving any monetary gain nor is he expecting any stock. He is an advisor. We want to thank him for the valuable help he has already given us. We shouldn't abuse his knowledge nor take advantage of his goodwill. There are personal reasons that he has confided to me. It is his decision as to whether he wants to share these issues with the group. Believe me the reasons are honorable and we should honor his request for anonymity if he so desires."

"Thank you J.P. I appreciate you're trying to keep my reasons confidential, but I think it is important that the team know these reasons. I say this because I know that my case is not unusual and if you know the reason it may help you with the battle, or rather the war. You are getting yourself into a war. Do not underestimate the situation."

Carl went on, "My reason for helping James could be classified as selfish."

J.P. started to interrupt, but Carl stopped him with a wave of his hand. "No, J.P., I understand where you are coming from and I again appreciate your efforts, but my reasons are selfish. I wouldn't be doing this if it were not for my son and myself. Let me explain. As you know, my son Carl, Jr. is a manager in the marketing department at James. He, in fact, works for Mandi. I think he has a great future with James. I do not ask for any special help for Carl, Jr., but I do want James to survive so that he has the opportunity to prove himself.

"Second, and this is what J.P. did not want to discuss. The fact is, I have been diagnosed as being in the early stages of Alzheimer's." The surprise in the room was audible. Carl, Sr. continued, "Yes, I am sorry for myself as well as mad. I have contributed a great deal to the free enterprise system and know I could contribute more in my older years. I will be deprived of participating in the future by a terrible disease. A disease that, as of today, has no cure. I see in the research that James is capable of conducting a chance for others who might have Alzheimer's to enjoy life to its fullest in their later years.

"Until it is time for them to leave this consciousness," he smiled to break the tension his remarks were causing, "I would be lying if

I did not have a slight wish that something could be developed by James and Bandai that could help me before it is too late. I realize that this is a remote possibility, but who knows?

"So, I want to help you to help James finish the research on the promise that Devil Tree bark may impart on JPC138 for all the people who have or will develop Alzheimer's. If I can help in any way, I will feel that I have made a final contribution to humanity." Again, in order not to leave his comments on a morbid note he laughed and added, "Whether the disease will allow me to remember or not to remember that I made the contribution." They all laughed nervously.

"Speaking for James," Phillip said, "I want to thank you from the bottom of our hearts. I hope and pray your disease will progress slowly and that the work of James and Bandai will help you to enjoy a full old age. With your help and the proposed relationship with Bandai Pharmaceuticals I feel that we have a better chance at success. And, not as an afterthought but as a statement, I do not know if you are all aware, but your son has already made his presence felt at James. He is, at present, rewriting the Lifeal market plan to reflect the creative ideas that he has developed through his market research activities. His ideas will provide Lifeal with a new start and prepare us for a time when we will be able to promote Lifeal as a prophylactic for arrhythmia. In fact the new Lifeal market plan will be part of our new James strategy.

"You should be very proud of your son as we are certainly proud to have him as an employee. I am certain that he has a bright future with James."

Nacheda took the opportunity to make his first remarks as a member of the team.

"I am new to the corporate world whether it be Japanese or American. I have heard and read many adverse stories about what really goes on in the executive ranks of a corporation. The Mrs. James situation validates those stories. I want to tell all of you and you especially, Mr. Manningham, that I am honored to be part of this team and potentially a member of the JamesBandai team. I know I speak for Dr. Nakasone, who is a very honorable man, Bandai

Pharmaceutical Company will do everything in their power to help you achieve your dream of a cure for Alzheimer's."

Everyone acknowledged Nacheda's statement and then J.P. spoke up to close the meeting, "My purpose is not to do the speaking for you Phillip, but we have a great deal of work to do before the annual meeting in May and you, Phillip, also have a company to run. I suggest I take charge of this war effort and, along with the team represented here at this meeting, we will keep you informed, seek your advice, your approval, and then give you friendly direction on how to act towards Evelyn and the current board. Is this tactic agreeable to you, Phillip, and to the rest of the team?"

"J.P., I could not think of a better suggestion." Phillip answered. "One thing I would like to know from either Brian or Carl."

"What is that?" Brian asked.

"I would like to know how much this proxy war is going to cost us and where will we get the funds?"

"Brian," Carl interjected, "I do not know where you will get the funds, but I do know roughly how much a firm of your size will have to pay to wage a proxy fight."

"Go ahead Carl. After your comments I will try and answer the question as to where we will get the funds," Brian said.

"First," Carl explained, "you must realize that a proxy fight is very expensive. Probably more than you realize. The problem is, everything has to be done formally, not informally. It is the formality that makes it so expensive. Over the last few years the Securities and Exchange Commission has been trying to change the proxy rules governing corporate shareholder battles. The SEC is caught between two groups, the top managers of large business firms and institutional investors. The institutional investors, mainly the retirement funds, want more communication leeway between investors. Presently, if there is communication between more than ten shareholders it can be viewed as a proxy solicitation. The institutional investment funds want to join together and influence management policy without the communications being considered a proxy fight by the SEC.

Management does not want this shareholder pressure from outside its corporate operations." Carl paused for effect.

"Now as for the cost, I can only give you estimates because each case is different. The total cost is also made up of what both parties have spent fighting with each other. The average proxy fight is just under ten million dollars   for both parties.

The team gasped.

J.P. spoke up quickly, Half of ten million is five million. Five million dollars to save a potentially five-plus billion dollar corporation! Not really that bad when you look at the situation from that perspective. The point here that cannot be overlooked is that it is James fighting James. So where does the money come from on both sides?

Well J.P., replied Brian, I am sure that somehow James, it's employees and shareholders will have to pay the full $10 million. The legitimate board is the one that is in place will recommend its own reelection. The new slate of directors will be represented by the James employees. It is ironic, but I think the employees will have to pay from their own pocket because the present board will not approve to pay for actions against itself.

Well that puts things in perspective, doesn't it? said Mandi. How are we going to get the employees to pay and still surprise Mrs. James?

There was silence in the room as everyone tried to think through this new barrier to success. The silence lasted a full five minutes.

Isn't there any other way, Carl? Phillip asked.

Not to wage a full battle, Carl answered in a matter of fact manner. It sounds like we should wage a limited war based on what funds we have to wage the fight. We can find a SEC law firm that will work on contingency. I think I can help find a good firm that will work with us. There are a few firms that owe me a favor.

That's great, Carl, J.P. said and continued, I can probably get a printing company to do the job on contingency and our time is free. All we require is the postage costs and other outofpocket expenses.

I can come up with $500,000 in funds from our emergency corporate funds, added Brian. The definition of emergency is left up to Phillip and I am sure that Phillip will designate this as an emergency.

It looks like we have a start, remarked Phillip. Once the fight starts I am sure we can ask some of our shareholders and employees to provide emergency funds.

Nacheda spoke for the second time today, Dr. Bradsmith, I will suggest to Dr. Nakasone that it would be to our mutual advantage to support your proxy fight. I will ask for a one million dollar fund be established and controlled at my discretion. Bandai Pharmaceuticals and Dr. Nakasone are dedicated to this agreement and we should share in the costs. If the NPC gains a foothold in the U.S. pharmaceutical market, then Bandai will not have the opportunity to be a player in the global pharmaceutical marketplace. This is a major objective of Bandai. I also don't think we could find a better partnership than James and Bandai. I would like to recommend that I undertake another assignment, J.P. I will work with Skip and our intelligence system to find out all we can about the NPC. We will report back to the team when we have meaningful information.

Good idea, Nachedasan, he replied.

Nachedasan we are very grateful for your vision and the financial demonstration of your commitment to our mutual objectives, Phillip continued. Now, J.P., if you could give us a quick summary of our pluses and minuses, maybe we can adjourn this meeting before we have dinner.

No problem Phillip, he answered. He got up from his chair and walked over to a blank flip chart page that he had brought from the office. He drew a line down the middle forming two columns. At the top of the left column he wrote the words Positive Factors. At the top of the right column he wrote, Negative Factors.

Let's list everything we can about the situation. After we finish we can prioritize the important issues and throw out the others.

Another hour passed before they had exhausted their thoughts. After an additional thirty minutes they had come up with a list that they felt they could work with in their war for control of James. The chart read:

POSITIVE FACTORS

Surprise

Bandai agreement Bandai funds

Bandai pure ingredient process New Devil Tree contract New Lifeal direction Carl, Sr.

Photographs of NPC connection Agreement with Bill Williams and Clintec

NEGATIVE FACTORS

Lack of sales and profit performance Mrs. James board control Potential NPC funds and investment Lawyers and finance board directors Shooting of Phillip Lack of funds

Limited material evidence against Mrs. James and the NPC Mrs. James' stock ownership Wall Street reports about James Time

A conspiracy usually cannot be proven

He summarized "Well, as we have surmised, the negatives outweigh the positives. This indicates a rough battle. Is everyone still agreeable to going ahead with the proxy fight?"

All the members of the team nodded their heads yes, but with less enthusiasm than what had been shown earlier in the afternoon.

Nacheda spoke up, "Dr. Bradsmith and J.P., under the circumstances I have two suggestions. One, that we continue to use extreme caution in all of our communications including using the security network that we had set up for the Bandai task force. Second, I shouldn't be seen near the Spectrum of Medicine Building or any other James facility or employee. I am certain that the NPC knows we have been talking. How could they not know? We should probably spread some misinformation about James and Bandai.

Another good idea Nachedasan. I will brief the team on the security system. We can communicate by phone through the system at Skip's Westwood Village condo.

Phillip stood up. He had a determined look on his face. He was ready to fight. He concluded the meeting by saying, The ball is in your court, J.P. Take it and run. I want to thank all of you for your faith in James and me. I feel honored to be part of this team. I know we will win, because it is right. I cannot imagine that all the work that we have put into this company will go for naught. James is too valuable to mankind and the quality of life. Thank you again. Remember, no notes and no conversation to anyone about what we're doing regarding the board or Bandai Pharmaceuticals. If what we are planning leaks out, our chances of winning are nil. We have all agreed that we are fighting an intelligent, albeit power-hungry, adversary. Please take your future direction from J.P. This meeting is adjourned.

3:00 P.M., THURSDAY, MARCH 16

JAMES FARM, GREYSTONE HALL SEAFORD, NEW YORK

"Hello?" he answered. "Well?"

"Nothing yet."

"Are you really doing something about the situation?" CCTJ.... _ •

I m trying.

"No you're not." CCT

I am,

"The hell you are!" she hung up the telephone.

He immediately called NPC, but no one answered. He called her back, but no one answered. He hadn't heard from the NPC since he saw Mr. Smith and gave him the 21st Century Plan. He had a funny feeling that he had been duped, but he was not about to tell her.

4:00 P.M., THURSDAY, MARCH 24

SPECTRUM OF MEDICINE BUILDING NEW YORK CITY

"Mrs. Evelyn PrestonJames sat at the large desk in her new office on the top floor, Phillip's floor. After Phillip returned to work from his convalescence at home, she had instructed him to construct the office. She claimed that she needed an office she could use when she visited the Spectrum of Medicine Building. Phillip had mentally listed the various nonoffice places he thought she could sit, but in the end he acquiesced and constructed an office from the open space that had been reserved for the expansion of the James museum. She had decorated the office in a very dark manner. There were dark Renaissance paintings and bookcases full of old books. The wall paneling and furniture were dark wood.

Mrs. James picked up the telephone and dialed his number. She felt great after what she knew was the greatest board meeting she had ever chaired. She knew that today things were absolutely going her way. She just knew the NPC had made contact. She needed a favorable report and she had to admit, the silence from the NPC was beginning to concern her.

"Hello?" he answered.

"Have you heard anything yet?" she asked in an upbeat tone.

"I'm sorry, Evelyn, nothing yet. I keep trying to call the NPC, but there is no answer. I even had the telephone company find me the number that Mr. Smith used to called me to set up our meeting in Pennsylvania. It was a western Washington exchange, but it has since been disconnected," he answered.

In an unusually calm voice, she said, "Well at least you are doing some thinking. That is a welcome change. Do you have any other ideas?"

"Not really. Remember, we are dealing with the Japanese and they work from their own schedule. They take a long time to make decisions."

"You don't have to tell me who we are dealing with." Her good nature was beginning to sour.

He felt her becoming angry again and tried to stop the tide by asking, "How was the board meeting?"

She brightened, "Great. I had good old Dr. Bradsmith by the balls. He is so incompetent it surprises me how Doc ever named him as his successor. He sat and took more verbal abuse than you can imagine. He hardly put up a fight. The shooting was a blessing in disguise. He is a broken man. We won't have any trouble implementing our plan if you would just do your job and get hold of Tanaguchi. We only have two months."

"Congratulations on the board meeting," he replied. He felt if he played his cards right he might be able to visit her at the farm. He ached. He went for the win, "Are you going to the farm tonight?"

"Of course." she answered.

"Do you.," he paused to gather up his nerve, "Do you think we could get together tonight?" he whispered.

She thought she would have some fun with him, "What for? We have nothing to discuss, do we?" she giggled.

He thought her giggle was seductive, "I don't want to talk, Evelyn." "What do you want to do?"

"You know."

She flushed excitedly and thought about the possibility of his visiting her bed tonight. If she gave in to him tonight her strong position with him would be weakened. He hadn't come through with any new information and that was the price of her body. No, she wouldn't give in to his needs or her own. She would wait and he would have to wait. She started to get angry again.

"You know the rules. No information, no sex. Now get in touch with the NPC. Do you hear me? Now!" She slammed the phone down.

"I'm trying," he said into the dead phone.

9:00 A.M., MONDAY, MARCH 27

SPECTRUM OF MEDICINE BUILDING
NEW YORK CITY

"Did you have a good weekend J.P.?" Phillip asked.

"As good as was possible with all of the legal work we are doing on this proxy issue and new strategic plan. Mandi and I had some free time to go to Lincoln Center Saturday evening. Did you recover from last Thursday's board meeting?"

"Your idea of my not coming to work on Friday was brilliant. I know I was acting on Thursday, but her tirades still bothered me. I think that if I had been in the office on Friday and had met her in the hallway I might very well have become violent. So you see J.P., you saved me from possible legal action and you enabled me to have a great weekend at home. Thank you."

"No thanks are necessary. By the way, I am checking out the Doylestown pharmacy today. Want to come along for the ride?" J.P. asked.

"No thanks. Janet has loaded me up with paperwork. I will be stuck here for the whole day. Have fun and let me know what you find out." "I'll see you tomorrow with a report."

12:00 P.M., MONDAY, MARCH 27
DOYLESTOWN, PENNSYLVANIA

J.P. drove his rented car over the Delaware River from Lambertville to New Hope, Pennsylvania using the old bridge. He disliked the relatively new US 202 bridge that by passed New Hope. He always left the by-pass to the truckers and tourists. For J.P., the area around New Hope always seemed to turn back time to the 18th and 19th centuries. The Delaware River, having been freshly replenished by the melting snow and spring rains was flowing swiftly on its trip to the Atlantic Ocean.

He didn't know what he expected to gain from this trip to Kuhn's Apothecary in Doylestown, but he had to close the loop concerning the copy of the 21st Century Plan. The adventure may have started in Doylestown, Pennsylvania, but he was sure it would end in the James Boardroom. If he could obtain proof of who had made the copy it would certainly help the cause. Perhaps nothing would come of this trip, but he had to make sure there were no loose ends. He still couldn't answer the question of why someone used a copy machine in Doylestown. His own research of company personnel records had shown that no one at James or connected with James lived anywhere near Doylestown.

He glanced in the rearview mirror as he crossed the bridge. The black Lexus he had noticed on Interstate 78 and US 202 was nowhere in view. He decided that he was still a little paranoid after his adventure in Southeast Asia. The car probably hadn't been following him, it was just someone else driving south on 202 the most direct route from New York City to Bucks County.

Everyone at James knew that J.P. was making this trip, he had made a great deal of noise the previous Friday about going to Doylestown. And at the staff meeting earlier this morning, he again announced that he was making the trip. He had quickly looked at all of the faces around the table to see if there was a reaction to his announcement. Nothing.

He drove up the little hill after the bridge and proceeded across the railroad tracks and over the Delaware Canal. New Hope was relatively quiet.

In the summer this area would be filled with visitors riding the railroad cars of the New HopeIvyland steam engine or the barges up and down the canal. The antique stores would have their old furniture on the sidewalks hoping that tourists would want to decorate their home in 18th19th century decor.

He headed northwest out of New Hope and again found US 202 two miles out of town. Here the highway was only two lanes and was called Lower York Road. The twenty-mile drive from New Hope to Doylestown was a beautiful scenic highway especially in the late spring or early fall. It was a little early for the full spring effect, but after the severe winter it looked like spring was going to be early this year. Many of the trees were already almost fully leafed. The dogwood trees were already full of their pink and white blossoms. Forsythia bushes were blooming bright yellows.

Nestled in the matted forest floor around the pines and blue spruces were multicolored flowered fields of tulips and irises. The drive to Doylestown with its forests and 17th Century period farms was like experiencing a moving panoramic painting. The countryside was rolling hills of farm land and horse paddocks. Homes had fences of Delaware Valley stone. The homes were constructed of stone, making them warm in the winter and cool in the summer.

He glanced in the rearview mirror, still no black Lexus. He turned to the sights of the countryside. He thought of Mandi and how much she would enjoy walking the trails of the Delaware River Valley. He would suggest a weekend escape with her to Bucks County for a day.

He passed through Lahaska with its 18th Century peddler village and the Cock and Bull Bar. The afternoon sun beat down into the left side of the car as he continued west. At Buckingham he made a right turn to the northwest again for the final leg of his journey to Doylestown.

As he made the right hand turn he glanced over his right shoulder and saw a black Lexus again. It was about five car lengths behind him. He wondered whether it was the same car or a different one. If it was the same car, it had to be following him. The New Hope by^pass was at least fifteen minutes faster than his trip through New Hope. The driver would have had to wait for him outside of New Hope and fall in behind him again after he passed. It occurred to him that perhaps his trip would be more eventful than he had expected.

There were no other cars between them. The reflection of the sun on the car made it impossible to make out any unique features of the driver much less the license plate number.

J.P. remembered that there was a stop light at on the outskirts of Doylestown at the intersection of the highway and Swamp Road. His plan was to time his driving so that he reached the corner while the light was red. He hoped that would be able to see something of the driver or observe some identifying mark on the Lexus. He would then take the back road into town by turning onto Swamp Road. If the Lexus also turned it would be pretty obvious that the car was in fact following him.

Ten minutes later he saw the traffic light at the intersection. He saw the light was green and slowed. As he drew nearer to the corner the light turned to yellow and then red. He stopped. The Lexus had anticipated neither J.P.'s slowing nor the stoplight. The

Lexus slowed and then made a small mistake. The car stayed back a good distance from J.P.'s car at the light, probably afraid of being seen. The distance between the cars allowed J.P. to easily read the New York license plate on the other car's front bumper, ZYN 103.

The light turned green and since there were no cars coming from the other direction J.P. stepped hard on the gas and made a fast left turn onto Swamp Road. He looked back over his left shoulder and noticed that the Lexus was still at the light. The car remained at the light too long for his liking and now J.P. was sure that a decision was being made inside the car. As he watched the intersection in his rearview mirror, the car proceeded through the intersection slowly and continued on along US 202.

J.P. made a right turn on Cherry Lane. Cherry Lane was a narrow, straight and hilly road. After he made the turn he slowed and watched the mirror for any sign of the car. Nothing.

As he was watching for the Lexus in his rearview mirror, a tractor pulled out onto Cherry Lane from a driveway on the right. He stomped on the brake pedal stopping just short of the cart that the tractor was pulling. If he had been going any faster there would have been an accident.

He sat there for a moment trying to regain his composure before proceeding along the road. This time he kept his eyes on the road, only making quick glances to the mirror. There was no sign of the black Lexus.

He made right hand turn onto Pebble Hill Road and entered Doylestown from the south. He hadn't been to Doylestown in over eight years. When he last visited they were in the process of restoring most of the town to its 18 th and 19th Century architecture. The Bucks County Historical Society was leading an exciting rebirth of the town. A Penn Central train now carried passengers directly from Philadelphia to Doylestown. The tracks ended in Doylestown after a one-hour commute.

As he passed the central intersection of town, a black Lexus swung in behind him. New York license plate, ZYN 103. This time he could see that the sole occupant was male. He wore a hat pulled down low over his brow to obscure his face.

J.P. continued his drive through town. At the memorial to all veterans and the memorial to Vietnam veterans, he angled right onto East Court Street. The Bucks County courthouse building was on his left. Finally, at the corner of Pine and East Court he found Kuhn Apothecary Shop, his destination.

He parked his car on Pine Street around the corner from the Apothecary's entrance and watched the Lexus cruise past as it continued along East Court Street. J.P. tried in vain to see the face of the driver, but he turned away as he passed his line of sight. He walked to the entrance of the store.

There was two Doylestown Historical Society brass plates on the wall next to the entrance. One was about the Kuhn Apothecary Shop and the other about the Gothic architecture style of the building.

GOTHIC TOWN HOUSE

44 East Court Street is an example of a Gothic Revival town house. The Gothic Revival is based on the medieval Gothic, was an introduction to the Victorian era. One of the chief charms was that it gave architects a great deal of freedom in developing a floor plan to meet a variety of individual needs. Planned from the inside out, it could be added to in many directions: wings, bays, projections of any kind together by an all embracing verandah. Gothic Revival homes were born of an age seeking fashion and closer connection with European culture. Victorians claimed that Gothic was "organic" and based on the same principles as natural plant growth.

This town house has a curious facade, with windows and doors of different shape and size tied together by the symmetrical design of dormers and roof. Trending to early Victorian, the first floor shows Federal design elements in the doorway with fanlights and sidelights and arch. The second floor has Gothic features.

Doylestown Historical Society February 19, 1966

The second brass plaque was very simple.
KUHN APOTHECARY SHOP

The original Ralph S. Kuhn Apothecary Shop opened in August, 1964. The reproduction was opened on the 30th anniversary of the original Apothecary Shop.

Doylestown Historical Society August, 1994

The store's entrance was slightly below street level. On the door was painted "G. Kuhn, Pharm. D." From the outside J.P. could tell someone had taken great pains to make the store look like an authentic colonial apothecary. He recalled walking by the historic building years before. Then it was used as an office building with a large asphalt parking lot in back. He noticed that a beautiful garden had since replaced the parking lot.

He opened the door and entered. A little bell sounded. He looked up and saw the little brass bell hanging from a brass rod attached to the doorframe. The door had a brass rod that hit the bell when the door was opened and closed. It rang a second time as he closed the door.

The inside was a beautiful reproduction of a very old apothecary. The waiting room was beautifully decorated and furnished. There was even a large fireplace. The prescription area was adjacent to the waiting room. A lovely woman who looked to J.P. to be in her mid-thirties greeted him.

"Good morning, sir, may I be of any assistance?"

She was 5'9" and on the thin side. She had short blond hair that framed a face with a great deal of character. The cheekbones were high and rounded. They were not sharp like a model, just nicely rounded, her brown eyes were searching. She wore a pharmacist smock and over the left pocket was an embroidered name badge which read, G. Kuhn, Pharm. D.

"Are you the proprietor of this fine apothecary?" he asked.

"Yes, I am," she replied with a strong sense of pride and conviction. She paused and with a quizzical look said, "You're the Dr. Koenig from James Pharmaceutical. You called yesterday for instructions on how to find the store and wanted to know if G. Kuhn would be working today, aren't you? Well I'm G. Kuhn, Dr. Koenig. The G stands for Gloria not Grant as it did for my grandfather who owned the original apothecary. And yes, I am the person who wrote Dr. Bradsmith about the copy of the secret page and sent it back with the letter. Over there," Gloria pointed to her right, "is the copy machine."

He followed her finger and saw the coin operated copy machine in the corner. It was beautifully enclosed in an antique cabinet. A modern instrument in a 19th Century environment.

"You were expecting a man, weren't you?"

J.P. answered her question truthfully, "I don't know why, but I guess I did think G. Kuhn was a man. Sorry."

Gloria laughed, "Don't apologize, you should have seen the locals when they heard that Kuhn's granddaughter was going to rebuild the apothecary. First they doubted that I could rebuild it and second they questioned whether I would be successful here on East Court Street's Lawyers Row, but I fooled them. I succeeded in doing both. Now, what can I do for you Dr. Koenig?"

"Please call me, J.P. May I call you Gloria?" "Please."

"I really don't know whether you can help me or not but I am trying to determine who might have made the copies. I would like to show you some photographs to see if you could identify anyone. I know it's been a long time since Thanksgiving, but I'm trying to find out why Doylestown was picked to make a copy of a secret James strategic plan."

Gloria just looked at him. Her body language was telling him she was beginning to get upset.

He nodded his head and said, "Yes, Gloria you do deserve more of an explanation than I have given. Sorry again."

He gave her a brief explanation of the reason for the 21st Century Plan and the importance it would have in the wrong hands. Gloria's stance eased slightly and he knew then that she would help as much as she could. As they talked he had been watching pedestrians walking past the store. He had seen an Asian wearing a hat walk by twice. Both times he had looked very hard at the window like he was trying to see something or someone inside.

J.P. was now anxious to get to the point, obtain his information, and leave. He had been there too long and if the man outside was the driver from the Lexus he had to be on the alert for trouble. He also did not want to involve an innocent person, Gloria, in the problems of James Pharmaceutical Company.

"Gloria, I have a set of photographs of possible people who had access to the plan. There are not many, please see if you can recognize anyone." He handed her a booklet with pictures of Phillip's staff, one level of management below the staff, and the board. She slowly turned each page. He watched her eyes to see if she paused unusually long on any one person. She methodically turned each page and stayed with each person the same amount of time. She finished and closed the booklet.

"Sorry J.P., I don't know any of these people."

"Okay, thanks for looking. One more favor. Think back, can you remember anything strange about that day? Did anyone come in for a prescription and then stay to make a copy. The person who made the copy would have had to stay at the machine for fifteen minutes to make a complete copy."

Gloria thought for a minute. He could tell that she was trying very hard to remember that day four months before.

"Well, as usual, Thanksgiving was a slow day. I'm only open in the morning, just in case someone really needs me. I would hate to have someone sick on a holiday. That Thursday, hardly anyone came in and there were no strangers that I can recall." She thought for a moment longer.

She seemed to become excited about something. She continued, "I don't know if this means anything, but I remember Tommy Crenshaw standing at the copy machine. I told him to get away from the machine, thinking he was just playing, but he said he was making a copy and not playing. To prove he was not playing he opened his hand and showed me two rolls of nickels. Tommy is a good kid. He is always hanging around the store. He's twelve and says he wants to be a pharmacist. I didn't remember him before because I considered him part of the apothecary.

"Now," her face lit up with recognition, "I clearly remember that Thanksgiving morning. It was unusual for Tommy to be using the copy machine, especially for such a long time. Do you think this is significant?" She ended her story with expectation in her voice.

"Gloria, it is something. Maybe Tommy was helping someone. Do you have Tommy's address?"

"Yes, but he's probably in school." She looked at her watch. "School is almost over and I have a deal with Tommy. Sometimes I have emergency prescription deliveries. I can call Tommy at home and he will come over to make a delivery on his bicycle. We have a large number of older people that can not always get out. I like to deliver to those customers. If you like, I will call and ask Tommy to come

by."

"Please, Gloria, it would be a great help to us. Tell him to come in through the back door. I can't tell you why but I think someone has followed me here and I don't want them to see Tommy. You're okay because you weren't part of whatever happened that day."

Gloria made the phone call and in fifteen minutes J.P. met Tommy in the back room. He was a good-looking kid. Tall for his age though not basketball tall. He wore jeans and a sweatshirt with Penn State written across the front.

"You wanted to talk to me, Dr. Koenig?" His voice cracked a little as it varied from soprano to baritone.

"Yes Tommy, sorry to pull you away from your after school activities, but this is important to James Pharmaceutical Company. Do you know James?"

"Sure, Dr. Koenig, I think they're a great company. Dr. Kuhn thinks they're the best and she is the expert." The boy's admiration for Gloria came through loud and clear to J.P.

"Do you remember making a copy of a report on Dr. Kuhn's copy machine for someone last Thanksgiving?"

Tommy did not pause "Sure, I remember it real well. The money I got for making the copy helped me buy my brother a bicycle for Christmas. It was his first bike."

"Great. Think carefully, Tommy. Who was it that asked you to make the copy."

"I remember very clearly it was an old lady in a old gray Volkswagen bug. She asked me if I would make a copy of a report for her. If I made the copy she would give me 20 bucks. 20 bucks is good money for just making copies."

"It sure is." J.P. replied.

"She sat in her car while I made the copy. She gave me three rolls of nickels to make the copy. After I finished, I brought both the original and the copy back to her car. She gave me the money and drove off. She even let me keep the extra nickels." He paused shifting back and forth on each leg, waiting for J.P. to respond.

"Anything else, Tommy?" he asked.

"She had a German accent, Dr. Koenig, which is not very unusual around here. But hers was different.it was heavy like she had just come to America or spoke more German than English. She also seemed to forget things because she said most things twice. I think she was very old, at least 80, but she looked like she was in good shape. I have seen her around town but I don't know who she is or where she lives. I have seen her driving her bug around town and at the grocery store."

Gloria spoke up, "I think I know who Tommy is talking about. She comes in here every month to get her cardiac prescriptions refilled. I can't remember her name, but I can sure find out." Gloria went back behind the prescription counter. Tommy started to follow her. J.P. stopped him.

"Tommy I want you to remain out of sight of the front window." He asked, "Why, Dr. Koenig?"

"Sorry pal, I don't have a good reason. I don't think someone wants me to know who made the copy so they could be watching me and I don't want them to see you.

"Okay, I understand."

Gloria came back around the prescription counter very excited and with a printout of a prescription record. "I got it, J.P., Mrs. Georg Schmidt. Her address is 211 Stoner Park Road over by Tohickon Creek. Next to the Ralph Stover State Park. It is about thirty miles from here. It won't be hard to find Stover Park Road, but her house might be hard to find." Gloria went on explain that most of the homes had been built a long distance from the road in the woods. She said the mailboxes wouldn't help much either because they usually weren't placed near the house they serve or even near the road to the house.

She then said, "Mailboxes are placed more for convenience of the postal delivery service than the people owning the homes. Visitors are supposed to know the location of the home they are visiting." She paused and looked at him questionably. "Are you going over to her house?"

"No, I don't think so. Just knowing who it is and their address is good enough for me," he answered.

J.P. lied when he answered her question, but he didn't want to involve her or the boy in what he was doing. He could only hope that he hadn't already endangered them by being seen in the apothecary. It seemed like the stakes in this game were getting higher and people were getting hurt and dying. So far no innocent bystanders had been hurt and J.P. didn't want these two to be the first.

"I think I'll head back to the city. Both of you have given me a great deal of help. We are very grateful. Tommy, I know having cash seems to be most important to you today, but college will be more important to you in the future. I'll tell you what. When I get back to James I'll see to it that we establish a scholarship fund named for Kuhn Apothecary Shop. It will be $4,000 per year for a Doylestown High School student who wants to attend a Pharmacy School. We will let Dr. Kuhn run the fund as long as you are the first recipient."

He stopped and looked at Tommy, "That is, if you want to attend pharmacy school."

Both Gloria and Tommy started to speak at once. Gloria was first. "J.P., that is very generous of you and James. I feel flattered and with the cost of a Doctor of Pharmacy degree what it is today this will really help a deserving student. I feel like this is too much for what we have done to help you."

"It is not just for what you have done. It is for caring about James Pharmaceutical Company and for being very observant. Both of you have done more than you will probably know. The least we can do is to help you to help yourselves. I couldn't think of anything else that will give the apothecary favorable public relations in Doylestown and help Tommy and others to go to school.

"Someone else will call you later this week to set up the scholarship. I must go now. If anyone asks you what we talked about tell them the truth. Everything is okay, there is no need for either one of you to get involved in this any further. Thanks again and good luck." He left by the front door.

He purposely made his exit through the front door. The last thing he wanted was for the driver of the Lexus to come in looking for him and get Gloria and Tommy more involved. He walked around the building to where he had parked on Pine Street. The half-acre garden in the rear of the apothecary was showing signs of an early spring. The bulb plants were beginning to emerge. Azaleas had small buds and the dogwood trees were one-third full of pink flowers. Gloria had not only done an excellent job on the pharmacy, she had made the outside a living landscape painting for all to share.

J.P. looked around, but couldn't see the man wearing the hat or the Lexus. J.P. wondered if he should let the Lexus follow him to Mrs. Schmidt's house or just try to lose him on the way. He thought about saving his visit to the Schmidt house for another day, but decided that he had to follow through. He decided that he would try to lose his escort along the way.

J.P. sat in his car and looked at the map until he found Ralph Stover State Park. He started the car and pulled away from the curb. He drove out of town into the rich farmlands of Bucks County.

As he drove along he checked his mirror. Still no Lexus. He was puzzled. Where was he? He used his cellular phone and called Gloria. She said nothing unusual had happened since he had left. Just the regular customers.

"Are you sure you aren't seeing things, J.P.?" she added with a soft laughter. He thanked her again for her help and hung up.

The scenery was magnificent. Patches of woods on both sides separated by fertile farmlands. Farmers were in the fields on their tractors preparing the land for spring planting. Finally, the road he was driving on turned into Stover Park Road and the rural woods on either side of him changed to dense forest.

He slowed and pulled to the side of the narrow road. He got out of the car and looked back in the direction that he had just traveled. The road was straight with small rises and falls. No Lexus, no cars at all. He got back in and slowly drove toward the Ralph Stover State Park looking at each mailbox for either 211 or Schmidt. He made one pass driving east. When he got to the park entrance, he turned around and started back. About a half a mile from the park on the north side of the road was a black mailbox with numbers 211 and the name Schmidt stenciled in white. A large pine tree had hidden the mailbox from J.P.'s view when he went by the first time. There was a driveway on the other side of the tree. He pulled into the dirt drive and looked down its length. He couldn't see the end of the drive.

Heavy trees lined the drive. The drive had two ruts that ran close together. Narrow enough to fit a Volkswagen bug but not the best driving conditions for his rented car. He decided to go ahead and drive along the rough driveway. He was banged around by the ruts and holes and hoped that at the end of the drive there would be a turnaround. It also occurred to him that it could be a trap.

The road seemed to become narrower and then suddenly it opened up into a clearing and before him was a beautiful, fairly new single story Tudor home with a circular drive. In front of the door was a gray Volkswagen beetle in beautiful condition. The sun bounced off its windshield and shining body finish.

He pulled counter-clockwise into the circular drive and parked on the left side of the bug. As he rounded the drive he could see that the house overlooked a canyon. As he started to get out of the car he heard barking and two large German Shepherds came running from behind the house. He stayed inside the car and closed the door.

The two dogs sat down close by the driver's door of the car. Their tongues hanging from their mouth from running. Their eyes were alert, but they looked calm. They weren't snarling just panting. They were on watch.

J.P. made a move to open the door and the tongues went quickly back into the mouth, eyes shifted to the occupant of the car, and their calm was replaced by a snarl. Not a good move, he decided.

He was about to blow the horn when the front door opened and a tall, dignified, elderly woman stood in the opening. The sun was directly in her eyes. She shielded her eyes from the sun with her right hand. She called out in German, "Rachel, Albert, *kommen sie hier.*" The two dogs obediently ran to her side and sat. She again called out, but this time to J.P., "You can come up to the door now." Her voice was strong and it was definitely a heavy German accent.

He slowly got out of the car while watching the dogs. He took the keys and left the driver side door unlocked and open just in case he had to make a quick return to the car.

"Good Day Mr.?"

"Dr. J.P. Koenig. I assume that you are Mrs. Schmidt? You can call me J.P."

"I will call you Dr. Koenig," she replied and turned to reenter the house.

"Please come in Dr. Koenig, the dogs will not bother you anymore. Sorry for the greeting, but we are isolated and I feel better with them on guard. What brings you into the forest to visit an old woman?"

She did not wait for him to answer her question. She turned and walked into the living room. She was about 5"10" thin and carried herself like an aristocrat. Her hair was silver and well kept.

The house was designed like a Bavarian Chateau. Everything was wood. The furniture was heavily padded leather and lacked color. Mrs. Schmidt showed him into the living room. On the far side was a large fireplace with a roaring fire. The ceiling went up two stories. On the walls were dark oil paintings. Two of the paintings were Prussian military officers. The others were scenes of Bavaria. That probably explained her aristocratic presence. She was of Bavarian aristocracy or at least she was putting on a good act. She looked to be in her eighties, but she seemed very healthy. Her silver hair was of medium length almost touching her shoulders. She had on a heavy brown sweater and pants.

She sat down in a leather chair and gestured to J.P. to sit opposite her on the leather couch. Two beautiful piercing pale blue eyes looked at him in a questioning manner.

They sat looking at each other. She picked up what looked like a sweater and started to knit. Her attention was completely directed to her knitting as though J.P. weren't in the room.

He cleared his throat, "Ah, em. Frau Schmidt."

"Ja? Hello. Mr.... ? What was your name?" she asked putting down her knitting.

"Dr. Koenig, Mrs. Schmidt. You just met me a few minutes ago. Are you okay?" he asked.

"Ja, Why do you ask?" "You forgot I was here."

"I'm very sorry Professor Koenig. Can I call you Professor Koenig?" "Ja, *bitte.*" he replied in German.

"Would you like some tea Professor Koenig?"

"Ja, vielen dank, Frau Schmidt. Mit creme, bitte."

"Ah, sprechen sie Deutshe? Das ist gut. Han!" she spoke to an unseen Han, "Zwei tees mit creme und brot, bitte."

"Jawohl, Frau Schmidt," Han answered from the direction of what J.P. knew must be the kitchen.

She looked at J.P. again not seeming to recognize him. He thought that they might have to go through introductions again, but she continued in German. He thought that if they continued to speak German that she would be able to better remain in a conversation.

In German she asked him, "What do you want Professor Koenig? I am sure this is not a social visit. I don't know you and I can not imagine how you know me." She was becoming very formal. Their conversation continued in German.

"I'll not go through a long explanation, Frau Schmidt, but you could be of great assistance to myself and to James Pharmaceutical Company my employer. I would like to ask you a few questions?"

"I do not know of any such company as James Pharmaceutical Company."

Her rapid reply was too fast. J.P. was sure that she had lied and had, in fact, heard of James. He settled back into the couch seat as Han, a tall blonde man in a suit, carried in a tray with a china teapot, two cups, and a plate with bite-size pieces of dark German bread. He set the tray down on a table between the two of them. The woman poured two cups of tea. She poured a small amount of cream into the tea. The cream was so heavy it sank to the bottom with out spreading on the surface. She slowly stirred the tea and cream. "Do you want any sugar?"

"Yes, two please."

She dropped two lumps into each cup and slowly stirred each cup again. She handed him one of the cups. J.P. reached forward and took the tea. He also took a couple of pieces of bread and settled back again. Frau Schmidt sat very rigid in her chair. She looked over at Han and with a silent signal from her, he left the room.

J.P. took his first sip of tea, while she watched his reaction. It was very strong German tea. Even though he did not enjoy strong tea, he forced himself to register pleasure. "This is very good. Thank you."

He continued by getting right to the subject. "I'm not surprised that you don't know of James Pharmaceutical Company. We aren't very large or well known, but we do manufacture the medicine that your cardiologist, Dr. Mueller prescribes for you." He had seen the prescription file that Gloria had printed out on Mrs. Schmidt. He saw Dr. Mueller's name alongside every prescription number and that he had prescribed Lifeal. He took a chance with a bluff.

"I realize that this information is confidential, but Dr. Mueller seemed to think it would be all right if I ask you if there had been any side effects from your medicine."

"No," she answered relaxing a little "No, I feel fine. No problem." All the time they had been talking, J.P. had been examining the room. Each table had photographs of what looked to be family.

He sipped the tea. He was actually grateful for the strong brew. He had a long drive back to New York City that evening. He saw a set of graduation photographs on the far side of the room below the picture window that looked out over the canyon and the creek running through it.

There were pictures of a man in a lab coat surrounded by beakers and other laboratory equipment. He decided that he had to get a closer look at these photographs. "Frau Schmidt that makes me very happy."

The look on her face became very concerned. "Should I not be feeling good? What is wrong with the product?"

"Nothing is wrong with the product." He then faked a surprise. "Oh, I am sorry I did not mean to frighten you. Nothing is wrong, we just do spot checks to ensure the patients taking our products don't experience unexpected side effects. Everyone I have visited has reported excellent results. No, don't worry." He got up from his seat. "You have such a wonderful view from the back of your house. May I look at your view and then I must leave."

"Yes, of course, *herr Doktor*," she replied with pride and pleasure in her voice. She placed her cup on the tray. She again picked up her knitting and seemed to J.P. to mentally check out.

J.P. walked alone to the large picture window that looked out over the backyard and canyon. It was just as well that she didn't follow him, he wanted to see who was in the photographs sitting on the table without her noting that his eyes were on the photos and not out the window.

He wasn't sure whether he was or wasn't surprised at what he saw in the photographs. If he really thought back over his activities of the last few months and the characters in the play that he was living, he would have come to the staff member whose photo he was looking at now. Whatever his emotions, he was now certain as to who made the copy of the 21st Century Plan and he had already begun to realize why.

He was looking at a photograph of Mrs. Schmidt and Helmut Walhters.

J.P. didn't know what the relationship was between Frau Schmidt and Helmut, but it was definitely Helmut in the photographs.

"The view is magnificent," he commented out loud, not knowing if anyone was listening. "I imagine in the spring and fall the view is a living painting."

"Yes, it is very beautiful. It is not Bavaria, but it is the best, next to Bavaria." he turned and saw that she had left her knitting and moved to his side. "Now you must go Professor Koenig, I have guests for dinner and I must help Han prepare the meal." She started walking to the front door and he followed. He decided to try a shock question and note her response.

"Frau Schmidt, last Thanksgiving you asked a young man to make a copy of a report. Could you tell me who asked you to make the copy?"

She paled and her straight stature slumped slightly. Her voice shook a trifle as she replied. "I don't know what you are talking about Professor Koenig."

In a few moments, she recovered her composure. "And I don't know what that question has to do with your visit. Now please leave my home. Don't worry about the dogs. Han has them tethered in the back. Good day to you, sir."

"Goodbye, Mrs. Schmidt," he said as he stepped outside. The sun was setting and it would be dark soon.

While J.P. had been inside talking to Mrs. Schmidt, the Asian had been working on J.P.'s car. He had parked his car down and off Stover Park Road so he could pull out and pursue J.P. when he left the house. He had walked up the long driveway to the house and checked in with Han and then went back to J.P.'s car.

While J.P. was in the house the Asian had slipped into the front seat of J.P.'s rental car through the open driver's side door. He crawled under the steering wheel and removed the gas pedal. He then had taken a pliable plastic material from his pocket and placed it around the gas pedal stem ^between the stem and the floorboard. The friction of the stem moving up and down against the floorboard would melt the outer layer of the pliable plastic. This would expose the next level of material that, with continued fiction and heat, would create a bonding agent. The end result would be to bond the gas pedal to the floorboard after about five minutes of normal driving. The purpose of the two-layer bonding agent was to allow the driver freedom of speed adjustment for a short period of time and then freeze the pedal at a significantly high speed resulting in a fatal crash and fire. The heat from the fire would melt the material and there would be no trace of tampering.

The Asian had finished his job and walked back down the driveway to his car on Stover Park Road to wait for J.P.'s car to appear.

J.P. left the house and walked to his rental car. The door was still open. He had the information he came to find. He knew the reason for making the copy of the 21st Century Plan was likely connected with the NPC activities and the James board.

He got back into his rental car and began his trip back to New York City hoping he had lost his tail but realize that the Lexis was part of the story. He would drive through Stover Park.

STOVER PARK OUTSIDE DOYLESTOWN, PENNSYLVANIA

Where was he and how did he get to where he was? All J.P. really knew was that his head hurt and he was beside a rock.

Slowly his brain began to put the pieces together. He had been to Helmut's home outside Doylestown and returning to New York City. Another piece of the picture slipped into place.

A car had followed him and forced him off the road and his brakes had failed. The picture was complete. He was in danger.

STOVER PARK, PENNSYLVANIA

After seeing the car go off the road and probably over the edge of the canyon the Asian stood at the wire mesh fence looking down at the explosion. He had examined the area. After a couple of visual sweeps of the general area where the car had made a trail through the forest and brush, he seemed satisfied that Koenig was in the burning car and assumed that he had burned to death. The Asian walked back to his car and returned to Frau Schmidt's house.

Back at the house he picked up the phone, and dialed an unlisted number in Osaka.

"Yes?"

"Hai, it is done. Koenig will no longer interfere with our project." "You are certain?"

"I took care of him myself. I used Plastoseal on his gas pedal and he went off a cliff and the car exploded in a river bed."

"It wasn't possible to find the body and ensure that he was dead." "What?"

"He could not have survived the crash."

"You will return to the scene. Do not call me again, until you are absolutely certain that this man is dead."

"*Hai,* Tanaguchisan, I will return to ensure he is dead and call you again."

The Asian hung up the phone and swore to himself in Japanese. Without another word he left the house and drove back to the place were J.P.'s car had gone over the cliff.

STOVER PARK, PENNSYLVANIA

J.P. began to slowly come out of his unconscious state and the flashback dream of how he had arrived wedged against the rock in Stover Park.

He looked around at his surroundings. He was on the downward slope of the cliff over the creek. It was a ledge just before the canyon dropped off straight to the bottom 100 feet below. There was a path along the fence to his right. To his left were the cliffs.

He could still hear was the noise of car burning in the creek bed, which told him that he had been out for tens of minutes instead of tens of hours. Except for the crackling of the fire, there was silence. It was now, almost totally dark except for a set of car headlights shining over his head out into the ravine. He looked at his watch, it had stopped at 6:15.

He quickly determined that the rock that he was wedged against had kept him from falling off the cliff. He checked his body. His head, shoulder, and ribs hurt, but the pain was tolerable. His knee on the other hand was badly hurt. He couldn't move his left leg without excruciating pain up and down his left side.

He didn't know exactly how long he had been wedged against the rock. He only knew that he had to get himself up to the road. Surely someone had seen the ball of fire. Then he remembered that he was surrounded by a county park, it was March, and a weekday. He doubted if anyone was around tonight. He strained to hear distant sirens. There were none.

When the Asian arrived back at the scene he was surprised to find that there were no other cars. He had hoped to find the police at the scene and then just wait around as an observer until the police found Koenig's body. Now, he wondered whether he should report the accident to the police by dialing 911.

He reconsidered, thinking that there might be an easy route to the riverbed. He could find Koenig's body and then get out of the area before becoming involved. If he was found with the body he could say he was trying to help the injured driver. No one would know the difference. He pulled the Lexus into the woods using the trail that Koenig's car had cut. He went to the edge of the canyon leaving his headlights shining over the cliff into the space above the ravine. He got out of the Lexus.

J.P. looked up at the headlights. His first thought was that it was about time someone showed up. He was getting cold and realized that shock was probably setting in. He looked up again to the car. The nose of the car was sticking out over the edge. The driver of this car was providing light. J.P. was about fifteen feet from the car. He was about to shout for help when he again looked up at the car. He could just make out the license plate, ZYN 103

J.P. hopes sank as he realized it was the driver of the Lexus, probably come to make certain that he was dead. It occurred to J.P. that the driver had probably had something to do with the gas pedal malfunction and if that was the case, then there was also probably a link to Helmut.

He went through his alternatives. One, sit there and remain undetected until he goes away. Two, make himself known to him and see if he could capture him and obtain some information. Or, three, kill him as quickly as possible and steal his car. There are probably other alternatives but he felt that he didn't have time to think them through.

J.P. watched as the Asian stepped to the edge of the cliff and looked down at the burning car. The Asian walked to the right. He was looking for a way down. He moved onto the path and out of the illumination of his headlights.

J.P. made up his mind. He figured the driver must think that he is dead or, at least, at the bottom of the ravine. He would not expect someone to steal his car. J.P. felt the pain in his back. Starting the car could be a problem. If he couldn't hot-wire the car he would release the brakes and send it to the bottom of the ravine. Two cars in independent crashes would confuse everyone.

J.P. crawled away from the rock. A few small stones tumbled over the edge. He froze. The stones made their bumpy ride down the cliff. Everything was quiet except that he could still hear the driver breaking twigs as he made his way down the cliff. Every once in a while he would swear in Japanese.

J.P. had an audible identification.

He crawled a little further up and out of his hiding place. He decided to try his leg. He pushed myself up using his right leg and arms. Because of the pitch of the slope, he could not get all the way to a vertical position. He pressed down on his left leg and a sharp pain shot up his entire body. He figured that his knee might be fractured. He carefully tore the sleeve off his suit coat and wrapped it tightly around his left knee. He decided he would drag himself up the slope, hoping that his adversary was far enough away that he wouldn't be able to hear.

J.P. dragged himself the fifteen feet to the car. He grabbed the left bumper and pulled himself up to stand on his right leg. He listened. It was almost totally quiet. The driver's door was slightly ajar. J.P. realized if the driver was on his way back after giving up his trip to the bottom of the ravine the inside car light would silhouette him if he opened the door. He bent down so that he wouldn't make a large target and opened the car door.

The door window above his head shattered and then J.P. heard another muffled report of a weapon with a silencer attached. The Japanese man had come back and had spotted him.

J.P. opened the door and quickly moved into the car. He shut the door and the inside light went off. He lay down on the seat and reached for the ignition and to his surprise and good luck, the key was in the ignition. The engine turned over with a laboring sound. The battery was not fully charged. The lights had drained the battery slightly. Another silenced shot and the left headlight went out with a small explosion. J.P. shut off the headlights. Another shot and the windshield cracked. Finally the engine caught. He put the car in reverse. The front wheels spun with the sudden acceleration and the car began its trip back up to the road. He managed to hit a few small trees but none seriously enough to stop the movement of the car. When he reached the road he turned the car around, shifted into drive, and sped south on Cafferty Road. He turned on the one remaining headlight.

He had made his escape. His leg or knee was injured and who knows what else was wrong internally, but he was alive and on his way back to New York City.

He looked at the clock on the Lexus' dash, 9:00 p.m. He figured he would be in New York City by midnight. This time he crossed the Delaware River using the new 202 bridge. He began to think through the story he would have to tell the rental agency about how he came to lose their car. Whoever owned the car he was currently driving would not report it stolen so he knew he was safe with this car. It came to him that he would report the car as stolen and let them take it from there.

He dropped the rental off in the New York City Port Authority parking lot. He spent the next fifteen minutes wiping fingerprints off the car. His leg was killing him and he could both feel and see the swelling under the leg of his pants. He berated himself for not stopping along the way to purchase ice for the swelling.

He called Roberto to drive him to the apartment. After Roberto saw J.P.'s condition, he called a physician friend who told Roberto that he would meet them at J.P.'s apartment.

The taxi pulled up the apartment door and doorman took a step back after seeing the way J.P. looked. "You look terrible Dr. Koenig."

"Really?" he stated with confidence and strutted into the lobby with his one good leg. His arm was draped over Roberto's shoulder and he was dragging his left leg.

When the elevator door opened, Mandi was standing in the elevator. The doorman had alerted her and she had evidently jumped into the waiting elevator and rode it down.

"J.P., what the hell has happened? You look like you have been in an accident or a fight or both."

He forced a smile and said, "Please Mandi don't say you were worried to death. In fact don't say anything. Your just being here is great. I will explain, but now I am in a great deal of pain."

Mandi and Roberto helped him into the apartment. As he passed the hall mirror he looked at his reflection. His suit was practically in shreds.

After reaching the apartment and finishing a painful effort of easing into a chair, the doorbell rang. Roberto open the door for his friend Dr. Rosinni. Roberto gave him the rundown on the events that J.P. had given him in the taxi and then left. Thirty minutes later Dr. Rosinni also left the apartment.

J.P. took inventory of himself. A large bump on the back of his head; one cracked rib, now bandaged; a bruised shoulder; and a strained left knee ligament, now also bandaged. Overall status, lucky. Dr. Rosinni had left him prescription a nonnarcotic pain killer, muscle relaxants, and sleeping pills.

Mandi helped him to bed and kissed his forehead. The next thing J.P. knew it was morning.

THE JAMES' FARM, GREYSTONE HALL
SEAFORD, NY

"Did you see the Wall Street Journal today, Helmut?"

She had turned onto her side to face her overweight lover. Just moments ago, he had satisfied himself and promptly fallen asleep. She shook him awake with her left hand and asked the question again.

"No," he grumpily answered after being suddenly awakened.

"You are worthless, Helmut. It is the most important time of our lives and you fuck and sleep and do not read the Wall Street Journal to see how rich we are going to be when we sell James." Her remarks were spoken for conversation only. She did not care about Helmut anymore and couldn't wait until the sale had been made and she could get rid of this wart that grew out of her body once a week.

Even though Thursday was their usual day at the cottage, she had suggested they meet again even though he hadn't heard from the NPC, for a couple of reasons. First, she needed sex and second because of the interest the financial analysts were suddenly giving James these days, interest that was causing the stock to start to climb.

She was attending many meetings explaining the recent success of the James stock including a meeting tomorrow with Bill Husted. She had no inkling of why the stock was going up, but she was a polished, optimistic spinner when required.

Thursday she had a meeting with investment bankers so she had commanded Helmut to spend Wednesday evening with her. He had jumped at her suggestion.

She had to get rid of him early. She wanted to be fresh for her meeting with Husted.

Husted, she thought. The meddling Wall Street Journal analyst was finally was going to be of assistance to her and her objectives. When the stock hit $125 earlier that day for the highest price in ten years, everyone was sure that James was on the rebound. The long lost hope had finally been realized. She had calculated her wealth after the proposed sale of her stock to NPC. It was the $125 times the 20% NPC bonus, which equaled $150 per share equaling $10,000,000. Not bad for a few years of work and too many nights with a fat slob.

Helmut had fallen back to sleep. He was not interested in the wealth they were earning on their James stock. There was no concrete reason for the growth of the share price. The rumor about the anti-arrhythmia use for Lifeal and the agreement with Clintec had leaked out to the marketplace and had some effect, but FDA approval of the prophylactic indications for Lifeal was at least five years away. It seems, some of the physicians had caught on to the prophylactic use and the Lifeal prescription rate had increased slightly, but nothing else had happened to warrant the increase from the $35 low after Phillip had been shot to that day's high.

Evelyn had been shocked when the market had reacted so negatively to the shooting of Phillip. She remembered thinking at the time that she had underestimated his importance to the company. He must be worth a lot more than she had given him credit. It was then that she decided that in order for her to succeed with her plan, she had to discredit him. She started her program in March and it was now, she concluded, beginning to pay off. The analysts were not crediting the growth of James stock to Phillip, but to Mrs. Evelyn PrestonJames. The credit for having good management sense was being credited to her because of her March board meeting decision to cut costs.

Even though Phillip had implemented the cost cutting program she made sure everyone in the investment community knew that she was responsible for the move and not Phillip. She was going to make sure Phillip wasn't as important as she and that Phillip was, in fact, dispensable. The proof was the fact that the media was now calling her for interviews and not Phillip.

She stretched, easily waking Helmut again. He had fallen into a lighter sleep since he had been awakened earlier.

"Yes, what is it?" he asked.

"Just me you old fool," she replied. She decided not to be as hard on him as usual because she was in such a good mood and didn't want to get herself worked up by yelling at him. She also knew that she had to get him out of her bed and out of the house as soon as possible. She wanted to be alone.

"I let you back into my bed and you haven't answered the twenty dollar question."

"What question?" he asked sleepily.

"Don't be coy with me. You know perfectly well what the question is.

Have you talked to the NPC lately?"

"No, but they said they would get back to me if there were any changes. As you well know, I have called them many times and they have chosen not to answer. As of this minute, they have not gotten back to me, so I guess there are no problems," he replied in a stronger than usual voice.

She noticed the irritation in his voice and let it go. "What was all the fuss about at your mother's place in Pennsylvania last Monday?"

She never ceased to amaze him. She seemed to know nothing and yet knew everything. "How did you know about that?" he asked with wonder in his voice and turning now on his side so that they were facing each other.

She looked him straight into his eyes and said, "None of your damn business. I have my ways and I will keep them my ways."

Her information came from an anonymous phone call she received last Monday. A man had given her the information. She had been so happy about the way things were going that the commotion at his mother's house had slipped her mind until a few moments ago.

"What about it?" she asked again and this time she let a little anger enter the tone of her voice.

Helmut knew Evelyn was going to go off the handle again and he just didn't feel like going through the degradation he felt from her cutting voice. He had about enough of her anyway. All the work he had done on her behalf and never a thank you. She was a good lay and would eventually be his ticket out of James, but to continue to take the verbal abuse when the James stock was souring, was more than he could take.

"Look, I have had about enough of your smart ass talk. Nothing of any importance took place at my mother's house. Someone tried to break in and that was it." But, that was not "it" he thought. That meddling J.P. had been snooping around and Helmut did not know why. The fact was, Koenig had been at his mother's house and the NPC people had seen him. There had been a chase and an accident.

In the first place he didn't like the fact the Japanese had set up headquarters in his mother's home. Why couldn't they have found someplace on their own? It also linked him with the NPC. He had not told Evelyn about NPC being in his mother's home nor the incident involving J.P. Neither had importance. The NPC representatives at the house refused to talk to him about the deal and the disturbance. As far as he was concerned, it did not have any importance and besides the stock was spiraling upward.

He now decided to tell her the whole story, just to piss her off and to show he was in control.

"Evelyn, I did not tell you because I did not want to bother you with details of implementing our plan. First, there is a little more to this incident than you already know."

"What?" she asked incredulously.

"Well, about a week after I had the meeting with Mr. Smith, my mother had a visit from some Japanese businessmen who showed her identification from the Nippon Pharmaceutical Council and said they were working with me. Before you ask, how they knew who I was and where my mother lived. It is beyond me."

Evelyn was slowly becoming furious and said to herself, and what isn't beyond you, you ignoramus. She continued showing him a weak smile so she could get him to tell the whole story.

He continued, "Mother called me at the office and I told her to ask them to come back that evening. After work, I drove out to her house. It had been about seven hours since her telephone call. I don't know if she told them to wait or what she actually said to them after she talked to me on the phone. All I know is what I saw when I arrived at about 7:00 that evening."

"What did you see?" she said pleasantly, but to herself she added, you idiot.

"Well," he said with a joyful tone. Feeling that he had her full attention and gaining some sense of respect, he continued in a laughing voice, "Can you believe the bastards had set up shop in the basement of my mother's house. They had a satellite communications station installed, extra telephones, and computers. They had a staff of five people. I asked my mother what had happened and where was Han." As a side remark he added, "You know I have Han there to take care of mother. Mentally, she isn't all there."

And you aren't all there either, Helmut, she thought, but said courteously, "Yes, I know. Please go on, what did mother say?" she added with a slight irritation she tried hard to keep out of her voice, but failed.

He paused and looked at her. His eyes questioning her last remark. Was she pulling his leg? No, he decided and went on. "Mother said indignantly that I had told her to tell these Asians to stay. Then she went on to berate me for allowing strangers in her house. I got her to calm down and again asked the whereabouts of Han. She answered that he disappeared just after they started to move in. I searched for Han and found him in his room bound and gagged. After my painful experience with Mr. Smith, I knew that these guys didn't negotiate their desires. Since mother had given them permission, a German valet wouldn't stand in their way. Han was bruised physically and emotionally, but not very badly. I heard his story, but told him not to interfere and just make sure mother is safe. He has done what he has been told." He paused waiting for her recognition of a job well done on a very touchy matter that could have blown the whole deal.

Evelyn continued her artificial smile, "Well, Helmut, that was some story you haven't felt necessary in telling me. Do you have any other gems you haven't told me about? Like, why you have been telling me you haven't had contact with the NPC when they have been living in your mother's home." She was trying hard to continue smiling and to remain calm, but her voice showed that she thought his actions were incredulous.

Helmut lay still. His mind was racing. He had hoped for congratulations, but she sounded like she was patronizing him and his efforts to help with the situation. He didn't know what to say. So he said nothing causing a long silence.

Evelyn broke the silence by calmly asking, "Well, why didn't the NPC tell you anything?"

"Oh," he was startled, "sorry, the Japanese guys refused to talk to me about the project. That is what they call us, the James Project. They were sorry there was a misunderstanding about moving into the house, but they were there and would stay out of my mother's way. They said I must continue to work with Tanaguchi and they were under his orders to just remain silent.

They were sure I understood the situation. Of course I didn't understand, but what was I to do? They wouldn't talk to me and Tanaguchi wouldn't answer my telephone calls. Would you have done any differently?" Irritation crept into his voice.

No, she said to herself, but she wasn't going to let this baboon know that she would probably have done the same to protect the James Project. In the end, what the hell is the difference, she would be rich. The ends do justify the means. Out loud to Helmut she answered his question now dropping the smile and raising her voice. "Dr. Wahlters, am I not the Chairperson of James Pharmaceutical Company?"

He didn't answer. He was staring again. She demanded, "Answer me, damn you!

"Yes," he said.

"Dr. Wahlters, am I not the creator and leader of what your new Japanese friends call the James Project?"

"Yes."

"So what in the hell were you thinking when you withheld this information from me?"

"I thought it wasn't important," he answered with conviction. "I don't pay you to think, Helmut."

Yes, that's right, he thought. You pay me for sex and to be a lap dog. Well, this has got to stop. He started to get angry instead of assuming his usual complacency. Before he could respond Evelyn verbally lashed out at him again.

"So, now smart scientist, please tell me about nosey Koenig?" she bitterly demanded.

Helmut had started to stare again and didn't respond.

"Hello, Helmut. Is there anyone in there?" she struck him on the forehead with the palm of her hand.

His response was swift and startled her. He grabbed her hand and gave it a slight twist. Not enough to do permanent damage, but Evelyn definitely felt pain.

"Ow! Damn you, that hurt!" She wrenched her arm away. "What in the hell has gotten into you?" Before giving him a chance to answer and trying to again gain control of the situation she repeated her question. As she spoke she moved ever so slightly backward to the edge of her side of the bed. Her voice was calm and contained a small amount of seductively. She didn't exactly know what to expect anymore, but she had to know everything that was going on with the NPC. "Helmut, why was Koenig at your mother's house?"

As if nothing had happened, Helmut replied, "J.P. was snooping around Doylestown and the NPC guys got nervous. Before you ask, I do not know why he was snooping around. There is nothing to find in Doylestown and nothing happened when he visited my mother's home. I hear through the corporate rumor mill, that he had an accident after he left the house, but, as far as I know, the NPC guys didn't have anything to do with the accident. I guess that he did have some kind of accident. He is walking around favoring his left leg."

What would J.P. be doing in Doylestown, she asked herself. J.P. was becoming a pain in the ass, but he was also very intelligent. She never really understood why Phillip had asked Koenig to consult at James, especially during this period of time. She had believed

Bradsmith when he said Koenig was at James to help with Lifeal. Lifeal was doing better, so she assumed that he was doing the job that he had been hired to do. But, then again, he kept turning up in odd places. She had learned that he was at the plantation with the woman from marketing and there was an unconfirmed rumor that there had been trouble. He had been in Doylestown and there was an unconfirmed rumor that there had been trouble. He had filled in for Bradsmith after Bradsmith had been shot. She sat up straight in the bed surprising Helmut with her sudden movement. Since she was almost on the edge of the bed, she almost fell off the bed.

She caught her balance, "Helmut, I believe there is more to this Koenig issue than we are giving credence. What do you know about him?" she asked with real interest in her voice. Her sudden change of tone to one of understanding and peer relationship threw Helmut another curve.

Helmut jumped to answer before she got upset again. "Look there is no need for concern. He is just an old friend of Bradsmith's and the company. He worked at James a long time ago and Phillip is just using him for special projects and for Lifeal."

"If he is just working on Lifeal marketing, he seems to be in a lot of convenient places that are more James oriented than just Lifeal."

"Only by coincidence, Evelyn. I tell you, there is nothing to be concerned about. He is a rich marketing guy with very little brains. He is not a problem and he is rumored to almost be done with his project."

"I don't care about your personal assessment. I think Koenig is a potential problem. I want you to keep your eyes and ears open to all of his activities. Everything is going beautifully with our plan and I do not want any outsider messing it up.

"I will, but in my opinion I don't think he will be a problem. We only have eight more weeks to go and then it will be over. What can he do in eight weeks to hurt us?"

"Yes, what can he do to hurt us?" she said pensively. She ran the thought through her mind. He can't do too much damage unless he started his meddling weeks or months ago. She turned from her sitting position and looked down at Helmut who was still lying prone on the other side of the bed. All of a sudden, fury engulfed her. The same fury that she felt all the previous nights after she tired of both his physical and mental capabilities. "Look, Helmut, I told you to keep an eye on him. I don't give a flying fuck about your opinion. When it comes to politics, intuition, and the implementation of this plan, I do not pay you to think. Now get out of my bed and out of my house." Her voice had continued to rise until she was screaming again.

He had had enough. He thought that he ought to respond to her threats, but he knew that arguing with her was not the answer. He was a realist. It was her bed and her house. Instead of protesting, he reached down and pinched the fat part of her right thigh. He pinched very hard and before releasing, twisted the skin. A deep blue bruise began to form almost immediately. Tomorrow morning she would have a very large and ugly bruise.

He rolled out of bed while she screamed from the pain of the pinch. "You arrogant bastard! How dare you play with me. You know I despise pain and people that inflict pain." She was screaming louder than he had ever head her scream.

He quickly dressed and walked out the door as she continued to scream obscenities. For the first time he got the feeling that she might be a little crazy. He would have to be more careful. Perhaps he should skip these Thursday nights or Wednesday nights as he reminded himself of the change of plans for that evening's rendezvous. The plan was working and when it was over he would find himself a real woman. He did not need Mrs. James.

He physically stopped in his tracks and for the first time realized that she didn't need him now and probably had never needed him. She had used him. Even after nights of making love he couldn't even think of her as anything except, Mrs. James. Once, months ago, he had the delusion that she loved him and would marry him.

"Bull shit," he said out loud as he walked out into the chilly night air. In the weeks ahead, he would have to be more careful with Mrs. James.

SPECTRUM OF MEDICINE BUILDING
NEW YORK CITY

"Well, Mrs. James, you must be very pleased with the performance of James stock," observed Bill Husted. He had taken a seat across the desk from Mrs. James. She was a very attractive mature woman he thought. Old Doc James had done all right for himself.

The interview between Mrs. James and Husted had just begun.

"Yes, we are very happy about the stock, but most of all we are happy about what the future holds for this company," she replied in a very pleasant business-like tone. She had dressed in a conservative dark business skirt and coat. She had chosen the suit to portray power but not hide the female attractiveness she knew she had. She wanted to keep Husted off balance.

"Do you attribute the share price growth to the management talents of Dr. Bradsmith?" he asked. He sat casually in his chair taking notes on a pad of paper lying on his lap. In the past he had tried small computers, but he had found there were three good reasons that computers did not work during the interviewing process. First, the noise of his typing on the keys threw off the person he was interviewing. Second, he could not use his own personal shorthand and third he could not watch the facial expressions of the person he was interviewing. He knew that some of the new handheld computers solved some of his problems, but he preferred his old tried and true method, a narrow reporter's pad.

He watched her reaction to his questions. He had learned he could find out more about how people really felt when he watched their facial and body reactions to his questions. Most interviewers looked at the questions written on a piece of paper, not daring to look the person in the eye when they were asking the question. His style was to memorize the major questions he wanted to ask and then adjust followup questions as the situation warranted.

To the question about Phillip, he saw Mrs. James bristle. It was just a slight movement of her lips and eyes. He had hit a sore spot, but of course he had known there was no love between the two of them. She did not blow up like she had done at the board meeting luncheon he had attended back in January.

Boy, you are cool, he thought. She did not know much about pharmaceuticals, but she seemed to be very knowledgeable about the politics of Wall Street. He had not thought of interviewing her, but recently it seemed that her name was being connected with the activities and new successes of James.

"Dr. Bradsmith is responsible for the day to day activities at James, but as you can see by the fact that I have an office here at the Spectrum of Medicine, I have begun to, how should I put it, participate." She smiled. Her smile was a very knowing sly smile that was not lost on Husted.

He wondered what Phillip would think about her answer. He decided to pursue this line of questioning to see how far he could go before she either shut him off or blew up.

"Why do you feel that you have to play a more active role in the running of James?" he asked. This time there was no change in her expression. She seemed to have adjusted to the tone of the interview.

"I, in accordance with the board of directors, felt that the demands of managing of a successful pharmaceutical company were more than one man could handle. Even more than a man as experienced as Dr. Bradsmith." She added. She had decided, before she started the interview, that this was the time to begin her strategy to discredit Phillip. Husted had conveniently played into her strategy. Her plan was to discredit him very slowly. Her reasoning was to prepare the shareholders for an NPC takeover. When the NPC took over James there wouldn't be an adverse shareholders' reaction to Phillip being asked to leave. She wanted the share price to stay high as long as possible. This was one of her tactics to protect herself against any unexpected events that might possibly drive the share price down and therefore reduce her financial win.

He noticed her practiced tone as Mrs. James statements moved to undermining Phillip's management. Husted, in his preparation for the interview, had anticipated that she would try the discrediting tactic. It was no secret to him and others that she didn't like Phillip and that she was stacking the board of directors against him.

What did surprise him was the fact that Phillip was not fighting back. He wondered if the shooting had taken that much out of Phillip. He remembered back to the days when Phillip was the wonder-boy executive of the pharmaceutical world. All of the companies wanted someone like Phillip on their team and when Phillip became president and CEO of James, the competitors saw his leadership potential as a treat to their business. The industry had concluded that James was sure to grow under Phillip and become a stronger competitor in the marketplace.

While that did not happen, no one blamed Phillip entirely. It was obvious Mrs. James was Phillip's obstacle and stumbling block. Her tactics had made him lose his focus on what was important to growing the company. Now, after hampering his potential success, she was setting Phillip up for a fall and herself as the person most responsible for turning the company around.

Husted knew the share price was improving, but he didn't really know why. He didn't even think Mrs. James knew what was causing the sudden turnaround in the company's success. She was an excellent politician and had more street sense than he had given her credit. She was riding the crest of a wave of increased interest in James. He thought to himself that she had additional hidden agendas, otherwise why go through the effort of discrediting Phillip?

Husted decided to see just how close Mrs. PrestonJames paid attention to the rumors of Wall Street. "Mrs. James, there is a rumor that the growth of the James share price isn't entirely the result of performance, but that James Pharmaceutical Company is an excellent takeover candidate and foreign interests have quietly been buying up the stock." Her expression changed a little, but he evaluated that she had been expecting a question about being a candidate for takeover.

She answered the question, "As you know, Mr. Husted, all successful companies are takeover candidates and I'm sure James is no exception. As far as the concern over whether the interested parties are foreign or domestic, there are SEC rules that cover this point. To date, no one has purchased the 5% of the outstanding shares that would require them to register with the SEC."

Husted then dropped the bomb that had just been released a few minutes before the interview had started. His office had paged him as he was coming up on the express elevator. He had called his office from Janet's desk. His office informed him that Reuters had just released some important information about James. The staff person on desk duty had read the release to Husted over the telephone. He had held it back from the interview until he felt that Mrs. James was feeling very comfortable with the course of the interview. He wanted to catch her off guard.

"Mrs. James, when I arrived here at the Spectrum of Medicine Building, I was paged by my office and given the following news release from Reuters. I am going to read the gist of it to you and I would like your comments.

"An unknown source today informed the Reuters International News Service that a physician in Germany is publishing a clinical paper on the use of Lifeal as a prophylactic for cardiac arrhythmia. The paper will state that over 50% of the patients in his study had arrhythmia while on the pharmaceutical Lifeal and the prophylactic indication didn't and wouldn't work. He concluded that all physicians should use caution when prescribing Lifeal and only to prescribe this potentially dangerous drug in approved dosages for the treatment when alternate courses of therapy didn't work. He definitely said that the product should not be used as a prophylactic.

Would you like to comment on this clinical report?"

"Proposed clinical report, Mr. Husted?" she immediately replied.

Husted noticed, for the first time during the interview that she was visibly upset, but her voice remained controlled.

She hadn't expected anything negative during the interview. She had thought that today, everything would be going her way.

He decided to dig in and see how she would react to tougher questions. He had nothing to lose. "You're right Mrs. James, it is reported as a proposed clinical report, but as we all know, Lifeal has had a less than glamorous history. Much of the stock gain has been attributed to the recent good news about Lifeal. I would assume this bad news will have some effect on the stock?" He noticed her face had begun to take on a different color. He had heard of her temper and wondered if he was going to see a firsthand demonstration.

"I say again, Mr. Husted, you said a proposed clinical report from an unnamed source. The paper hasn't been published nor does the report specify the name of the physician that has made this wild clinical pronouncement." Her voice began to rise in tone and loudness. "It is just like someone in the media to jump to conclusions. Things are going well here at James, so you have to make things look bad. Don't your kind ever look at the bright side of things?"

"Mrs. PrestonJames," he emphasized his use of her formal name, "I only report what has been given to me. I don't make up stories. You know Lifeal has failed to reach the marketshare, sales, and profit objectives that James has set for these important success criteria. The reasons given for failure have always been that the product never received approval for being a prophylactic. Now we have a report saying Lifeal doesn't work in prophylactic situations. You haven't given me a satisfactory answer to this Reuters report."

Her face turned red as she tried to control her emotions. Husted caught every reaction in her face and noted them on his pad. He concluded, as he had in the past, that he didn't like this woman. She again began to complain that he had jumped to a conclusion and was putting too much emphasis on it being an actual clinical report when in fact it wasn't.

He stopped her in mid sentence by asking a new question, "Would you like for me to call my desk and ask them to give me the current price of the James stock?"

This question seemed to catch her off guard. She was expecting more questions on the clinical trial not the quick switch to the share price. She was quiet for a second. He didn't know what was going through her mind.

She felt her inner strength weaken. All of a sudden she realized that rumors like this could affect her selling price to the NPC. She wanted desperately to know whether the price had dropped, but she also didn't want to seem overanxious to Husted. She now knew she could not trick him into taking her position in her war with Phillip. She had to be careful. Discrediting Phillip wasn't going to be as easy as she had planned.

She finally replied, but she had returned to her original soft and business voice again. Her anger had been brought under control. "Yes it would be interesting to find out. You may use my phone if you would like."

Husted picked up the phone and dialed his office. After a cryptic minute-long conversation with the person at his office, he replaced the phone and resumed his seat across from Mrs. James.

"James Pharmaceutical stock closed yesterday March 29th at $125 per share."

"Yes, I know that." Irritation had crept back into her voice. She didn't like playing games with the member of the media.

"As of this moment," he looked at his watch to prolong the announcement and then watching her expression, "exactly ten thirty, on March 30th, the stock is now $120. Down five points."

Her expression went blank. She was calculating what the $5.00 loss had cost her. She was not paying any attention to him. He continued to watch her very closely.

She came to the conclusion that although she had just lost more than $300,000, she still had plenty. Besides the clinical report on Lifeal was just a rumor and what went down could just as easily come back up. She decided to be very calm. She took more time before answering.

"Well, that doesn't seem that bad on a nasty rumor," she answered emphasizing the word nasty.

Husted knew he couldn't push things any further. It was time to end the interview. He had gotten a private inside look at this woman and the way she handled herself. He would have to spend more time on the James story. The annual meeting was coming up in May. He would pursue some of the rumors and see what was behind the growth in the share price. He ended the interview and left her office. He was sure that when he left she had been shocked because of his abruptness.

8:00 A.M., FRIDAY, MARCH 31

NPC CONFERENCE ROOM OSAKA, JAPAN

"*Ohayougozaimasu*, gentlemen, may we please have a roll call of the Board of Directors of the Nippon Pharmaceutical Council? Director Hideo Okamoto, would you please read the names?" Tanaguchi, the chairman of the council, requested of his council secretary sitting to his right.

"*Hai*, Chairman Tanaguchi." Okamoto paused and then read off the names of the other eight men who were gathered at the Osaka headquarters of the NPC and made up the ten-man NPC board of directors.

Each answered the reading of his name with the customary morning greeting, " *Ohayougozaimasu*, Chairman Tanaguchi," and then bowed their head slightly in the direction of Tanaguchi who sat at the head position of an oval-shaped, dark mahogany conference table. The names of the directors were read clockwise from Chairman Tanaguchi's left. Director Sataru Otani Director Koichi Miyazana Director Hiroshi Kawaguchi Director Morihiro Akai Director Ichiro Fujinami Director Tsutomu Oe Director Hajime Umeta

Tanaguchi opened the business meeting, "Well, gentlemen, our rumor plan was implemented a week ago. Please report on the results to date." Then to ensure he had communicated clearly, he ordered in a strong and authoritative voice, "Status report."

The first man on Tanaguchi's left was the first to report. "Chairman Tanaguchi," said Director Sataru Otani, "over the last two weeks we have purchased 3% of the James Pharmaceutical Company stock. Our percentage of ownership has been low, but our impact on the share price has been high. Our intention was to purchase more than 3%, but rumors of foreign investment began to result in an inflated price. We will now begin to buy short, which will help drive down the share price. The timing of our subsequent purchases will be in concert with the rumors created by our fellow director, Director Kawaguchi. The rumors will provide the rumorsusceptible Wall Street stock analysts with a great deal of misleading information on James. I fully expect to have 15% under our control before the annual meeting in May." He smiled.

"Otanisan," Tanaguchi asked, "you have a funny story that you wish to tell the group?"

Softly Otani answered, "It is only a funny thought, Mr. Chairman." He didn't know whether the authoritative and humorless Tanaguchi was trying to embarrass him for smiling during a serious discussion or whether Tanaguchi wanted to hear the story.

Tanaguchi must have been in a pleasant mood for he asked Otani to describe his thought. "Please, Otanisan, describe your thought to the group."

At this point Otani had to respond. "Chairman Tanaguchi, I visualized how we have handled Mrs. PrestonJames and her lover. We have acted as fishermen spreading our nets to cause entrapment. Then we threw them a hooked fishing line to bring them into the NPC boat. They have taken our hook and we let them run freely under the false security that they were free. Now," he cautiously smiled, "we are reeling them into the NPC boat. I see them flipping wildly across the troubled waters as they discover they weren't secure and have, in fact, been hooked." He then smiled freely. He had determined a way to remove himself from this potential Tanaguchi trap. Otani continued, "It will be your artistry and leadership Chairman Tanaguchi that will gently reel them and James Pharmaceutical Company into our boat without damaging our future newly acquired company."

The rest of the group watched Tanaguchi for his reaction. He started to laugh. The rest of the directors determined that he was in a good mood and joined him in laughing out loud with Otanisan and his vision.

"Thank you, Director Otani." Tanaguchi paused and then looked to the second man to his left.

"Chairman Tanaguchi," Koichi Miyazana addressed Tanaguchi, "I have, as you know, placed into, what the Americans call the rumor mill, a number of very optimistic reports about the future of James Pharmaceutical Company. The objective was to drive up the share price. As Director Akai will report, we have been more than successful in our goal of inflating the share price to provide," at this point he looked to his right at both Otani and Tanaguchi for silent approval, "Director Otani's fish, secure seas of optimism." Tanaguchi smiled, but did not laugh. "Mr. Chairman, that is the conclusion of my report and my specific responsibilities in the implementation of Project James."

"Thank you, Director Miyazana. You have done extremely well in spreading optimism. Please assume your advisory role for the remainder of the project." Tanaguchi paused, "Now Director Kawaguchi your report on turning optimism into pessimism."

Director Hiroshi Kawaguchi bowed slightly in Tanaguchi's direction. "Mr. Chairman, I am honored to be part of this project." He paused and then started his report. "Yesterday I placed a rumor with the Reuters International News Service in Switzerland. The rumor announced a proposed clinical report showing that Lifeal does not work as a prophylactic for arrhythmia. The report, of course, is unfounded. As for the future, over the next weeks we will provide different news services with appropriate rumors. There will be at least one rumor every week from now until the James annual meeting in May. Our objective is an overall lowering of the marketplace confidence in James. In our moving from optimism to pessimism we will exercise caution so only the confidence in James management is destroyed and not the future of JPC138."

Kawaguchi paused to let the caution statement sink into the Director's conscience memory. He continued, "We will spread the rumors across the entire James product line and all of the James executives. I have no doubt that we will drive the stock down at least fifty percent from today's opening of $120.00"

"Thank you, Director Kawaguchi. Your work is very important to our success. Please keep us informed of problems if they should occur between our meetings." Tanaguchi paused and looked to the director on Kawaguchi's left. "Director Akai, your report please."

"Chairman Tanaguchi, sir," Director Morihiro Akai replied with a slight bow, "I am happy to report that the stock of James had risen on the first day of our project to a high of $125.00 caused by Director Miyazana's optimistic rumors. As Director Kawaguchi just reported, the stock has fallen 4% from

$125 to $120 just on the one rumor he inserted into the press. As we calculated, the stock high did not have enough foundation and it was easy to begin the toppling. In my humble opinion, we will have no problem in driving the stock down to whatever level we desire."

"Very good gentlemen, are there any problems that we have not discussed or identified?" Tanaguchi asked.

"Director Fujinami, in charge of security, Chairman Tanaguchi," Ichiro Fujinami answered. *"Hai,* I would like to report on a situation that occurred with our forward people deployed in Doylestown, Pennsylvania." "Proceed, Director Fujinami," Tanaguchi replied cautiously.

"Dr. Koenig, the James consultant has again become a nuisance. Last Monday, Dr. Koenig showed up at our temporary headquarters located in the home of the mother of Dr. Helmut Wahlters in Doylestown. We tried to take a positive elimination action, but we weren't successful. I want to assure you that there will not be any repercussions, Chairman Tanaguchi. I consider this incident just an unfortunate event and nothing to worry about." Fujinami concluded hoping the simple explanation was enough for Tanaguchi and he wouldn't have to go into a full explanation.

Tanaguchi was both pleased and upset. He was pleased because his feedback system had worked. When the NPC associate that was following Koenig telephoned him, he had been made aware of the Koenig situation. Tanaguchi had chosen not to tell any of the other directors to see if they were on top of all of the NPC situations. It was evident in this case that the directors were informed. He was upset because Koenig hadn't been eliminated as he had instructed. His premonition about Koenig being a problem was slowly coming true. Koenig now knew too much to be eliminated. The elimination would draw too much attention and quite possibly an investigation might lead to the NPC. Who was this Dr. Koenig who always seemed to be around every situation where the NPC had planned to obtain an advantage? He needed to know what happened after he talked to the NPC associate in Doylestown, so he decided to ask Fujinami.

"Director Fujinami. Your explanation isn't complete. How do you know there will be no repercussions?" Tanaguchi asked.

Director Fujinami then went over the same informaton that the NPC associate had told Tanaguchi on the telephone.

Tanaguchi couldn't stop Fujinami's narrative because this would disclose the fact that he had spies within the NPC organization. As Fujinami droned on, Tanaguchi worked hard to prevent showing Fujinami and the other directors his impatience. Finally Fujinami came to the part after Koenig left the house.

"The NPC associate returned to where Dr. Koenig's car had gone over the cliff. He tried to find Koenig, but was unable to walk down to the bottom of the ravine to see if Koenig was still in the car. He then returned to his car to find Koenig in the car. There were some gunshots and then Koenig took off in the car. The car was located the next day. It was found abandoned in the New York City Port Authority parking garage on the New York City side of the Lincoln Tunnel. We then called the rental company of the car that Dr. Koenig left at the bottom of the ravine. The rental company said that Dr. Koenig had reported that he had been in an accident with the car. He told them that it was just a case of two cars going too fast on a narrow winding road. He didn't mention any foul play to the rental company or in the subsequent accident report. We have determined that he doesn't want any investigation and therefore, we won't have any repercussions. Mr. Chairman, we will appreciate any of your wisdom."

"Director Fujinami, I agree with your assessment," Tanaguchi answered. Tanaguchi was quiet as he thought about the situation. The directors waited for his direction. Tanaguchi turned to the director in charge of internal affairs, Director Tsutomu Oe.

"Director Oe." he said.

"Yes sir, Chairman Tanaguchi?" responded Oe. He answered sitting straighter in his chair and slightly bowing his head towards Tanaguchi.

"Director Oe, what is the status of the murder of our NPC associate and the escape of the peasant?"

"I am very sorry to report that there is no further information. Our murdered guard was turned over to his family and the police are investigating. We have decided not to take an active part in the investigation so as not to implicate NPC. At this point in time there is no direct connection between the murder and NPC. We are investigating the underground through our connections. At this point in time, there is no new information."

Tanaguchi didn't respond. He stood up and abruptly adjourned the meeting.

3:00 P.M., MONDAY, APRIL 10

SPECTRUM OF MEDICINE BUILDING
NEW YORK CITY

To J.P., the days were both dragging and speeding, if that was possible. They were dragging because everything seemed to take longer to resolve than planned. Speeding because the April board meeting was only a week and a half away. There were no noticeable actions coming from Mrs. James. He began to wonder if perhaps she hadn't become overconfident. If she had, he knew it would ultimately help their case.

Over the weekend, he and Mandi had gone up to Stowe, Vermont for spring skiing. The winter had been good to the skiers. The heavy snows had left a snow pack that allowed this ski season to be one of the longest in New England history.

The drive up to Stowe was even more beautiful than the trip he had made to Doylestown. Spring in the lower altitudes had arrived early and flowers were in bloom everywhere.

Mandi had made the suggestion to go spring skiing. J.P. had never tried spring skiing in New England, but he was a ready and willing companion. Mostly he had wanted to get away from the city and the James situation. Mandi had arranged to rent a house through some friends of hers.

They were able to put James behind them and just have fun together. For some reason they didn't even talk about their possible future together. He felt that they had come to an unspoken conclusion that whatever happened was fine.

So they both sought to ensure that every minute together was precious and filled with fun, love, and happiness. A complex formula, but it had been achieved over the last few weeks of work and now over the two-day ski weekend.

J.P. leaned back in his chair and looked out the window. He tried to get his thoughts back to James. It was a beautiful spring day in the city. The days were now getting longer and the warm afternoon sunlight filled his office. The ringing of the phone interrupted his daydreaming.

"J.P., Nacheda here. Do you have time to talk? Is this line clear?" Nacheda's voice came across strong, but J.P. sensed the urgency and caution in his voice.

"Good morning, Nachedasan." It was Tuesday morning in Japan. He had spoken many times to Nacheda since the team meeting in his apartment on St. Patrick's Day, but most of the conversations were just status reports. The day after their St. Patrick's Day meeting Nacheda had flown to California to work with Skip on the NPC project.

"I have time to talk Nachedasan, but I don't know if the line is clear." "J.P., take out the scrambler I gave you on my last visit. Hook it up and call me back at the Bandai office." He disconnected.

J.P. retrieved the black box from his briefcase and hooked it up to his phone. He dialed Nacheda's number at Bandai. Nacheda picked up on the first ring.

His voice took on the scrambled digital tone. Technology had improved beyond the garbled voice days of the eighties, but J.P. could still tell the voice he was hearing was being processed through a scrambler. It was a little higher in pitch than the normal voice and it seemed to make a person sound like they were talking faster than normal.

"How are you Nachedasan?" he asked.

"I am fine," he answered in an almost normal voice. Now that they were talking, the urgency in his voice seemed less.

"I have been confirming the information that Skip and I developed from our recent sessions with SAM."

"What have you found?"

"Plenty, J.P. First, after our meeting, Skip and I decided to call the task force and once again put them to work. At first they were reluctant, but after I told them about Joe Berger they were more than happy to assist our project. By the way, Skip, Reiko, and Annie send their regards. You had better call Annie. She thinks you've dropped off the face of the earth. She laughingly stated to Skip that she has put your house up for sale, considering that you don't live there anymore."

"That's Annie. I had better call. Knowing Annie, the joke could turn into a reality just to punish me for not calling her every week as I promised. Please go on, Nacheda."

"Well, after the team did their preliminary research and sent the information into SAM, Skip and I had a long talk with SAM."

"And what did SAM have to say?"

"SAM feels the James situation is just the tip of the iceberg when it comes to the activities of NPC. We input all of the members of the NPC whose names have been published. SAM ran a worldwide search. He came up with some very interesting employee profiles. I will provide a copy of the report when we meet this weekend. Suffice it to say we are not dealing with a mere bunch of Japanese pharmaceutical executives. We are dealing with some of the most powerful men in Japan. After learning this fact, I felt it was necessary to return to Bandai and discuss the entire situation with Dr. Nakasone. As you know, he has been in the pharmaceutical industry for a very long time and knows his competitors. I thought I would seek his counsel and give him a briefing on our proxy fight with Mrs. James."

"What did Dr. Nakasone have to say about the NPC?"

"Nothing good. He wished I had informed him about the NPC earlier. The NPC was one of the reasons he had taken his company to Bandai and not located it in Osaka or Tokyo. He felt the people that made up the NPC weren't up to any good and he didn't want to have anything to do with their underhanded methods. He believed in honorable competition and also in basic research. They didn't believe in either. They believe in gaining control of the marketplaces in which they compete in any manner possible, using the quickest method. After Singapore, you and I can attest to that strategy ourselves.

"Dr. Nakasone told me about the Japanese pharmaceutical industry and their long-range plans."

J.P. had heard most of this story before. In the early seventies, when it was almost a certainty that the Japanese would eventually try to take over the US, and subsequently global, automobile industry the financial power groups of Japan analyzed the profitable US markets. Their objective was to target the next market that they were going to control. It wasn't surprising that these powerful global Japanese executives determined the US healthcare pharmaceutical industry was very attractive and fit their profile of a potential controllable industry. The US pharmaceutical industry was large and focused with only a relatively few large companies. Most importantly, the companies were very profitable.

Since the Japanese were good at heavy industry markets that required bending metal they didn't go directly to the pharmaceutical market. The first step in the healthcare market was to go after the healthcare capital equipment market. Toshiba and Hitachi made the marketing thrust into the imaging and clinical chemistry markets. They were relatively successful but could not take over the market from the major US and European companies. Their biggest problem was their inability to keep up with emerging technologies.

They wanted a steady long-term manufacturing line, but the US entrepreneurial spirit foiled their strategy. The start-up companies would leap frog technologies into newer generations before the Japanese could realize a profit from the steady production of the older model. The US and European companies would purchase the small entrepreneurial companies and the Japanese could never catch up. Japanese managers in America kept faxing and then emailing the Japanese home offices demanding new models in order to compete. The Japanese home office refused to retool to a new model before the old model was profitable, therefore they were always behind and never gained a controlling marketshare.

While the Japanese were fighting G.E., Siemens, and Phillips, the US pharmaceutical companies like Abbott, Merck and others were beginning to make inroads into the backyard of Japan, the Japanese pharmaceutical market. This market was ripe for the taking by US and European pharmaceutical companies.

Until a several years ago, there were very few pharmacies in Japan. The closest to a pharmacy that they had were pharmaceutical herbal shops. The physicians in the United States heavily influenced most of the Japanese physicians. The Japanese physician wanted to prescribe US pharmaceutical products for their patients. Since there were no pharmacies, the Japanese physician prescribed US pharmaceuticals for their patients and did their own dispensing. The Japanese government allowed the US and European countries to enter the pharmaceutical market because they couldn't deprive their citizens from having the best healthcare.

American companies loved the opportunity to enter the Japanese pharmaceutical market. The market for pharmaceuticals there was as large as the US market and the population was only half as large. The reason for the large pharmaceutical market was because Japanese physicians generally over prescribed. The physicians were paid for their professional services and for the pharmaceuticals they sold to their patients. There is a definite profit incentive to over prescribe.

Over prescribing by the physician for personal financial gain, is the reason the US government protects the pharmacy laws. The pharmacist is considered a check and balance on the physician and the physicians' potential profit from dispensing pharmaceuticals to their patients. In many ways a physician prescribing and selling is a conflict of interest.

On the other hand, Japanese financial powers were very angry that the US companies were beginning to control one of Japan's largest markets. So the Japanese set out to gain a strong foothold in the US pharmaceutical market in any way that they could.

Ever since the Thalidomide tragedy and until recently, the FDA has made sure new pharmaceuticals took a long time before they are approved, marketed, and eventually become profitable. A company has had to live with erratic FDA decisions for years when a product is going through the approval process. In recent years the approval mechanism has smoothed out a little, but it is still years before a product has the possibility of making a profit. Pharmaceutical companies in the US also have to live with the ups and downs of the investment community.

Japan took care of both of these problems. The Japanese government encouraged pharmaceutical research by financially supporting the clinical studies of their pharmaceutical companies. In the US the pharmaceutical company has to pay for clinical studies of unapproved products.

Nacheda continued, "Japan provides incentives to the large Japanese chemical and brewery companies to develop products and enter the US pharmaceutical marketplace. The Japan Pharmaceutical Manufacturers Association was the legitimate arm of the industry and within the Japanese culture ethics, they were playing an ethical role in the development of the Japanese pharmaceutical companies and how these companies would approach overseas markets.

"The NPC, on the other hand, was the cast off organization. The borderline companies that were not going to be a success the honorable way decided to break away and buy their way into the US market. The members are less than honorable executives that feel it is their right to be in the global market and will exercise that right anyway they can. These NPC member companies are financially backed by the Japanese investment bankers and stockbrokers who don't want to wait for the legitimate Japanese pharmaceutical industry to grow. They want their return on investment faster. With large investments from financial investors, the NPC has the money to buy whatever and whomever they need in order to succeed. Until the James opportunity came along, the NPC couldn't find an American candidate. They had made approaches to purchase U.S. and European ethical pharmaceutical companies, but with no luck. The romanced companies didn't buy into the NPC story.

"The NPC didn't have the know-how to form a task force like the Bandai task force that found James. The NPC witnessed Dr. Nakasone's lack of support for the JPMA and concluded that he was a rebel. They decided to watch Bandai's actions to see if they could steal any expansion ideas from Bandai.

"You know the rest, J.P. The NPC executives are ruthless and will strive to establish control of James at all costs. If they are in direct contact with Mrs. James, Dr. Nakasone doubts they have been honest with her and he feels there is a very good possibility that the NPC is working to achieve a different agenda than that of Mrs. James. I agree with Dr. Nakasone's assessment. What is the other agenda? We can only guess, but I would imagine that it doesn't include Mrs. James and bodes ill for the James Pharmaceutical Company."

"I think you are also saying that not only will our group have to defeat Mrs. James, but we will have to take on the NPC." J.P. paused for the answer, but none was forthcoming. He continued, "Nacheda, I don't think we have the resources to undertake a project of fighting the NPC."

"I agree. That is exactly what I told Dr. Nakasone." "What did he say?"

"Dr. Nakasone is an old man. He is probably over eighty years old. He has accomplished much in his life and he doesn't want his work destroyed. He believes in what we are doing and he wants to help us as much as he can."

J.P.'s mind suddenly came alert. What had started as a joint venture between two friendly companies now was beginning to smack of a takeover situation. He immediately jumped to a number of conclusions. Phillip's group could not come up with the funds to fight both Bandai and the Mrs. James/NPC alliance. The only assets their side of the evolving James scenario had was the James Pharmaceutical Company itself. So, he concluded, James would be taken over by either the NPC or Bandai. If it had to be one or the other, Bandai would certainly be the preferable choice, but it would still be a takeover. J.P. became heartsick at the possibility of James being owned and operated by anyone other than the James family of employees.

"J.P., do you understand? Nacheda asked. "J.P., are you there?" Nacheda asked again.

J.P. had grown silent as his thoughts had considered the negative possibilities. "Yes, I am here. Sorry, what was it you asked?" he finally replied.

"I asked if you understood what I was saying?"

"Yes, I'm afraid I do understand. We will likely have to give up control of James to Bandai in order to pay for the support Dr. Nakasone will graciously provide us." His voice now completely reflected the depression that he felt about the whole James issue. What started as a simple industrial espionage mystery to discover who had stole a strategic plan, was now going to be a major proxy fight between Mrs. James, the NPC, and the survival of Phillip's team.

"Nachedasan, what does Dr. Nakasone want us to do?" he asked wearily.

Nacheda started laughing. J.P. started to tell him to go to hell and hang up the phone when Nacheda said, "You have it all wrong J.P."

"Have I?" he responded.

"J.P., calm down. Even with your voice coming through the scrambler I can tell by the sound of your voice that you don't understand. I called because I have good news, not bad news. Now, as we used to say in the Army, listen up."

"Okay, Nacheda. I'm listening."

"Thank you. I want to tell you that Dr. Nakasone doesn't want to take over James, he wants James to take over Bandai Pharmaceuticals and all of its resources. He believes in what Phillip and the team are fighting for and feels that it will be better for both companies and the patients they serve that James is the surviving company." He paused and sensed that he had to emphasize the point in order for J.P. to believe him.

His senses were accurate, what J.P. was hearing was too good to be true. "J.P., Dr. Nakasone will fight with and for us and he will help us to finance our fight."

8:00 P.M., THURSDAY, APRIL 13

THE JAMES' FARM, GREYSTONE HALL
SEAFORD, NY

"Helmut laid in Evelyn's bed faking sleep. It was no good. Each Thursday he wanted to tell Evelyn PrestonJames to go straight to hell and yet when the appointed time arrived on their Thursday evenings, he would dutifully drive to her house and climb into her bed. He would satisfy a physical need that, only a few months before had died in both his mind and body. She, at least brought him back to life, he thought to himself. Satisfying his physical needs had cost him mental peace and almost all of his pride. But, he reminded himself that if all of their dreams came true, he would be rich.

What was it Dostoevsky had said in Crime and Punishment? "Yes," he said out loud and then to himself, "the ends will justify the means."

"What?" came the reply from the other side of the bed in a loud and irritating voice. "I thought you were in your usual after-sex stupor."

"Nothing, I said nothing. You must have imagined hearing voices," he weakly replied. To himself he repeated, "I am going to be rich."

"I did not imagine anything you old fool. I heard you say, yes, and then mumble something unintelligible. Was that a delayed post-orgasmic response after your usual twenty-minute brain delay. Perhaps you should sign yourself up for the JPC138 clinical trials?"

He didn't answer her. He reminded himself that in a short six weeks he would be rich and sleeping with this woman would be finished. With the money he would be able to buy anything his heart or crotch desired. He smiled.

She was watching him. His eyes were shut as he lay there on his back with his hands folded across his ever-growing stomach. Hell, she thought, he had to lie on his back, he could not lay on his stomach, he was too fat. She lifted the sheet that covered her body and looked down at her own nude body. At 43 she was trim and tan. Her breasts were still firm and her abdomen was flat and toned all the way down to the tops of her thighs.

"What in the world am I doing in bed with you, you ogre?" Quickly she answered herself, "Because I need him to complete the plan." Also, Helmut was her conduit to the NPC.

The completion of her plan was moving in the wrong direction, away. The stock had taken a slight downturn. It closed at $110 the day before. She told herself that she had been too greedy when the stock was at $125, rationalizing the money she had lost on paper since the March 31st close. Then there was the NPC 20% bonus, which brought the stock from $110 to $132. She began to smile to herself. She would be able to buy any man that she wanted after this was over.

The two of them, lying in her bed smiling for basically the same reason, were brought back to consciousness by the ringing of the telephone.

She grabbed the phone in irritation. "Who would be calling me at this time of night?" Her question was quickly answered when she heard the voice on the other end.

"Mrs. James, did I disturb you?" Tanaguchi asked. "If so, I am very sorry, but something has come up that I wish to discuss with you. Do you have time to talk?"

"Yes, of course," she answered. Her voice sounded to her as though she was in a large, empty ballroom. "Do you have me on a speaker phone Mr. Tanaguchi?" she asked cautiously.

NPC CONFERENCE ROOM OSAKA, JAPAN

Tanaguchi smiled at the group around the conference table. They all knew the chances were almost 100% that Dr. Wahlters was in bed with Mrs. James when she had answered the telephone. They intentionally had called her during their Thursday night liaison. It would keep her off balance. The speakerphone was a new touch. The object was to make her feel as though she was on display.

"Yes, Mrs. James. Do you mind? The other members of the NPC board are with me and we are quite concerned about the recent drop in the James stock price and stories in the U.S. press. The Japanese media has picked up the stories as well." He inwardly smiled at the Japanese media comment. In truth, the Japanese did not care about James, but she didn't know he had fabricated the story.

"We think the subjects of these reports are serious enough to be discussed with you personally, as you Americans say.... ASAP," he paused to give the impression that he had to struggle with the slang. "If this isn't a convenient time we can call back next week." He paused again for some response. There was none forthcoming. He added, "You do know it is Friday here in Tokyo?"

"No, not next week. It is convenient right now," she quickly replied knowing that they knew very well that it was not a very convenient time to talk. She forced herself to use her best charming voice and attitude. She continued, "No, I don't mind the timing of your telephone call nor the fact that I am on your speakerphone. I was, in fact, just preparing to go to bed. Of course, Mr. Tanaguchi, I don't have my brief case in front of me so I'll only be able to answer your questions from memory."

The men around the table all smiled and each seeing the others' smiles were having a hard time suppressing outward laughter.

"Mrs. James would you please provide us with some idea as to why your stock price is sliding. This morning, on the Tokyo exchange, the James stock slid another 20 points. This slide was based on a late Thursday report from New York saying the clinicals for JPC138 were being stopped by the FDA because of an unreported side effect stating that there is a possibly an excess of brain activity."

There was silence on the phone. Tanaguchi looked around at the other members. These late night phone calls to the United States were a stroke of genius by Director Kawaguchi. He had to reward Director Kawaguchi. He had tied together the Lifeal side effect, the shooting of Dr. Bradsmith and JPC138. Helmut had dropped the name of Ralph Wilson's cardiologist to one of the NPC associates during a conversation when he had made one of his frequent visits to his mother. The NPC associate leaked the information to one of the potential JPC138 clinical trial physicians.

He had called the physician posing as a James research scientist and told the physician there would be a further delay before the start of the JPC138 clinical trials. The NPC associate further suggested the physician might call one of the New York daily papers and mention the delay and that the call was from a concerned physician who was supposed to be conducting the clinical trials.

The sound of Mrs. James voice came from the speaker. Her voice had a cautious tone and seemed to be uncertain. "I'm very sorry Mr. Tanaguchi, but I'm not familiar with the press report that you are talking about. I was very busy this evening and didn't read the evening newspaper." Again the group of directors smiled and one of the men whispered to the man next to him, "I'll bet she was busy."

Tanaguchi saw the two men whispering and gave them a very stern look.

There were no more side conversations.

"I will, of course look into this article first thing tomorrow morning. Do you want me or Dr. Walhters to phone you back with a report?"

"No, that won't be necessary Mrs. James. We are very concerned over our potential," Tanaguchi emphasized the word potential, paused, and then continued, "James investment. A question keeps going through our minds. Would you like to know the question, Mrs. James?"

"Yes," she answered too quickly.

The directors smiled again at how well Tanaguchi controlled the woman.

"The question is this, is the James Pharmaceutical Company and it's stock worth the high value we initially placed upon it and will we still be able to keep our promise of a 20% premium?"

There was a prolonged silence on the speaker. The overseas satellite background noise seemed to be amplified. The directors around the table knew the woman had been taken aback by Chairman Tanaguchi's question about the 20%. Like most Americans this woman chairman didn't realize the Japanese negotiating rules. The negotiations were never over until a contract was signed. In her case, the NPC directors didn't feel the negotiations would be over until the NPC had actually purchased her stock and had control of James. Until then, everything was open to negotiation and change. They knew she had calculated the 20% into her winnings. She had come to the wrong conclusion.

Mrs. James was stunned into silence, she had seriously miscalculated the NPC and had let optimism take control of her better judgment. The 20% bonus hadn't been a certainty and in the worst case was probably a negotiable term. Now, after this press release the bonus was probably in jeopardy.

"Are you saying," Mrs. James voice came over the speaker with a distinct quiver, "the 20% is open to further negotiation?"

Tanaguchi did not answer immediately but let the question hang in the air. Again the background noise filled both the conference room and Mrs. James ear. Then, with finality to his voice he answered her question, "Everything is always open to negotiation Mrs. James. This is especially true when things aren't what they seem. Your sliding stock value and the rumors surrounding the viability of your products seem to paint a much different picture than what you wished us to believe. Please pay better attention to your business, Mrs. James. We don't want to work with someone who doesn't know the day to day activities of their business. We will be in contact. Enjoy your evening." He paused and then concluded. "I believe you require a document from us for your proxy statement. It will be faxed to you this weekend for your review and approval. Please don't try and negotiate the terms of the agreement. We aren't in a negotiating mood." Tanaguchi broke the connection.

Tanaguchi lifted up his finger from where it had pushed the button to break the connection. He had a very pleased smile on his face. The group then broke up into laughter.

"A brilliant strategy, Chairman Tanaguchi. She is probably very upset with herself. She will undoubtedly vent her frustrations on poor old Dr. Wahlters." Director Otani said.

"I believe we have won this deal, Chairman Tanaguchi. I propose at the end of today's business we meet for dinner and celebrate our successful activities," stated Director Hajime Umeta, the youngest member of the group.

The table all of a sudden grew silent. Mr. Tanaguchi glared. Everyone knew that Tanaguchi had been Umeta's mentor ever since Umeta had been appointed to the NPC board last year. All eyes watched the mentor as he glared at his charge for his impropriety.

Tanaguchi finally spoke. His voice was soft, but stern. "Director Umeta, you are young and we don't expect you to know the workings of this business. You must have patience and, just as Mrs. James can't go to the bank on the 20% premium, we can't celebrate a win that hasn't been won. Many things can happen on the road to success. We must not reach the end of the road in our minds when a distance remains stretched out before us. A distance with many curves and hills. Do you understand Director Umeta?"

Umeta's face flushed from the scolding given by Tanaguchi. Umeta was one of the new-generation Japanese that considered themselves the birth of the new Japan.

Umeta began to think to himself. He had earned his way to membership in this prestigious group it wasn't a gift. He was as good as the rest of these directors. In his mind he felt he was better. The brains of these old men were filled with outdated history and the ancient culture of Japan.

He was filled with thoughts of winning and making money in a global commercial war. But, he reflected, it wasn't time to argue with his mentor. He was a member of the group and he would serve their needs until the time was right for him to take a stronger position. He remembered the humility his father taught him and made his apology for his insubordination.

"I am very sorry, Chairman Tanaguchi. I apologize to you and the rest of the directors. My enthusiasm clouded my mind and obscured the lessons you have been teaching this inexperienced man. Please except my humble apologies and I will restrict myself to only those issues that are of value to the group and for which I am trained to comment." While he was speaking to Tanaguchi, his head was bowed to a point where his forehead was almost touching the table. His voice was slightly muffled as he spoke into the table.

Mr. Tanaguchi was impressed with Umeta's apology as were the rest of the directors. They knew Umeta as an opportunist. He had earned his way on to the group by rising to the head of a start-up Japanese pharmaceutical company based in Hong Kong. Tanaguchi felt that perhaps the influence of the group had begun to favorably influence the young man and perhaps his scolding had been a little too harsh, but he remained silent. Tanaguchi didn't acknowledge the apology. A lesson was being learned and he wouldn't interrupt the lesson by softening his scolding by responding to the apology.

"Now gentlemen, please the status report on the James project." Tanaguchi commanded.

"Chairman Tanaguchi," Director Otani began, "we have purchased 5% of the stock. The stock ownership is in the name of ten people who don't know one another. I still expect to have 15% ownership under our control before the annual meeting in May."

"Thank you, Director Otani. Director Kawaguchi. Your report please." Tanaguchi indicated to the next man around the table.

"Mr. Chairman, the rumor you just related to Mrs. James will take affect tomorrow. We have seeded the press with nine rumors. The press is now alerted to the James situation and is hungry for more adverse news. The press is even finding things that we haven't reported. The fact that the stock was so high and that the annual meeting is getting closer has fueled the interest concerning James. To set your minds at ease, there has not been any true reports that would change our minds as to the viability of James as our acquisition candidate to enter the US pharmaceutical market."

"Thank you, Director Kawaguchi. Director Akai."

"Chairman Tanaguchi, sir. Again I am happy to report the share price has been slowly dropping. Mrs. James has helped us a little with her very poor interview with the Wall Street Journal analyst Mr. Husted. I project the stock will be under $100 by next Thursday's April James board meeting.

"Are there any security problems, Director Fujinami?"Tanaguchi asked.

"None to worry about Mr. Chairman. We have been keeping track of Dr. Nakasone and Mr. Nacheda of Bandai Pharmaceuticals. Nacheda is back in Bandai after stopping at the condominium in Westwood. There seems to be an increase in activity between Bandai Pharmaceuticals and Dr. Koenig, but as yet, there doesn't seem to be any connection with James.

There is that man, Koenig again. Tanaguchi jokingly commented to no one in particular.

Otani spoke up trying to suppress a laugh, Perhaps since this Koenig fellow is failing with James he is trying to drum up new consulting business. The group broke out in laughter. The mood was light. Even with Tanaguchi's scolding of Umeta still ringing in their ears the group could smell the win.

Perhaps so, Director Otani, Fujinami continued, but we must wonder why, after so much work was done by Nacheda's task force in Westwood that there is no direct connection between James and Bandai. Remember the report that Lonewolf provided us. Bandai was looking to work with James. The only direct connection has been the trip to the plantation where Lonewolf met his death.

We continue our visual outside Doylestown at Dr. Wahlters mother's home. Nothing new has happen since the incident I spoke about at our last meeting. Since the plan is coming to a conclusion in six weeks I have increased surveillance of all the players. With all due respect, Mr. Chairman if I may offer an opinion, I feel confident that our project has gone too far to be stopped.

Director Oe, any word on the escaped peasant? asked Tanaguchi.

"Hai, Chairman Tanaguchi. We located him in Hong Kong. He was living and working under a false identity. We questioned him at length about how he left Japan and made the trip to Hong Kong. We tried to trick him into telling us who had helped him, but since he had been one of our best questioners before his mistake, he knew he was going to die whether he gave us the information or not. He chose to die without disclosing the information."

"Very well, thank you. Directors, we will meet again on April 24th, the day after the James April Board of Directors meeting." A slight smile curled from the corner of his mouth. "Perhaps we will again talk to Mrs. James at her home. Now, this evening at 6:00 we should meet at Noguchi Steak House for dinner." He looked over at Umeta and gave him a very small knowing wink.

Umeta nodded ever so slightly towards his mentor.

12:00 P.M., FRIDAY, APRIL 14

EDGAR ALLAN POE STREET NEW YORK CITY

J.P. left the Spectrum of Medicine Building early to prepare for the proxy team meeting later that afternoon at his apartment. It was a beautiful spring day in New York City so he decided to walk back to his apartment rather than take a cab.

When he arrived at the apartment he went straight to the dining room, or what used to be the dining room. After the first April meeting of the proxy group, he had transformed it into a makeshift war room. As they followed their battle plan they gave each project a status board created from large flip pads that were arranged around the walls of the room. The meeting that day would be particularly important. Things had to come together for their first announcement at next Thursday's board meeting when Phillip would ask Mrs. James and the rest of her directors to resign.

Nacheda would arrive sometime around 2:00, when the meeting was scheduled to start. J.P. hadn't talked to Nacheda since Monday when he had called with the brief report on the NPC and Dr. Nakasone's offer of resources.

Mandi arrived at 1:30 and they discussed the agenda. By 2:00, Phillip, Brian, Carl Sr., Peggy, and Allen had arrived. J.P. called the airline and learned that Nacheda's flight had been on time so he would be arriving soon.

"Let's wait another fifteen minutes for Nacheda," he announced to the group seated around the dining room table. The group was apprehensive. This was the first real decision point. Did they have enough information and support to pursue the fight? The stock was gradually going down and today's announcement on the JPC138 clinical trials had sent the stock down another 5 points. Mandi and J.P. had tried to figure out where all the reports were coming from, but to no avail. Their thought was that someone on the team might know or that together they might be able to come up with some idea of who was feeding the press. Assuming Mrs. James' goal was to sell out at a high price, it almost certainly wasn't her.

They were about to start when the doorman phone rang. "Good Day Dr. Koenig, a Mr. Nacheda and another gentleman are on their way up to your apartment."

"Thank you, Jim."

The front door bell rang and he went to open it for Nacheda. He was pleasantly surprised when he saw that the other gentleman was, in fact, Dr. Nakasone.

"Dr. Nakasone, what a pleasant surprise. We are honored to have you as our guest. Nachedasan you should have told us."

"Dr. Koenig, a pleasure to see you again. Do not blame Nachedasan for not telling you that I was coming. He was following my instructions. I will explain later this afternoon why I am here and why I didn't want my presence announced."

"I understand, Dr. Nakasone. Nacheda-san, good to see you again," J.P. said taking his friend's hand.

"Thank you, J.P. Now we must start the meeting. We don't have much time. Dr. Nakasone will have to fly back to Bandai tonight," Nacheda responded with concern in his voice.

"Fine, follow me." They walked to the war room. J.P. announced Dr. Nakasone and introduced him to everyone around the table. He gave him the seat to the right of Phillip.

"J.P., you have changed your beautiful dinning room into a war room.

Quite impressive." remarked Nacheda breaking the awkward silence.

"Yes, I felt our last meeting was a little too comfortable. As you remember, we were sitting in easy chairs." Everyone smiled, but didn't laugh. "Okay, well, welcome to the proxy team meeting. Today, we have a great many decisions to make before the April board meeting next Thursday. Since we have been in a secret mode of operation, we haven't had much opportunity to exchange information. I therefore recommend that we each brief the group on his or her activities since the last meeting. We must keep these briefings short. Dr. Nakasone and Nachedasan have to fly back to Bandai this evening. The major decision we have to make is whether we follow through with our plan to ask Mrs. James and her board members to resign. Remember, we must have positive proof of her involvement in actions detrimental to the survival of James. We must also decide whether we can follow up our request that she resign with a legal suit claiming that she has hurt James.

"Does everyone understand our objectives for this meeting?" he concluded his opening statement. Everyone in the room either nodded or said yes.

"We welcome Dr. Nakasone as a member of the team. Also present who were not present at the last meeting are Dr. Allen Strong and Dr. Peggy McCleary of the James research department. They have been brought up to date on what we are doing, but aren't and won't be permanent members of the proxy team. I therefore ask them to be the first to brief the group. That is unless Dr. Nakasone, you wish to be the first."

"No, Dr. Koenig, I would prefer to be the second to last to speak. I believe this places me just before Dr. Bradsmith," he replied bowing slightly to Phillip.

"Is this sequence of events okay with you, Phillip?" J.P. asked. "No problem, J.P. Please proceed," Phillip replied.

"Allen and Peggy you're on," he gestured to them to begin.

"Thank you, J.P. I will begin and Allen will summarize," Peggy replied then continued with her report. She moved to the head of the table at the opposite end from where Phillip and Dr. Nakasone were sitting. She had on a Navy blue blazer with a white silk blouse. Her skirt was a different shade of blue complementing her blazer. She carried herself very well and spoke withconfidence.

"Our objective was to determine whether Dr. Helmut Wahlters is purposefully delaying JPC138 and get some concrete evidence as to his involvement with Mrs. James and or the NPC." Peggy paused. "We were moderately successful in the three weeks that we had to accomplish our objective. We do feel we will have more evidence before the annual meeting.

"The information we have today concerns the toxicology and pathology sections of the FDA filling. We were to have filed this information with the FDA in February. All of the researchers associated with this section of the filing had completed their work by mid-January. The report was given to Helmut on January 23rd for final editing and then he was to do the actual filing the first week in February, the Monday after our meeting with J.P. and Mandi."

"At the research staff meeting I innocently asked Helmut how the filing was going for JPC138. He had quickly replied, very well. With my questioning I had created an interest in the group for a better answer. The head of Tox/Path, Dr. Milton Ansley, spoke up and reminded Helmut that he had given him the final report and draft of the FDA submission in January, but hadn't seen the filing report. He then asked Helmut specifically what day the report was mailed to the FDA and he wanted to know when the FDA had acknowledged receipt of the report. Helmut just gave Ansley an angry look and then changed the subject without answering the question. Ansley tried to bring up the subject again, but was always thwarted in his attempts to obtain an answer. On the third attempt Helmut ended the meeting.

"After the meeting I visited Dr. Ansley and asked him what was going on with JPC138. Milton gave me an earful for almost a full hour. He told me about Helmut's delays and his meddling in the JPC138 filing. His summary of the situation was that Helmut doesn't want to see JPC138 go to clinical trial. I asked him if he knew why? He replied, that he didn't know what agenda Helmut was working toward, but it wasn't Phillip's agenda. I asked him if he had any proof of Helmut's actions. Milton surprised me by opening a file drawer and pointing to a row of files. He told me that once the delays started he was afraid he would be blamed for the fact that JPC138 wasn't going to go to clinical trial on time. Milton had decided to document all of the conversations that he had with Helmut. He had been doing so ever since January. His standard procedure would be to write up the minutes of their meetings and then send Helmut a copy. Helmut had never responded to any of the memos. I told Allen...Dr. Allen Strong...about my conversation with Milton. Allen then visited Milton."

Allen addressed the team from his chair, "Milton gave me a copy of all of the files after I told him that Phillip had asked me to investigate why JPC138 was going so slowly." Allen reached down into his brief case and pulled out a stack of files about a foot thick. I have read all of these files and even though there is no direct evidence to implicate Helmut, Milton has documented numerous delays and non-responses from Helmut. I am sure that Milton would testify to the fact that Helmut is purposefully delaying JPC138. Peggy."

"Thank you Allen," she responded. "Since my meeting with Milton, we have tried to find the research logbooks. These valuable books are usually kept in the R&D safe. They weren't there when we looked. Considering all aspects of our investigation we have every reason to believe the logbooks have been taken by Helmut. We can't prove that, but I would bet they are in his possession at his home. He would never destroy them, he is too much of a researcher. A good researcher never destroys the logs.

"Allen then asked Helmut to file the JPC138 Tox/Path the first week in April. To date, Helmut hasn't attempted to make the filing. Allen has one other piece of information. Allen." Peggy took her seat.

Allen stood up and walked to the end of the table. "The two subjects I will talk about are sensitive. I have taken some risks on behalf of James. I am wholly responsible for my actions. I believe with all my heart in James research and what we can do for the future of mankind. I was very enthusiastic about what J.P. and Mandi told Peggy and I about the Bandai process. I decided that Helmut and

Mrs. James could not stand in our way to possibly achieving a treatment for Alzheimer's." He looked over at Phillip. Allen was tall and of medium weight. He looked very dignified in his double-breasted suit. They all waited as he addressed himself to Phillip.

"Phillip, I hope I did the right thing. Two weeks ago I hired a reputable private detective agency to watch Helmut's actions. I also authorized them to monitor telephone calls because I felt who he talked to would be of benefit to the proxy fight. I then had the phone numbers traced and the persons who called identified. This morning they gave me their report and copies of the recorded taped conversations. But, I am getting ahead of myself.

"In an effort to save time I will summarize my conclusions. Conclusions drawn upon my personal experience with Helmut, the detective's report, and the tapes.

"The last two Thursdays Helmut has gone to Mrs. James Long Island home where they almost immediately have gone to bed to have sex."

The room was stunned.

"Are you sure of your information?" it was Phillip that asked the question.

"Yes sir," Allen replied. "I also believe that the Thursday night arrangement has been going on for a long time. Remembering back over the months, Helmut always left work a little early on Thursdays and never could attend a function on Thursday nights. He always had an excuse."

"What about the phone call or calls?" It was Carl Sr. who asked the question.

"Last night their bedroom activities were interrupted by an international phone call. The detective agency bugged her telephone. I will play this for you, it is not very long.

Allen punched on the portable tape player he had brought with him.

"Mrs. James did I disturb you? If so, l am very sorry, but something has come up that I wanted to discuss with you. Do you have time to talk?"

"Yes. Do you have me on a speakerphone, Mr. Tanaguchi?" Mrs. James asked.

From the group came an audible gasp. J.P. looked around and saw that Nacheda had a smile on his face. The tape continued.

"Yes, Mrs. James. Do you mind? The other members of the NPC board are with me and we are quite concerned about the recent drop in the James stock price and the stories in the U.S. press. The Japanese media has picked up the stories as well. We think the subjects of these reports are serious enough to be discussed with you personally, as you American's say….ASAP. If this isn't a convenient time we can call back next week. You do know it is Friday here in Tokyo?"

"No, not next week. It is convenient right now. No, I don't mind the timing of your telephone call nor the fact that I am on your speakerphone. I was, in fact, just preparing to go to bed. I of course, Mr. Tanaguchi, don't have my briefcase in front of me so I'll only be able to answer your questions from memory."

"Mrs. James would you please provide us with some idea as to why your stock price is sliding. This morning, on the Tokyo exchange, the James stock slid another 20 points. This slide was based on a late

Thursday report from New York saying the clinical trials for JPC138 were being stopped by the FDA because of an unreported side effect stating that there is a possibly an excess of brain activity."

There was silence.

"I'm very sorry Mr. Tanaguchi, but I'm not familiar with the press release you are talking about. I was very busy this evening and didn't read the evening newspaper. I will, of course look into this article first thing tomorrow morning. Do you want me or Dr. Walhters to phone you back with a report?"

"No that won't be necessary Mrs. James. We are very concerned over our potential James investment. A question keeps going through our minds. Would you like to know the question, Mrs. James?"

"Yes."

"The question is this, is the James Pharmaceutical Company and its stock worth the high value we initially placed upon it and will we still be able to keep our promise of a 20% premium?"

There was a prolonged silence.

"Are you saying," Mrs. James voice, "the 20% is open to further negotiation?"

"Everything is always open to negotiation Mrs. James. This is especially true when things aren't what they seem. Your sliding stock value and the rumors surrounding the viability of your products seem to paint a much different picture than what you would have us to believe. Please pay better attention to your business, Mrs. James. We don't want to work with someone who doesn't know the day to day activities of their business. We will be in contact. Enjoy your evening."

Allen then punched the stop button. He had sort of a sly look on his face and stood waiting for the groups reaction.

"Well done, Allen," J.P. said. "We have now tied in Mrs. James to the Nippon Pharmaceutical Council and Helmut into both Mrs. James and the Nippon Pharmaceutical Council. I know the tape is not admissible in a court of law, but it can and will be used. Let me assure you, it will be used."

Allen jumped in, "We confirmed that the phone call came from the NPC headquarters. My private detective had the number traced and it was from Osaka, Japan. He then called a friend of his in Japan. The number is listed as the Nippon

Pharmaceutical Council. The NPC. J.P., how did you know NPC was the Nippon Pharmaceutical Council?"

"I am sorry Allen, I jumped to a conclusion. I was not certain the NPC was the Nippon Pharmaceutical Council, but independent to your investigation we have determined the NPC is an interested party in the future of James. When you said the call was from Japan, I jumped to the conclusion that it was the Nippon Pharmaceutical Council."

"Dr. Koenig, you are correct," Dr. Nakasone spoke up. His voice was soft and the group physically moved forward in their chairs to hear better. "Mr. Tanaguchi is the chairman of the Nippon Pharmaceutical Council. He is a very ruthless man. He is a Samurai who made his money at other people's expense. His money came from real estate investments. After he became rich he then decided to enter the healthcare business. Since he has no formal training in healthcare he purchased his way into the NPC and was elected chairman."

"Thank you Dr. Nakasone for your insight." Phillip replied respectfully. "Carl, do you understand the significance of the 20%?"

"I'm not positive, but there is usually an incentive associated with a major shareholder selling their stock. If Mrs. James is selling her stock to the NPC it is possible that she is doing it for 20% over market value. Since it would be a private transaction then it is legal," Carl answered.

"Dr. Bradsmith," Dr. Nakasone again joined the conversation, "I apologize for my continued interruption, but I must agree with Mr. Manningham's conclusion about the 20%. In Japan, the usual starting point for negotiations on stock purchase bonuses is 25%. The 20% is already lower than the normal. It seems to me after hearing the tape that Mrs. James' 20% is in jeopardy. I can't determine the reason, but I would imagine that Mr. Tanaguchi is somehow putting the squeeze on Mrs. James. This should eventually be to our advantage."

"Thank you again, Dr. Nakasone," Phillip commented.

"Allen and Peggy, is there anything else you want to add to your report?" J.P. asked.

"No, not at this time. With your permission we will continue with our project of watching Dr. Walhters," replied Allen.

"We can't condone your private detective's work, Allen. As far as collecting evidence on Helmut holding up the filing of JPC 138, please do continue." J.P. silently hoped that Allen would continue the surveillance of Helmut and Mrs. James. "Thank you Allen and Peggy. We appreciate what you have done. We will keep you informed."

Allen and Peggy left the apartment.

"Brian, would you please give your report."

"Thank you, J.P. I have been doing two things since our last meeting. First, I have managed the funds for the proxy fight and second I have been working with Carl, Sr. and our trusted lawyers to develop the paper work for our own proxy statement. As far as the money is concerned, to date we have spent approximately $100,000 on legal fees to develop the proxy statement. If Mrs. James doesn't resign next week, the expenditures will accelerate until the annual meeting. I have projected that, worst case, the fight will cost $1.5 million. As I stated at our last meeting, we only have $500,000 at our disposal from the James emergency fund."

"Brian, has Mrs. James spent any money on the annual meeting?" J.P. asked.

"Nothing out of the ordinary. The proxy statement has been printed along with the ballots. The package is ready to be sent out after the board ratifies the contents at the next board meeting. This normal expenditure has cost James $500,000. The meeting itself will cost another $200,000. Both of these expenditures were budgeted. I have been watching for unusual requests for funds from Mrs. James, but to date there has been nothing out of the ordinary."

"Carl, how is the content for our proxy statement coming along?"

"It is coming along fine, J.P., but we are missing two very important elements. We don't have a written strategic plan or a board director slate."

"The plan will be on Brian's desk on Tuesday. It will have Phillip's approval," he responded.

"I will tell you about the new board by next Tuesday," Phillip announced. He continued by asking J.P., "What is the plan for next Thursday's board meeting?"

"The plan is not very complex, Phillip. You will have to tolerate Mrs. James and whatever she will come up with to challenge your capabilities. I hope," he smiled to make sure that the group knew he was kidding, "that you will not let yourself get so angry that you get kicked out of the meeting." The others smiled, but did not laugh. He continued, "You must endure the pressure until the new business section of the meeting. At this point you will present your case for the resignation of Mrs. James and her directors. Your accusations will be made to Mrs. James. We don't know what her cronies have done in support of her activities, nor do we know their involvement. We don't want to directly implicate them, but insinuate their involvement by association.

"We might obtain some unplanned support from the lawyers and accountants among her directors. With the legal responsibilities of board members becoming more and more complex, they might want to bail out at the first sign of trouble. On the other hand, they have a great deal of cash to lose if they bail out. She has chosen her board well. They aren't the most respected professionals, but they aren't the worst either. We will have to wait and see. We will have resignation letters prepared for each of the board members, including those whom we feel are your supporters. Carl has advised us that they must also be given a chance to resign before the proxy fight. If you can get any of her supporters to sign their letter of resignation, you must do so. They don't all have to resign. We will take what we can get.

"We will also have prepared for you, a dossier on Mrs. James and the activities that she has taken, forming the basis for our asking her to resign. The reason will be because of performance detrimental to the survival of James Pharmaceutical Company. We won't provide you with the actual proof. Originals of the proof will be held in a safety deposit box in case she doesn't resign. Our strategy is for her to resign before the proxy fight. If she and the directors resign then we will use our platform for the shareholders to vote on and not the one Mrs. James is preparing. If she doesn't resign then we want our platform to be as strong as possible. So we won't give away our secrets before the annual meeting so she can plan a defensive strategy.

"Evelyn knows what she is doing. We feel that a strong hint that we know everything will push her and the board over the edge to resignation. If Evelyn and her directors are in a fighting mood and want to protect the game they think they have won, then, no matter what we show them in April encouraging them to resign, they will stubbornly resist."

"Remember," Carl interjected. Every person in the room shifted their attention to the resident expert on the SEC and matters of proxy fights. "Not to rain on our parade, but in my expert opinion I still think we don't have a chance in hell in getting her to resign and only a fifty percent chance of winning the proxy fight at the annual meeting."

Carl and Brian had become friends during the time they had spent working together over the new proxy statement. Brian spoke up with humor in his voice, "Old gloom and doom has brought us back to reality." Everyone laughed, but not freely. Brian continued, "I agree with Carl, but I also feel that we have a better chance now than we did after our last proxy team meeting. As far as I'm concerned, this favorable trend is good enough for me. As long as we keep getting stronger then I feel we have a chance."

The other members of the team all acknowledged Brian's feelings as representing their own feelings.

"Dr. Bradsmith," Dr. Nakasone acknowledged the leader, "I apologize, but I'm not familiar with the ways of a US corporation.

We, of course, in Japan follow, without question the corporate chairman. We don't argue with their plans for our future. As far as Bandai is concerned, I am sure that no one would speak out against the direction I want to take the company. In fact, they would not expect me to tell them where I am going to take the company. The employees and shareholders feel the fact that I am chairman, gives me the right to direct the company as I see fit for the general welfare of the company and the community. You would call this a blind faith in the leader's judgment. I'm not going to discuss whether this philosophy is right or wrong. I'm just stating a cultural fact.

"You must understand a discussion, such that we are having here today, wouldn't take place in Japan. What Mrs. James, as the chairman, does or doesn't do isn't the business of the other corporate shareholders. The chairman's word is accepted, without question, as the best strategy for the company." He paused as if thinking about what he had said and what he was going to say.

"I would imagine," Dr. Nakasone paused to find the right words, "that this Japanese corporate tradition is why we have a Mr. Tanaguchi in a high position. A person that can have a major influence over both of our corporate philosophies."

Dr. Nakasone continued with more of an upbeat tone in his voice, "I do feel honored to be a member of this group and look forward to finishing our negotiations with Dr. Bradsmith on how Bandai and James will work together. Working together to research and develop products for humanity. I know there isn't one of you sitting here today that feels they are here to do Mrs. James harm, rather we are here to work for the best for James Pharmaceutical Company and the patients of James products. Bandai employees feel the same about the Bandai Pharmaceutical Company. I know James and Bandai will make good partners. I know you will like the Bandai people and the combination of James and Bandai talents will make wonderful medicine.

"Now, if you will permit me, Dr. Koenig, I would like to speak to Dr. Bradsmith in private. May we use one of the other rooms in your beautiful home? After we speak, I must return to the airport and catch my plane back to Bandai, before I am missed. Thank you for allowing me to share this experience with you and I look forward to working with you."

"Thank you Dr. Nakasone," Phillip responded, "I think the team would be very willing to move into the living room while we talk in this room." He gestured for them to leave the room. "Please, if you all would be so kind as to leave Dr. Nakasone and I in private so we can talk. Thank you, we will reconvene our meeting once Dr. Nakasone leaves."

They all moved to the living room and left the two men alone to their own discussion. Once in the living room they continued preparing for the Thursday Board of Directors Meeting.

After thirty minutes the two presidents joined them in the living room.

Phillip addressed the group, "Dr. Nakasone, has discussed some wonderful things with me. We have found, in a short period of time, that our visions of the future of James and Bandai fall along the same path and we have decided that the two companies should work closer together. What I now am going to tell you is secret and to be discussed only with the people in this room. This information is very important to our winning the May proxy fight. You can't breath a word to anyone, as Carl, Sr. will tell you, you are now privy to corporate insider information. If the information ever leaks out or you use the information for personal gain, you may be prosecuted for being in violation of SEC laws. If any of you feel uncomfortable with these conditions and can not participate in what I am going to say, then please excuse yourself."

No one left the room.

"Thank you for your confidence." he paused. "I am very happy to announce to you that Dr. Nakasone has very graciously offered to merge the two companies into one global pharmaceutical company. The name to be decided upon. He has also made an offer to James Pharmaceutical Company, which I feel is so wonderful that I wish Dr. Nakasone to tell you himself. Dr. Nakasone, please."

"Friends, I call you friends because of my discussions with Nachedasan have brought me to know you and respect what you represent. I welcome being one of your friends. I'm an old man and I have seen many of my dreams come true. But, I believe some of the decisions I have made to make Bandai a good company will also keep Bandai from becoming a great pharmaceutical company. Bandai and its people have to have a broader view of the global healthcare market in order to fulfill their destiny. Bandai can't accomplish this alone. I can't continue to be their only vision because my vision is becoming limited with the broadening of science and genetic engineering. James and Bandai are unique in that they both believe in the natural ingredients of pharmaceuticals. Basically, we are both herbal companies with genetic engineering to be used to further herbal pharmaceuticals.

"The other pharmaceutical companies work with chemicals and other forms of genetic engineering. As I said, we are unique. Our uniqueness will fail if we work alone or just as joint venture partners. We must be fully integrated. I believe this integration must be made with James the controlling company. Therefore, if you win your proxy fight with Mrs. James I will donate all the shares of Bandai

Pharmaceutical Company to James Pharmaceutical Company. The Japanese government won't like what I am doing, but they won't be able to do anything about it. The Japanese laws are all based on selling, not giving.

"I do have a few minor stipulations, but they aren't difficult and Dr. Bradsmith has agreed to them in principle. Nachedasan will return to New York next Friday to be briefed on the results of the board meeting. He will work out the details of this merger with Dr. Bradsmith or his designate and assist you in your fight for control of James. I wish you success in what you are doing for both the employees of Bandai and James. You should be very proud of what you are doing and I look forward to June when we can put these problems behind us and move our new company ahead."

There was silence and then Carl began to clap. The rest of them joined in and for a small group the noise was loud and the feelings were high.

Dr. Nakasone and Nacheda put on their coats and walked to the door. At the door Dr. Nakasone again thanked the group and said he would see us at the annual meeting in May. He closed the apartment door and was gone. Everyone had been standing and now sat down in the closest chair and reflected upon what had happened.

Mandi was the first person to speak. "Well, I for one, am very happy to be part of James and to be part of its potential future. I say potential because we still have to perform. I don't know the full extent of what Dr. Nakasone has done, I don't know the Japanese culture well enough to speculate. I do know that what he has proposed is different than anything I have read and experienced within the Japanese business culture. I believe that he is taking a big chance in what he has proposed and he has done this based on what Nacheda-san has told him about us and James. He also left the ultimate conclusion in our hands. Phillip, can you share with us the stipulations he has placed on the gift?"

"Yes, I can Mandi. By the way, thank you for starting the conversation. I was at a loss for words. What he has proposed is so far from what I had ever imagined could happen to us that, to tell the truth, my mind is unwilling to accept the proposal. I know it is true, but it seems to be so terrific that it can't be true. Do you know what I mean?"

They all nodded their heads in the affirmative.

He continued, "As far as the stipulations, I don't think we will really have to discuss any of them. First, he wants royalties paid to the Bandai employees for whatever they develop. He wants any inventions from Bandai to be registered in all of the Bandai employees' names so they earn royalties from any products produced from the use of their patents. This will be the Bandai bonus plan. The royalties can't be lower than 6% of the patented products net worldwide sales.

"Second, he wants James to assure the Bandai employees that they will have employment for life just as they would under Dr. Nakasone's leadership. He doesn't believe in the employment for life concept to its fullest, but he does believe in management working as hard as possible to ensure corporate life for the company. He suggests we consider the Bandai operation a secured loan that has to be paid before any other person or party is paid. If the James corporation doesn't survive in the future, we are to do everything to ensure the Bandai research operations and its people survive.

"Third, he stipulates that Nacheda-san become the president of the Bandai operation and Nacheda-san and any subsequent president of the Bandai operation under James, sit on the board of directors of the new James Pharmaceutical Company.

"Fourth, that Dr. Nakasone be a member of the James Board until he is not capable of performing as a working board member or he decides to resign.

"That is all. If these stipulations are approved then James will receive all of the stock and assets of Bandai including the available cash. As for the cash situation he has given us access to a bank account that he has established here. We can use this money for the proxy fight. Nachedasan will manage the account. He has placed five million dollars in the account. He feels that since the Bandai assets will be James assets we will use the money in the best manner to achieve the victory for the new James plan.

"Finally he recommends that we don't release this information to the public until we are in control."

"What does that last statement mean, Phillip?" J.P. asked.

"He means, we can't use any of what I just told you to win the proxy fight. Yes, we can use the money, but not the merger of the two companies. One of the reasons for his stipulation is simple. The merger is dependent upon us winning the proxy fight. It is a sort of Catch 22. We might not like this stipulation, but we have to live with his decision.

"We can use the possibility of a license of the Bandai process to help JPC138 in the proxy, but we can't use the stock gift. He wants to protect Bandai and himself from being placed into jeopardy if we don't win the proxy fight. If what he has offered us or is willing to do for us becomes known to outsiders and we don't win the proxy fight, he and Bandai will probably be forced out of business for making such a radical agreement with a foreign company.

"You must all swear to secrecy. Dr. Nakasone took a chance in telling the whole group. After he told me his plan he asked me if he should tell the group. I said I would trust each and every one of you with my life. That was good enough for him and now you are part of an arrangement that could change the nature of business between our two countries and perhaps the world. Profit reinvested into the future as well as a reward for the shareholders and employees. Sound unusual? It shouldn't. That was what the free enterprise system was set up to do in the first place. The stock market has gotten a little out of hand in the last decade or two with non-product operational manipulators, but we have the chance to at least start making things right. Are you all behind us?"

"Absolutely" came the response.

"Okay, J.P., let's get on with our plan and be ready for our first step next Thursday."

"We have a tough job ahead of us especially when we can't use to win our fight, the wonderful gift of merger that Dr. Nakasone has given James. But, if we can't pull this thing off then I don't know if James deserves his gift. We must also not forget Nachedasan's role in this merger. He has helped James from the beginning. Even though most of you don't know him, I want you to know that he is an outstanding person and I hope represents great things for the future of this company.

"If no one else has anything to add to this meeting we will adjourn until next Friday. Meet here at 2:00. Brian, Mandi, and I will meet with Phillip in his office at two o'clock on Tuesday to review the material for the Thursday board meet^ing.

6:00 P.M., FRIDAY, APRIL 14

EDGAR ALLAN POE STREET NEW YORK CITY

By six o'clock everyone had left J.P.'s apartment except for Mandi. They had decided two weeks before that Mandi would move into the apartment until the project was over or they decided otherwise. The second alternative was never talked about, but understood. Their relationship had reached new levels of mutual respect and love. They had reached a mental and physical awareness that neither of them had ever experienced. Presumably, the only problem between them was where the relationship would go. The problem had first emerged in Hawaii. Since then the subject had never come up between them, but it was always there simmering in their minds.

It wasn't about love, for both of them knew that love was not an issue. They loved each other. Love was a fact that was respected by both of them.

The issue was of future, careers, families, and geography. The cause for delay in discussing the subject was that while they had one another, they also had the James proxy fight to consume their focus and energy. The future of Mandi and J.P. would have to wait until June. Today the plan was to enjoy each other and work hard.

"Let's have dinner here tonight, J.P."

"Sounds good to me. I'm still in a slight state of shock over Dr. Nakasone's proposal. I would like to talk about it some more, do you mind?"

"Nope, as long as you feed me and promise me that we will have some quiet time together later on this evening."

"I have a better idea. I've changed my mind," he said.

"Boy, talk about women changing their minds. I do believe that you change your mind quite often, Dr. Koenig. And what is it that your heart desires? No, don't answer that question. I know what you really want and you can't have any until you satisfy my stomach." She laughed. "Okay, enough teasing, now tell me your plan."

"I don't know about you, Mandi. You are getting to know me a little too well. Anyway, how about dinner, then after dinner drinks to get our creative juices flowing and then a dip in the hot tub to see if we can come up with anything new concerning the proxy fight?"

Mandi moved into his arms and whispered into his ear. "I am disappointed. I thought when you said come up with something new, it was going to be something other than work. But, since you want to be creative, okay. I reserve the right to alter the sequence of events anytime I want, agreed?"

"You deserve the right and have the privilege to alter any event." Again she whispered in his ear, "I love you, Jean Paul."

"I love you very much, Amanda. If we don't get to the task of feeding you, we will end up on our backs looking up at the beautiful spring evening sky a little earlier than we had planned."

"Okay, mister business."

Two hours later, after their meal and with drinks in hand, they were sitting in the hot tub with their arms wrapped around one another. Prokofiev's Romeo and Juliet was softly playing in the background.

Again Mandi's lips found their way to J.P.'s right ear. "You like?" she whispered as she ran her hand down his abdomen.

"I like," he whispered back.

She pulled away, "Well you can't have." "Why?"

She pulled completely away and sat down opposite him in the tub, "Because I have an idea about how we can help our chances with the proxy fight," she said, teasing him. "Don't you want to listen to my ideas, J.P. Aren't my ideas good enough for you? Aren't you interested?"

"You know I think your ideas are the greatest. Now stop teasing me with your words and body. So let's hear it."

The music hit a couple crescendos and Mandi began to talk about her idea.

"J.P., remember we talked about asking the employees to help us by purchasing shares of stock. I have been thinking about how we might go about making that happen. Today the stock closed down five points from yesterday. This was mainly on that false rumor about the JPC138 clinical trials. As a side note, we should do some brainstorming about who is feeding the market with the false rumors."

J.P. started to respond, but Mandi cut him off with a quick motion of her right hand across her neck.

"Not now, J.P., tomorrow. Going on with my idea. Most of the employee stock options are at between $50 and $60 a share. I checked Thursday, and found out that there are just over a million shares of options yet to be exercised. Between Phillip and Mrs. James' board cronies they make up over 750,000 of that million. Two conclusions. First, 250,000 is not that many votes and second, the people who have the 250,000 option shares probably can't afford to buy them or borrow the money to exercise their options. My conclusion is that we have to find another source to purchase stock."

"As usual my dear, you are on top of an important point that no one else has considered."

"Thank you, sir, for the compliment," Mandi replied and then went on with her idea. "There are two groups of people that, over the years, have been very supportive of James and other pharmaceutical companies in their time of need. You can now probably guess who they are."

"You are a genius, Mandi." he replied enthusiastically, "The pharmacist and the physician."

"Correct, Dr. Koenig. These two groups have been known to purchase a few shares of pharmaceutical stock. If the grand lady James does not resign next Thursday, I think a public relations campaign should be started by a third party organization to purchase James stock. I don't know the legal ramifications about how we do this, but I am sure that Carl can tell us. I know it can be done because

I have seen it done before with advertisements in the newspapers. What do you think, J.P.?"

Mandi's voice lost her confident and humorous tone. It was replaced by a voice seeking approval. J.P. thought it was a great idea and the timing was perfect.

"Mandi, you are truly a genius. The idea is outstanding and I'm sure there will be a way to implement a plan to purchase stock. What I think is illegal is the selling of stock. The SEC doesn't want companies hawking their own stock. Brokers can recommend their clients to buy and the news media can recommend persons to buy. The employees can ask for help from the company shareholders to support one management position or another. That is what you have seen in the newspaper."

"Great, J.P. We should assume that Mrs. James and the others won't resign and that we will have to release our proxy plan to the shareholders. That will give us license to ask for support. Monday we can develop a multiphased marketing program to hopefully obtain support and indirectly new shareholders."

J.P. knew that Mandi was warming up to her idea and program. In the four months that he had known her, he had always enjoyed her when she was involved in a program. Her enthusiasm was contagious. She was a good marketer. She was creative, detailed, comprehensive, and she was an implementer. She was good and J.P. felt that James was lucky to have her on the corporate team. His heart sunk a little at the thought about James' need for her and her need to be a truly successful marketing executive. He looked over at her and was pleased to see that she hadn't noticed or felt his mood change.

Her voice was excited and she spoke in a clear and enthusiastic manner. "You know, now that I think about it, we shouldn't wait until Thursday's results. Bandai has given us the money to fight. We all know she won't resign. If we don't proact now we will lose the opportunity to use the money except in retaliation to her plan and we have been doing too much reaction already. Do you agree?

You're right on track Mandi. What should we do?

We should move quickly. First we'll develop ideas for a series of newspaper ads. I'll contact the communications firm that we use and get them to establish a series of positive press releases. We'll get our media friends to interview Phillip. You need to work on Mr. Husted to establish a better corporate relationship with him. Slip him something he can use and I'll bet he'll listen. And, finally, how about if we hold a meeting of the employees' association with you and Bill Husted as outside speakers?

She concluded, I'm not clear as to the last point and whether that is selling stock or not.

Go on with your thought, Mandi, he encouraged.

Well, we have an employees' association. We should assume that when the two proxy plans come out, they will want to support our plan. This will then be the forum to run the newspaper ads promoting their position, which will also be our position. You and Mr. Husted can give your opinions.

For your information Mandi, I called my voice mail and I had one message. It was from Bill Husted. He wants to talk to me on Monday. I'll call him tomorrow and see if we can talk before Monday.

That's great, J.P. Hopefully we can get started tomorrow. What do you think?

Again her voice sought approval. Mandi, the idea and plan are brilliant.

As the leader of the proxy team I assign you to be in charge of this project. Do what you think is necessary to implement the plan. Just keep me informed and also set up some measurement gates so we can determine the effectiveness of the program. Have it ready to implement next Friday. We will give you the word to go or not go at our team meeting next Friday afternoon. You should have everything in place before then. If she resigns we can cancel. If she doesn't then we will be ready to implement and catch the opposition off guard. Again Mandi, the plan is very good and was well worth my staring at you across this tub for the better part of an hour.

I am sorry, sweetie, I got so excited about the plan that I forgot where we were.

No need to apologize. Remember the plan to come up to the hot tub to be creative and talk about our fight plan was mine. I also didn't expect the outcome to be as good as your idea.

Mandi slowly slid down into the water and disappeared, emerging again between his legs. Her long red hair covered her face as she rose up. Water dripping, she took her hands and parted her hair to reveal her beautiful face. She then draped her arms over his shoulders and pressed her lips to his. His arms enfolded her and brought her body up to hold against his.

10:00 A.M., THURSDAY, APRIL 20
SPECTRUM OF MEDICINE BUILDING
NEW YORK CITY

"Will the James Pharmaceutical Company Monthly Board Meeting please come to order," Mrs. James said in a very strong authoritative voice rapping the gavel on the small wooden tray that had been placed there to protect the table from dents. "Note in the minutes that all eleven members of the board are present. Mr. Secretary have the minutes of the last meeting been amended?"

"Yes, Madam Chairman, the minutes have been corrected. There were no major corrections. I make a motion the minutes be approved as amended," Brian spoke as he played his role as secretary.

"Do I hear a second to the motion that the minutes be approved as corrected?" Mrs. James asked as the formality of the meeting began. During the formality of the first thirty minutes Phillip was silent except for his president's report. He was very matter of fact and was somewhat surprised when neither Mrs. James, nor any of her other aligned board members, asked him any questions. He wondered what they were up to.

"Under old business, I would like to discuss the sorry state of affairs with this company and the performance, or lack thereof, of the current James management." Mrs. James' voice began to increase in volume. She had been lying in wait for the moment when old business was to be discussed. Phillip could see that she was barely able to contain herself. Her tan skin took on a reddish hue and her neck strained a little at the edge of her buttoned white silk blouse.

Phillip felt good about what the proxy team had prepared for him. He now had more confidence about winning the fight. In fact he felt good about everything. The fight was now going to come out into the open. No more backroom discussions and best of all no more defensive measures or getting pounded by Mrs. James. Today was the beginning of his offense. If Mrs. James' adrenaline was pumping, his adrenaline was pumping harder. He had to keep himself under control. The phrase, silent but deadly, kept creeping into his thoughts. Mrs. James still controlled the board and he didn't want to be shut off like last month. He wanted to make sure his comments were placed in the board minutes.

Mrs. James looked to where Phillip was sitting at the other end of the table. He usually wanted to sit in the middle of the table so she didn't look directly at him. Today he wanted to sit at the end so in essence there were two heads of the table. If they got into one of the heated exchanges the other directors would have to swing their heads back and forth between Mrs. James and Phillip. He wanted everyone to see him as her equal.

Mrs. James stared the length of the 15-foot conference table and continued in a very accusing voice, "Your president's report, Dr. Bradsmith, was completely unacceptable. I didn't comment on the report at the time it was given because I wanted to see if you were going to explain yourself and your performance before old business. Much to this board's surprise, you have chosen to remain silent. A great strategy for you, but unacceptable to this board and to its chair. Your silence won't allow this board to forgive you for the continued mismanagement of James." Her face was getting red and an accusing finger was being pointed at Phillip. She turned to Brian and said, "Mr. Secretary, I want you to record every word that I say in the minutes of this board meeting."

Brian looked up from his computer notebook where he had been typing the notes, "Yes, Madam Chairman. I would request that you speak a little slower and not shout. I will be able to concentrate on your exact words a little better. I certainly don't want to miss recording any of the words spoken at this meeting," he said with about as much seriousness that he could muster.

Brian then made a quick glance over at Phillip. Brian was sitting to the left of Mrs. James. Phillip realized that Brian was trying to help him through the tough part of the meeting. Phillip warmed inside at the loyalty that he felt with the majority of his staff.

Mrs. James was not smiling. She looked directly to her left and at Brian. "Mr. Secretary, are you mocking me?" she asked shaking an accusing finger.

In a much more serious tone than even Phillip thought was possible from Brian, he said, "No, no, Madam Chairman, I was not mocking you. I do want to remind you that, at your request, this meeting is being taped so that every word is recorded for inclusion in the transcript of the official minutes."

The other members of the board began to speak all at once. They did not know that the meeting was being taped and were offended that she would order something like taping a board meeting without their knowledge and permission. Her own board members were shocked.

Mrs. James started pounding her gravel on the wooded tray and then on the conference table itself. Dents were forming all around the disk and her yellow pad of paper where she wrote her notes of the meeting. She kept pounding and saying, "Order, order, order." Everyone went silent, but she continued to pound and yell. Suddenly she stopped and looked around at the surprised and alarmed faces of all of the men at the table. Tears came to her eyes as she stared at the silent group.

Mr. Hammond one of her lawyers spoke, "Madam Chairman, I recommend that we take a 20 minute recess to have a cup of coffee."

Phillip almost spoke up and said he didn't think a coffee break was necessary, but then decided it would look better in the meeting minutes if he wasn't taking aggressive action.

"Yes, yes...a twenty minute recess." She pounded her gravel once more and this time hit the wooden disk.

Twenty minutes later everyone was back in their chairs. Mrs. James had recovered her composure. "I apologize to the board for my uncharacteristic outburst. I have instructed the secretary to remove the tape recorder. The minutes will be taken as usual, by the secretary using his computer. We were discussing old business and the performance of Dr. Bradsmith as the president and CEO of James Pharmaceutical Company."

Mrs. James spent the next thirty minutes bringing up past issues and the rumors of the last three weeks. She also accused Phillip of causing the decline in the stock price from $125 to $98 at the close of the markets the day before. Throughout the entire thirty minute tirade Phillip remained silent and by all appearances, calm. After he saw how ridiculous she had looked when she blew up before the break, Phillip decided he would be professional at all costs.

When she finished, one of the old board members, Mr. Simpson, asked her why she was so destructive of the current management. Was there a motion she wanted to place before the board? If not, he didn't understand the personal assassination of Phillip's character.

Mrs. James replied that she didn't want to make a motion, but that she felt the board should think seriously about the changes that have to be made to management in order to turn James around.

She stopped talking and every head turned to Phillip expecting him to blow up and defend himself and James as he had done in previous meetings.

He was silent for a prolonged period of time. He calmly looked at Mrs. James as if he were expecting her to say something else. The faces down both sides of the table continued to look at him and just as they were about to give up on Phillip and return their attention to Mrs. James, he spoke. His voice was calm and filled with his new assurance of ultimate success.

"For the record, Madam Chairman, are you asking me for my resignation?" Phillip asked.

All of the directors showed surprise in their faces at his question. They all swung their heads back to Mrs. James to hear her answer.

She replied with one word, "No," and then she continued without taking a breath, "if there is no additional old business we will continue to the next topic, New Business. Is there any new business?"

Phillip raised his right hand to be recognized. Mrs. James recognized him with a wave of her left hand, almost in dismissal. Her hand hit the edge of Brian's laptop computer screen and snapped it down on his typing hands.

"Ouch!" Brian exclaimed and raised the screen to begin typing again. He knew that Phillip would now drop his own bomb. He poised his fingers for Phillip's next words.

"Mr. Secretary, I will proceed very slowly with the subject of New Business to enable you and the directors to hear every word and for the secretary to type each of my words in the official minutes of this meeting. It is a shame that we have removed the tape recorder. I'm sure that some of you will want to hear what I have to say again at a future date. The subject is important, because it is possible that there might be legal ramifications to what I am going to say.

"I also have a written report from which I will verbally summarize. I will submit the written report to the secretary to be attached to the official minutes of today's meeting."

"What is going on here?" one of Mrs. James' lawyers, Mr. Harman C. Coontz, IV asked as he pushed back his chair and stood up. "First, with due respect to Madam Chairman, we have accusations without penalty that are being made by Mrs. James. Then we have unapproved use of tape recording, again by Mrs. James. Now we are going to have a legal report by a Ph.D. Again I say, what is going on here?"

Phillip thought to himself, the issues are getting hot and mister know-itall lawyer is getting a little uncomfortable.

Phillip stared directly at Coontz and in a very firm and authoritative voice said, "You know nothing about healthcare, much less James Pharmaceutical Company. You are only on this board to do the chair's bidding. If I told you what was going on with pharmaceuticals you wouldn't understand what I was talking about, so sit down and shut up." The confident voice of authority coming from a person everyone at the table thought was a defeated executive had its desired affect. Coontz sat down and the rest of the board sat stunned and silent. Including Mrs. James whose tan had noticeably faded.

"Now," Phillip continued in his positive authoritative tone of voice, "all of you just sit back and listen to my presentation. It is not long, but it is important. I'm only going to say what I have to say once and then I will make a board resolution. I'm going to make some accusations that will not have material evidence to back them up included in the report. Be assured that the accusations are backed up with facts and evidence. Depending on the outcome of the vote on the board resolution, I will make the decision of when I will release the hard evidence. I will not, under any circumstances release the evidence before the vote. The reasons for this unorthodox approach will be evident when I make my resolution. Does everyone understand?" He looked up from his prepared notes and saw a shocked group of faces looking back at him and they were nodding their heads that they understood. Phillip glanced over at Brian who gave him a knowing wink. He purposefully avoided eye contact with Evelyn Preston-James.

"Mrs. James….Madam Chairman, it has come to the attention of the president and CEO of James Pharmaceutical Company, namely myself, Phillip T. Bradsmith, Ph.D., that you and your appointed members of the board have conspired to commit injurious harm to James Pharmaceutical Company that threatens the survival of the company."

The six board members that had been appointed by Mrs. James jumped up from the table. They were all speaking at once. Words and phases came through the overall noise. Phillip could hear phrases like, "crazy bastard," "incompetent," "false," "liar," "you have no proof," "I don't have to listen to this," and just shouts of, "no, no, no!"

Over the ruckus, Mrs. James surprising steady voice could be heard along with her pounding her gavel on the wooden disk. "All of you sit down," she paused until all heads had swung back to her end of the table and their eyes were focused on her. She then completed her sentence, "Now!"

"Thank you Madam Chairman, shall I continue?" Phillip asked and then proceeded before she could answer. "To continue, I was saying, Mrs. James and her appointed members of the board have conspired to commit injurious harm to James Pharmaceutical Company that threaten the survival of the company." Again, Coontz started to protest. Mrs. James took the gavel by the hammer end like a pistol and pointed the handle at him. He remained quiet.

"This acquisition is based on the following five points," Phillip then looked up from his report and looked directly in the eyes of each person one by one. Going from his left to the end of the table and ending locked onto Mrs. James eyes. As their accuser, he wanted to memorize the changes in their faces and wanted to look them directly in the eye when he made his accusation. As he spoke each charge. They lowered their eyes in order not to look directly into his.

He spoke the charges, "One, that Madam Chairman and certain board members knowingly passed on secret company property, the 21st Century Plan to outsiders for the purpose of selling shares and the shares of your friends to an association owned by foreign companies for personal gain.

"Two, that certain board members were given stock options that have been exercised in order to gain more control of James and to personally profit by the sale of said stock when the company is sold to the foreign association.

"Three, that Madam Chairman and certain board members have been working on a plan to sell James Pharmaceutical Company since at least November.

"Four, that Madam Chairman and certain board members have encouraged the head of research, Dr. Helmut Walhters to delay work on the new pharmaceutical JPC138.

"And, five, that the association that Madam Chairman and certain board members plan to sell their stock is the Nippon Pharmaceutical Council. A group that represents Japanese interests and not those of James."

There was not a sound in the room except the low hum of the fresh air system.

"In light of these charges, I make the following resolution," Phillip looked down to read from his type written resolution. "That Mr.Hammond, Mr. Coontz, Mr. Alexander, Dr. Wickersby, Mr. Weinstein, Mr. Rogers, and the Chairperson, Mrs. James resign immediately from the board, and today each one of you sign a document that you will not sell your stock for one year unless you have a personnel emergency and then only with the permission of the board of directors."

Phillip looked up from his report. "I repeat what I said earlier, these charges are backed up with documentation. I don't feel documentation is necessary due to the fact that you know you are guilty and to be openly exposed would do more harm to James and your personal reputations than unexpected resignations. I will present the documentation to you after you have resigned. If you don't resign and insist on claiming to be innocent, others and I are prepared to enter into a proxy fight with you for control of James. A proxy fight will not help James, but will ensure the future of a great pharmaceutical company of which you," he pointed to the accused group, "are all prepared to destroy for purposes of your own greed." Phillip folded his papers.

The silence from the group continued. Then from his right came the strong voice of Mr. Simpson, one of Doc James' oldest friends, "I second the resolution and call for the vote."

Silence. Mrs. James' board members were looking at her for direction. They had knowingly set up the selling of James. To their benefit, they probably didn't know what NPC was doing to gain control. They were in the deal for a monetary gain and had not thought of what the outcome would do to James the company, its customers, or its patients.

Finally Mrs. James spoke. Again Phillip was surprised at how calm she was. He thought that she was either the coldest woman he had known or had downed a couple of tranquilizers during the break. He thought it was probably the latter.

Phillip, Brian, and the directors on Phillip's side waited. He thought, if she votes yes for the resignation resolution, then it was done. The others will follow. If she votes no, the others will also vote no and the resolution will be defeated and we will go into a proxy war. Phillip thought to himself, so be it... we are prepared. In his heart he wished she would say yes to the motion, but he knew she had too much at stake and she was a gambler or she wouldn't have started the series of events that had led them to this time and place.

She would call his bluff and vote no. Since she was calm and not irate, he knew he had lost round one.

"Dr. Bradsmith, I won't honor your remarks with a long answer. In fact the answer is just two letters.no! I vote no to the resolution that we resign."

She had expected an immediate response from the others of her group. What she got was a yes from Phillip and additional yeas from the four board members who were not in her control. Silence from her board members.

Brian summarized the voting, "The vote on the motion to have Mrs. James and other board members resign is five yeas and one nay." Brian's voice reflected that he was enjoying the moment.

Mrs. James looked over at Brian as she reflected upon shooting the messenger. Then she looked at her five board members and shouted, "Well? Vote damn you!"

The five, in unison, meekly said, "Nay."

Mrs. James then looked at Brian and said, "Okay, big shot read the vote now."

Brian, still with confidence in his voice said, "The vote on the resolution to have Mrs. James and other board members resign is five yeas and six nays. The resolution does not carry."

"Now, Dr. Bradsmith, you will have to back up your charges, which I doubt you can do." She thought for a second and a sly smile came to her lips as she concluded, "See you at the annual meeting. This meeting is adjourned." She got up from the table without waiting for the proper motion to adjourn and the subsequent vote. She walked out of the boardroom. The outside board members remained in their chairs, stunned. As Phillip picked up his papers, Brian folded his computer and they walked out together.

8:00 P.M., THURSDAY, APRIL 20

THE JAMES' FARM, GREYSTONE HALL
SEAFORD, NY

"Can you believe the guts of that bastard?" Mrs. James commented. She was with Helmut in the living room, which was a change from their usual routine. They were discussing the board meeting.

Earlier in the day, during their post board meeting telephone conversation, they decided to discuss the day's events and the next month's annual meeting before beginning their bedroom exercise.

After the board meeting had adjourned and she had walked out she had returned to meet with her board members. After two hours of discussions she had convinced them that Phillip didn't have a case and everything would be fine. She was sure he didn't have hard evidence and that he was dealing with conclusions built around rumors and assumptions. The group had reviewed the proxy statement they would send to the shareholders that weekend. They felt the document reflected their collective opinions.

On Monday the NPC had faxed an agreement to Mrs. James at her farm. She had sent a copy to her board members who incorporated it into the proxy statement.

The proxy statement outlined the agreement with Nippon Pharmaceutical Council. The agreement stated that the NPC would finance research for JPC138 with an additional ten million dollars in working capital. For the $10 million working capital they were asking the shareholders to allow the selling of an as yet to be determined number of shares of stock from the company's treasury of unissued shares. The number of shares depended on the average stock price during the five business days before the annual meeting. This would result in a stock dilution.

The proxy statement talked about the new vision that the NPC investors would bring to James. The board members on the ballot included Mrs. James, her five current members, Phillip, and five new members. Four of the five new members were old friends of Mrs. James and would be loyal to her. The fifth new member was Mr. Tanaguchi of the NPC.

Four of the new members had the same stock option deal that the previous four members had received from Mrs. James. The new members were investment bankers, lawyers, and healthcare association officials. Their credentials were impressive. Their knowledge of running a pharmaceutical company was almost zero. The common shareholder didn't know the difference between board members that did and did not know healthcare. They would vote for the management ballot. To them the James proxy statement and ballot were very impressive and they would be glad such prestigious executives would be on their board, protecting their share value.

Mrs. James wasn't going to tell the James shareholders about her hidden agenda. The fact that an additional sale of stock would take place between Mrs. James, the board members, and the NPC. Or that Dr. Bradsmith would be asked to resign after the annual meeting to be replaced by a president and CEO of NPC's choice. This was a secret between Mrs. James and the NPC.

The sale after an annual meeting was not illegal, but knowing about it before the meeting took place and not disclosing it in the proxy statement was withholding information. The reason it was wrong was the simple fact that management wasn't allowing the shareholder to make a decision based on all of the known corporate activities at the time of the writing of the proxy statement. This was illegal, but would be difficult to prove.

During the afternoon meeting, Mrs. James' group had come to the conclusion that Phillip's effort to get them to resign that day was just a nuisance. They would not change their plans. They were still in the driver's seat.

After sitting in the living room and discussing the situation with Helmut, he had agreed with Evelyn's assessment of the board meeting. They also agreed that they wouldn't have their usual weekly session in bed. Although they did not say so out loud, both were relieved that they wouldn't have to face the drudgery of sex together that night.

Just as Helmut was about the leave the farm, the phone rang. They stopped talking and looked at the phone. Helmut spoke after the third ring, "I'll bet it's Tanaguchi."

"I agree. What do we tell them about the board meeting?" she asked Helmut. Even though the relationship was deteriorating and after next month's annual meeting she wouldn't need him, she still respected his mind.

Helmut was taken aback. It wasn't very often she asked his advice. "Nothing happened, so you don't have to say anything."

"Yes, I agree." She picked up the telephone. "Hello?"

Mr. Tanaguchi's voice, "Good evening, Mrs. James. How was your day?"

As hard as she tried to be relaxed, little beads of perspiration popped out on her brow. She looked over at Helmut for support. He just stared at her from his chair. "I am just fine Mr. Tanaguchi," she replied in a calm voice. "How are you this afternoon?" She knew it was early Friday afternoon in Japan. She tried to impress him with this knowledge.

1:00 P.M., FRIDAY, APRIL 21
NPC HEADQUARTERS OSAKA, JAPAN

Tanaguchi was not impressed. Before answering her question, he looked around the table. The NPC board was assembled as previously announced at the previous month's meeting. The mood of the group was high. Things were going along exactly as planned. No hitches.

"I am fine Mrs. James. How was today's board meeting?" he asked.

He listened as she went through the board meeting. She told him that Dr. Bradsmith's president's report was unsatisfactory and that she had told him that his work was unacceptable. She told him that Dr. Bradsmith didn't have a satisfactory explanation for any of the press stories and why the stock price was falling.

"Is everything on schedule for the annual meeting?" Tanaguchi suddenly asked in the middle of her board meeting report.

She told him everything was going as planned. There would be no problems. She then asked him if he was going to attend the meeting.

"I have given it a great deal of thought and I have discussed the issue with my advisors. As of today I am planning to be at the meeting. Do you have a problem with my attending?"

She told him that she thought it would be a good idea if he would attend. "Fine," he said. He then became silent for a prolonged period of time.

He was listening to Mrs. James. He had a small smile on his face so the rest of the men around the table didn't become concerned with the long message that Mrs. James was apparently giving Mr. Tanaguchi.

Every minute or so he would say, "yes" to acknowledge that he was listening to her dissertation. It was a full ten minutes before he again spoke into the mouthpiece.

As he began his side of the conversation, the NPC board listened attentively to the one-sided conversation. "Yes, Mrs. James, I understand your concern over the James stock, but I don't know what this has to do with our arrangement. In fact, with the terrible press reports that are being printed about James, my board is concerned about whether we have aligned ourselves with the right company and perhaps we should reconsider our deal. No, no, no, please Mrs. James, let me finish." The attention of the group sharpened. She must have tried to interrupt Mr. Tanaguchi. He went on, "Although conditions look very bleak, Mrs. James we are sticking by you and your team. We are sorry that the stock has tumbled below $100. As I have mentioned in the past, the reduction of stock price concerns us just as much as you say it concerns you."

There was another pause. "Yes, we are sticking with our 20% bonus on the purchase of your stock. He listened. "Yes, and of your chosen board members. But I must tell you Mrs. James that I can't hold the 20% if the stock continues its downward movement. My board is beginning to question the real value of the James stock. We felt the stock was overpriced when it was at $125. We wondered whether someone was promoting the stock in order to get it to the high level. The stock is still thirty times earnings. That is very high multiple, Mrs. James." He listened. "Yes, Mrs. James I understand the unknowns of the New York Stock Exchange, but our business arrangement was predicated on a different set of conditions than what exists today. I most strongly urge you to keep the James stock price up by refuting the press stories." He listened. "I am sorry to inform you Mrs. James that my board has instructed me to reduce our bonus from 20% to 15% if the James stock goes below $75 a share and to 10% if it goes below $50 per share."

Again he listened to Mrs. James response to his statement. "Yes, I know you could interpret this reduction in bonus percentage as going the opposite direction of what you and your board desire and this might jeopardize the business arrangement between our two boards. But, like you, Mrs. James, I must abide by the directions from my board. Financial conditions are very tough in Japan, Mrs. James. The interest rates are climbing and our export trade is not as high as projected."

He smiled to his board. Yes, the interest rates were up, but the rates were still below US interest rates. Rates for obtaining funds to make investments in acquiring overseas assets was lower than they had been for years. He knew that to Mrs. James and her American ear, she would interpret Tanaguchi's statement as a very bad omen. There was a good chance she might weaken in her negotiating position. He had nothing to lose.

Export trade wasn't up to Japanese projections, but the projections were placed 20% higher than the prior year's actuals. Again Mrs. James would probably misinterpret the situation and might weaken her position.

The NPC board watched in silence as Tanaguchi listened to Mrs. James plead with him to keep the 20% bonus. This short dialog with Mrs. James would probably save NPC 10% of the bonus no matter what the actual stock price was when the deal was signed. They all knew that the deal wouldn't be signed until after the annual meeting.

"Yes, Mrs. James, I hear you, but as you Americans say, that's the way it is. I am very sorry. I will call you the day before I leave for the annual meeting. I should like to meet you in person. If anything comes up that requires my attention then please call me at the number I gave Dr. Wahlters. My assistant will keep you informed of my travel arrangements. Now, Mrs. James I must get back to work, you know it is just Friday afternoon here and there is work to be done.

Please continue what you were doing. Good day," and he pressed the disconnect button.

He turned his attention to the group, "Well, gentlemen, the plan unfolds as we desired. Now, please, your status reports.

"Mr. Tanaguchi," Director Sataru Otani began to speak, "we have purchased 12% of the stock. Ownership is in the name of the original ten people and five additional new investors. Again, they don't know one another. Our goal to have 15% ownership under our control before the annual meeting in May is on track."

"Thank you, Director Otani. Director Kawaguchi," Tanaguchi indicated to the third man around the table. He skipped Miyazana because his job of spreading optimistic rumors was finished.

"Mr. Chairman, we are interjecting the US financial press with stories at the rate of two per week. The stock continues its downward trend. We will continue to feed stories until the Monday before the annual meeting when we will stop and let the US press generate their own stories."

"Stock situation, Director Akai."

"Mr. Tanaguchi, sir. As you so ably told Mrs. James, the James share price has continued to drop. As I predicted, the stock was below $100 for the April board meeting. The $50 level at the annual meeting is within reason given the current trend line and my esteemed associate Director Kawaguchi's success with false news releases."

"Director Fujinami, any security problems?" Tanaguchi asked.

"None of any major importance. We thought we had lost track of Dr. Nakasone last week, but he was slightly ill for two days. He was back at work on Monday. There doesn't seem to be any activity between James and Bandai. We have come to the conclusion that the reason there is no activity is because of the fall of share price and the rumors in the press. We have, quite possibly scared Bandai off of James. We continue to watch, but with the time left before the annual board meeting it doesn't seem they could make any arrangements that would negate our plan."

"Thank you gentlemen. I see no reason to detain you any longer. I will call you if there is reason for us to get back together before the Friday before the annual meeting." He consulted his notes, "That date is May 19th. Any problems with this date?" He looked at each of the men at the table. "Very well then, this meeting is over."

EDGAR ALLAN POE STREET NEW YORK CITY

The entire team was assembled in the dining room that had been converted to a makeshift war room. Nacheda had quietly arrived in New York City the same way he and Dr. Nakasone had done the week before.

J.P. could feel the excitement in the room. The real fight, that everyone had worked so hard to be prepared for, was about to begin. The group was a little disappointed that Mrs. James and her cronies had not chosen to resign at the board meeting, but down deep they were happy. They didn't want her to get off with an easy resignation. Phase two would start that day with the release of the Dr. Bradsmith's proxy statement and his slate of directors.

"Brian," J.P. said seriously, trying to calm the euphoria of the moment, "perhaps you can give us a status of the Mrs. James proxy statement and how it compares to our own. After you have finished I would like Carl to comment on the filing process. Brian."

"Thank you, J.P." He paused and looked down at his papers. He had four stacks of printed documents. Two sets of proxy statements and ballots. One set for Mrs. James' platform and one for the Dr. Bradsmith platform. He handed one of each set to the members of the team.

"First," he began, "let's look at the Mrs. James platform. There is really nothing new or unexpected in her platform. She has added five additional board members of her choosing. When I received this document early this morning I did some background checking on the new members. They are just routine members. Nothing positive and nothing negative. As far as she is concerned they will be safely on her side in all of the issues. Their credentials are impressive, and the shareholders will be very impressed, but they won't provide the board with any new expertise. They look like they are just interim members until the NPC places their directors on the board.

"On the other hand, the section on the strategic plan announces an agreement with Nippon Pharmaceutical Council that would provide the working capital to accelerate the research on JPC138. The amount for JPC138 isn't specifically earmarked for research, but there is an additional $10 million in working capital above the funds required to operationally run the company. They, the NPC, will provide the funds to James by purchasing common stock. The number of shares and the value of those shares hasn't been determined." He looked up at the team and added a comment, "As you know, this will depend on the average share price." He looked back to his notes and continued. "They have chosen the five business days before the annual meeting as the time period to be used in determining the price. As a side note, if the stock continues its slide and we don't win, the NPC will realize a great bargain. There is nothing in the proxy statement that indicates the NPC is going to purchase Mrs. James' stock. With the current stock price they are going to get a very good deal on the stock purchase because there is no minimum purchase price."

Brian again looked up from his papers and addressed the team. The tone of his voice turned from business. He took on more of a questioning, wondering tone, as if he were asking himself the question rather than the group. What he said had significance.

"This brings up an interesting point. I have been thinking about the ambitions of the NPC since this morning when our stock took another hit from the rumor announced in last night's New York Evening Herald. This is a matter that I think we should discuss, if not now then later." He stopped to formulate the words in his mind before speaking them out loud. "Perhaps the NPC is feeding the marketplace with these rumors. The reason behind this strategic move by NPC would be to drive down the stock price in order to get a better price on the James stock." He stopped and looked around the table. The eyes of the team were staring back at him. Then one by one they started nodding their agreement.

Mandi then added to Brian's postulation. Her voice was excited as she started to add her own thoughts. "I think that Brian has hit on something. I have had to pay close attention to these rumors and acquisitions because I have had to provide answers for our sales representatives to use in selling situations. They have been inundated with questions from physicians. To us, each item is one event. To the sales organization and their physicians the events have a cumulative effect on their reception in the physicians' offices. Carl, Jr. was in my office the other day and informed me that both the new and refill prescription rates for Lifeal have started to decline. I asked the VP of sales, Jake Crossfire about Lifeal sales. He said he is definitely seeing a slow down this quarter compared with last quarter. Spring is usually a good new prescription period. People are starting to feel like they have to get back in shape for the summer and exercise too quickly which leads to cardiac problems."

Carl turned to Brian and asked him a specific question. "Brian, you watch the stock buys and sells. Would you please see if you could answer a few questions?" Without waiting for Brian to answer he stood up and listed the questions on a blank piece of flip chart paper.

"Have you noticed any unusual selling? Have you seen large blocks being sold or purchased? Have you seen any increase in selling short? When the share price was increasing was there an increase in buying long? Are there any new large shareholders?"

Carl, Sr. went on, "I will assume that no new shareholder has declared themselves to us as owning more than 5%, as the SEC requires. The reason I'm asking these questions is that we might have a possible hostile takeover attempt happening at the same time that Mrs. James is playing her games. She is taking all of our concentration and there is a possibility that we are not seeing the macro situation. There is a scenario where NPC is purchasing stock to increase their control of James beyond what Mrs. James is able to sell to them. The NPC not only wants control, but they also want to make money when the stock goes back up to its correct earnings ratio share price.

From what I have heard about the NPC, I wouldn't discount them in trying to force the stock price down as low as they can without totally ruining the James reputation. NPC has everything to gain and nothing to lose by using this tactic. I bet this is their strategy… to make the $10 million they said they would invest in James. A neat strategy, I might add. What do you think Brian, or anyone else?"

"Carl, you have just put together all of my scattered thoughts," Brian replied. "I have been wondering about a lot of little nagging issues, but couldn't put them into any cohesive answer. You just did. Let me try and answer your questions. I will answer your second and last questions first. There hasn't been any large block selling or buying or large new shareholders. But, there has been some funny shifting in stock ownership. I received the first quarter stock movement print out last week. I analyzed this information plus the April movement up though yesterday. I also talked to Husted at the Wall Street Journal, who, by the way, is an expert on James and becoming very interested in what is happening. His interest isn't from an adversarial point of view, but supportive of what he sees as the Phillip Bradsmith cause. He wonders where all the announcements are coming from especially since they are all adverse. He said this is very unusual. Usually someone or the company starts to fight back. He wonders why James is not fighting back." Brian smiled. "Monday he will find out why and then he will see us fight back. Right?" He pounded his large fist on the table.

The assembled group jumped and unconsciously said, "Right!" Brian smiled. "Nice to see that I can get a rise out of this astute group."

He went on, "Anyway, here is the interesting part of my analysis. There has been a movement of stock from institutional block investors to private investors purchasing shares. No single investor has holdings of over 5%, but we have a few new 3% investors. We have a tracking report that provides us with a heads up when a person or group gets to a 3% share level. Any corporation that believes it may be a potential candidate for a hostile takeover has this tracking system. Phillip wisely, asked me to implement this system last fall.

"Since the beginning of the fourth quarter of last year, when I started watching for new 3% shareholders there had been zero. That is zero until the April report. Since the first of April there are four new 3% shareholders. That isn't the only interesting fact. They all have addresses in the United States, but they also all have Japanese last names. They all purchased their shares through a discount brokerage house and hold their shares in their own names.

There is a broad geographical distribution...almost too much distribution. There is one in the Northeast, one in the South, one in the Midwest, and one in the West.

"As for selling short, I can't answer that question, but the reason that Husted was calling me was to ask me whether I knew of a reason why people would be selling short. I answered no and then he commented that a number of stockbroker friends had been calling him to ask him why there was a new trend to sell James short. Husted's comment didn't register with me until Carl wrote down his questions."

The expressions on the faces of the team were quizzical and slightly alarmed. J.P. tried to sum up their concerns. "What we have is a situation where there might be another player in our proxy party or NPC is not playing entirely up front with Mrs. James."

Nacheda answered the question, "I think it is safe to assume that the culprit is the NPC. From everything I have learned about them and the executives that make up the council, this type of action would fall into their style of managing situations. I am sorry I didn't see this happening before today. I should have anticipated this move. They only play by their rules. We should always assume that they are doing more than what they seem. A council that would hire and send Berger to the plantation wouldn't stop at anything to achieve their goals. I must apologize for my fellow countrymen, but all cultural societies have their good and bad points. Greed is a terrible driving force. We see it in Mrs. James, her friends, and the NPC. The religions of the world try to address the adversities of greed, but to no avail. We must watch for greed at every step in our process to win."

He concluded by saying, "We must conclude that it is the NPC that is trying to obtain more stock and they are using associates in the US to purchase stock for their takeover plans. The stock won't be registered in the NPC name, but you can be assured that the shares are controlled by the NPC. If there are four new shareholders with 3% that equals 12%. I would imagine that they are going for 15 to 20% ownership through this method."

J.P. spoke up, "Adding these shares to the shares Mrs. James and her lawyers control and we have a 40 to 50% obstacle to overcome in our proxy fight." The mood of the group was now distinctly down and was starting to take on an attitude of defeat.

"Look, everybody, we knew this battle was not going to be a slam-dunk. What we have heard today is just additional difficult obstacles to overcome with our own plan. We have a good plan. We have to believe in our plan or change what we are planning to counter Mrs. James. Our plan will be launched this weekend when we place advertisements supporting our position in the Sunday papers. Our plan will begin to turn the situation around and start to move things our way. Whether we get enough votes to win won't be decided until the annual meeting. Today some new obstacles have been placed in our path, but they have all been what I call unethical, not illegal. Both Mrs. James and the NPC are formidable competitors, but so are we and we haven't even begun to play. So cheer up and let's get on with the implementation of our plan. We have some fun days ahead of us and whether we win or lose we want them to know that they have been in a great proxy war and they have met a formidable player. Does everyone agree?" The faces hadn't brightened, but J.P. saw in their faces a firm determination to win.

9:00 A.M., TUESDAY, APRIL 25

NPC HEADQUARTERS OSAKA, JAPAN

Tanaguchi picked up his phone to call Mrs. James in her office at James as soon as all of the members of the NPC Board were assembled for this emergency meeting. The news of the ads by James had hit his desk yesterday. They had been emailed by five different NPC-employed James shareholders. Tanaguchi had called an emergency meeting of the NPC board to discuss the new turn of events. He had acknowledged the emails and asked that the shareholders send him a copy of the second set of proxy statements and ballots. They were to save the ballot they were going to use to vote. They were instructed to send the documentation to him as soon as possible.

It was 9:00 a.m., Tuesday in Japan and 4:00 p.m., Monday afternoon in New York City. Tanaguchi dialed Mrs. James' private office number and waited. As soon as Mrs. James picked up the telephone handset he placed the conversation on a speaker.

Before she could say anything he said, "Good afternoon, Mrs. James, I have again placed you on the speaker. I have the NPC board members here in the room where they can listen to our conversation and ask questions." Without waiting for a response, he moved rapidly along. "We would be most interested in what is going on back there concerning the two proxy statements and why you didn't inform us of this situation before we had to call you. You have our telephone number, do you not?" He continued again not giving her a chance to respond. "I also assume you have seen the other," the word other had a very spiteful tone to it as he spoke, "proxy statement and ballot and have sent either the original or a copy to us." He stopped abruptly and waited.

Mrs. James was either thinking about her answer or waiting for him to continue and she didn't answer immediately. When she did answer there was noticeable anger, frustration, and uncertainty in the voice that came from the speaker.

"I..I was just informed of the second proxy statement myself on Saturday morning. I am sorry, but I didn't think to send a copy to you. I will have one sent via courier service this afternoon. I didn't inform you because I am trying to assess the situation and wanted to give you a complete report when I called." Her voice was taking on a more confident tone as she continued. "I was planning to call you within the hour, but since you called I can give you and your board the situation report. Is that satisfactory?" Now her voice was very confident and a little on the authoritative side.

The first thought Tanaguchi had was to immediately berate her. He had second thoughts and then decided to let her talk. He wanted to find out what was happening as soon as possible in order to make decisions on what NPC should do with the James Project. Do they cancel the project, take their losses and start again with another pharmaceutical company, or should they stick with the investment they had made in James? The second proxy statement had done a better job of driving down the James stock than anything Director Kawaguchi could have planted in the press. The stock opened Monday at the Friday close of $95, by afternoon it had dropped to $85. His US purchasers were still buying. He had not shut them off, for the moment. But after this conversation with Mrs.

James, the NPC board would make a new resolution on stock purchases.

Tanaguchi said, "Please go ahead with your assessment, Mrs. James."

"I have come to the conclusion that they are doing too little, too late. We already have 30% of the stock committed with my shares and the board members who support us. All we need is an additional 21% and we are winners. My lawyers advise me that for the other party to get 51% of the shares without a starting major block of stock is nearly impossible. This group of rebels doesn't have enough money to exercise their own stock options. Besides their options would not equate to more than 8%."

Tanaguchi did a quick calculation. Her 30% plus the NPC 15% was 45%, yes he could feel confident in her getting 51%. Another five plus percentage was easy. Surely she would get that many votes from the common shareholders.

Tanaguchi interrupted her, "Very well, Mrs. James that is all well and good, but who is the 'they' that you keep referring to in your explanation?"

"I apologize again, Mr. Tanaguchi, I forgot that you didn't know who comprises the other side."

Stupid woman he said to himself and was sure the rest of the board was thinking the same thing. He was glad that after this was all over she would be out of the picture.

Mrs. James' voice was droning on over the speaker about how there was no worry and then she gave the names, "Dr. Bradsmith is, of course, the key member of the opposition. He is being helped by the VP of Marketing, Mrs. Amanda Hayes and Dr. J.P. Koenig, a consultant. I really don't think they can sustain this proxy fight. They just don't have the resources. They are using the James Employees' Association as a forum to gain support. You were able to see that in the newspaper advertisements."

"Was there any mention of Bandai Pharmaceuticals Company in the other proxy report?" A note of concern was in Tanaguchi's voice, but Mrs. James missed the inflection in her desire to please him.

"There was a small mention in the plan that James was going to receive a license to use a Bandai Pharmaceuticals Company extraction process for the Devil Tree bark alkaloid. I didn't think this announcement was important to our plans because of the NPC strength in Japan. I had thought that this license could be re-negotiated after the annual meeting. In fact I thought this was an advantage to us. We, Dr. Wahlters and I, weren't aware of this discovery." Tanaguchi looked around the table and the other members were shaking their heads in the negative. They hadn't heard of the new Bandai process.

"Well Mrs. James, you have made a good assessment. Could you please tell me who are the people the other side has placed up for election to the board of directors?"

"Yes, yes, I have the names right here." Her voice reflected her desire to please and pride that she had anticipated his question. "They are not very important people. There is, of course, Dr. Bradsmith and Dr. Koenig. Then there is a group of seven prominent physicians, pharmacists, and regulatory professionals. They aren't the best in their fields, but I have been told that they are recognizable names to people in the industry. The final person is from Bandai Pharmaceuticals Company, you know, the company I mentioned. His name is Dr. Nakasone. Do you know him?"

"Yes, Mrs. James, we know him." His voice sounded like he was talking to a small child. "He is well known here in Japan, but thought of as an outsider. He will be of no concern to us. The others don't concern you or your lawyers?" He formed the last statement as a question.

"The only concern my lawyer friends had," her shallow laughter was heard over the speaker, "was that there were no lawyers in the group. They said that was stupid of them. I personally think it was smart of them to include customers. In the future, when this is all over I think I will remove some of my lawyers and finance people in favor of customers. I think it was a good move, but the thought behind the move will be lost on the shareholders. We have no concern over their proposed board."

"Fine, Mrs. James, thank you very much. Keep us better informed next time," Tanaguchi said as he broke the connection.

He looked around at the rest of the board and said, "Well, you heard the same thing I did. Do we have a problem?"

Director Hideo Okamoto, who had hardly said anything in the previous meetings was the first to request to be heard. He was the president of a small biomedical company south of Nagasaki. He was a quiet man, but well respected. If the truth were known, he was the most respected of the NPC members. He had tried to obtain a position on the Japanese Pharmaceutical Association board or at least on one of their powerful committees, but the JMA elders felt that he was too young and didn't have the correct family background. They had remarked to themselves that he should be required to wait for a few years. They told him that certainly in the future he would be given the opportunity to be on one of the committees, but not anytime in the foreseeable future. Okamoto dropped his company's membership in the JPA and joined the NPC. This surprised the conservative JPA. It surprised them more when the NPC gave him a position on their board. The move was quickly rationalized that both Okamoto and the NPC were good for each other, both were radical outsiders to the industry. The JPA reputation was intact.

Director Okamoto spoke in a quiet, but authoritative voice. When a person first heard his voice they were surprised at how well the voice carried in a room and how much authority it seemed to command. Every other member quickly stopped trying to get Mr. Tanaguchi's attention and let Okamoto have the floor.

I do not pretend to know as much about international business as you gentlemen, but I would recommend that we take positive action to ensure our success.

Do you have any suggestions, Director Okamoto? Tanaguchi asked.

Okamoto carefully folded his hands in front of himself. They were carefully laid on top of his stack of notes. If anyone bothered to look at his notes they would have found that the characters were very precise. The margins were precisely even all the way down the paper. They were not aligned by a printed margin, but by Mr. Okamoto himself.

"*Hai, doumoarigatou* Chairman Tanaguchi. I think we should counter the advertisements of the James Employees' Association. They are probably painting the NPC as the knight on the black horse and not the savior that we know we are to James Pharmaceutical Company. We know Mrs. James isn't good for James. We aren't sure of the other officers and there are always good people that are casualties of every war. We must inform the shareholders about NPC and what we are capable of doing for James. We must have our own public relations program." Again he went silent.

"What do the rest of you think of Director Okamoto's idea?" Tanaguchi asked the others on the council board.

After a short discussion they all agreed that the idea was good. Even though subconsciously they knew they weren't going to provide James with very much actual support. They did know that the James Project would provide a vehicle to earn a great deal of money for the members of the NPC.

"Director Okamoto you are designated as the board member in charge of this project. You have a budget of 500,000 yen. Please keep me informed and I will keep the rest of the board informed.

"Are there anymore comments or changes from last Friday's meeting?" Tanaguchi asked.

"Chairman Tanaguchi," Director Otani, the man in charge of the stock purchases, asked to be acknowledged, "do you wish us to continue to purchase James stock?"

"Ah, thank you, Director Otani. I suggest we keep to our objective of achieving 15%. With the price dropping more rapidly, we should benefit by purchasing at a lower average share price. To every disadvantage, there is an advantage, eh?" and he chuckled to himself. No one else thought it was funny.

"Sir," Kawaguchi, in charge of the rumors, asked for Tanaguchi's attention and then continued, "I will work with Director Okamoto on the public relations program." Kawaguchi was inwardly insulted that Okamoto had been given the project. He knew he had done a very good job with the rumor press releases. He should have received the honor of implementing the public relations program. He thought to himself, the least he would do is assist Okamoto and perhaps steal some of the honor of success in this effort as well as the recognition that he had already earned with the press release rumor project.

"As you wish," replied Tanaguchi.

"Chairman Tanaguchi, sir," spoke up Akai, the director in charge of watching the stock price. "With the announcement of the proxy fight, Monday's stock price dropped again. I would predict the ultimate price we will pay Mrs. James could go as low as $40." To patronize Tanaguchi, he added. "As you would say Chairman Tanaguchi, another advantage, eh?"

As a rebuke Tanaguchi answered "I am sorry Director Akai, but I don't agree. A share price below $40 would be more of a disadvantage. Everyone has a lower level. She might not want to sell if the stock goes too low. Then, Director Akai, we will have to pay a higher bonus. You have to think through the entire issue Director Akai, and not jump to the easy conclusion."

Tanaguchi looked away from Akai's reddening face and looked to Fujinami, "Any security problems, Director Fujinami?"

After the rebuttal to Akai, who now had his head bowed so low his forehead was hovering over the table, Fujinami thought it was best to keep quiet.

"None sir," was all Fujinami said.

"Thank you gentlemen for coming to this emergency meeting. Perhaps the meeting wasn't necessary, but upon hearing about the second proxy, I was suspicious that Mrs. James had a situation she hadn't expected and had no counter plan. I now see my suspicions were true. She didn't expect, nor had she a plan, to overcome these most recent developments, but it is obvious that we are still in control and have a share advantage that the opposition can't very easily overcome. I will call you if there is a reason for us to get back together before our next scheduled meeting of Friday, the 19th of May. Good morning." He got up from the table and left the room.

After he left there was a great deal of conversation around the proxy fight issue. The topics centered on whether the NPC was doing the right thing with the James Project. Again Okamoto spoke up and everyone turned to listen.

He stood up and said three words, "We are winning," and he left the room.

Akai turned to Fujinami and said, "Man of few words!"

"Weird," the young Umeta interjected and they all left the room to return to their companies and allowed the running of the council up to Chairman Tanaguchi.

8:00 A.M., THURSDAY, MAY 24

SPECTRUM OF MEDICINE BUILDING
NEW YORK CITY

J.P. stared out the window and looked down at the park along the Hudson River. The large oaks, ashes, and maples were taking on a green hue caused by their budding leaves. The dogwoods and cherry trees were all in bloom. The view from the eighth floor was a mint green, pink, white, and brown collage. The grass was still slightly on the brown side and there were many brown areas in the tree foliage where the leaf buds had not started. The day was very clear without even a light haze. The day before there had been a series of showers move through and cleaned the city. It was even warm for a late May morning. The temperature was already 50 degrees.

Earlier that morning Mandi and he had decided that it was such a beautiful morning that they would walk to work. He had called Roberto and told him that they would walk to work. Over the last few months, Roberto had become Mandi and J.P.'s chauffeur. Whenever either of them needed transportation they called Roberto who responded almost immediately.

The walk to the Spectrum of Medicine building had been invigorating, but also slightly depressing for the two of them. Mandi and he had walked hand in hand, but quietly. They were both aware that his work on the James project was coming to an end. All that remained to do was wait for the final outcome of the shareholders vote.

It had been a month since the ballots had been sent to the shareholders. The shareholders who hadn't already voted by proxy would cast their ballots that afternoon and be counted along with the proxy ballots. At 2:10, Brian, acting as the Secretary of James Pharmaceutical Corporation, would announce the members of the new board of directors. No matter what the outcome, his original two-month project would end after four months.

As they neared the building they could see the large circus tent that had been erected on the grass mall between the Spectrum of Medicine Building and Westside Highway. The city of New York provided the tent for the James annual meetings as part of their thank you for the James headquarters remaining in the city. It was a very large circus tent and was rumored to have belonged to the Barnum and Bailey Circus when they had held their tented circus in Central Park before moving to Madison Square Garden.

J.P. turned to Mandi, "Would you like a small piece of trivia?" He realized that he must have intruded on her inner thoughts, because she reacted in a startled manner.

"What? Huh? What did you say?"

"I said, would you like a small piece of trivia?"

"Well," Mandi turned to him and smiled, "as long as it is a happy piece of trivia."

"You knew the tent was from the Barnum and Bailey Circus, right?"

She nodded her head in agreement. Her long red hair bounced from her shoulders. She was wearing a navy blue blazer and matching skirt under her tan raincoat.

"Well, P.T. Barnum grew up in Bridgeport, Connecticut where he became famous. The P.T. Barnum festival is still held annually in Bridgeport. Our annual meeting tent was borrowed from Bridgeport."

"Really, J.P., I will cherish that piece of trivia for the rest of my life," she said sarcastically. Then she added, "I wonder what manner of fools will emerge from today's meeting. Will it be us or Mrs. James?"

"I wish I knew, but whatever happens we put up a good fight," he answered squeezing her hand.

She squeezed back and they lapsed back into silence.

As they walked towards the Spectrum of Medicine building, they could see that the tent was huge and commanded their view. The morning sun had played its rainbow trick off the Spectrum of Medicine Building. The colors of the rainbow were reflected onto the tent turning the canvas into gigantic pyramid movie screen. The tent was ablaze with color. P.T. Barnum would have loved the effect, as would old Doc James. James Pharmaceutical Company needed Doc James today to hold his company together. The outcome wasn't going to be a rainbow of colored beauty like the spectrum that bounced off of the building and tent. It was going to be black or white. There wasn't going to be a compromise, no shades of gray and certainly no rainbow. Fights didn't produce rainbows except in the minds of the defeated after they had been severely beaten.

As J.P. sat looking out the window of his office, his thoughts turned from memories of earlier that morning to what was to come later that day. So much had been done in a short period of time. When the team meeting ended the day after the April board meeting the proxy fight began. Mrs. James learned about their counter plan on the Saturday after the board meeting when Brian telephoned her. He told her that on Monday there would be two sets of proxy statements and ballots to be sent out to the shareholders. She had demanded an explanation. Brian responded that the SEC had instructed him that this was the procedure for a company when the shareholders had to choose between two sets of board of directors. She had asked for the second slate of directors and he replied that he would send her a copy of the two sets by messenger and then hung ᵘp.

Since that Monday in April, there had been no communication between the two sides. Their Employees' Association plan had kicked in on Sunday, April 26th. They had taken a chance that the association would side with Phillip. Mandi had bought, with J.P.'s own money, a half-page advertisement in the Sunday <u>New York Times</u>, <u>Chicago Tribune</u>, and <u>Los Angeles Times</u> business sections. She had two announcements ready. One was an announcement to James shareholders from James Pharmaceutical Company that they would be receiving two proxy statements and ballots. The shareholders were to read each of them carefully before voting. The second was the same announcement, but it was from the James Employee Association (JEA), not the James Pharmaceutical Company. It gave the same information but also said that the JEA supported the James plan as presented by Dr. Bradsmith and they definitely didn't support the Nippon Pharmaceutical Council plan for James. The strategy was to attack the NPC Japanese connection as having a controlling influence over the future of James.

On the Monday evening after the meeting at the apartment, Mandi had set up a special meeting with the association. By then the employees knew something was happening with James management. They didn't know what, but the rumor mill had churned up enough interest that when Mandi had the president of the JEA call an emergency meeting for Monday night, all officers and a large quorum of members were in attendance.

When Brian had informed Mrs. James of the two plans on the previous Saturday, he had also asked her to attend the 7:00 p.m. Monday JEA meeting. She had declined. That had left the task of explaining the two plans up to Brian, the secretary of the corporation. Brian did the best job anyone could have done considering the situation. Under Carl's advice, they recorded the meeting. Under the deepest scrutiny, no one could accuse the secretary of being biased towards one plan or the other. In fact, he oversold the NPC plan as Mrs. James' plan was now being called.

At 8:00 p.m. the James Employees' Association approved a motion to support the James Plan and reject the NPC Plan. They would support the James Plan by advertising in the news media and encourage all shareholders to vote for the James Plan. On Tuesday, a new advertisement was run in three New York newspapers, the <u>Wall Street Journal,</u> and every newspaper in the US with a circulation over 500,000. The advertisement was addressed to James Pharmaceutical Company shareholders and customers. It went into detail about the two plans. It even had a matrix comparing both plans. Addressing the advertisement to shareholders and customers was about as close they could get to asking customers to purchase James stock and vote. Since it was the employees and not the company itself, then they could make the subtle sell to the customers. Brokers and customers picked up on the hint.

The JEA campaign went on until mid-May. The effects of the public relations program weren't readily apparent to anyone. Brian had reviewed the stock movement daily and could only come to the conclusion that there was heavy volume movement with the James stock. In fact over the last two weeks, the James stock had been one of the top five in share volume movement.

When J.P. had asked Brian whether the plan was working. Brian had replied that he honestly didn't know and that he wouldn't be able to obtain copies of the shareholder printouts until after the annual meeting.

The downward trend of the stock had slowed over the last month and it had closed at $60 the day before. This quieted the doomsday sayers who said that the stock would go below $50 by the annual meeting.

Mrs. James had started her own public relations campaign. It was mostly to do with the advantages of the pending NPC-James agreement and what the NPC could do for James. The feedback had been mixed to negative. J.P. had met with Jack Husted the week of April 30th. He gave Husted a copy of a secret report that he had written on all the activities of Mrs. James and the NPC. He made the journalist promise not to divulge the source of the information, but otherwise told him to use the information in any ethical way he desired.

Husted had been stunned by the sequence of events and was pleased to have hard information. J.P. had included copies of the pictures that Nacheda had provided. Jack had asked why James wasn't using the information to fight Mrs. James and the NPC. J.P. had answered his question by saying that they felt that by disclosing the information, the fight would turn into a dirty proxy fight of lies and half-truths. As it was, the proxy fight was going to be hard enough on James' future. No matter who won it was most important for the company to survive. They felt the criminal information would be too much for James corporate reputation to withstand. Therefore they had decided to use only positive information in selling the James Plan as the right plan.

Husted felt that they should have used some of the information especially when it contradicted the information that was fed to the New York Evening News. On Thursday, April 27th, Husted's column in the Wall Street Journal was a masterpiece. This article and many more that followed between that date and the present more than justified J.P.'s decision to let Jack Husted in on the total picture. Husted became an unbiased ally and helped James gain back some of the corporate credibility that had been lost within the financial world. The brokers regained confidence and helped to sell stock to their customers.

J.P. still had a copy of Husted's column on his desk. He picked it up and began reading it again.

Over the last number of weeks numerous articles have been printed by the general press concerning the James Pharmaceutical Company. Many of my readers were surprised that the initiator of the articles was a paper new to the New York newspaper scene and that I had not written the articles. They wrote I had probably lost contact with the current events of the pharmaceutical industry. I must tell you that at times the information was so dramatic that I began to question myself.

Last Saturday an independent consultant contacted me. He requested that I keep my sources anonymous. He provided me with a report documenting numerous activities that make up, what might be called the true James story. This information isn't insider information, but events that have taken place over the last few months and tell a different story than what has been written in the general press.

I haven't decided how to use this information, but you will be able to decide for yourself as I tell the story as best I can without betraying the source of the information.

Today I want to write a different column. The remainder of this column will be what would be classified in today's industry, a negative story.

This reporter always investigates everything before I write my column. That is why you didn't see any response from me concerning the rumors about James. Yes, that is what they were, rumors. Some of my readers either purchased or sold stock based on these rumors. You either made or lost money and, as the future unfolds, your decisions will be judged as good or bad. The outcome is important, but the outcome isn't important to the issue in this column. The issue is, you made your buy or sell decision on rumors spread and given credibility by reporters trying to sell newspapers.

The SEC, ethical financial reporters, and the ethical financial media don't report rumors, they report facts. If it's not a fact, they will inform the reader in the written text what the information is based upon. Many times the WSJ will be late with dramatic information because we have to do our homework. Others and ourselves don't jump at information that isn't verified letting time prove or disprove what was written.

I don't entirely blame the reporter or the newspaper in question. They were trying to establish themselves in a highly competitive media market. I give them some credit because they did enough research to give the stories credence. My research, on the other hand, went way beyond the other reporters research activities.

When I researched the stories, I couldn't find the hard core proof that I felt I had to have before giving the story credibility in my column. I also blame the investor and those that give the investor advice. You jump too soon. If you know you are taking a higher risk than the SEC intends for you to take, that is your choice, but then don't blame the financial industry for your loss.

I want to thank my benefactor for giving me the opportunity to print the truth about the James stories in my upcoming columns.

Over the next three weeks Husted published six columns on the James story. They weren't all favorable articles, but they were the truth. His articles helped to keep the stock from a total slide to below $50.00. He also included information on what was currently going on with the proxy fight. His articles didn't exactly help the James plan, but more importantly they didn't help Mrs. James or the NPC. His articles were able to paint a different picture of the NPC than what Mrs. James' public relations program was trying to paint.

Husted's articles talked about the potential of JPC138 with the combination of the James capability and the Bandai isolation process. They highlighted the agreement with Clintech, Bill Williams' company, and how the diagnosis of arrhythmias was going to help Lifeal. J.P. thought the most positive message concerned the true feelings of the employees and how they felt that the James Plan, as presented by Dr. Bradsmith. Husted noted that he felt that this plan was the best for the James customers, patients, and employees.

As for a likely outcome, J.P. was still unsure about that. He knew that Mrs. James had too much of a lead on them and too many shares for J.P. to feel comfortable or confident regarding their chances. If their assessment of the NPC purchases was correct, the NPC now had five holders of 3% each for a total of 15%. Added to Mrs. James' 30% and they had 45% in the bag.

There was still a chance to win. As long as there was a chance, J.P.'s team decided to go for the win. Last weekend Mandi and he had spent hours going over the plan and the final week of the fight. They wrote two speeches for Phillip. One was in case they were winners going in and the other was a final ditch effort. The one chance they had was that the deciding votes would be cast from the audience. There were a large number of shares still unaccounted for and many large shareholders had told them that they would attend the meeting and cast their votes after listening to Phillip and Mrs.

James. If anything, J.P. figured that they had stopped Mrs. James and the NPC from having a slam-dunk.

J.P. looked at his physical reflection in the window and noted that he had gained a little weight since leaving Mammoth in January. Not much chance to have a routine exercise program, he rationalized. He decided that he was still trim for an executive his age. His usual tan was barely evident. His mental state was in great shape. Probably the best shape in years, maybe the best in his life. He attributed this to his relationship with Mandi and the project that they had lived with for the past several months. He had met a person in Mandi whom he loved dearly and yet remained a friend and business associate. She was many people in one person. Their personal characters matched as perfectly as he had ever experienced.

He started to wonder about what would happen to their relationship after the annual meeting? What would be their career goals and where will the goals fit into their personal lives.

"I'm too old for her," he muttered out loud.

Then he realized that he was simply using the answer that all mature men use when they fall in love with a younger woman.

"I belong in Mammoth and Mandi belongs here."

He stopped himself. He was making decisions for both of them and that wasn't fair. It was also not what they had agreed to last Sunday night lying in their bed discussing the dreaded subject of what would become of them after the annual meeting. They had decided that the decision that they made had to be a joint decision and that it was okay to delay that decision. J.P. liked the last option. He wasn't ready for a decision even though he knew, in his heart that a decision had to be made.

He looked at his watch, 11:30. Two and a half more hours before the outcome of all of their work would be known. He went downstairs and left the building. Everyone else was occupied preparing for the annual meeting. There was nothing he personally had to do except wait. He was troubled over Phillip's insistence that he be a director on the new board if they won. He really didn't want to be on the board.

He left the building and started walking towards Central Park. The sidewalk was crowded. He always enjoyed spring in New York City. Everyone took walks whenever they had the time and the city seemed more alive than any other time of the year.

His plan for lunch was to purchase a couple of New York City sidewalk hot dogs with kraut and mustard and drink a Yahoo. After eating he decided he would walk around the park until about 1:30 and then make his way back to the tent by two. He figured that he would arrive back at the tent at just about the time that everyone had taken their seats.

After getting his lunch from a cart on the Avenue of the Americas, he walked to Central Park and sat beneath the nearest tree. At the base of the tree he spread out his handkerchief and sat down. The Central Park trees were as beautiful looking up from ground level as the Hudson River park trees had looked from the eighth floor of the Spectrum of Medicine Building. He bit into his hot dog and savored the flavor of the juicy fat. New York street corner dogs were some of the best hot dogs in the world. He finished his hot dogs and leaned back against the tree. There was a slight breeze and he felt free. Free for the first time in months.

He dozed off. The next thing he knew, his chin bumped his chest and he suddenly awoke. When he looked at his watch it was 1:20. He quickly got up, picked up the lunch trash, and his handkerchief. He noted a trash bin a reasonable distance away and took a quick jump shot to deposit the trash. He started his walk back to James and to the shareholders decision as to who was going to run James.

2:00 P.M., THURSDAY, MAY 24

MEETING TENT OUTSIDE THE SPECTRUM OF MEDICINE BUILDING NEW YORK CITY

J.P. slipped into the back of the large tent and remained standing in the rear. He looked around the tent. There was seating in the tent for 500 people and it looked almost full. The bright afternoon sun made the inside of the tent very light inside.

He was surprised and happy to see Nacheda, Dr. Nakasone, and the rest of the proxy team. He couldn't find Carl, Sr., but remembered that Carl had told him that he didn't know if he should be present. He saw Jack Husted and Bill and Janet Williams. Most of Phillip's friends were sitting on the left side of the tent. On the right side, J.P. could see Dr. Helmut Wahlters sitting with a dignified-looking Japanese man. He wondered if this was the infamous Mr. Tanaguchi.

At the far end of the tent was the dais on which the current board was seated in a line separated by the lectern, which was positioned in the middle of the dais. The group on the dais was split into two groups. Mrs. James was to one side of the lectern with her appointed board members. On the other side of the lectern sat Phillip and his board members. At the far end of Phillip's side sat the corporation secretary, Brian. The dais seating matched the way the audience was seated with Phillip's supporters on one side of the tent and Mrs. James' supporters on the other side.

J.P. noted that there were more people on Phillip's side of the tent, which he decided was to be expected because he had more individual shareholder support, but his supporters had fewer shares than Mrs. James' shareholders.

At exactly 2:00 p.m., Mrs. James got up from her chair and moved to a position behind the speaker's lectern. She brought her gavel down on the wooden surface of the lectern.

Mrs. James looked the part of a corporate chairperson of the board of directors. Her shoulder length blond hair was pulled back and wound in a bun behind her head. She had a very stylish navy blue hat that matched her navy blue suit. The jacket was double breasted and she had on a white silk blouse with a navy blue scarf that was loosely tied around her neck. The buttons of the jacket were gold.

"The annual meeting of shareholders of James Pharmaceutical Company is officially called to order. My name is Mrs. Evelyn PrestonJames. I'm your chairperson of the board of directors. I want to welcome our many shareholders to this annual shareholder meeting. Once we conclude our official business and adjourn the formal meeting, I would be very happy to answer any pertinent questions. Please, if possible, save your questions until then."

Like most annual meetings, the James annual meeting had two sections. The first was an official board meeting and the second, an informal question and answer period. J.P. found an empty chair in the last row and sat down to await the shareholders' verdict.

Mrs. James went on, "Notice of this meeting was duly given to stockholders of record as of April 21st of this year. A copy of the notice and the accompanying proxy statements are inserted in our Corporate Minutes Book along with a copy of the Certificate of Mailing. The meeting, therefore is lawfully and properly convened.

"Mr. Brian Smith, our chief financial officer and secretary of the corporation has been appointed to act in the capacity of inspector of elections for this meeting. Mr. Smith would you please tell us whether or not a quorum is present?"

Brian stood at his place behind the dais, "Yes there is, Madam Chairperson.

At 2:05 she said, "Mr. Secretary would you please present the financial report.

Mrs. James sat down and Brian moved to the lectern. Brian had on a double-breasted black thin pinstriped suit with a lavender tie that complemented his light lavender pinstriped shirt. He looked very dignified.

He addressed the shareholders, "Madam Chairperson, board directors, Dr. Bradsmith, James Pharmaceutical Company shareholders. The James board of directors and the accounting firm of Thomas and Thomas of New York City have reviewed the financials. They were certified and sent to shareholders of record as of April 21st of this year. If there are any questions the board and officers of the company will answer them during the period following the official board meeting." He then returned to his seat and sat down.

J.P. looked at Brian's facial expression to see if he could get any indication of how the shareholders vote had gone. He actually looked pleased.

Compared to the rest of the board, who looked so serious that it was depressing, J.P. thought that Brian looked relaxed and actually had a slight smile.

At 2:07, Mrs. James again assumed her position at the lectern and addressed

Brian again, "Mr. Secretary, would you now read the results of the shareholder vote for proposal number five, ratification of appointment of independent audits tors.

"The board of directors, upon a recommendation of its audit committee, has reappointed the accounting firm of Thomas & Thomas as James' independent auditors for the coming fiscal year. Are there any comments?" Mrs. James' and Brian's eyes scanned the room.

Seeing no hands raised for comment, Mrs. James said, "If not, I would be pleased to entertain a motion for ratification of the reappointment of Thomas & Thomas as independent auditors for James Pharmaceutical Company."

From the middle of the room came the voice of one of the James employees, "I make the motion to reappoint Thomas & Thomas as our independent auditors."

Mrs. James said, "Thank you. Do we have a second to this motion?" Again from the audience came a voice, "I second the motion."

"What is the voting on this motion?" Mrs. James asked turning to Brian for the answer.

Brian answered, "The motion is carried."

Mrs. James said, "The appointment of Thomas & Thomas as independent auditors for the coming fiscal year is hereby ratified."

At 2:09 p.m., she paused and confidently went on, "Now we turn to the item of business today and that is the election of directors for ensuing years. The company's proposed slate, as set forth in the corporate developed proxy statement sent to shareholders of record as of April 21st, consists of James board of directors. At the same time and within the bylaws of the corporation a second proxy statement was mailed which listed management's proposed slate of directors.

Mr. Smith will you please report the results of the voting," and sat down in her chair next to the lectern.

As Brian again moved to the lectern, J.P. tried to compare the two groups on the stage. They all looked very serious, but to his eyes, the Mrs. James group looked more confident. Brian reached the lectern. The moment had arrived. J.P. looked at Phillip seated up on the dais. His eyes were staring directly ahead. He had probably fixed them on some distant object at the back of the tent.

"Ladies and gentlemen shareholders," Brian began. Almost immediately there was a murmur from the audience. He was starting his report of the vote count as though he were going to give a speech. He continued in a very official manner, "I have been asked by the shareholders representing institutional investment groups to exercise paragraph 23 of the James Pharmaceutical Company corporate bylaws."

Mrs. James started to get up to protest the change in format. Brian, lightly placed his left hand on her right shoulder and kept her from rising.

"Please, Madam Chairperson, this request is within the bounds of the corporate bylaws of which we must abide." She slumped back into her chair to listen to the secretary read paragraph 23. Her members of the board were hurriedly trying to find paragraph 23 in their copy of the corporate bylaws.

"Paragraph 23 reads as follows, any shareholder with due cause may exercise his or her rights to retract or withhold their vote for the board of directors and demand a discussion of the issues before again submitting said votes. Due cause has to be submitted to the secretary prior to the commencement of the annual shareholders meeting and it is the secretary's duty alone to evaluate the validity of the due cause request before taking action. The chairman of the board may call for a vote of the shareholders present to determine whether the request for discussion should, in fact, go forward. If 20% of the shareholders present vote to go to discussion, then discussion shall take place. The secretary will lead the discussion." As he was reading the paragraph I could see the amazed interest on the faces of Phillip and his side of the dais. Mrs. James was staring at Brian as if she could not believe her ears. Her lawyer board members were madly reading the bylaws and her financial members were just staring forward, not looking very interested in the events that were taking place around them.

Just then, Mrs. James started to get up again. "I'm sorry Madam Chairperson, but unless you want to contest the bylaws that you have duly sworn to uphold when you took the position of chairperson of the James Pharmaceutical board, you haven't been recognized by myself, the secretary." She again slumped even farther into her chair.

Brian went on, "The secretary recognizes Dr. Petersburg, Director of the American Association of Retired Teachers Retirement Fund. Dr. Petersburg." Brian's hand again restrained Mrs. James and added, "Dr. Petersburg, please proceed to one of the microphones in the aisles. Thank you."

A very dignified gentleman who looked to be over sixty years of age began his slow walk to one of the many microphones that stood on stands in the middle of the aisles. They had been placed in the aisles for the question and answer session. Dr. Petersburg was thin and tan. His silver gray hair and gray speckled beard gave him a look of knowledge and experience. As he made his way to the microphone J.P. again looked at the board members sitting on the dais. Mrs. James was red faced. Her lips were pressed together. She was definitely holding back her anger. J.P. knew that her plan had just hit a bump in the road.

Dr. Petersburg adjusted the microphone to his height. He stood straight and didn't lean down to the microphone like many tall men tended to do when speaking into a microphone. He knew how to command presence. "Ladies and gentlemen, fellow James Pharmaceutical Company shareholders." The people in the room made an audible sound. His voice was a very clear bass with a slight academic accent.

"I represent the American Association of Retired Teachers Retirement Fund. We have at our disposal more than two billion dollars of investments that we control for our retired teachers.

"I also represent the following other institutional shareholders and their votes....Dr. Goldsmith, Director of the American Chemical Scientists Retirement Fund. Dr. Myerson, Director of the American Pharmacists Retirement Fund. Mr. Ponchinelli, Director of the Allied Chemical Workers Retirement Fund. Mrs. Hamerschmidt, Director of the Retired Nurses Retirement Fund.

"I believe that the secretary has verified our credentials. Is that correct, Mr. Secretary?"

Brian, still standing behind the lectern replied, "That is correct Dr. Petersburg. I met with each of the five representatives and verified their credentials and the reported number of shares and votes that each of them represents." He remained standing. He continued to prevent Mrs. James from taking over the lectern and microphone.

Dr. Petersburg continued, "In accordance with paragraph 23 of the bylaws, I must show just cause in order in invoke a shareholder discussion as to the issues surrounding the voting for a new board of directors and what they represent. My justification is as follows, on April 1st of this year the share price of James was $125.00. Today the price is $60.00 a drop of $65.00 or 52 percent. Converting this to shares of the five retirement funds that I am representing here at this microphone it is a substantial loss to people who have, in general, lost their individual earning power and must live on social security and the earnings from their retirement funds. If this isn't just cause enough for discussion we must demand to know what is going on between the two James groups and to demand that they discuss their plans for the future in this forum. With the stock at its present low level we don't want to sell our holdings, but we must do so if we don't have confidence in the future of James. The risk is too great for our retirees who want us, the fund directors to make conservative investments. A 52% drop in share price in almost two months on top of a proxy fight is anything but conservative.

"We the directors of these funds withdraw our block votes for the Mrs. James slate of directors and will hold our vote until we hear from both sides of the proxy fight. I think Robert's Rules of Order requires a motion at this point. I make a motion that there be an open discussion on the two platforms presented to the shareholders and that the shareholders present have the opportunity to resubmit their vote once the discussion has concluded. Thank you Madam Chairperson and Mr. Secretary." Dr. Petersburg then returned to his seat and sat down.

Brian spoke into the microphone. "The group of shares that Dr. Petersburg represents equates to 20% of the shares of James Pharmaceutical Company."

"Mr. Secretary, Mr. Secretary may I please be recognized?" A middleaged woman, slightly on the heavy side was standing next to a microphone half way back on the left side of the tent.

"Yes, Mrs. Little, you are recognized."

"Madam Chairperson, Mr. Secretary, fellow James employees and shareholders, I am Mrs. Jeanna Little, president of the James Employees' Association. As the name suggests, we represent 1,000 employees of James. We second the motion for a discussion of the different plans. Thank you." She returned to her chair.

All at once there were hundreds of hands waving to be recognized. There was no noise, just hands waving in the air. From J.P.'s perspective from the back of the room it looked like a cornfield with the stalks waving back and forth with the wind.

Brian calmly leaned toward the microphone and announced, "If the requests for recognition are to encourage a discussion of the issues between the two plans, I hereby ask for a vote by a show of hands. All those in favor of the motion for discussion, raise your hands." Nearly every hand in the tent went up. "Thank you. Those opposed, please raise your hands." About twenty people raised their hands. "Thank you, the vote for discussion carries." There was a sudden outburst of applause.

Brian continued, "I have researched the procedure on discussion and there is none specified. The discussion period is left up to the secretary. As the secretary, I set the following discussion protocol. I will ask Mrs. James and Dr. Bradsmith to present their views and plans in a talk that will last no longer than thirty minutes each. I defer to Madam Chairperson her choice as to who will go first. Madam Chairperson?"

J.P. couldn't hear her reply, but her face showed anger. Brian spoke into the microphone, "Mrs. James chooses to follow Dr. Bradsmith. Madam Chairperson, I, as the corporate secretary, ask that you announce a thirty minute recess to allow you and Dr. Bradsmith an opportunity to prepare your presentations."

One hand was waving for recognition and the man was saying, "Mr. Secretary, Mr. Secretary, a question of protocol please."

Brian recognized the man. He stayed next to his seat and asked, "My name is Mr. Stark and I only own 100 shares, but I am interested in the future of James because my grandfather has Alzheimer's. Will there be a real discussion after the presentations?"

"No sir. As an explanation, the word 'discussion' as stated in the context of the Corporate Bylaws, means presentation with no discussion. You will have to make up your mind on how you will vote after hearing from the two speakers. Discussion will take place after the formal board meeting is adjourned. I am sorry, but this is the way the rules read." Brian paused.

"Before a recess I would like to clarify the voting procedure. If you voted by proxy and are in attendance you can resubmit your vote. Those not in attendance will have their votes counted as filed by mail. After the discussion and when the vote is called for, I will be prepared to change any votes as long as the person changing the votes shows proper credentials. I will ask a representative of each of the two groups to bear witness to the credential certification and voting. Each shareholder changing their votes will be asked to sign the computer sheet indicating a change in vote from their proxy vote. If there are any questions I will try and answer them during the thirty-minute break. The time is now 2:30. Please be back in your chairs and ready for the discussion at 3:00. There are refreshments outside in the rear of the tent. The refreshments were planned for the after-meeting reception, but I'm sure that there is enough for this unscheduled recess as well. Madam Chairman, you may now temporarily suspend the board meeting for thirty minutes." Brian moved back to his chair at the end of the dais.

Mrs. James stood up and took up the gravel. Her face was red and taut with tension. Her voice was steady, but it wasn't the same polished voice that had started the meeting just a short thirty minutes before.

She pounded the gravel and announced, "The James Pharmaceutical Company annual meeting is recessed for thirty minutes, please return at 3:00 p.m. Thank you."

Mrs. James dropped back into her chair as if exhausted. She then looked at Phillip who had not moved. He slowly felt her eyes and turned towards her and smiled.

She started to talk, "You bastard," but stopped herself. She had forgotten to turn off the lectern microphone. The words "you bastard" were barely audible because she had been sitting down when she spoke them and wasn't speaking directly into the microphone, but the words were heard by many of the shareholders in the room. Mrs. James jumped up and turned off the microphone and while standing, looked down at Phillip, who now had a very noticeable smile. She said something else to Phillip and then stomped off the dais to join her lawyers, Helmut, and Mr. Tanaguchi who had all gathered at their end of the dais.

J.P. got up from his chair and decided to see if Phillip needed his help. Phillip had gotten up from his chair and was presently talking to Brian. They were laughing together and looked very relaxed. By the time J.P. had walked through the mass of people who were going the opposite direction to get to the refreshments, Phillip and Brian had stepped down from the dais and were now talking to Dr. Petersburg. Brian was just introducing Phillip to the doctor. J.P. stopped and decided to wait until he finished talking to Dr. Petersburg. He looked around and found that he was standing close to where Dr. Nakasone was still seated and looking at the people around the room. J.P. walked up to his row of seats and sat down next to him.

"Good morning, Dr. Nakasone. Did you have a comfortable flight from Tokyo?"

"Good Morning, Dr. Koenig. Yes, thank you very much. The JAL flight recommended by Nachedasan was an excellent choice. Plus it gave me the opportunity to meet and talk to that beautiful young woman with whom Nachedasan seems to have fallen in love."

"She is a delightful person. Does it bother you that Nachedasan has fallen in love?"

"On the contrary, Dr. Koenig. I am very supportive of this relationship. Nachedasan will require a strong woman as he continues to climb the corporate ladder. Reiko seems to be the logical person. She is beautiful, intelligent, and loves to travel...a perfect combination. Best of all she is modern Japanese. Too many of our traditional women don't meet the needs of a modern Japanese family. They are too instilled in the old subservient culture of the past. Nacheda requires a modern partner and Reiko looks to be the perfect choice. I'm in full support of their relationship."

He paused and looked around the room again and then exclaimed, "Amazing!

"What is amazing, Dr. Nakasone?"

"The process you use to get other peoples' opinions. First, in Japan there wouldn't have been a proxy fight in the first place. If by some slim chance there was a disagreement between the shareholders, the chairman would have uttered a command and the disagreement would have been ended. The chairman is lord in Japanese business. We talk about the groups working together as a team in Japan. That is true at lower levels, but not as far as corporate direction is concerned. The chairman or his equivalent sets the policy and strategy and the employees acting as teams implement the chairman's wishes. You Americans really take a chance with your freedom to express ideas. Don't get me wrong, Dr. Koenig, I love your system. It's the best for mankind, but it is unusual for Japan."

He stopped and pointed a thin finger at the Mrs. James group. "Look at Mr. Tanaguchi, he is both bewildered and angry. I can hear him now. He will be telling Mrs. James that she should not have let this happen. She is the chairman and she is the boss. He is scolding her. In the back of Tanaguchi's tortured mind he will be saying that this wouldn't have happened if the chairman had, if fact, been a man and not a woman." He smiled at her predicament.

"Do you think we will win, J.P.?"

The question and the use of his initials threw J.P. off for a moment.

"I really don't know, Dr. Nakasone." he answered and then thought he would take a risk. "Dr. Bradsmith will need all the help he can get."

He was silent for a moment.

"You are telling me that I should allow Dr. Bradsmith to tell the entire JamesBandai arrangement here today in his thirty-minute presentation?" His voice was soft and pensive.

"He has a very good speech, Dr. Nakasone. It is strong and has a great deal of substance. I think he has a good chance of winning, but not a 100% chance. I think we should help him to win. For this company to be under the control of that group of people," J.P. said waving a hand towards the group gathered around Mrs. James, "would be disastrous. James will not be James and Bandai will not want to work with the people operating James. Bandai and James, as they are now structured, are made for each other. Under Mr. Tanaguchi's leadership and whomever he chooses to be the President, will not be a good fit for Bandai. The new company won't be the ethical global pharmaceutical company that we envision. The company won't specialize in herbals. Sure they will want your isolation process, but probably for a different use than JPC138. JPC138 is years away from making a commercial profit. Mr. Tanaguchi won't wait that long, will he?"

Nakasone did not speak for what seemed to J.P. to be minutes, but probably was only seconds. "No, he won't wait that long." he responded. He then sprung up from his chair. He had made a decision.

"Come with me Dr. Koenig," he said, pulling on J.P.'s arm.

J.P. got up from his seat and followed him to where Phillip had been holding audience with many of the shareholders. It looked as if Phillip had used the break to try and align votes for his James plan. J.P. looked over at the Mrs. James group. They were huddled around the end of the dais table madly writing. They looked to be writing Mrs. James' speech.

Dr. Nakasone reached Phillip with J.P. in tow. He interrupted Phillip's conversation with a shareholder. Phillip introduced Dr. Nakasone and then excused himself to talk to Dr. Nakasone. Phillip then saw J.P., "J.P., where the hell have you been all day?"

"I was playing scarce. I know you, my friend, and you probably would have wanted to change something. I knew we had done all there was to do to in preparation for today. No changes were required, just time to let things play out," he replied.

"You are right as usual, J.P. I would have wanted to change my speech and as it turns out the second speech is right on. If I had changed anything it would have missed the target. How did you get to be so smart, J.P?" He humorously remarked.

"Pardon me, Dr. Bradsmith for interrupting your conversation, but Dr. Koenig and I have been talking and I think we should make a change in your presentation."

Phillip became very attentive and looked over at J.P., assuming that the change would come from him. "Change, J.P.? I thought we agreed we were spot on." Phillip had a slight edge to his voice.

"Don't look at me, Phillip. Hear Dr. Nakasone out, I think it is good news," he replied.

"Dr. Koenig reminded me of what you Americans call the winning edge, Dr. Bradsmith. I have thought things over and I now give you approval to release the JamesBandai agreement, contingent, of course, on your board being voted in and giving its approval to the plan. I also give you the right to state to the shareholders that Bandai will not work with the Mrs. James-NPC controlled board. I give you my hand as a guarantee that I will abide by what I said in your apartment on April 21st."

During Nakasone's announcement Nacheda had joined the small group and was acknowledged by each of them with a slight nod of their heads.

After finishing, Dr. Nakasone reached out his hand to Phillip. "Dr. Koenig and Nachedasan can be witnesses to what I have said."

Phillip immediately responded to Dr. Nakasone's outstretched hand and placed his hand in Dr. Nakasone's hand. Their hands stayed locked together as Phillip spoke in genuine sincerity, "Dr. Nakasone, I vow that you will never be sorry that you have taken this step. I will protect our faith in the James-Bandai merger. We are setting new rules for people to work by. I hope others will follow and seek higher grounds of moral global businesses together. Whatever the vote, we have won. Whether we ever have the opportunity to see our vision achieved depends on the people here in this tent. The four of us can see the vision. The future of our vision has been given the opportunity to become a reality by the people in this room demanding a resubmission of their votes. It's now up to me to ensure the voters assembled in this tent vote for our plan. I was ready, thanks to J.P. and Mandi, to convince them to go our way before your generous offer. Now I feel prepared to provide the coup de grace. Whatever the outcome, I love you all for what the team has tried to accomplish. Our lives won't be the same after this meeting. Pray we can hold our ideals after the vote. Thank you. *doumoarigatou . Dr.* Nakasone."

Phillip turned and walked confidently back to the dais. The others returned to the seats that they had previously occupied.

At exactly 3:00, Mrs. James rapped her gavel and called the annual meeting back to order. She had regained her confidence and looked as if nothing had or would happen. She spoke, "As presented before we recessed, Mr. Secretary will chair the discussions. Mr. Secretary." She laid the gravel down and Brian made his way to the lectern.

"It was decided that Dr. Bradsmith would be the first to make his presentation to the shareholders. Dr. Bradsmith, you have thirty minutes. It is almost 3:05. You have until 3:35 at which time I will ask you to stop and I will again take control of the microphone."

Phillip jumped up from his chair eager to start. The enthusiasm Phillip showed for his task wasn't lost on the shareholders.

"Ladies, gentlemen, shareholders, customers, business associates, and friends of James Pharmaceutical Company. First, I want to thank you for giving me the opportunity to present our plan for James clinical and economic growth. You have read the proxy statement. This document gave you the broad outline of the plan that my proposed board of directors slate has approved. What wasn't in the proxy statement was the profound difference between the two plans. Doc James, the founder of our company and an associate of mine for fourteen years until his untimely death a few years ago, was famous for giving titles to everything. Thus, we have names of buildings like the Spectrum of Medicine Building, and the Plan for the Latter-Twentieth Century, and more recently, my own 21st Century Plan."

It had been J.P.'s idea to throw in the reference to Doc James. He figured that Mrs. James would use him to her advantage and he wanted everyone to know that Doc James was Phillip's associate before there was a Mrs. Evelyn PrestonJames.

Phillip continued, "I will follow one of Doc James' traditions and label the two plans. I will try to make the titles as neutral as I can in order not to have bias in your minds that may influence your vote." There was a small titter from the shareholders. "I will title the plan I am presenting, The James Vision and the other plan, The James Tragedy." The tittering turned to laughter.

He continued, "I know you are saying to yourself that the names of these two plans are not neutral. Well, fellow shareholders, I am up here to tell you that the two plans are not neutral. They are as different as their titles suggest. I will use the next twenty minutes or so of your valuable time explaining the difference between a James Vision Plan and a James Tragedy Plan.

"A vision is something that you can build upon. A vision has to have substance and a foundation as strong as the granite of the island on which we are meeting today. A vision isn't built upon wishes and sand. The James Vision Plan has substance. The major substance is our knowledge of the James market and James technology. Sure we have had setbacks over the years, but we have never lost our focus. As an example, Lifeal. To date we haven't met our expectations, but we haven't given up on our patented pharmaceutical. We will come out of the generic doldrums and into unique product differentiation.

Some of the newspaper press that reports rumors has reported that we were having problems with Lifeal in its use as a preventative to arrhythmia. Mr. Husted, in his column in the Wall Street Journal, refuted this terrible rumor. In fact I am very happy to announce that just yesterday, Mr. Williams the President of Clintech, our partner in the clinical diagnosis of arrhythmia, informed James that he has completed one successful clinical trial on his Lifeal blood test with a 98% correlation."

There was a scattering of applause. "We were expecting 95%. This encouraging news will enable us to start four new clinical trials next month. James Vision Plan builds on the strength of Lifeal and in our vision, we don't give up on a product for which we hold patents. Through our hard work and focus, we found a better way to use Lifeal to serve mankind, and yes, to make a profit.

"The James Tragedy Plan. What would they have done if they were in control of Lifeal? First, if you read their plan, you saw very little mention of Lifeal. Why? Mrs. James and her research advisor Dr. Helmut Wahlters have given up on Lifeal. In fact Dr. Wahlters placed roadblocks in the way of continued research into Lifeal and Mrs. James cut the research budget.

"What does the James Tragedy Plan have to replace the potential profit from a successful Lifeal product? They say they have new, as yet unidentified products. Wishes and sand. Not substance and vision.

James has a tradition of knowledge of pharmaceutical herbs. Doc James built the company on herbal research. Our most successful products have been based on herbs. The basic compounds for Lifeal and JPC 138 are from the bark of the Alstonia spectabilis tree, more commonly known as the Devil Tree, grown in Indonesia. Dr. Allen Strong and his team have developed a process that changes the properties of the bark. This gives JPC138 the capability to clinically enhance human memory brain cells. As reported in Mr. Husted's column, we have completed the toxicology and pathology reports with JPC138 and will enter clinical trials as soon as the FDA gives us approval." More applause came from the shareholders.

"This has been done without the help of Dr. Wahlters who has chosen to delay the approval process every chance he has had." The shareholders became quiet.

Phillip went on, "Included in the proxy statement, was the announcement that we have tentatively signed an agreement with Bandai Pharmaceutical Company of Bandai, Upper Honshu, Japan. The agreement is to use their patented alkaloid isolation process. This process will provide James with the capability of isolating the pure active ingredient, in this case the alkaloid." The applause grew louder with the Bandai announcement. "The isolation process will free the raw material from all impurities that cause unwanted side effects. Side effects of the type that caused Mr. Ralph Vandermere to attempt the murder of myself after he had purposefully taken an overdose of Lifeal. He had ignored the directions provided by his personal pharmacist. The pharmacist, himself a Lifeal.. James shareholder, is present at today's annual meeting." More applause.

Mandi and J.P. had written Phillip's speech so the applause breaks would come closer and closer together building up to a strong conclusion.

Phillip's presentation continued, "I am happy to announce that Joseph Marshall our VP of operations has signed a lifetime agreement with Mr. Ming Chang for the exclusive rights to the Devil Trees from which we harvest Alstonia spectabilis bark. No restrictions or conditions apply to this contract. James Vision Plan guarantees material substance in the agreements with our vendor partners. Vision in what JPC138 will do for Alzheimer's disease.

"What about JPC138 and the James Tragedy Plan? We have proof that the Nippon Pharmaceutical Council tried to acquire the rights to the Alstonia spectabilis bark by force. If it had not been for Mrs. Amanda Hayes and two members of the board that I am recommending be voted in as directors today, namely Dr. Koenig and Mr. Nacheda of Bandai Pharmaceutical Company, the NPC would control the entire world's supply of the Alstonia spectabilis bark and we would be held ransom for our basic raw material for both Lifeal and JPC138." Jeers came from Mrs. James side of the tent because Phillip was making unfounded accusations. Phillip held up his hand to quiet them. "I know, I know, I have made an accusation for which you haven't seen substantive proof. I don't ask you to make your decision based on just this single fact but on the complete story behind the James Tragedy Plan. If proof of this incident is what you want before you vote,

Mr. Chang the owner of the plantation is here today as a James shareholder. He has pictures of NPC employees at his Devil Tree plantation and a sworn affidavit from the Indonesian government as to what happened at the plantation last February 28th." Again applause stopped the speech.

"As for the agreement with Bandai Pharmaceutical Company, the executives of the NPC will tell you that they will make the same agreement on the Bandai isolation process. These gentlemen don't know Dr. Nakasone, chairman of the Bandai Pharmaceutical Company very well. He has given me permission to state to the shareholders of James, that he will never allow NPC or any associate of the NPC the rights to the Bandai isolation process." The audience murmured.

"On the issue of JPC138 research, we have proof that Dr. Helmut Wahlters has purposefully delayed the filing of the toxicology and pathology data to the FDA, and that Mrs. James has cut the budget for this valuable product. Valuable….crucial….to both the clinical and financial success of James. Not to mention how much the product will be missed by the millions of worldwide Alzheimer's patients. The James Tragedy Plan? Wishes of deception and plans of sand."

Phillip took his water glass and took a few small drinks. He picked up his speech and tapped the pages into a neat pile and laid them back down onto the lectern. J.P. looked at his watch. Phillip was halfway through his thirty minutes. He looked over at Mrs. James and the others on her side. They were expressionless, staring straight ahead.

Phillip began to speak again, "The James Vision Plan! I am extremely happy to make the following announcement. It is an announcement of global consequences because it is a change in the way that American and Japanese companies conduct business together.

I stress the word, together." He paused. "Last month Dr. Nakasone, the chairman and single shareholder of Bandai Pharmaceutical Company, swore myself and a number of my close associates to secrecy on the plans he envisioned between James and Bandai. During the refreshment break, in front of witnesses, Dr. Nakasone gave me permission to make the following announcement to you, the shareholders of James.

"Before I make the announcement I must first tell you that during the recess, we notified the SEC that all sales of James stock are to be suspended until next Monday. The decision to do this was based on the following announcement because it will have an effect on the share price."

Phillip smiled, "Now all the risk investors and brokers that had started to make their way out of the tent with their cell phones, can sit back in your chairs knowing that someone won't beat you to purchase or sell stock depending on your interpretation of my announcement."

There was laughter by almost all of the audience. Three people returned to their seats. J.P. looked over at the Mrs. James side and the faces were not as expressionless as they were a minute ago. In fact there was genuine interest on their faces. He remembered that they were also James shareholders.

Phillip looked up from his prepared speech and seemed to look everyone in the tent directly in their eyes as if speaking to each of them individually. With real emotional sincerity he stated, "Dr. Nakasone and myself have discussed many wonderful things about herbal pharmaceuticals and how biogenetic engineering and other technological advances will increase the use of herbs as cures to today's and tomorrow's diseases. We feel it would be in the best interest for both companies and the patients they serve to work closer together. It is with the deepest respect that I announce to the James shareholders that we, therefore jointly announce, contingent on today's vote and the approval of the slate of directors that I have proposed, the merging of the two companies into one global pharmaceutical company." People started to applaud, but Phillip stopped them by raising his hands, saying, "Please wait, please wait." He continued, "Please wait, let me continue by quoting Dr. Nakasone's own words."

He looked down at his notes and quoted what Dr. Nakasone had said at the April 21st proxy team meeting. "I quote, 'James and Bandai are unique in that they both believe in the natural ingredients of herbal pharmaceuticals. Basically we are both herbal companies with bio-genetic engineering to be used to further the promise of herbal pharmaceuticals. The other pharmaceutical companies work with chemicals and other forms of genetic engineering. Our uniqueness will fail if we work alone or just as joint venture partners. We must be fully integrated. I believe this integration must be made with James as the controlling company. Therefore, if you win your proxy fight with Mrs. James I will give all the shares of Bandai Pharmaceuticals Company to James Pharmaceutical Company.' end of quote." The tent erupted with applause and cheers. Almost everyone was standing except those on the Mrs. James side of the dais. Their interest had turned to disbelief. Mrs. James started to get up, but thought better of the idea and sat back down.

Again Phillip asked the shareholders to be silent and let him finish. They obeyed immediately. "Thank you. There are a couple of other stipulations that I want to tell you about, not because they are bad or difficult to meet, but because they illustrate the heart of this great man. I have spoken harshly of the NPC and what they represent. I can't even go into the accusations that I could make about the NPC. I have summed up my feelings in the title, the James Tragedy Plan. I want you to know that the situation we find ourselves involved in is not a Japanese cultural issue. This is an issue between the honor of two groups of people. One group, the Bandai-James group comprised of myself, the people I represent at James along with Dr. Nakasone and the people he represents at Bandai. And the other group, the NPC-James group comprised of Mrs. James and her non-healthcare lawyer and financial consultant directors and the members of the Nippon Pharmaceutical Council, the NPC. The NPC is an organization of Japanese pharmaceutical companies that operate on the fringe of the Japanese healthcare industry with only a profit motive." He stopped for a second to bridge from the bad to good. The audience did not move. All that could be heard was the breeze gently flapping the sides of the tent.

"I again quote Dr. Nakasone, 'I'm an old man and I have seen many of my dreams come true. I believe that what I have done to make Bandai a good company will keep it from becoming a great company. Bandai and its people have to have a broader view of the global healthcare market in order to fulfill their destiny. They can't accomplish their destiny from Bandai alone. I can't continue to be their vision because my vision is becoming limited with the broadening of science and genetic engineering.' end of quote. As you have likely deduced he isn't asking for any money for the Bandai shares, they are a gift to James." The shareholders who hadn't yet figured this out began to applaud again, which led to everyone applauding. This time Phillip let it go on for many seconds.

"The other stipulations are as follows. First," Phillip proceeded to explain the four points that Dr. Nakasone had given him on April 21st concerning patents, royalties, employment, Nacheda's presidency, and the director position for himself.

When he finished the tent again erupted with enthusiasm. Mrs. James' group sat looking downcast and defeated.

Phillip looked down at his notes for his summary statement. "Shareholders of James, the road to success is long and difficult. Accomplishments never come as fast as any of us would like for them to come. We have been late with some of our plans, but we have never given up. I believe the time is right for James with the implementation of the James Vision Plan. A plan that has been developed with the vision of the future in mind. A future that you, our shareholders, will participate in as long as you hold shares of our company. What is most important are the clinically viable products that James will research, produce, and market to our patients. This will, in turn, produce a profit margin that will enable us to research more herbal pharmaceuticals and return to you a reasonable return on your investment. Our intention isn't to be spectacular, but to be the very best in what we do for our shareholders, physicians, pharmacists, and patients."

Phillip looked up from his notes and again looked into the eyes of the audience. "I want to leave you with two short statements. We have spoken of the Devil Tree and its role in Lifeal and JPC138. It's interesting," he paused for effect, "that the tree that can bring so much happiness to ill people has the word, devil, in its name. So here is the first statement: The Devil Tree can bring us tragedy when in the hands ofpeople who don't understand the fact that we are in the business to cure people who are ill. In the hands of those with vision and heart the Devil can be made to work wonders."

He paused, "I wouldn't be a good marketer unless I asked for the order, so my second statement is, please vote for the James Vision Plan. When you vote this afternoon, I promise you, we aren't miracle workers, but we will do the very best we possibly can. Thank you for your time, attention, and support."

There was silence and then the audience broke into a thunder of applause and cheers. The noise lasted for five minutes.

J.P. looked at his watch when Phillip finished, 3:35, thirty minutes exactly.

The reception to Phillip's presentation was more than he ever had expected. It seemed like everything was now going their way, but they still had to get over fifty percent of the shares and the fact that the Mrs. JamesNPC coalition controlled forty-five percent.

Brian moved to his place behind the lectern and started to wrap the gavel for attention. After numerous attempts he bent the microphone down to where the gavel hit the wood and made one hard hit. The tent went quiet.

He stared at the shareholders trying to get them back into a serious mood for Mrs. James. "Thank you. We will now hear from Mrs. James. Madam Chairperson, the lectern is yours for the next thirty minutes or until 4:10." He then moved back to his chair and sat down.

Mrs. James slowly got to her feet. She had a small pile of yellow legal papers in her left hand. She stood tall behind the lectern as she laid her notes on the slanted surface. Brian had left the microphone pointed down where he had left it after his last gavel hit. Mrs. James reached for the microphone holder arm and straightened it so she could speak directly into the microphone. The noise of the straightening was enormous. The room had been completely silent, showing a restrained respect for Mrs. James. The live microphone amplified the noise of the coiled metal microphone arm.

There was a brief moment of silence, and then laughter broke out in a far comer of the room and then there was pandemonium. The tensions of the day had been building up over the last hour and a half, was suddenly vented. Vented not directly at Mrs. James, but at the microphone, an inert object.

J.P. looked at Mrs. James and immediately saw that she thought the laughter was directed at her. She began to bang the gravel to get attention and then she began to shout, "You have to give me a chance, everything was planned so well. You have to give me a chance, it was planned so well. You have to give me a chance, it was planned so well. You have to give me a chance, it was planned so well." She had started loud and by the fourth time she had repeated herself she was whispering in a pathetic voice, while still pounding on the lectern. The gavel swing was wider and harder each time until the gavel handle broke and the head went flying out into the shareholders. Almost simultaneously with the breaking of the handle, the audience saw what was going on and went silent.

They stared at the woman at the lectern as she murmured one last, "You have to give me a chance, it was planned so well."

J.P. almost felt sorry for her, but he quickly remembered all the things she had done and intended to do to James. For a brief moment, he actually thought she was making a pathetic scene on purpose, but that would be giving her more credit than he thought that she deserved. She looked out at the audience and seemed to receive strength from the emotional pity she was receiving from the shareholders. She slowly straightened up as the silence grew longer. J.P. looked down at his watch and found that almost ten minutes had gone by since Brian had turned over the lectern to Mrs. James. He watched her seize the moment. There was a slight curling of the comers of her mouth.

In a whisper she said, "Thank you, thank you. I apologize for my gravel pounding, but I have so much to tell you and so little time. Now I have even less time." Her last sentence was strong and under control.

Phillip's attention was now on Mrs. James. She was going to have the last word. Would enough shareholders remember Phillip's talk to carry the vote? In less than thirty minutes the mystery would be over.

Mrs. James looked down at her notes and she began her hastily prepared speech. "Ladies, Gentlemen, guests, and shareholders," she began. "You have just heard the longest dissertation on nonsense that I or any intelligent investor has ever heard."

For the next ten minutes, Mrs. James gave a formidable speech on the facts of James cash finances and how management under Dr. Bradsmith would continue to be a failure. "An investor has only to look to the current stock price to determine what investors thought of the James performance," she quipped. "And, as for the Bandai deal, to coin an old TV ad for a fast food chain, 'Where's the beef?'

Indeed, where's the cash? James requires cash to do all of the amazing things that Dr. Bradsmith has promised you. Without cash and sales you don't have a James." She paused for emphasis, "No, you don't have a James Pharmaceutical Company. Even though the company might have a cure for Alzheimer's, an active ingredient process, and a life long contract for the Devil Tree that doesn't mean that there will be a James. With our plan, which has been referred to as the James Tragedy Plan, there is cash and new products. Dr. Bradsmith said the new products were wishes and sand. These products are real. They are already on the market in Japan and they are selling a the rate of hundreds of million yen per year."

J.P. noted that she had neglected to point out that FDA approval might take years. She also said the word, yen very softly hoping that everyone only heard hundreds of million and subconsciously added their own dollar sign.

Mrs. James ended her presentation by mimicking Phillip's second statement, "Our illustrious president, Dr. Bradsmith gave you two statements. One was a little deep for me to understand its relevance. The other statement was very relevant so I will steal it from him and use my prerogative as chairperson to change a few words. I wouldn't be a good Chairperson unless I asked for the order, so my final request is, please vote for the James Tragedy Plan when you place your votes this afternoon. I promise you a much higher and quicker return on your investment and that is really what we are here for isn't it? Thank you for your time and attention." She sat down. She had a confident look on her face. She felt she had done well.

The shareholders were giving her a good ovation. J.P. looked at the other members of her group. They didn't look as confidant. They had probably caught some of the subtle mistakes that she had made in her presentation. Still, Mrs. James didn't need very many votes to win the proxy fight. The vote would be very close.

Brian moved to the lectern and the audience went quiet. "Now you must cast your votes, change your vote, or stand with what you voted on before the meeting. I have a table set up at the left side of the dais." He pointed to his right. I will have a representative from our share clearinghouse as well as a member of each of the two sides to witness to all changes. I would appreciate your giving me the last name of the person or institution in which your stock is registered. Then give me the number of shares you wish to vote. You will have to be prepared to show me your credentials to prove you have the right to vote the shares. I would like to thank you in advance for your cooperation. After voting, or if you aren't voting, refreshments are again being served outside the rear of the tent. I hope to have the vote count within thirty minutes." He looked at his watch, "That would be 4:45."

The thirty minutes of voting went by very slowly. The line to change votes was very long and never seemed to stop. After thirty minutes there were still shareholders standing in line. At 5:00, the last shareholder voted and Brian moved to the lectern. "I am sorry, but there were more changes than I had expected. The clearinghouse representative will now count the votes. It should not be more than fifteen minutes."

The room fell silent. People that had gone for refreshments began to wander quietly back to their chairs. Once they had found their chair they sat down and didn't speak. They just waited. Thirty minutes went by. It was 5:30 when Brian again stood at the lectern.

"We have a new board of directors and I am afraid that it was not as close as I expected. The new board is the board headed by Dr. Phillip T. Bradsmith."

The tent went wild. It was like someone had let air out of a balloon by punching it full of holes. The shareholders were moving all around the tent talking and congratulating one another. Over the din of the shareholders, Brian's voice could be heard saying, "Will the new directors please take their seats at the dais."

J.P. made his way to the dais. As he approached where Nacheda and Dr. Nakasone were sitting, he asked them to join him on the dais as new directors of James. He looked over at Mrs. James. She was still sitting in her chair on the dais. Phillip moved his chair to be close enough to her to speak. J.P. knew what he was telling her. She still had a large block of stock that she could blackmail the new board with whenever she saw fit. The proxy fight team had all agreed that the resignation agreement that had been presented to her and the other members of her board would be re-worded as a sale of stock agreement. She would now have to sign the document or the new board would take her questionable James activities to the SEC. If the SEC ruled in favor of James then she would lose all profits from the sale of her stock. If she signed the sale of stock document then she could sell her stock in two years and keep the profits.

As Phillip kept talking, J.P. could see that Mrs. James was not enjoying the conversation. Her face was contorted. The stress of the moment was really getting to her. She grabbed the stock sale document and pen from Phillip's hand and signed the paper. J.P. knew that with her signature, the others would follow. The presentation of the stock sale document had to be worded just right for the lawyer and financial directors. As Phillip finished talking to Mrs. James, he moved his chair back to its original position. Tanaguchi and Helmut approached her, both with dour looks on their faces. They stopped across the dais from Mrs.

James. By then the new board had taken their positions behind the dais table. Mrs. James still had not moved.

Helmut, was the first to speak. All of the Thursday nights on Long Island came to a focus. Helmut had seen the dream of money fly out of the window and it was all because of her. In fact, there was a good chance he had lost his job at James. When he spoke there was venom in his voice. He was so mad, the German accent that he had worked so many years to cover came through.

"Ja, you are a bitch. Old Doc James, he vould never have allowed this to happen." He got himself under emotional control. He continued without accent, "You are as bad in business as you are in bed. Your incompetence has destroyed me."

Mrs. James focused on the two men in front of her. She knew one intimately and the other from the humbling and degrading international phone conversations that were conducted over speakerphones. She looked at Helmut with hate in her eyes. The skin around her eyes had taken on added folds and had turned red. In the comer of her mouth was a small amount of white spittle. She began to speak to Helmut in a venomous tone, at the same time coming up out of her seat and lunging at him. Mrs. James was suddenly spread across the dais table and her hands were on Helmut's shirt and necktie. She then grabbed his necktie and spoke.

"You sanctimonious fat son of a bitch. My husband and I made you, you bastard. Don't you tell me how I am in bed, you are nothing do you hear me, you are nothing. You have nothing I have ever wanted or needed. I used you, you useless old fool. Aren't you smart enough to realize that I used you. Without me you are useless, now get out of my sight."

Helmut listened, her words were the same she had always used, in one form or another, to command him to leave her bedroom and house.

In Helmut's mind she had always humiliated him and he had always whimpered away like a beaten puppy. No more he thought.

He brought his right arm up from his side where it had been resting. His fist was clinched into a ball. Those around saw what was beginning to happen, but they were late in reacting because the bizarre scene stunned them. Helmut's right fist hit Mrs. James squarely in the jaw. Her head had been at the level of his face as she tightly held his necktie verbally berating him. The force of the blow and the tightness of her grip on his tie had an unusual effect. First the force of the blow turned her head towards the lectern and broke her lower jaw. The crack of bones was so loud that those who were not involved in the scene now turned to the noise and were appalled at what happened next. The fist continued raising her head up and back. With her lock grip on Helmut's necktie she pulled him slightly up and off his feet, the force of her backward movement yanked the necktie tighter around his neck. Mrs. James fell back off the table and onto her chair. The quick force from her fall backward lifted Helmut up and onto the top of the table. The upward movement of the necktie crushed his windpipe.

He lingered a brief second, gasped, and then started to fall off the dais to the floor. Mrs. James never let go. Her hand around his necktie seemed to be locked in place.

Helmut's knees buckled in oxygen starved faint. His fall started to pull Mrs. James up out of her chair and across the dais table. One of the new board members tried to stop her from falling over the table. He couldn't see Helmut's plight. He grabbed her around the waist to keep her from going over the table. He held her steady on the table as Helmut began his fall to the floor. Mrs. James never loosened her grip on his necktie.

Helmut's head jerked back as the tie tightened around his neck. Blood was flowing from Mrs. James mouth and began to cover her hand, the necktie, and now Helmut's face. Helmut's heavy weight was contributing to the tightening of his necktie noose and his crushed windpipe was too much for the man's heart.

His dead weight was too much for Mrs. James to hold and the grip around her waist too firm to allow her to fall over the table.

The necktie gradually slipped through her blood soaked fingers and Helmut fell into a dead heap on the floor in front of the dais table.

A few of the frozen observers flew into action. The new board member who had Mrs. James by the waist was Dr. Wickersby, a family physician from Milwaukee. He quickly went to work on Mrs. James broken jaw. Her adrenaline was still running at a high rate and she started to talk, yell, and scream at the same time, but only gurgling would come out of her mouth. Her jaw flopped from her head. Dr. Wickersby stopped the bleeding and worked desperately to keep the blood out of the back of her mouth to prevent her from drowning in her own blood.

A cardiologist who had attended the meeting reached Helmut as his head bounced on the floorboard of the tent. He quickly assessed the situation and took a pocketknife from one of the other shareholders and performed a tracheotomy to allow Helmut to breathe. He then commenced CPR and pounded on Helmut's chest. His efforts were in vain and after a few minutes he leaned back from his sitting position on Helmut's girth and shook his head. Helmut was dead by strangulation and a failed heart.

Paramedics swarmed into the tent. They had been stationed outside just in case of an emergency. An emergency such as an old shareholder having a heart attack. One set of paramedics took over from Dr. Wickersby and was able to get Mrs. James under control, outside to the ambulance, and on the way to New York Medical Center. The other paramedic group placed Helmut's body into a body bag. His size was so great they could not zip the bag up tightly. They had to put the blood soaked dais tablecloth over him out of respect for the dead.

During the entire tragic event the people who weren't participating in the scene were transfixed to the spot they had been standing when Brian had announced the new board.

J.P. looked at his watch. The events they had just witnessed had taken less than ten minutes. He looked over at Phillip. He was ashen. J.P. thought that he was probably having some sort of flashback from when Ralph Vandermere had tried to kill him and then had turned the gun on himself. J.P. walked over to Phillip and put his arm around his friend's waist. "Are you all right Phillip?"

His head turned toward J.P. For a second, his eyes were a little glassy and then they cleared up.

"Yes." he suddenly replied. He continued, "Here, take this for safe keeping. I have to get this meeting under control." He thrust the signed stock sale documents into J.P.'s hands and went to the lectern microphone.

In a calm, strong authoritative voice Phillip said, "Ladies and Gentlemen, please may I have your attention. A terrible tragedy has happened here, but everything is now under control. I am sorry to report that Dr. Helmut Wahlters, James VP of research has died of a heart attack. Mrs. James was injured and has been taken to the hospital. She is in stable condition."

As Phillip was talking, J.P. tried to find Tanaguchi. He had been a witness and almost a participant in this tragic scene. He spotted the Japanese businessman walking quickly down the side aisle of the tent. J.P. knew if he didn't stop him, he would escape his involvement in the situation. Suddenly, he remembered that Tanaguchi still controlled a 15% share of James stock. Once the Bandai news hit the street this devious bastard was going to make a handsome profit for NPC off his aborted attempt to acquire James.

Again the bad guy, who in the background and had caused the events that had culminated that day was going to escape and make a profit.

"Over my dead body," J.P. said aloud.

He jumped off the dais and exited the tent through a flap behind the dais. Once outside he ran down the outside of the tent to the main entrance. He met Tanaguchi just as he stepped outside from the tent.

"Mr. Tanaguchi, we haven't had the pleasure of officially meeting, but I am Dr. Koenig and we have some unfinished business."

"I know who you are, Dr. Koenig," he said with bitterness in his voice. "I don't know of any business we had together that would have to be completed. Now if you will excuse me, I have had enough of this American tragedy. My limo is waiting. I have to catch a plane back to a sane country."

"I am sorry, Tanaguchi, but we do have unfinished business and I don't give a damn about your limo or your plane. As far as the sane country concept, you caused today to happen and, by God, you aren't going to profit from these events," J.P. spoke directly into his face.

Tanaguchi tried to get past him, but J.P. kept moving sideways blocking his path. He was prepared to get Tanaguchi's complete attention with a blow to his soft midsection when a voice behind him said, "Is there any trouble here, Mr. Tanaguchi?"

Tanaguchi stared into J.P.'s eyes. The fear that J.P. had seen a moment ago had been replaced with a confident smile. He snarled, "Is there any trouble, Dr. Koenig?"

J.P. knew that at least one of his bodyguards was behind him. He felt that he had no choice but to get out of Tanaguchi's way and let him escape to Japan where he would give the order to sell his stock on Monday or Tuesday, or whatever day he desired. He started to move and let Tanguchi pass when he heard the sound of expelled air and yelp of pain.

He heard the familiar voice of Nacheda, "No problem behind you, J.P. Proceed with your business."

Tanaguchi's expression changed again to fear and he made another attempt to get to his car. This time J.P. hit him a solid blow to the stomach. Again the sound of expelled air could be heard. J.P. held him upright as he began to fall. To a casual observer, they were just talking.

"You aren't going anywhere, Tanaguchi, until we have a signed agreement from you concerning the James stock that NPC owns."

"What James stock?" he gasped. He then added with more alarm and fear on his face, "You are a crazy man. You won't get away with this.. .this...this is extortion. I am a Japanese citizen and you can't touch me." With his last statement he had gained back some of his confidence.

J.P. took on a commanding voice and looked directly into his eyes. "Look, Tanaguchi, I'm going to say this just once and you had better remember what I've said. Then I will ask one of my lawyer friends and Mr. Husted to join us for a short chat. Then you will step into your limo and catch your plane back to the

Japanese hole from which you crawled. There, back in your sane country, I am sure, you will continue to carry out your dishonest strategies." He stopped talking to collect his thoughts. A plan had gradually come to mind on how the disadvantage of his leaving could be turned into an advantage.

Just as he was about to resume his conversation with Tanaguchi, Mandi exited the tent. She read the anguish on his face. "J.P., do you need any help. I noticed you had suddenly left the dais. I see Nachedasan has already come to your rescue. Can I help?"

"Yes Mandi. Please find one of Phillip's lawyers and Mr. Husted. We require the lawyer as soon as possible and ask Husted to join us in fifteen minutes." She started to go back into the tent when Nacheda also asked her to find a security guard. She smiled and turned to go back into the tent.

J.P. turned back to Tanaguchi and condescendingly placed his hand on his left shoulder. "Okay, Tanaguchi, here are your choices. After I give you the choices and you make the right choice, I will dictate a legal statement for you to sign. It will be a statement that will make you a hero, which is more than your organization deserves. First, to let you know where you, the NPC, and James stand in relationship to each other. We know all about your activities concerning James. We know about Lonewolf, the attempted kidnapping at Raffle's in Singapore, the purchases of James stock by your people in the US. We even know their names."

Tanguchi's face reflected the realization that they had more information on him and the NPC than he had thought. His arrogance had been replaced by fear.

J.P. continued, "We know about your involvement with the plantation incident and have pictures to prove your activities. We know of your association's activities outside of Doylestown, and the false rumors that your board fed the press to influence the James stock. I'm sure that once Mrs. James recovers and stops drinking her meals through a straw that she will be able to tell us a great deal about you and the NPC. Everything I have just told you is in a written report. Hard evidence that you and the NPC have engaged in murder, illegal activities, and stock manipulation. Copies of the report are in sealed vaults in five different locations. All are under control of various law firms. Copies of the document are located at Bandai Pharmaceutical Company in Bandai, Bank of Tokyo, James Pharmaceutical Company, Citibank in New York City, and the Swiss National Bank in Zurich. They will never be released to the press unless you renege on the document I'm going to give you to sign. So," he paused, "are you ready to listen to the proposition that will allow you to save precious face, keep you out of jail, and quite possibly make you a hero?"

"*Hai,*" was all that he said. He was defeated.

"You will sign a document saying that you are going to immediately sell the James shares that are owned by you, NPC, and your associates. The total amount of the sale will, in turn, be donated to the Alzheimer's Foundation. The only condition of the donation is that the donation be given to the James Pharmaceutical Company for their research of Alzheimer's. You will specify that the funds will be used to help the patients participating in the JPC138 clinical trials. Any funds left over will be used at the discretion of the director of the Alzheimer's Foundation. A report on the usage of these funds will be provided to NPC and to James on a quarterly basis. This signed document will be stored with the report that I previously mentioned on the NPC activities.

"After you finish with the legal statement, you will be interviewed by Mr. Husted of the Wall Street Journal. He will write an article about your interest in Alzheimer's disease. I would also recommend that you conduct an interview in Japan, but I will leave that up to you. Only after you have accomplished these two objectives will you be allowed to leave. Do you understand?" he tightened his grip on Tanaguchi's shoulder.

"Hai."

Just as he had spoke, Michael Thom one of Phillip's board lawyers emerged from the tent. He took in the scene with a quick glance and turned to

J.P. "Mandi said you were in the need of some legal help. Amazed as I was at your strange request, I decided I should follow her suggestion and here I am, legal pad in hand and ready to do your bidding."

"Thank you, Mr. Thom." He turned Tanaguchi around so both Thom and Tanaguchi were facing each other. "Mr. Thom, I would like to introduce you to a most wonderful man, Mr. Tanaguchi, the chairman of the Nippon Pharmaceutical Council or NPC." They shook hands. J.P. continued addressing himself only to Thom, "Mr. Tanaguchi would like to make a statement about selling the NPC-owned James stock. Then he would like to sign the statement making it legally binding. Mr. Nacheda, Mandi, and myself will be witnesses to the wonderful gift that Mr. Tanaguchi is going to make to the Alzheimer's Foundation. If you require a notary public, I am sure we can find one somewhere in the tent. By the way how are things going in the tent?" He released his grip on Tanaguchi's shoulder and pointed towards the tent.

"J.P., they couldn't be going better," the lawyer responded. "Phillip has complete control. Dr. Nakasone has already proven he is a great man. This is in direct contrast to the man of questionable honor that stands before us. The James official board meeting has adjourned. Before adjourning they passed motions on the

Bandai stock gift to James and the wonderful stipulations that Dr. Nakasone has placed on the gift. His international business foresight is bound to be written about in the press and duplicated by other companies who want to have global business and not just play lip service to the global strategy while racking up profits for their own greed and country.

"The shareholders were very appreciative of the meeting's outcome. To use a political term, I believe Phillip has a mandate to carry out his plan. I'm sorry that you missed it, J.P. I could see the

J.P. stamp on what happened today and over the last few months. We owe you a great deal of gratitude." He stopped talking to J.P., turned to Tanaguchi, and became serious. "Now that all of the good news has been spoken, what is it you want me to do with this gentleman you just had me shake hands with?" he said wiping his hand across his suit coat.

Tanaguchi's face turned red with anger. He suddenly and quite unexpectedly verbally lashed out at Thom, "I don't have to take this abuse from you white barbarians." Looking directly at Thom he yelled, "You are a lawyer. You know my rights. You must stop this charade immediately. You must protect me. I'm a citizen of a respected country and I should be protected while I visit your country. Tell these crazy people to release me immediately and let me return to Japan. They have done both mental and bodily injury to me and I wish to sue them."

Thom looked back at Tanaguchi and directly into his eyes. The stare was so intense that Tanaguchi could not hold the stare and after fifteen seconds lowered his eyes to stare at Thom's chest.

All Thom said was, "Go to hell."

J.P. grabbed Tanaguchi's arm and wrenched it behind his back and pulled him off to the side of the tent where no one could view what was happening. Thom and Nacheda followed. J.P. released Tanaguchi's arm and brushed off his suit. Tanaguchi knocked J.P.'s hand away and tried to look dignified.

"Nacheda," J.P. asked, "are any of Tanaguchi's NPC cronies around?"

Nacheda smiled, "I don't imagine there will be any interference from this person's bodyguards. I neutralized Tanaguchi's personal guard by handcuffing him to the steering wheel of his limo. If there were other bodyguards in the vicinity they have disappeared not wanting to be involved in the activities. I'm sure the area is secured."

"Thank you Nachedasan."

Once they were off to one side of the tent and out of view of most of the attendees. J.P. dictated to Thom the statement that Tanaguchi would sign.

When asked, Tanaguchi readily signed the statement. They all witnessed the signing. Thom didn't feel that a notary public was required.

Just as they finished witnessing the statement, Jack Husted and Mandi came out of the tent. Nacheda saw them looking around and hailed them from their hidden position. They joined the group.

Husted was very jovial, "J.P., a great meeting. I will have enough information on James, Japanese international trade interference in US corporations, international teamwork, and Alzheimer's to last me for months. I'm very glad the result of the voting went to the James Vision Plan." He then looked over at Mandi, "Your creative input into James marketing and Lifeal was justifiably rewarded. Congratulations on your promotion to executive vice president of marketing and strategic planning for James Pharmaceutical Company. I don't know of a more deserving and talented person to help take the new James to the top. J.P., what was it you wanted to see me about?"

Mandi was stunned. If someone had looked at J.P. they would have seen the same stunned face, but everyone was looking at Mandi. Mandi was staring at Husted and then she looked at J.P.

She addressed her comment to Husted, "I don't have clue about what you're talking about."

"That's right, you guys haven't been paying attention to the meeting. You've been out and about cleaning up the mess left behind by this creep," he said pointing to Tanaguchi.

Tanaguchi didn't react. He was used to the abuse by now and just wanted to get out of New York City. In fact his mind was contemplating what was going to happen to him once he was back in Japan. What would the NPC board do to him when they found out what happened to the James Project and their financial investment? Tanaguchi shivered. Two options, glory or suicide. He would have to do everything in his power to make sure that glory was the winning option. Including turning the opportunity he now had with the arrogant Husted to his favor. Tanaguchi was planning his survival. He wasn't listening to Husted's answer to Mandi's remark.

Husted went on with his explanation of what was going on in the tent. "Phillip just announced the reorganization of James and Mandi's promotion. I guess there was no reason for you to know what he was going to do. Your group was too busy working on the proxy fight to worry about reorganization. Mandi, your promotion is much deserved and earned. It looks like you and I will be having some chats about the future of James. I look forward to our meetings. How about lunch next Wednesday?" He smiled and looked at the group. "I thought I would close the order while I had the chance." He waited for Mandi's answer.

She hesitated letting the question sink in and then replied enthusiastically, "Yes, Yes, Bill. It's a date. Give me a call on Tuesday and we'll firm up the time and place."

J.P.'s realized that his friend and lover was on her way up the corporate ladder. His thoughts were mixed. He wanted her to succeed, but he also knew that success might tear them apart.

Husted interrupted his thoughts, "Thank you, Mandi. I look forward to Wednesday. Now what did you guys want me for?"

"Mr. Tanaguchi of the Nippon Pharmaceutical Council would like to provide you with an exclusive statement. He has witnessed some great events here today. He is sorry that his plan to work with James didn't work out, but he is happy about the results of the election. He has explained to us that one of the major reasons that the NPC had been interested in James was their work on Alzheimer's. He feels the choice of Bandai as a working partner was excellent and he would like to show his appreciation. He and the other members of NPC have great feelings for Alzheimer's patients and would like to demonstrate their desire to help. Isn't this correct Mr. Tanaguchi?" J.P. asked, squeezing Tanaguchi's arm.

Tanaguchi suddenly came to life after reaching an internal decision. He began to tell Husted everything about he and NPC's dedication to Alzheimer's research. To back up his dedication he was going to make a major contribution. He then proceeded to explain the material that was contained in the agreement without ever hinting that he was being forced to give the stock proceeds. What could have been a short forced statement lasted fifteen minutes. Husted was delighted. After Tanaguchi finished Nacheda and

J.P. escorted him to his limo. Nacheda released the guard after Tanaguchi had given the guard a signal that everything was all right.

J.P. assisted Tanaguchi into the back seat of the limo in what would seem to onlookers to be a friendly gesture. He took his seat next to the door.

J.P. bent over and sat back on his haunches.

He looked into the limo and directly into Tanaguchi's eyes. Once their eyes locked in a common stare Tanaguchi closed his eyes and lowered his head.

"Don't you close your eyes to me, look at me." J.P. commanded. Tanaguchi opened his eyes. J.P. continued, "I will assume that I will never see you again in my lifetime. I encourage you never to attempt to enter the US marketplace with your unethical tactics. You bring shame on an honorable profession and the Japanese people. It is you and your associates' type of business conduct that keeps the world on the edge of trade warfare. You hide behind your honored culture and the free enterprise system when greed and power alone motivate you. You use immoral techniques to gain what you want to control and then you throw our business honesty back into our faces. Learn from today, Tanaguchi. Learn from Dr. Nakasone and Mr. Nacheda. They do your industry and Japan proud. Not because James is seemingly the winner here, but because ethical human beings and honesty won. James only seemed to win because it was logical to have the name James retained. Next time good people work together, the company name could be Japanese. You probably don't understand a word that I am saying so I will end my short lecture with a final warning. Stay out of my way."

J.P. started to rise, but to his surprise Tanguchi responded. "The answer to your comments Dr. Koenig is, I understand, now goodbye." The driver had moved around to the rear limo door and now began to close the door.

J.P. stood up from his squatting position and stepped back. The driver closed the door with a sharp snap, moved around to the driver's side of the car, got in, and slowly drove off. Nacheda and he were left standing on the curb.

"J.P.," Nacheda responded, "he may say that he understood, but don't count on him to necessarily agree to change his business style or heed your warnings."

Nacheda saw the anger quickly come to J.P.'s eyes and smiled. "Not to worry. Tanaguchi is a proud and intelligent man that has made his way in the world by using power. I'm sure he won't trouble you in the future. He had to say what he said to you to save face. If not for himself, then for the benefit of the driver and NPC.

At that moment, the tent flaps where thrown back by the annual meeting ushers and the James shareholders started streaming out of the tent. They were laughing, joking, and moving towards the refreshment tables for the third time that afternoon, this time to celebrate.

Husted and Mandi wandered over to where Nacheda and J.P. were standing. Husted summed it up in twenty six words, "Like most days today was both a good day and a bad day but the important fact was, this day ended up as a good day."

CENTRAL PARK NEW YORK CITY

Mandi and J.P. were sitting in the same location where they had built their island in the snow months before in January.

This place was now special to both of them. The day was another beautiful cloudless spring day. The temperature was in the sixties and was expected to climb into the seventies. They had packed a lunch at the apartment and called Roberto to drive them to their spot in the park.

As Roberto pulled up to the curb, he sensed that this was an important moment and that his two favorite passengers might be saying goodbye. They assured him that it wasn't goodbye, but the project that J.P. had been working on had come to an end and things would almost certainly be different. They talked about the last four months and their times together in his cab. Finally, they said goodbye to Roberto. Mandi and J.P. had already decided that they would walk back to the apartment. As an afterthought, J.P. said that he would call Roberto when he came into town for James board meetings. They both knew that he probably wouldn't call him.

Roberto simply said, "Great, see youse then," and drove off.

The days after the annual meeting had been filled with stress-relieving fun. There had been many meetings all day Friday. J.P. hadn't been asked to attend nor had he expected to attend. He was now a board director and was not expected to interact with daytoday business activities. He used the time to pack up his personal things and clean out his office. He had lunch with Carl Manningham, Sr. and his son. He thanked them for their help and wished them well.

Mandi had promoted Carl, Jr. to the Director of Market Planning. Carl, Sr. was very proud of his son. J.P. had a moment alone with the elder Manningham. He thanked him for all of his help and wished him good health. The lawyer had tears in his eyes when J.P. wished him good health.

"I only hope that James can work fast on JPC138 before it is too late for me."

J.P. answered that he thought things would move much faster without the interference of the unfortunate Helmut and with the combination of the James and Bandai research departments.

Brian was promoted to an executive VP as well as securing his hold on CFO.

He thought of the day before. Everyone had wanted to carry over the Friday night proxy team party into Saturday night. They had started out Friday night at J.P.'s apartment with before-dinner cocktails. There was Phillip and his wife Sandi, Brian and his wife, Nacheda, and Mandi and J.P. Reiko had flown in late Friday afternoon. Skip and Annie, on a whim flew in on Friday. They were just in time to join in on the victory celebration. Carl Sr. couldn't attend because of a previous commitment and Dr. Nakasone wanted to be back in his Bandai office before the Tokyo exchange opened on Monday. He wanted to talk to his employees and tell them what had happened at the James meeting.

After cocktails at the apartment they moved the party to the Four Seasons on 57th Street for dinner. They were nearly kicked out of the Four Seasons for making a ruckus. After dinner they went to PJ Clark's and drank until after midnight. Finally, at 2:00 a.m., the group returned to the apartment.

No one wanted the night to end. They talked all night about James and the future for the company and their group of friends. They decided to meet next year at Mammoth for skiing as well as other future trips that they would make together. J.P. hoped that all of their dreams would come true, but he knew that reality would set in on Monday and he was sure most of the fun activities of getting together would be canceled for one honest reason or another.

Mandi and he wanted to spend their last day and night in the apartment together and alone. The group asked them about their Saturday plans and they dodged every question with silly answers. Saturday night they had front row seats for a concert in Central Park.

It had been a very warm evening in the park and a good way to end their period of living together. When the concert was over they walked back to their apartment. They adjourned to their favorite refuge, the hot tub outside the bedroom. Mandi had leaned back against him as they stared up at the sky.

After a while she turned her body and was sitting on his lap. Their bodies joined together and they rocked until they couldn't hold back any longer. They hugged one another as tightly as they could, afraid to let go for fear that they wouldn't ever be as close as they were at that moment. Neither wanted to be the first to break the hug.

After a long time, Mandi said, "Okay, so who is going to be the first to unhug. I know it won't be me, even though I am beginning to freeze right here," she nodded her head towards her breasts. Their upper bodies had been above water and the temperature difference between the hot tub water and warm room temperature had caused her to chill.

"If you don't make the move to unlock then lets please move off this beautiful tub love seat and slide into the water so the warm water can rejuvenate my body."

J.P. slid them both deeper into the warm water. Their lips met again and they kissed. Their lips and tongues seeking and finding the deep recesses of the other's mouth. They stepped out of the tub, dried each other off, and went to bed.

After they had slid under the sheets they tried to talk about their future together. They had not spoken about futures since Hawaii. Again, as in Hawaii, the words didn't come easily. Every time a conclusion was going to be made, one of them would turn it into a joke and that would be the end of that communication attempt. Sunday morning was spent talking about the past and individual dreams. There was more loving with small naps inbetween.

It was during one of the nap periods, that J.P. remained awake and watched Mandi sleep. Her bare breasts rose and fell with her breathing. The blanket was pulled up just above her stomach. He marveled at her beauty. He knew that she was ideal for him, but he honestly didn't know how ideal he was for her. He knew that she would be angry with him for even thinking such thoughts and would sternly tell him that the decision as to who was best for her was her decision alone. As he watched her, she moved from a position of lying on her back to a fetal position facing away from him. Her cold feet came to rest against his right leg.

J.P. was brought back to Central Park from his memories of that morning by Mandi's stern voice, "J.P., you are staring at me and not talking. What were you thinking J.P.? I hope your thoughts weren't negative thoughts or foolish things like we must end this relationship. If you are, I am going to hit you."

She moved around to lay with her head on his chest as she had in January. They were both in Levi's and sweaters. Her right leg was thrown over his and her crotch was pressed into his right thigh. Her right arm was thrown across his chest.

"If you don't stop rubbing against my right leg we are liable to have a Central Park public sex incident."

Mandi raised up, smiled seductively, and then nibbled at his ear. He pulled her body on top of his and they kissed.

"Mandi?"

"Oh, no you don't Jean Paul Koenig," Mandi replied and pulled herself to a sitting position. She sat back on her heels and folded her arms across her chest. Her tight Levi's and a bulky sweater hid her figure under cloth.

In a scolding voice she commanded, "No profundity, please, J.P."

He replied softly, "Nope, no profundity, love. Today is a special day. We are now going to leave our spot in the park, walk home, and probably make love. I will take my suitcase to the door and leave, take a limo to the airport and fly to Los Angeles on the late flight. From Los Angeles I will go to my plane and fly back to my home in Mammoth. I will be flying the Owens Valley by moonlight thinking of you all the time. I will probably be so wound up after my flight that I will probably go to my jogging room and run a half marathon. After running to exhaustion, I'll go to bed without you. I will not sleep very well and in the morning I'll wake up alone.

"Mandi, I don't care how much we want to ignore facts, but tomorrow will be different. We can continue to ignore this fact and I am willing to do so, but."

Mandi broke in, "Huh, what was that middle part again… something about walking home and making love?"

"But," J.P. insisted, "you must be allowed to fly and I must be allowed to get on with my writing."

"You know, that's not the first time you've used that phrase about me flying. What do you mean I must be allowed to fly?" there was the beginning of a slight edge to her voice.

"You are a beautiful, intelligent, capable, wonderful woman and executive. James and Phillip need you now and for the foreseeable future. You must be allowed to have your future. I have had my day in the spotlight. You deserve your day."

"Yes, but.," she paused. "Now you have me saying buts," she replied with a choke in her voice and tears in the corners of her eyes.

"But, you also need me, don't you?" Her tears were now running down her checks.

"I need you more than you will ever know." Tears had welled up in his eyes and were now running down his cheeks. Mandi sprung off of her heel sitting position into his arms. They held each other as tightly as they had the night before and cried together like children.

After a while, the tears subsided and they kissed. Their salty tears washing down their cheeks and lips, mixing in their mouths.

"Let's go back to our apartment," he concluded.

"Yes," was all she said.

They walked back in silence their hands locked together. Every few seconds they would squeeze the other's hand or move their thumbs back and forth in a soft caress.

Once back in the apartment, they made soft and quiet love and Mandi feel asleep. At 6:00 p.m., he got up and went downstairs to the desk and wrote her a note.

Dear Mandi,

I am sorry that I must leave tonight, but I have to get back and tonight is as good as any night. In fact there are no good nights to leave you. But, (there is that word again) it had to happen one day. We will only be apart for a short three weeks. Phillip wants me to come back to New York the Monday before the board meeting. I will plan to be back on that Friday afternoon so that we can have the weekend together. How about a weekend trip to Newport? I can also stay the weekend after the board meeting.

In fact, for some reason, our friend Phillip wants me to continue to consult for James one week a month. So you see, my darling things will work out.

I know you will be mad at me for writing this note and not waking you up, but since it is not goodbye, I thought I would let you sleep. No matter what that pretty head of yours will think, today is not goodbye, but just a short parting. You have to go to your work tomorrow and I have to go to my work.

I will call you when I get home. Home in Mammoth sounds funny. Home is really wherever we are together. It's not the apartment that we have enjoyed so much over the last four months, but our home is within ourselves. See you soon. I love you very much, Amanda.

He signed the note Jean Paul and then folded it and inserted it into an envelope. He heard a noise behind him and turned to find Mandi standing there in her silk robe. The late afternoon sun was behind her exposing her beautiful body in a seductive xray.

He smiled, "You better get away from the sun streaking though your body from behind or I will never catch my plane."

She was not smiling and said in a soft sleep voice, "You didn't intend to sneak out of here and leave me a goodbye note did you, J.P.?" There was a touch of indignity in Mandi's voice.

"Don't we know each other yet, my love. In answer to your question, of course not. I just wanted to leave you a happy love note for you to read after I left. Believe me. This is a moment that could be sad because we will be separated for awhile, so I decided to write a happy note. I was going to go back upstairs and give you a kiss and a squeeze and then leave for the airport. I will call you when I get to LA and I will see you in a couple of weeks."

"Two weeks, I thought that you would not be back until the board meeting in three weeks."

I took her into my arms and whispered in her ear, "It is all in the note. Now let me go. I love you very, very much Mandi. I will see you soon. Now go back up to bed and sleep tight.

Everything will be okay and somehow Mandi and J.P. will work things out. Two talented healthcare executives can surely work out a relationship."

He picked up his bag, gave Mandi a long deep kiss, and turned to leave. As he walked to the door he looked back over his shoulder. She had not moved from the position of standing in the sunlight. He smiled and waved. There was nothing more that he could say. He didn't say goodbye.

EPILOGUE

It had been four months and ten days since J.P. had been called to New York City by Phillip to work on the 21st Century Plan project. So much had changed, yet nothing had changed. He was still a writer, a consultant, and a detective for healthcare companies who think they are being hurt by others stealing their ideas or products. With his bonus shares of James stock, he was a little richer.

The James and Bandai road to market success will be long and hard, but at least it will be a road built on two well matched international pharmaceutical companies working together to help their physicians to help patients. In four months they had changed the way companies should look at how they work together and they saved the Devil Tree and its use in medicine.